Butterworths Guides to Information Sources

Information Sources in the
History of Science and Medicine

Butterworths Guides to Information Sources

A series under the General Editorship of
  D.J. Foskett, MA, FLA
  and
  M.W. Hill, MA, BSc, MRIC

This series was known previously as 'Information Sources for Research and Development'. Other titles available are:

Information Sources in Agriculture and Food Science
  edited by G.P. Lilley

Information Sources in Architecture
  edited by V.J. Bradfield

Information Sources in Education and Work
  edited by E.H.K. Dibden and J.C. Tomlinson

Use of Biological Literature (Second edition)
  edited by R.T. Bottle and H.V. Wyatt

Use of Chemical Literature (Third edition)
  edited by R.T. Bottle

Use of Criminology Literature
  edited by M. Wright

Use of Earth Sciences Literature
  edited by D.N. Wood

Use of Economics Literature
  edited by J. Fletcher

Use of Engineering Literature
  edited by K.W. Mildren

Use of Management and Business Literature
  edited by K.D.C. Vernon

Use of Mathematical Literature
  edited by A.R. Dorling

Use of Medical Literature (Second edition)
  edited by L.T. Morton

Use of Physics Literature
  edited by H. Coblans

Use of Reports Literature
  edited by C.P. Auger

Use of Social Sciences Literature
  edited by N. Roberts

Butterworths Guides to Information Sources

Information Sources in the
History of Science and Medicine

Editors

Pietro Corsi, DPhil
Ricercatore, University of Pisa

Paul Weindling, MA, PhD
Research Officer, Wellcome Unit for the History of
Medicine, University of Oxford

Butterworth Scientific
London Boston Durban Singapore Sydney
Toronto Wellington

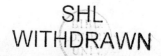

First published 1983

© Butterworth & Co (Publishers) Ltd 1983

British Library Cataloguing in Publication Data

Information sources in the history of science and
    medicine.—(Butterworths guides to information sources)
    1. Medicine—Information services
    2. Science—Information services
    I. Corsi, Pietro   II. Weindling, Paul
    610′.7   R118.2

ISBN 0–408–10764–2

539116

13921325

Typeset by Scribe Design Ltd, Gillingham, Kent
Printed and bound in Great Britain by Cambridge University Press

Series editors' foreword

Daniel Bell has made it clear in his book *The Post-Industrial Society* that we now live in an age in which information has succeeded raw materials and energy as the primary commodity. We have also seen in recent years the growth of a new discipline, information science. This is in spite of the fact that skill in acquiring and using information has always been one of the distinguishing features of the educated man. As Dr Johnson observed, 'Knowledge is of two kinds. We know a subject ourselves, or we know where we can find information upon it.'

But a new problem faces the modern educated man. We now have an excess of information, and even an excess of sources of information. This is often called the 'information explosion', though it might be more accurately called the 'publication explosion'. Yet it is of a deeper nature than either. The totality of knowledge itself, let alone of theories and opinions about knowledge, seems to have increased to an unbelievable extent, so that the pieces one seeks in order to solve any problem appear to be but a relatively few small straws in a very large haystack. That analogy, however, implies that we are indeed seeking but a few straws. In fact, when our information arrives on our desks, we often find those few straws are actually far too big and far too many for one person to grasp and use easily. In the jargon used in the information world, efficient retrieval of relevant information often results in information overkill.

Ever since writing was invented, it has been a common practice for men to record and store information; not only facts and figures, but also theories and opinions. The rate of recording accelerated after the invention of printing from movable type, not because that in itself could increase the amount of recording but because, by making it easy to publish multiple copies of a document and sell them at a profit, recording and distributing information became very lucrative and hence attractive to more people. On the other hand, men in whose lives the discovery or the handling of information play a large part usually devise ways of getting what they want from other people rather than from books in their efforts to avoid information overkill. Conferences, briefings, committee meetings are one means of this; personal contacts through the 'invisible college' and members of one's club are another. While such people do read, some of them voraciously, the reading of published literature, including in this category newspapers as well as books and journals and even watching television, may provide little more than 10% of the total information that they use.

Computers have increased the opportunities, not merely by acting as more efficient stores and providers of certain kinds of information than libraries, but also by manipulating the data they contain in order to synthesize new information. To give a simple illustration, a computer which holds data on commodity prices in the various trading capitals of the world, and also data on currency exchange rates, can be programmed to indicate comparative costs in different places in one single currency. Computerized data bases, i.e. stores of bibliographic information, are now well established and quite widely available for anyone to use. Also increasing are the number of data banks, i.e. stores of factual information, which are now generally accessible. Anyone who buys a suitable terminal may be able to arrange to draw information directly from these computer systems for his own purposes; the systems are normally linked to the subscriber by means of the telephone network. Equally, an alternative is now being provided by information supply services such as libraries, more and more of which are introducing terminals as part of their regular services.

The number of sources of information on any topic can therefore be very extensive indeed: publications (in the widest sense), people (experts), specialist organizations from research associations to chambers of commerce, and computer stores. The number of channels by which one can have access to these vast collections of information are also very numerous, ranging from professional literature searchers, via computer intermediaries, to Citizens' Advice Bureaux, information marketing services and information brokers.

The aim of the Butterworths Guides to Information Sources is to bring all these sources and channels together in a single convenient form and to present a picture of the international scene as it exists in each of the disciplines we plan to cover. Consideration is also being given to volumes that will cover major interdisciplinary areas or what are now sometimes called 'mission-oriented' fields of knowledge. The first stage of the whole project will give greater emphasis to publications and their exploitation, partly because they are so numerous, and partly because more detail is needed to guide them adequately. But it may be that in due course the balance will change, and certainly the balance in each volume will be that which is appropriate to its subject at the time.

The editor of each volume is a person of high standing, with substantial experience of the discipline and of the sources of information in it. With a team of authors of whom each one is a specialist in one aspect of the field, the total volume provides an integrated and highly expert account of the current sources, of all types, in its subject.

D.J. Foskett
Michael Hill

Acknowledgements

The successful completion of this volume involved the help of many historians of science and medicine, librarians and publishers. The project was initiated at the suggestion of Professor Margaret Gowing and of Butterworths. Both Professor Gowing and Glen Hughes provided much help and encouragement throughout the project. The editors are also greatly indebted to their colleagues at the Wellcome Unit for the History of Medicine, Oxford, for frequent assistance. Besides those who have contributed to the volume, Dr R. Cooter and Mrs J. Loudon have been particularly helpful.

Many librarians have given expert advice. We are especially grateful to S.A. Jayawardene for generously placing his breadth of bibliographical learning at our disposal. The staff of the Library of the Wellcome Institute for the History of Medicine have given frequent and prompt assistance. The staffs of the Bodleian Library and Radcliffe Science Library, Oxford, the University Library Cambridge, and the Whipple Science Museum Library, Cambridge, helped with many inquiries. Especial thanks are due to K. Andersen, Aarhus; J.L. Biss, of the Medical Library Association; Dr G. Cantor; the Council of Botanical and Horticultural Libraries; Dr J. Cule; Ms M. Dunn, Ontario; Dr J. Erlen, Dallas; J. Gaston, Southern Illinois University; S. Gibbs of the Center for Polar and Scientific Archives, Washington; Dr I. Grattan-Guinness; Dr F. Greenaway; Dr S. Kohlstedt, the History of Science Society; M. Lafollette, MIT; the Philosophy of Science

Association; Dr M.E. Ring; E. Talkès of the *Bulletin signalétique*; the Secretary of the American Association of the History of Medicine. Much assistance was also provided by Marica Corsi and Julia Taplin.

Preface

The history of science and medicine has been developing rapidly during the past ten years. New priorities have meant that it has been changing perhaps faster than many sciences. There has been a considerable increase in publications, particularly monographs and periodicals, and a need has arisen to present a balanced survey of the literature and of underlying changes in interpretation.

The aim of the present survey of literature, methods and concepts is to provide a series of succinct assessments of important areas of the history of science and medicine. The division of the volume into four parts is designed both to produce a reference work with readily accessible bibliographical and historical information, and to present essays that are readable and also of interest to specialist groups concerned with particular disciplines and themes. General chapters consider not only the development and main features of the history of science and medicine, but also relations with associated areas: anthropology, philosophy, religion and the social sciences. The second section of the book deals with general literature and major institutions, and provides an outline of research methods. This is followed by essays dealing with historical treatments of a range of modern sciences and developments in medicine: the physical sciences, mathematics, chemistry and the life sciences, as well as scientific instruments and medicine since 1500. This organization reflects recent developments in many respects. History of medicine is accorded independent status, so that medical developments are treated primarily as distinctive problems relating to the health of past societies and not just as appendages of scientific innovations.

A substantial section of the book, mainly but by no means exclusively Part IV, reviews studies of non-European developments. A case-study is included on the rapid expansion of science in the United States and on aspects of medicine in America. In contrast there are chapters on Indian, Islamic and Chinese cultures. MacDonald's analysis of anthropological approaches includes African examples. These are areas of study receiving increasing attention.

Contributors discuss the many available approaches and assess the most important features of particular fields. Bibliographies have been so constructed that major works of reference and basic studies are included, which when consulted will provide further material. This has allowed space for historiographical and critical discussion of the development of studies in particular areas, evaluation of major works, sources and problems requiring investigation, and assessments of the best standards appropriate to each area. As a guide not only to information sources but also to conceptual and historical problems, this volume is thus intended to generate further research into and discussion of subjects of great intrinsic importance.

Pietro Corsi
King's College
Cambridge

Paul Weindling
Wellcome Unit for the History of Medicine
Oxford

Contributors

David Elliston Allen
Lesney Cottage, Middle Road, Winchester, Hants, SO22 5EJ

Edward H. Beardsley
Department of History, University of South Carolina, Columbia, S.C. 29208, USA

William H. Brock
Victorian Studies Centre, The University of Leicester, LE1 7RH

Pietro Corsi
Istituto di Filosofia, Universita' di Pisa, Piazza Torricelli 2, 56100 Pisa, Italy

Christopher Cullen
Clare Hall, Cambridge CB3 9AL

Gian Arturo Ferrari
Universita' di Pavia, Corso Strada Nuova 65, 27100 Pavia, Italy

Margaret M. Gowing
University of Oxford, Faculty of History, Broad Street, Oxford, OX1 3BQ

L.J. Jordanova
Department of History, University of Essex, Colchester, Essex CO4 3SQ

S.A. Jayawardene
42 West Park Avenue, Kew, Surrey TW9 4AL

Michael MacDonald
Department of History, University of Wisconsin, Madison, Wisconsin 53706, USA

Arnold Pacey
53 Millway Close, Upper Wolvercote, Oxford OX2 8BL

T.J.S. Patterson
University of Oxford, Wellcome Unit for the History of Medicine, 47 Banbury Road, Oxford OX2 6PE

Margaret Pelling
University of Oxford, Wellcome Unit for the History of Medicine, 47 Banbury Road, Oxford OX2 6PE

Simon Schaffer
University of London, Imperial College, London SW7 2AZ

Emilie Savage-Smith
Gustave E. von Grunebaum Center for Near Eastern Studies, University of California, Los Angeles, California 90024, USA

Charles B. Schmitt
University of London, The Warburg Institute, Woburn Square, London WC1H OAB

G.L'E. Turner
University of Oxford, Museum of the History of Science, Broad Street, Oxford OX1 3AZ

Mario Vegetti
Universita' di Pavia, Corso Strada Nuova 65, 27100 Pavia–Italy

Charles Webster
University of Oxford, Wellcome Unit for the History of Medicine, 47 Banbury Road, Oxford OX2 6PE

Paul J. Weindling
University of Oxford, Wellcome Unit for the History of Medicine, 47 Banbury Road, Oxford OX2 6PE

Paul B. Wood
Division of History and Philosophy of Science, Department of Philosophy, University of Leeds, Leeds LS2 9JT

Contents

Preface
Pietro Corsi and Paul Weindling   xi

PART I

1 History of science, history of philosophy and history of
   theology
   Pietro Corsi   3

2 The historiography of medicine
   Charles Webster   29

3 The history of technology
   Arnold Pacey   44

4 Anthropological perspectives on the history of science
   and medicine
   Michael MacDonald   61

5 The social sciences and history of science and medicine
   L.J. Jordanova   81

6 The history of science, politics and political economy
   Margaret M. Gowing   99

7 Philosophy of science in relation to history of science
   Paul Wood   116

PART II

8 Guide to bibliographical sources
   Pietro Corsi   137

9   Periodical literature and societies
     Paul Weindling   157

10   Research methods and sources
     Paul Weindling   173

     PART III

11   Science, technology and medicine in the classical
     tradition
     Gian Arturo Ferrari and *Mario Vegetti*   197

12   Recent trends in the study of medieval and Renaissance
     science
     C.B. Schmitt   221

13   Scientific instruments
     G.L'E. Turner   243

14   Mathematical sciences
     S.A. Jayawardene   259

15   History of physical science
     Simon Schaffer   285

16   History of chemistry
     W.H. Brock   317

17   Life sciences: natural history
     David Elliston Allen   349

18   Experimentalism and the life sciences since 1800
     Margaret Pelling   361

19   Medicine since 1500
     Margaret Pelling   379

     PART IV

20   The history of American science and medicine
     Edward H. Beardsley   411

21   Islamic science and medicine
     Emilie Savage-Smith   437

22   Science and medicine in India
     T.J.S. Patterson   457

23   Science and medicine in China
     Christopher Cullen   476

     Bibliography of journals   501
     Index   509

Part I

1

History of science, history of philosophy and history of theology

Pietro Corsi

Historians of science of every major historiographical school have been concerned with the relationship between modern science, philosophy and theology. One group has stressed the opposition between science and theology or metaphysics. The contrary thesis, defended by historians of philosophy, religiously oriented historians of science and sociologists, has emphasized the strong – even though problematic – links between religion, science and philosophy.

This important debate has been at the centre of the discipline during the past decades, and indeed since the second half of the nineteenth century. This chapter will concentrate on features of the problem most relevant to current historiographical debates. Particular attention will be paid to developments in French philosophy and epistemology during the first half of the twentieth century that considerably influenced post-Second World War history of science in Britain and USA. It is the aim of this brief survey to point out the cultural roots of theses defended by Alexandre Koyré and Gaston Bachelard. The 'discovery' of the epistemology proposed by the latter among young historians of science in the English-speaking world makes it important to take note of the intellectual context and priorities that led Bachelard to stress the epistemological features of scientific discourse (Gaukroger. 1976). Mention will also be made of the contribution of general historians to widening the intellectual horizons of the history of science.

Consideration of the thesis of the close relationship between Puritan theology and the rise of modern science put forward in 1938 by the American sociologist Robert K. Merton will lead to a survey of two major contemporary historiographical debates: the conflicting interpretations of what has been defined as the scientific revolution of the seventeenth century, and the more recent discussion of the role of theology in the development of English and American natural sciences of the nineteenth century. (Chapter 7 below is devoted to discussing recent developments in the philosophy of science and their impact upon the historiography of science.)

The debate on positivism

The view that the methods of science represented a fundamental step forward in the history of humanity was forcefully propounded by the French philosopher Auguste Comte, in his famous *Cours de philosophie positive* (1830–42). Comte regarded the history of Western culture as characterized by three stages of development: the theological, the metaphysical and the positive. Each stage corresponded with particular concepts of nature, which changed with man's increasing capacity to understand and master natural phenomena. The positive stage, represented by the experimental and theoretical achievements of modern physico-mathematical sciences, signified the abandonment of theological and metaphysical approaches to nature. Men renounced the dream of investigating the animistic, theological or conceptual 'causes' of phenomena, and resorted to the only method possible in science – the study of the laws connecting natural phenomena as observed by man or subjected to his experiments.

Theological and mystical tendencies in Comte's thought, as well as the increased pace of progress in late nineteenth-century physical sciences, caused many supporters of positivism fundamentally to revise the teaching of the French philosopher. Yet, even though Comtean positivism never became a dominant epistemological or philosophical component of French and European culture, it should be pointed out that in the later decades of the nineteenth century a broadly 'positivistic' approach to science was defended by scientists and philosophers alike. Epistemologists and philosophers of science stressed the progressive and cumulative nature of scientific knowledge, its anti-metaphysical implications, its experimental, a- and anti-philosophical approach to nature. Physical scientists merely reflected and investigated the succession of natural phenomena. They avoided unprofitable questions such as those concerning causes of phenomena or the structure of reality.

In his widely read *La Science et l'hypothèse* (1906), the French scientist Henri Poincaré maintained that the language of science was free from philosophical or theological concepts. Rather it was a conventionalist systematization of everyday and technical language, which helped men organize information gathered from experience of natural phenomena.

Ernst Mach, the influential Austrian scientist and philosopher, was convinced that scientific statements only *described* natural phenomena. Scientific theories represented simplified and 'economic' summaries of observations and experiments conducted over the course of centuries. Science developed in opposition to philosophical or theological constructions of nature, whose supporters failed because they pretended to provide comprehensive and unified views of reality and its inner structure. Mach's *The Science of Mechanics* (1893) was an impressive historical survey. He did not deny that many scientists of the past were deeply religious, or that they regarded their theological views as relevant to their science. Mach conceded that theological concepts were at times responsible for the formulation of viable scientific hypotheses. He nevertheless concluded that 'the theological proclivities which these men followed, belonged wholly to their innermost life' (1893: 450).

The physicist and historian of science Pierre Duhem was the distinguished follower of Mach in France. He subscribed to many of Mach's views on the 'economic' nature of scientific theories, and accepted Poincaré's conventionalist view of scientific language, albeit with further critical insights. Duhem was convinced that science merely systematized and expressed in mathematical terms man's experience of natural phenomena. Yet he concluded *La Théorie physique* (1906) by maintaining that the choice of hypotheses in science had been determined historically by extra-scientific factors. The history of science showed that new theories were rarely accepted by supporters of older ones. There was no 'scientific truth' that compelled assent by practitioners of science, just as there was no *experimentum crucis* that had historically settled a scientific dispute (Poirier 1967). It was thus the proper task of the history of science as conceived by Duhem to examine the factors – philosophical and theological in particular – that favoured the formulation of successful scientific hypotheses (Bosmans 1921; Baudot 1967). Duhem considered Aristotelianism, and even astrological doctrines, as systems of thought that provided science with working ideas and concepts.

Le Système du monde (1913–59), Duhem's ambitious attempt to write the history of Western physical sciences, put forward the idea that modern science was generated in the course of debates on Aristotelianism in the French universities of the thirteenth century. In order to prove his point, Duhem, a fervent apologist of Catholicism, went to extreme lengths. He thus maintained that modern science was born on 7 March 1277, when Etienne Tempier, the Bishop of Paris, condemned 219 philosophical and scientific propositions as contrary to the Christian view of nature. Tempier denied naturalists the right to think that the world was finite, that there was only one world, or that there was no void in the universe, since these Aristotelian tenets contradicted the dogma of God's omnipotence. Aristotelians were thus forced to revise many of their assumptions and concepts: the stage was set for the development of modern astronomy and physics (1913–59, vi: 21–30). Duhem's 'continuity thesis', as his approach has been defined in historiographical debates, has represented the source of inspiration and information for recent generations of historians of science, even though the limits of his historical reconstructions have been often pointed out (Maier 1949–58; Agassi 1963; Zambelli 1965; Martin 1976; Schmitt chapter 12 below).

However, attempts by Duhem or by his positivist critic Paul Tannery to substantiate their at times opposing views on the philosophy of science by concrete historical research were not pursued by French philosophers and historians concerned with science. Sympathizers and critics of Duhem's standpoint concentrated instead on the epistemological and broadly philosophical analysis of crucial developments in early twentieth-century physical sciences. The dramatic succession of physical theories and experiments announced by Einstein, Born, Heisenberg, Millikan and others between 1900 and 1930 appeared to French philosophers and epistemologists as clearly indicating that 'science' was undergoing a deep conceptual revolution, which Duhem's disciples and critics had failed to understand. Philosophers of various schools and tendencies stressed the need to come to terms with contemporary 'scientific' categories. Traditional positivistic approaches to the historical development of science were regarded as insufficient to explain the new 'scientific revolution' (Lecourt 1969; Redondi 1978). Indeed, modern scientific development was seen as a powerful challenge to traditional concepts of knowledge, requiring a fundamental revision of classic philosophical categories.

The exclusive focus on the intellectual, rational component of scientific theorizing characterized the work of philosophers following different and at times opposite traditions. Léon Brunschvicg

(1912, 1922), a French historian of philosophy and the proponent of 'critical idealism', wrote on the history of mathematics and physics, two disciplines that to him showed the capacity of the human intellect to build powerful conceptual structures. Thus, the history of science, as well as the history of philosophy and of religion, provided the philosopher with material relevant to the study of the human intellect and its creativity. Idealism was better defended by studying the actual rational product of the human mind, rather than by analysis of subjective cognitive procedures (1912: 5).

Emile Meyerson (1908, 1927), patron and friend of the historian Alexandre Koyré, also maintained that the history of science was the perfect laboratory of the philosopher (see Koyré 1939; La Lumia 1966). Meyerson primarily considered the conceptual and mathematical dimensions of contemporary science, as did Abel Rey (1907, 1927), another influential representative of French thought between the two wars. The latter, who opposed conventionalist and positivistic approaches to science, was concerned only with 'pure' science, and regarded the history of science as the historical unfolding of epistemologies. Rey was the founder of the journal *Thalès* (1934–40), and cooperated with the Italian historian of science Aldo Mieli in establishing the Comité International et Centre International d'Histoire des Sciences at the Centre International de Synthèse (see *Archeion*, Vol. 8, 1927: 155; Vol. 9, 1928: 498–509).

Even though the direct impact of Brunschvicg, Meyerson or Rey on the development of the history of science was limited in the long term, the effect on the discipline of Gaston Bachelard, a renegade pupil of their school who regarded research in the history of science as exclusively guided by epistemological priorities and preconceptions, cannot be underestimated.

Bachelard represented an important influence in contemporary French philosophy. He sanctioned an approach to the history of science that has produced suggestive insights, as well as strongly reductive interpretations of the task of the historian of science. Bachelard was critical of French idealistic, spiritualist and positivist philosophy of science, as well as of the reluctance of scientists to reflect upon the philosophical import of their work, although it is appropriate to point out that his perceptiveness in relation to the philosophical dimensions of contemporary science tempted Bachelard into showing less than adequate appreciation of the problems of interpretation of the historical data. Bachelard's merit was his stress on historical discontinuities in science and epistemology. He was impressed by the dramatic developments in contemporary physics, and categories such as the idea of 'epistemological break' introduced by Bachelard to indicate revolutionary conceptual changes in science have found great favour in many areas of history (Bouligand *et al.* 1957; Dagognet 1965a; Barreau *et al.* 1974; Gaukroger 1976). Thus the philosopher and the epistemologist dictated to the historian of science how and what to study (Bachelard 1934, 1938, 1951). As Bachelard's pupil Dominic Lecourt approvingly commented, 'if epistemology is historical, then the history of science is necessarily epistemological' (Lecourt 1969: 9). Bachelard also predicted that the history of science needed to be rewritten whenever a significant conceptual change occurred in physico-mathematical disciplines. The task of the history of science, a discipline he never pursued systematically, was to consider the present state of science and epistemology, and to trace the discontinuous path that historically led to the 'discovery' of contemporary scientific ideas. The history of science was thus seen as the history of just a few scientific ideas and concepts. Moreover, the definition of science itself was determined by modern disciplinary boundaries and criteria.

Alexandre Koyré

As has often been the case with the evolution of the history of science as an academic discipline, important and fruitful developments were fostered by practitioners of allied disciplines, in particular the history of philosophy. Alexandre Koyré, probably the most influential French historian of science of the last four decades, was trained as a historian of philosophy and of religious thought. A pupil of the German philosopher Edmund Husserl and a convinced Platonist (Spiegelberg 1960: 225), Koyré studied in Paris under the supervision of Brunschvicg and was a close friend of Meyerson. Like his teachers, Koyré was convinced that the history of science was the laboratory of the philosopher wishing to understand the achievements of the human intellect. Koyré offered many and masterly exemplifications of Brunschvicg's idea that philosophy, theology and science had to be studied as part of closely interrelated historical developments of man's attitudes to nature and knowledge (Koyré 1922, 1929, 1933).

Koyré's first specific study in the history of science, the *Études Galiléennes* (1939), gave convincing proof of the potential of his approach, which he defined as 'conceptual analysis'. Koyré, like the majority of his colleagues, regarded science as a purely intellectual activity. Technology and scientific instruments only represented the embodiment of a theory, and had no crucial relevance to the development of modern science. Thus, he argued that the history of astronomy owed little to the telescope, and Galileo was denied a place in his history of astronomy from Copernicus to Borelli (1961; Taton 1965).

Koyré's contribution to widening the cultural horizons of the history of science has been outstanding. Through detailed investigations and sophisticated historical reconstructions, he proved that the history of science could not dispense with the philosophical, theological and general cultural context of scientific theories. An analysis of Renaissance Platonism, or of the philosophy of the Cambridge Platonist Henry More, was shown to be essential to the understanding of Galileo's and Newton's work. Koyré's effort to extend the intellectual scope of the history of science was however characterized by well-defined limits. The controversy with the American historian Henry Guerlac well illustrated the aims and priorities of Koyré's method. In an impressive paper on 'Some historical assumptions of the history of science' (1963), Guerlac praised the contribution of conceptual analysis to the history of science, but also warned that the approach favoured by Koyré severely restricted the concerns of historians: negligible attention was paid to the technological, social and political dimensions of science. Guerlac courageously defended the contributions to the history of science of scholars writing from a Marxist perspective, and showed little patience towards those who denounced on *a priori* grounds the investigation of the relationship between science and economic or social conditions. 'It is fallacious', he concluded, 'to make an arbitrary separation between ideas and experience, and to treat ideas as if they had a totally independent life of their own, divorced from material reality' (Guerlac 1963: 811). Koyré's reply concisely stated the views that guided his investigations in the history of science. Science was 'essentially *theoria*, a search for truth'. As he often repeated, science was man's *itinerarium mentis in veritatem*, and its history had to be confined to the description of the path that led to scientific truth (Koyré 1963: 856–7). Within the limits pointed out above, Koyré's analysis of seventeenth-century European physical science still represents an important contribution to the analysis of the historical relationship between science and philosophy.

The cultural dimensions of the history of science in Britain and the USA

The traditional dominance of neo-positivist and logical approaches to scientific theories and their history in British and American culture did not favour the widening of the horizon of the history of science in the first half of this century (Wood, chapter 7 below). Contributions to the journal *Philosophy of Science* during the late 1930s and the early 1940s well illustrated the attitude of leading philosophers of science like P.P. Wiener, O. Neurath or P. Frank to the history of science. According to Frank, the physics of Galileo and Newton 'put an end to the animistic period' (1937: 49). Wiener viewed the history of science as 'a synoptic view of the major doctrines... incorporated in the progress of science' (1937: 388).

Philosophy of Science also printed less dogmatic contributions. G.K. Chalmers, for instance, argued (1937: 76) that Gilbert's theory of the magnet 'involved metaphysics'. J.D. Irving conducted a polemic against Wittgenstein and his followers, and pointed out that philosophical systems of the past were historically 'something more than myths and fancies' (1936: 214). The *Journal of the History of Ideas* (1940–) also helped to put forward a broader concept of the history of science (Wilson 1981).

Notwithstanding his scholarly, 'humanistic' dedication to the history of science, George Sarton, the distinguished Belgian–American founder of *Isis*, stressed the teleological nature of the discipline. The history of science was the history of man's conquest of truth. Modern science developed in opposition to superstition, astrological doctrines, Hermetic beliefs and other 'deviations' (Thackray and Merton 1972). Thus, for instance, Gilbert's 'metaphysical fancies' only illustrated the 'queer limitations of genius' (Sarton 1957: 97–8). Sarton, during his early philosophical training, had become deeply absorbed in the French debates on science described above. This was probably the reason why, paradoxically, his approach to science and its history shared many of the assumptions on which Bachelard's opposed and arguably more sophisticated analysis of science was based. Sarton, contrary to Bachelard, was a convinced proponent of the continuous, cumulative development of science – 'the gradual unveiling of truth and the conquest of matter by mind' (1957: vii). He was however convinced, as was Bachelard, that the progress of physico-mathematical science had to lead to a revolution of philosophy. Moreover, as with Bachelard, Sarton considered the history of science as the history not only of truth but also of mistakes; indeed, the history of mistakes was seen by both as extremely instructive, since it helped in understanding the history of truth. Sarton also shared with Bachelard the belief that the history of science had to be rewritten following the progress of science (1913: 26–7).

These various and at times opposite traditions of philosophy and historiography point to science as pure theory and truth, or at least the highest form of knowledge accessible to man. The task of the historian of science is thus a relatively simple one. The conclusions of his investigations are already drawn by contemporary scientists and epistemologists. The historian has only to dramatize the succession of events inevitably leading to contemporary scientific truth. Philosophical, theological, political or social beliefs regarded by scientists of the past as part of their intellectual scheme of reference are excluded from the legitimate concerns of historians of science. Even Koyré's sophisticated conceptual reconstructions of philosophical, theological or cosmological systems of the period 1500–1700 were in the final analysis the description of the conditions that made it possible for Western culture to achieve *veritas*.

New perspectives in the history of science, religion and philosophy

The overriding preoccupation with contemporary epistemological and scientific issues, and their bearing upon the history of science, did not prevent general historians from widening the scope of the history of science. Fifteen years before the publication of Koyré's *Études Galiléennes*, E.A. Burtt published *The Metaphysical Foundations of Modern Science* (1924). He expanded upon the relationship between Newton and the Cambridge neo-Platonists, and stressed the metaphysical dimensions of Newton's thought. The history of philosophy and the history of theology were seen by him as essential components of the history of science. Burtt (1924) indeed paid tribute to positivistic views of science; he agreed with many contemporary epistemologists that 'mathematical science' was 'the most stupendous conquest of modern times'. Thus, his inquiry into the relationship between cosmological views and the birth of modern science had well-defined limits. He regretted, for example, that Kepler's cosmology embodied 'crude inherited superstitions which the most enlightened people of his time had already discarded'. Yet Burtt's (1912, 1922) pioneering reconstruction of the relationship between philosophical, theological and scientific concepts in seventeenth-century Britain should be remembered as a stimulating contribution to the discipline.
Burtt's work did not initially have direct influence on the history

of science, and was long opposed by philosophers of science (Burtt 1943). However, many of the points to be found in Burtt's writings were later made by Koyré. It was the superior sophistication of Koyré's conceptual analyses that convinced many American and British historians of science that it was time to reconsider traditional methodological guidelines of the discipline. During the Second World War, Koyré emigrated to the United States, where he helped to establish the École Libre des Hautes Études of New York. His contacts with several American centres for the history of science and personal friendships with distinguished historians had a significant impact on the history of science in the United States and Britain. He was also well received by the group of intellectual historians gathering around Arthur Lovejoy and the *Journal of the History of Ideas* (Gillispie 1964).

A contribution by a general historian to the history of science deserves mention. This is Butterfield's *The Origins of Modern Science* (1949). It is well known that Koyré regarded this book as the best general work in the history of science (Rossi 1964). Butterfield was critical of Sarton's preoccupation with precursors of modern scientific ideas and opposed Marxist and, in general, economic and sociological interpretations of science. He also criticized historians of civilization who rarely if ever mentioned the role of scientific ideas in society and culture. Butterfield accepted elements of Duhem's continuity thesis, and referred to 1277 as the year in which 'a religious taboo operated in favour of freedom for scientific hypotheses' (1949: 9). He too, however, considered the history of science from the point of view of the results achieved in modern times. Butterfield stressed the need to take account of 'the misfires and mistaken hypotheses of early scientists'. Yet he did not consider the study of alternative scientific cultures of the past as part of the history of civilization, except in so far as these 'had their effect on the progress of science in general' (1949: 9).

The historical reconstructions offered by the representative figures of Burtt, Butterfield and Koyré undoubtedly contributed to arousing interest in the role of philosophy and theology in the development of modern science. It is however necessary to point out that theological and philosophical debates of the past were investigated only in so far as they represented the preconditions for important developments leading to the formulation of modern scientific theories. The definition of science implicit in the works examined was determined by the boundaries of contemporary disciplines and by contemporary epistemological debates on physico-mathematical theories. Inquiries into the social, institutional or even technological dimensions of scientific cultures and practices of the past were regarded as unprofitable and irrelevant to the understanding of progress towards modern science.

Puritanism and science

In the mid-decades of this century, intellectuals of the English-speaking world elaborated alternative approaches to the history of science that were to some extent independent of epistemological and modern philosophical priorities. A major, provocative contribution to the study of sciences in history, and their relation to social and religious movements, came from the sociologist Robert K. Merton. This American scholar approached scientific developments in seventeenth-century England from the point of view of the religious affiliation of leading recruits to science. He was not concerned with proving or disproving epistemological points, and his interests were clearly at odds with those of the traditional epistemologically oriented historians of science (Merton 1936, 1938). A paper by Stimson, considering the relevance of moderate Puritanism to the development of science in mid-seventeenth-century England, had already attracted some attention (1935). It was however Merton's thesis that started, albeit after some delay, a historiographical debate that is still involving leading scholars of the scientific revolution.

Merton exploited views on the relationship between social ethics, theology and economic development put forward by Max Weber, R.H. Tawney and Ernst Troeltsch. He took note of Irene Parker's pioneering study *Dissenting Academies in England* (1914). Merton also relied on the idiosyncratic listing of Protestant scientists compiled in 1873 by Alphonse de Candolle, and stressed that the majority of participants in the scientific movement of the seventeenth and eighteenth centuries subscribed to one of the forms of Protestantism. He concluded his study by positing a direct causal link between Puritan views of man's place in nature and of God's dispensation, and the expansion of scientific investigation and education in seventeenth-century Britain.

It could be claimed that for the first time in the history of science, and owing to the work of an outsider, the interpretation of a crucial period in the history of modern science attracted widespread attention from historians and social scientists. It soon became clear that Merton's thesis was regarded as a provocation by historian apologists of Catholicism or defenders of the pure, areligious nature of scientific enterprises. Thus F. Russo (1957), the bibliographer of the history of science discussed in chapter 8, argued that historical evidence did not prove the thesis of the alleged Protestant superiority over Catholicism in the development of modern science. In his controversial paper 'Merton revisited', A.R. Hall commented in 1963 on leading contributions to the debate between 1938 and 1962, and concluded with a firm, albeit critical, defence of Koyré's conceptual approach to the rise of modern science (Hall 1963; in Russell, 1973). Hall pointed out that Merton had failed to cope with the technical and conceptual features of scientific discourse in the seventeenth century.

Studies on the intellectual origins of the English Revolution by Hill (1964, 1965), and the debate on the relevance of scientific and technological developments to the utopian and political programmes put forward by various factions of the Puritan movement, added further dimensions to the discussion (Turnbull 1947, 1953; Webster 1979). A series of important papers contributed to *Past and Present* in the 1960s and early 1970s provided new ammunition for historians denying and affirming the causal link between Puritanism and the scientific revolution of the seventeenth century (Webster 1974).

Historians who, like Hall, were prepared to admit the profitability of inquiries into the relationship between science, philosophy and theology in the seventeenth century were not inclined to concede that religiously inspired utopian technological programmes had any significant relevance to the scientific revolution (Hall 1972). Other historians concentrated their investigations on the origins of the Royal Society, and claimed that significant steps forward in scientific theorizing took place at the Restoration (Purver 1967; Mulligan 1973). After 1660, Anglican latitudinarian naturalists and disillusioned supporters of parliamentary rule found ideal conditions for the pursuit of science (Purver 1967; compare Webster 1967). Further statistical evidence on the religious affiliations of members of the early Royal Society suggested to Mulligan that Puritanism, as well as latitudinarianism, played no significant role, since the majority of Fellows appeared to subscribe to royalist and conservative Anglican creeds (1973; in Webster 1974: 317–39). Mulligan did however conclude that in the final analysis Anglican and political conservatism were not relevant factors in the development of modern science, and stressed the progressively areligious, purely 'scientific' priorities dominating the ideological concerns of the Fellows of the Society.

Reading the papers collected by Russell (1973) and Webster (1974), as well as recent contributions quoted below, gives the impression that the debate was characterized by traditional assumptions about the uniqueness of the scientific enterprise, in particular its 'truth' value. Since the seventeenth century witnessed a scientific revolution of permanent value and import to the history of Western cultural and economic civilization, then there had to be a well-defined and coherent body of factors that led to, or could explain, the birth of modern science at that time and in that particular country. To some, the causal link was Puritanism; to others it was Anglican latitudinarianism; and still others pointed out the demise of the religious view of nature.

The very vivacity and at times the very polemical heat of the debate helped to highlight important episodes and figures of seventeenth-century science. The debate has also provided convincing evidence that traditional historical accounts of the scientific revolution dominated by scientific or epistemological priorities offered a very limited view of the complex network of philosophical and theological beliefs and programmes relevant to seventeenth-century scientific debates.

A synthesis of the evidence brought to light by scholarship in the preceding twenty years, and wide coverage of previously disregarded manuscript and printed primary sources, was produced by Webster (1975). *The Great Instauration* represents an innovative contribution to the discussion of Puritanism and science in the seventeenth century, bringing new historiographical perspectives into the study of the cultural role of science. Webster argued that the concentration on issues traditionally investigated by historians of science – chemistry, astronomy, theories of matter, etc. – inevitably led to reductive and misleading interpretations of mid-seventeenth-century debates on science and society.

Critics have suggested that *The Great Instauration* represents a renewal of the Merton thesis (Mulligan 1980; Jacob and Jacob 1980; compare Webster 1975: 484–5). Reading the book does not confirm this view. Webster was concerned neither with the rise of modern science, nor with proving that the Puritan ethic was the major or the only factor responsible for it (Webster 1975: 520, ch. six). Indeed, long sections of the book are devoted to analysing the approach to natural sciences, anatomy and physiology by authors such as Harvey and his group or conservative representatives of Cambridge neo-Platonism, who opposed parliamentary rule and radical Puritanism (1975: 115–51). Webster pointed out that, even within the Puritan group, the plurality of theological, philosophical and political standpoints defies clear-cut definitions. He warned against analysing the variety of approaches discussed in mid-seventeenth-century Britain in terms of simplistic definitions –

Puritanism, Anglicanism, royalism, etc. – that would make historians lose sight of the historical dynamics of contemporary scientific, theological and political debates. Philosophical and theological considerations bearing upon scientific debates are thus shown in their concrete historical dimensions.

Webster strongly stressed the inadequacy of single-factor explanatory models. As he pointed out: 'it would be totally unrealistic to write the history of the emergence of English science in the period 1560–1660 in terms of monocausal derivation from Protestantism, Anglicanism or Puritanism.' It would be equally unrealistic to argue that the various factions of the Puritan movement taking part in the debate on natural knowledge had no role in the process (Webster 1981: 31).

The science–Puritanism debate represents a further development in the history of the study of the relationship between science, philosophy and theology. Philosophy and theology are not now always investigated as providing contextual dimensions to the progressive accumulation of scientific knowledge. Moreover, fundamental problems have emerged concerning the historical analysis of theological and philosophical traditions, for instance questioning the tendency to consider individuals as personifications of theological, philosophical and scientific ideas, and not as historical actors reshaping traditions or stressing elements of their cultural heritage that appeared to them most suited to interpret or to change the reality they lived in. The historical understanding of Puritanism, Calvinism, Anglicanism or Catholicism, as well as of Baconianism, neo-Platonism or Newtonianism, is hardly furthered by first defining what each term means in abstract, theoretical terms – if such definition is indeed possible – and then listing historical actors fitting the requirements of the definition.

Religion and science in the nineteenth century

For a long time historians of science inspired by diverse methodological priorities have agreed that the scientific revolution of the seventeenth century represented a turning point in Western thought. Comte's doctrine of the three stages of man's intellectual development was tacitly endorsed even by opponents of the positivistic school. 'Science' in the nineteenth and the twentieth centuries was seen as a body of 'mature' disciplines free from theological, philosophical or political assumptions and implications. From a state of timid independence from or indeed of subservience to philosophers and theologians, scientists painfully achieved the splendid autonomy of modern science. The aggressive anti-clerical and lay liberal ideologies that characterized political and philosophical debates at the end of the last century and at the beginning of the twentieth produced histories of freethought and science, in which the history of science and of philosophical radicalism were seen as the epic celebrations of the victorious fight of reason against clerical persecution and the clouds of superstition (Benn 1906; Robertson 1929; Draper 1874; White 1896; Fleming 1950; Moore 1979).

As far as nineteenth-century science was concerned, commentators focused on the struggle by geologists and biologists to free their disciplines from theological tutelage. Doctrines like geological uniformitarianism put forward by Charles Lyell (1830-3) or the evolutionary synthesis produced by Darwin (1859) were regarded as crucial episodes in the final battle between science and religion, although, in the last twenty years, commentators have pointed out that opposition to Lyell or to Darwin was motivated by logical, philosophical and 'scientific' reasons, and not by mere theological or clerical obscurantism as hitherto assumed (Rudwick 1970, 1972; Bartholomew 1973, 1976; W.F. Cannon 1960a,b; S.F. Cannon 1976; Limoges 1970; Vorzimmer 1972. For studies in the history of geology see Challinor 1971; Porter 1977; Sarjeant 1980). Investigations of the relationship between science and religion in the nineteenth century revealed the theological and broadly cultural dimensions of contemporary science. In a pioneering study of early and mid-nineteenth-century debates on geology and the Bible, Gillispie (1951) analysed the apprehensive reaction within religious circles to modern investigations of the natural history of the earth. He questioned the thesis that geological research was opposed by theologically inspired polemicists, and pointed out the contribution to geology by Anglican clergymen such as William Buckland, the first Reader of the discipline at Oxford, or his Cambridge colleague Professor Adam Sedgwick.

In a series of papers published in the 1960s and 1970s Susan F. Cannon approached the wider issue of the relationship between the development of various scientific disciplines and British theological and religious movements of the decades 1800–1860 (1960a,b, 1962, 1976, various papers reprinted 1978). Cannon argued that the major instigators of scientific progress in early and mid-nineteenth-century Britain were a group of Cambridge dons and students inspired by liberal or, according to a contemporary label, Broad Church theological doctrines. Her thesis that Broad Church ideas provided the active theological basis for a sympathetic attitude towards science and its organization has been accepted by various scholars (Morrell 1980; Thackray 1980). The study by Morrell and Thackray (1981) on the early years of the British Association for the Advancement of Science – established in 1831 – emphasized the role of Broad Church leaders in creating a harmonious relationship between the scientific movement and important sectors of the contemporary theological spectrum. It should however be stressed that the category 'Broad Church' is difficult to define in theological and historical terms. Indeed, the label was introduced by mid-nineteenth-century commentators to indicate individual standpoints that often had little in common but a supposed and indeed generic 'liberal' approach towards science, philosophy and modern theology. Moreover, individuals designated as leaders of the 'movement' strongly denied any sympathy with liberalism and the Broad Church. Some also opposed what they regarded as unsound scientific developments, such as Darwin's theory (Corsi 1979).

Increasing attention has also been paid to the role of natural theology traditions in fostering acceptance of a view of nature as a system of natural laws providentially designed by the Creator. The series of eight essays known as *The Bridgewater Treatises* published between 1833 and 1836 has been seen as the celebration of the reconciliation between the truth of science and the truth of religion (Hooykaas 1959; W.F. Cannon 1960a; Young 1973; Limoges 1970). Further research has however pointed out that early and mid-nineteenth-century natural theology cannot be taken as a coherent and systematic body of doctrines upheld by a significant majority of participants in the debate on science and religion (Yule 1976; Brooke 1979; Corsi 1980). Historians have often overlooked the fact that natural theology was part of the theological debate, and that the plurality of standpoints that characterized the latter was of significant relevance to the former. Attitudes towards science – geology and natural sciences in particular – as well as towards natural theology were subject to deep changes during the first half of the nineteenth century. The outcome of debates on the philosophical foundations of scientific investigation also produced a variety of interpretations of the reliability of scientific results. As a consequence, various brands of natural theology, or standpoints opposed to the design argument, presupposed different and often contradictory epistemologies (Corsi, to be published). Thus the historiographic assumption that natural theology represented a unified view of science and religion is misleading on many accounts.

The idea put forward by Young (1969, 1973) that the description of developments within the scientific movement of the nineteenth century requires reference to wider social and political debates has still to be thoroughly investigated. However, as noted when discussing the issue of Puritanism and science, the historiographical debate on science and religion in the nineteenth century is clearly beginning to recognize that monocausal explanations cannot find adequate and satisfactory historical substantiation.

Finally, mention should be made of the growing concern of historians of Darwinism with the relationship between Darwin and contemporary natural theology, and religious thought in general. Historians accepting the Darwinian doctrine as the turning point in natural sciences – away from metaphysics and theology into the positive stage – have disregarded and misconceived the entire issue of the philosophical and theological roots of Darwin's thought. The publication and discussion of Darwin's early manuscripts, and in particular of the notes, notebooks and essays written between 1837 and 1844, provided scholars with a mass of documents pointing to Darwin's early ideas and his evaluation of contemporary scientific and cultural trends.

In a pioneering study of 1970, Limoges argued that Darwin's theory developed out of a systematic critique of natural theological concepts of adaptation. Gruber (1974), the editor of Darwin's notebooks on man, mind and materialism, dwelt upon Darwin's philosophical and theological preoccupations. A further study by Manier (1978) investigated the 'cultural circle', or, in other words, the authors and topics Darwin saw as related to his research programme in natural history. This has further confirmed Darwin's critical awareness of contemporary philosophical and theological debates. (See also Schweber 1977; Green 1977; Ruse 1979; Corsi 1980.)

In the last few years historians of Darwin subjected the actual relationship between the natural theological concept of adaptation and the development of Darwin's early manuscripts to thorough investigation, and produced revealing insights into Darwin's painstaking process of rethinking and critically evaluating the concept of organic adaptation he found in the works of William Paley. Ospovat (1980, 1981) expanded upon Kohn's work (1975, 1980), and analysed the relationship between Darwin and the Paleyan tradition until 1859. Ospovat made ample use of manuscript notes for the years 1844–59 hitherto disregarded by Darwin scholars.

Moore's massive *Post Darwinian Controversies* (1979) strongly emphasized Darwin's debt to what the author defined as 'orthodox natural theology'. This book represented the first attempt to offer a synthesis of recent studies on the relationship between evolutionary theories and debates and contemporary theological thought. It is Moore's belief that Darwin's theory stemmed from the Christian 'orthodox' view of nature, which he regards as a uniform body of doctrines untouched by historical development. Moore's free use of categories such as 'orthodox Christianity' and 'orthodox natural theology' to characterize a variety of historically diverse theological and philosophical standpoints constitutes a serious limitation of his study.

The volume of essays planned for the occasion of the centenary of Darwin's death in 1982 and the 1982 conference by the British Society for the History of Science on the relationship between science and religion in the nineteenth century provide further insights into the relationship between science and religion in contemporary natural sciences.

This selective survey of major methodological and epistemological trends in the history of science, and of approaches to the issue of the connection between philosophical and theological assumptions and 'scientific' investigation and theories has emphasized the extensive change of perspectives within the discipline. The great majority of historians quoted with reference to the debate on Puritanism and science, or on theology and natural sciences in the nineteenth century, avoided taking sides in the methodological and epistemological discussions described below by Wood in chapter 7. The names of Popper, Kuhn or Lakatos feature decreasingly in recent historical production. Practitioners of the discipline are increasingly aware of the historical specificity of the problems they are investigating. A definition of science in modern terms, based on disciplinary and conceptual demarcations characteristic of contemporary science, does not necessarily help in disentangling the maze of assumptions, beliefs and social and political preoccupations that characterized 'scientific' activities of the seventeenth or the nineteenth centuries. Moreover, the investigation of economic, political or sociological features of theological, philosophical and scientific movements of the past should make historians of science increasingly reluctant to limit the sphere of their concern to a few texts, ideas and personalities selected for their relevance to contemporary priorities. Rigorous historical scholarship is necessary to promote the understanding of scientific cultures and activities of the past. Philosophical and epistemological training, as well as private theological beliefs, are certainly and inevitably part of the cultural equipment of the historian of science. But his work cannot be reduced to investigating the past as the repository of suitable examples proving or disproving contemporary views of science, philosophy or religion.

Bibliography

Agassi, J. (1963). *Towards an Historiography of Science.* History and Theory
Studies in the Philosophy of History, Vol. 2. The Hague; Mouton

Bachelard, G. (1934). *Le Nouvel esprit scientifique.* Paris; F. Alcan

Bachelard, G. (1938). *La Formation de l'esprit scientifique. Contribution à une
psychanalyse de la connaissance objective.* Paris; J. Vrin. 4th edn (1972)

Bachelard, G. (1951). *L'Activité rationaliste de la physique contemporaine.* Paris;
Presses Universitaires de France

Barreau, H. *et al.*, Ed. (1974). *Bachelard. Exposés.* Centre International de
Cérisy-la-Salle. Paris; Union Générale d'Editions

Bartholomew, M. (1973). Lyell and Evolution: An Account of Lyell's Response to
the Idea of an Evolutionary Ancestry for Man, *British Journal for the History of
Science*, Vol. 6, 261–303

Bartholomew, M. (1976). The Non-Progress of Non-Progression: Two Responses
to Lyell's Doctrine, *British Journal for the History of Science*, Vol. 9, 166–174

Baudot, M. (1967). Le Rôle de l'histoire des sciences selon Duhem, *Les Études
Philosophiques*, Vol. 22, 421–433

Benn, A.W. (1906). *The History of English Rationalism in the Nineteenth Century.*
2 Vols. London; Longmans, Green

Bosmans, H. (1921). Pierre Duhem (1861–1916): notice sur ses travaux relatifs à
l'histoire des sciences, *Revue des Questions Scientifiques*, Vol. 53, 30–62, 427–448

Bouligand, G. *et al.*, Ed. (1957). *Hommage à Gaston Bachelard. Études de
philosophie et d'histoire des sciences.* Paris; Presses Universitaires de France

Brooke, J.H. (1977). Natural Theology and the Plurality of Worlds : Observations
on the Brewster–Whewell Debate, *Annals of Science*, Vol. 34, 221–286

Brooke, J.H. (1979). The Natural Theology of the Geologists: Some Theological
Strata, in *Images of the Earth. Essays in the History of the Environmental
Sciences.* Ed. L.J. Jordanova and R.S. Porter. The British Society for the History
of Science Monographs, Vol. 1. Chalfont St Giles; The British Society for the
History of Science, 39–64

Brunschvicg, L. (1905). *L'Idéalisme contemporain.* Paris; F. Alcan

Brunschvicg, L. (1912). *Les Étapes de la philosophie mathématique.* Paris; F. Alcan

Brunschvicg, L. (1922). *L'Expérience humaine et la causalité physique.* Paris; F.
Alcan

Burian, R.M. (1977). More than a Marriage of Convenience: On the Inextricability
of History and Philosophy of Science, *Philosophy of Science*, Vol. 44, 1–42

Burtt, E.A. (1924). *The Metaphysical Foundations of Modern Science. A Historical
and Critical Essay.* New York; Harcourt Brace. 2nd revised edn (1932; reprinted
1967). London; Routledge and Kegan Paul. Quotations from the 1967 reprint

Burtt, E.A. (1943). Method and Metaphysics in Sir Isaac Newton, *Philosophy of
Science*, Vol. 10, 57–66

Butterfield, H. (1949). *The Origins of Modern Science 1300–1800.* London; G. Bell
and Sons. New revised edn (1957). London; Bell

Butterfield, H. (1964). The History of Historiography and the History of Science,
in *Mélanges Alexandre Koyré*, Paris; Hermann, Vol. 2: 37–68

Cannon, S.F. (also known as Cannon, W.F.) (1976). Charles Lyell, Radical
Actualism, and Theory, *British Journal for the History of Science*, Vol. 9,
104–120

Cannon, S.F. (1978). *Science in Culture. The Early Victorian Period.* New York;
Dawson and Science History Publications

Cannon, W.F. (also known as Cannon, S.F.) (1960a). The Impact of Uniformitarianism. Two Letters from John Herschel to Charles Lyell, 1836–1837, in
Proceedings of the American Philosophical Society, Vol. 105, 301–314

Cannon, W.F. (1960b). The Problem of Miracles in the 1830s, *Victorian Studies*, Vol. 4, 5–32

Cannon, W.F. (1962). The Role of the Cambridge Movement in Early 19th Century Science, in *Proceedings of the Tenth International Congress of the History of Science*, 317–320

Cannon, W.F. (1964). Scientists and Broad Churchmen: an Early Victorian Intellectual Network, *Journal of British Studies*, Vol. 4, 65–88. Expanded version (1978) in *Science in Culture*. New York; Dawson and Science History Publications, 29–71

Challinor, J. (1971). *The History of British Geology. A Bibliographical Study*. Newton Abbot; David and Charles

Chalmers, G.K. (1937). The Lodestone and the Understanding of Matter in Seventeenth Century England, *Philosophy of Science*, Vol. 4, 75–95

Comte, A. (1830–42), *Cours de philosophie positive*. 6 Vols. Paris; Bachelier. New edn (1975). Ed. M. Serres, F. Dagognet, A. Sinaceur, J.-P. Enthoven. 2 Vols. Paris; Hermann

Corsi, P. (1979). Sciences in Cultures, *Isis*, Vol. 70, 593–598

Corsi, P. (1980). Essay Review of Manier (1978), *Annals of Science*, Vol. 37, 673–678

Corsi, P. (to be published). *Revelation and Science: Anglican Theology and the Scientific Debate in England, 1800–1860*. Cambridge; Cambridge University Press

Crombie, A.C., Ed. (1963). *Scientific Change. Historical Studies in the Intellectual, Social and Technical Conditions for Scientific Discovery and Technical Innovation, from Antiquity to the Present*. Symposium on the History of Science, University of Oxford, 9–15 July 1961. London; Heinemann

Dagognet, F. (1965a). *Gaston Bachelard. Sa vie, son oeuvre avec un exposé de sa philosophie*. Paris; Presses Universitaires de France

Dagognet, F. (1965b). Brunschvicg et Bachelard, *Revue de Métaphysique et de Morale*, Vol. 70, 43–54

Darwin, C. (1859). *On the Origin of Species by Means of Natural Selection, or the Preservation of Favoured Races in the Struggle for Life*. London; John Murray

Draper, J.W. (1874). *History of the Conflict between Religion and Science*. London; H.S. King

Duhem, P. (1905). Physique du Croyant, *Annales de Philosophie Chrétienne*, Vol. 1, 44–67, 133–159

Duhem, P. (1906). *La Théorie physique: son objet, sa structure*. Paris; Chevalier et Rivière. New edn (1954). *The Aim and Structure of Physical Theory*. Trans. P.P. Wiener. Princeton; Princeton University Press

Duhem, P. (1913–59). *Le Système du monde. Histoire des doctrines cosmologiques de Platon à Copernic*. 10 Vols. Paris; Hermann

Fleming, D. (1950). *John William Draper and the Religion of Science*. Philadelphia; University of Pennsylvania Press

Frank, P. (1937). The Mechanical versus the Mathematical Conception of Nature, *Philosophy of Science*, Vol. 4, 41–74

Gaukroger, S.W. (1976). Bachelard and the Problem of Epistemological Analysis, *Studies in History and Philosophy of Science*, Vol. 7, 189–244

Gillispie, C.C. (1951). *Genesis and Geology. A Study in the Relations of Scientific Thought, Natural Theology, and Social Opinion in Great Britain, 1790–1850*. Cambridge, Mass.; Harvard University Press

Gillispie, C.C. (1964). Elements of Physical Idealism, in *Mélanges Alexandre Koyré*, Paris; Hermann, Vol. 2: 206–224

Green, J.C. (1977). Reflections on the Progress of Darwin Studies, *Journal of the History of Biology*, Vol. 10, 1–27

Gruber, H.E. (1974). *Darwin on Man: A Psychological Study of Scientific Creativity.* Transcribed and annotated P.H. Barrett. New York; E.P. Dutton. London; Wildwood House

Guerlac, H. (1963). Some Historical Assumptions of the History of Science, in *Scientific Change.* Ed. A.C. Crombie. London; Heinemann, 797–812. Reprinted in H. Guerlac (1977). *Essays and Papers in the History of Modern Science.* Baltimore and London; Johns Hopkins University Press, 27–39

Hall, A.R. (1963). Merton Revisited: or, Science and Society in the Seventeenth Century, *History of Science*, Vol. 2, 1–16

Hall, A.R. (1972). Science, Technology and Utopia in the Seventeenth Century, in *Science and Society, 1600–1900.* Ed. P. Mathias. Cambridge; Cambridge University Press, 33–53

Hill, J.E.C. (1964). *Society and Puritanism in Pre-Revolutionary England.* London; Secker and Warburg

Hill, J.E.C. (1965). *Intellectual Origins of the English Revolution.* Oxford; Clarendon Press

Hooykaas, R. (1959). *Natural Law and Divine Miracle: a Historical–Critical Study of the Principle of Uniformity in Geology, Biology and Theology.* Leyden; Brill

Hooykaas, R. (1972). *Religion and the Rise of Modern Science.* Edinburgh and London; Scottish Academic Press

Hunter, M. (1981). *Science and Society in Restoration England.* Cambridge; Cambridge University Press

Irving, J.A. (1936). Leibniz's Theory of Matter, *Philosophy of Science*, Vol. 3, 208–214

Jacob, J.R. (1977). *Robert Boyle and the English Revolution.* New York; Burt Franklin

Jacob, J.R. and Jacob, M.C. (1980). The Anglican Origins of Modern Science: The Metaphysical Foundations of the Whig Constitution, *Isis*, Vol. 71, 251–267

Jacob, M.C. (1976). *The Newtonians and the English Revolution 1689–1720.* Ithaca, NY; Cornell University Press. Hassocks, Sussex; Harvester Press

Kohn, D. (1975). Charles Darwin's Path to Natural Selection, University of Massachusetts PhD Dissertation

Kohn, D. (1980). Theories to Work by: Rejected Theories, Reproduction and Darwin's Path to Natural Selection, *Studies in History of Biology*, Vol. 4, 67–170

Kohn, D., Ed. (1982). *The Darwinian Heritage.* 2 Vols. Wellington, New Zealand; Nova Pacifica

Koyré, A. (1922). *Essai sur l'idée de Dieu et les preuves de son existence chez Descartes.* Paris; E. Leroux

Koyré, A. (1929). *La Philosophie de Jacob Boehme. Étude sur les origines de la métaphysique Allemande.* Paris; J. Vrin

Koyré, A. (1933). Paracelse, *Revue d'Histoire et de Philosophie Religieuse*, Vol. 13, 46–76, 145–163

Koyré, A. (1939). *Études Galiléennes.* 3 Vols. Vol. 1, *À l'aube de la science classique*; Vol. 2, *La Loi de la chute des corps, Descartes et Galilée;* Vol. 3, *Galilée et la loi d'inertie.* Paris; Hermann. Vol. 3 printed (1940)

Koyré, A. (1955). *Mystiques, spirituels, alchimistes du XVIe siècle allemand; Schwenckfeld, Seb. Franck, Weigel, Paracelse.* Paris; A. Colin

Koyré, A. (1961). *La Révolution astronomique. Copernic, Kepler, Borelli.* Paris; Hermann. Trans. (1973) as *The Astronomical Revolution.* London; Methuen

Koyré, A. (1963). Comment on H. Guerlac (1963), in *Scientific Change.* Ed. A.C. Crombie. London; Heinemann, 846–857

La Lumia, J. (1966). *The Ways of Reason. A Critical Study of the Work of Emile Meyerson.* New York; Humanities Press

Lecourt, D. (1969). *L'Epistémologie historique de Gaston Bachelard.* Paris; J. Vrin

Limoges, C. (1970). *La Sélection naturelle. Étude sur la première constitution d'un concept (1837–1859).* Paris; Presses Universitaires de France

Lyell, C. (1830–3). *Principles of Geology, being an Attempt to Explain the Former Changes of the Earth's Surface, by Reference to Causes now in Operation.* London; John Murray

Mach, E. (1893). *The Science of Mechanics. A Critical and Historical Exposition of its Principles.* Trans. T.J. McCormack. Chicago; The Open Court Publishing House. 1st edn (1883). Leipzig; F.A. Brockhaus

Maier, A. (1949–58). *Studien zur Naturphilosophie der Spätscholastick.* 5 Vols. Rome; Edizioni di Storia e Letteratura

Manier, E. (1978). *The Young Darwin and His Cultural Circle. A Study of the Influences which Helped Shape the Language and Logic of the First Drafts of the Theory of Natural Selection.* Dordrecht and Boston, Mass.; D. Reidel

Martin, R.N.D. (1976). The Genesis of a Medieval Historian: Pierre Duhem and the Origins of Statics, *Annals of Science*, Vol. 33, 119–129

Mélanges Alexandre Koyré. Publiés à l'occasion de son soixante-dixième anniversaire. L'aventure de l'esprit (1964). 2 Vols. Paris; Hermann

Merton, R.K. (1936). Puritanism, Pietism and Science, *Sociological Review*, Vol. 28, 1–30. Reprinted in R.K. Merton (1957). *Social Theory and Social Structure.* New York; Free Press of Glencoe, 574–606

Merton, R.K. (1938). Science, Technology and Society in Seventeenth Century England, *Osiris*, Vol. 4, 360–632. Reprinted with new introduction (1970). New York; Howard Fertig. Paperback edn (1978). New York; Humanities Press

Meyerson, E. (1908). *Identité et realité.* Paris; F. Alcan

Meyerson, E. (1927). *De l'explication dans les sciences.* Paris; Payot

Moore, J.R. (1979). *The Post-Darwinian Controversies. A Study of the Protestant Struggle to Come to Terms with Darwin in Great Britain and America 1870–1900.* Cambridge; Cambridge University Press

Morrell, J.B. (1980). Savants and Clergymen, *History of Science*, Vol. 18, 39–45

Morrell, J.B. and Thackray, A. (1981). *Gentlemen of Science. The Early Years of the British Association for the Advancement of Science.* Oxford; Oxford University Press

Mulligan, L. (1973). Civil War Politics, Religion and the Royal Society, *Past and Present*, No. 59, 92–116. In Webster (1974), 317–346

Mulligan, L. (1980). Puritans and English Science. A Critique of Webster, *Isis*, Vol. 71, 456–469

Neurath, O. (1937). Unified Science and its Encyclopaedia, *Philosophy of Science*, Vol. 4, 265–277

Ospovat, D. (1980). God and Natural Selection: The Darwinian Idea of Design, *Journal of the History of Biology*, Vol. 13, 169–194

Ospovat, D. (1981). *The Development of Darwin's Theory: Natural History, Natural Theology and Natural Selection, 1838–1859.* Cambridge; Cambridge University Press

Parker, I. (1914). *Dissenting Academies in England; Their Rise and Progress and Their Place among the Educational Systems of the Country.* Cambridge; Cambridge University Press

Paul, H.W. (1976). Scholarship Versus Ideology: The Chair of the General History of Science at the Collège de France, *Isis*, Vol. 67, 376–397

Paul, H.W. (1979). *The Edge of Certainty: French Catholic Reaction to Scientific Change from Darwin to Duhem.* Gainesville; University Presses of Florida

Poincaré, H. (1906). *La Science et l'hypothèse.* Paris; Flammarion

Poirier, R. (1967). L'Epistémologie de Pierre Duhem et sa valeur actuelle, *Les Études Philosophiques*, Vol. 22, 399–420

Porter, R.S. (1977). *The Making of Geology: Earth Science in Britain, 1660–1815.* Cambridge; Cambridge University Press

Purver, M. (1967). *The Royal Society: Concept and Creation.* London; Routledge and Kegan Paul. Cambridge, Mass.; MIT Press

Redondi, P. (1978). *Epistemologia e storia della scienza. Le svolte teoriche da Duhem a Bachelard.* Milan; Feltrinelli Editore

Rey, A. (1907). *La Théorie de la physique chez les physiciens contemporains.* Paris; F. Alcan

Rey, A. (1927). *Le Retour éternel et la philosophie de la physique.* Paris; E. Flammarion

Robertson, J.M. (1929). *A History of Freethought in the Nineteenth Century.* 2 Vols. London; Watts

Rossi, P. (1964). Sulla storicita 'della scienza e della filosofia, *Rivista di Filosofia,* Vol. 55, 131–153

Rossi, P. (1968). *Francis Bacon: From Magic to Science.* London; Routledge and Kegan Paul. Chicago; University of Chicago Press. 1st edn (1957). Revised edn (1974). *Francesco Bacone: dalla magia alla scienza.* Turin; Einaudi

Rudwick, M.J.S. (1970). The Strategy of Lyell's *Principles of Geology, Isis,* Vol. 61, 5–33

Rudwick, M.J.S. (1972). *The Meaning of Fossils. Episodes in the History of Paleontology.* London; Macdonald. New York; American Elsevier

Ruse, M. (1979). *The Darwinian Revolution.* Chicago and London; University of Chicago Press

Russell, C.A. (1973). *Science and Religious Belief: a Selection of Recent Historical Studies. The Open University.* London; University of London Press

Russo, F. (1957). Rôle respectif du catholicisme et du protestantisme dans le développement des sciences aux XVIe et XVIIe siècles, *Journal of World History,* Vol. 3, 854–880

Sarjeant, W. (1980). *Geologists and the History of Geology. An International Bibliography from the Origin to 1978.* 5 Vols. London; Macmillan Reference Books

Sarton, G. (1913). L'Histoire de la science, *Isis,* Vol. 1, 3–46

Sarton, G. (1924). The New Humanism, *Isis,* Vol. 6, 9–134

Sarton, G. (1957). *Six Wings: Men of Science in the Renaissance.* London; The Bodley Head. Bloomington; Indiana University Press

Schweber, S.S. (1977). The Origin of the *Origin* Revisited, *Journal of the History of Biology,* Vol. 10, 229–236

See, H. (1932). *Science et philosophie dans la doctrine de M. Emile Meyerson.* Paris; F. Alcan

Spiegelberg, H. (1960). *The Phenomenological Movement: A Historical Introduction.* 2 Vols. The Hague; M. Nijhoff

Stimson, D. (1935). Puritanism and the New Philosophy in Seventeenth Century England, *Bulletin of the Institute for the History of Medicine,* Vol. 3, 321–334

Strong, E.W. (1936). *Procedures and Metaphysics; A Study in the Philosophy of Mathematical–Physical Sciences in the Sixteenth and Seventeenth Centuries.* Berkeley; University of California Press

Taton, R. (1965). Alexandre Koyré historien de l'astronomie, *Revue d'Histoire des Sciences,* Vol. 18, 141–146

Thackray, A. (1980). History of Science, in *A Guide to the Culture of Science, Technology and Medicine.* Ed. P.T. Durbin. New York; The Free Press. London; Collier Macmillan, 3–69

Thackray, A. and Merton, R.K. (1972). On Discipline Building: The Paradoxes of George Sarton, *Isis,* Vol. 63, 473–495

Turnbull, G.H. (1947). *Hartlib, Dury and Comenius: Gleanings from Hartlib's Papers*. Liverpool; University Press of Liverpool

Turnbull, G.H. (1953). Samuel Hartlib's Influence on the Early History of the Royal Society, *Notes and Records of the Royal Society of London*, Vol. 10, 101–130

Turner, F.M. (1974). *Between Science and Religion: The Reaction to Scientific Naturalism in Late Victorian England*. New Haven, Conn., Yale University Press

Vorzimmer, P.J. (1972). *Charles Darwin, The Years of Controversy. The Origin of Species and its Critics 1859–82*. London; University of London Press. Also (1970). Philadelphia; Temple University Press

Webster, C. (1967). The Origins of the Royal Society, *History of Science*, Vol. 6, 106–128

Webster, C., Ed. (1974). *The Intellectual Revolution of the Seventeenth Century*. London; Routledge and Kegan Paul for Past and Present Publications

Webster, C. (1975). *The Great Instauration. Science, Medicine and Reform, 1626–1660*. London; Duckworth

Webster, C. (1979). *Utopian Planning and the Puritan Revolution. Gabriel Plattes, Samuel Hartlib and Macaria*. Research Publications, No. 2. Oxford; Wellcome Unit for the History of Medicine

Webster, C. (1981). Puritanism and Science. Paper read at the International Conference on Christianity and Science: Two Thousand Years of Conflict and Compromise. Madison, Wisconsin. Proceedings to be published, Eds D.C. Lindberg and R.L. Numbers

White, A.D. (1896). *A History of the Warfare of Science with Theology in Christendom*. 2 Vols. London; Macmillan

Wiener, P.P. (1937). Review of F. Enriques and G. de Santillana, *Histoire de la pensée scientifique* (Paris; Hermann, 1936–9), *Philosophy of Science*, Vol. 4, 387–390

Wilson, D.J. (1981). *Arthur O. Lovejoy and the Quest for Intelligibility*. Chapel Hill; North Carolina University Press

Wilson, L.G. (1972). *Charles Lyell. The Years to 1841: The Revolution in Geology*. New Haven, Conn.; Yale University Press

Young, R.M. (1969). Malthus and the Evolutionists: The Common Context of Biological and Social Theory, *Past and Present*, No. 43, 109–145

Young, R.M. (1973). The Historiographical and Ideological Contexts of the Nineteenth Century Debate on Man's Place in Nature, in *Changing Perspectives in the History of Science*. Ed. M. Teich and R.M. Young. London; Heinemann Educational. Boston, Mass.; D. Reidel, 344–438

Yule, J.D. (1976). The Impact of Science on British Religious Thought in the Second Quarter of the Nineteenth Century, University of Cambridge PhD Dissertation

Zambelli, P. (1965). Rinnovamento umanistico, progresso tecnologico e teorie filosofiche alle origine della rivoluzione scientifica, *Studi Storici*, Vol. 6, 507–546

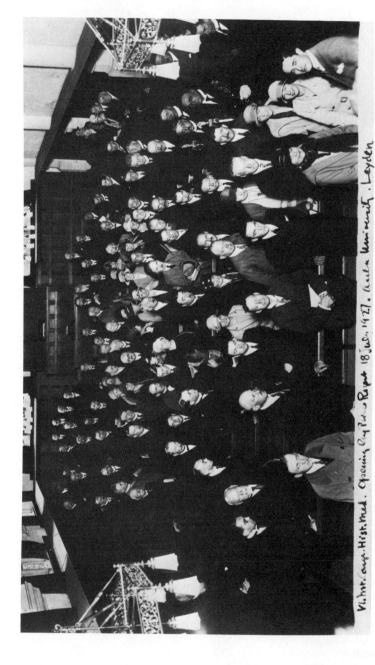

Plate 1. The VI International Congress for the History of Medicine, Leyden, 1927. Mieli, D'Arcy Power, Singer, Sudhoff and Welch were among those present. By courtesy of the Wellcome Trustees

2

The historiography of medicine

Charles Webster

The idea of progress is a fundamental tenet of modern Western thought. The experimental sciences provide exemplary support for this idea with their continuous development and record of innovation, which has been consistently maintained from the time of the scientific renaissance of the sixteenth century. Accordingly, histories of science assume the role of the natural and most authentic record of the idea of progress, thereby contributing to the high estimation of science in Western society.

Medicine is a field in which progress has been less spectacular, and in which the idea of linear development is much less tenable. But kinship with the sciences is undeniable, and it is not surprising that historians of medicine have absorbed the ethos of the history of science and have cultivated a sense of medicine's unity with science. Their histories of medicine run parallel to and interdigitate with histories of science, thereby carrying over into medicine the idea of progress advanced by the more successful partner. The history of medicine as a professionalized discipline has derived a strong directive influence from the history of the biomedical sciences. If anything this bias has become more pronounced as the present century has progressed. The history of medicine is to a large extent now regarded as a subdivision of the history of science. Aspects of medicine lying outside the scientific horizon are regarded as of subsidiary importance.

General histories of science and medicine have tended to reinforce this perspective. Because general surveys retain their position as major works of reference, and because they reflect often undisclosed changes of perspective in their subject, this review will briefly discuss the major standard histories of medicine, before concluding with a reference to possibilities for the realignment of the subject. Throughout its whole development modern medicine has been accompanied by a running historical commentary actively contributed to by some of the leading medical thinkers. Monographs in the history of medicine to a large degree reflect the tone of historical comment in the historical introductions that were until recently conventionally included in all types of medical treatise. Because historical reflection was taken more seriously in the past by the leaders of the profession, older histories of medicine must be treated as serious documents in view of their ostensible historical comment, and by virtue of their value as records of contemporary opinion. The older literature is thus by no means obsolete, or entirely superseded by modern workers. Indeed it contains discussions of many matters that have fallen into neglect, and that are only now recapturing interest. The great body of general histories produced before 1900 constitutes one of the important neglected resources of medicine. Rather than attempt any detailed listing, comment will be restricted to those works that are more substantial, original, influential or accessible. Many of the others not discussed deserve consultation for specific purposes; while a final large residuum comprises commercial productions devoid of intellectual seriousness. By contrast with the substantial comment on individual leading historians of medicine and their work, no author has attempted a detailed review of the modern history of medical historiography. The most adequate consistent interest in the broader subject is the virtual monopoly of one author (Heischkel 1931, 1938, 1949), who was concerned almost exclusively with the German contribution in this field.

Before 1700, many scientific treatises bore the title *Historia*, although such works were surveys of the present rather than the past. For the early modern period historical data and interpretation derive from every type of writing, but more specifically from collections of lives of scholars or from cumulative bibliographies. From an early date during the scientific revolution certain major authors developed a taste for such compilations. For instance, Otto Brunfels, author of the pioneering *Herbarum vivae icones* (1530–6) also compiled a *Catalogus illustrium medicorum* (1530). Of greater importance, Conrad Gesner, author of the huge *Historia animalium* (1551–87), also produced an impressive *Bibliotheca universalis* (1545) containing biographical notes, as well as a detailed bibliography concerning medical writers from the ancients onwards. Gesner remains an invaluable source, especially concerning Renaissance and Reformation authors. With the emergence of such works as *Vitae Germanorum medicorum* (1620) by Melchior Adam, the patriotic motive entered the history of medicine, and it was never again to recede in importance, in the history of either science or medicine. Thus one detects something of an inconsistency when finding in histories pronouncements on the universality of science and the fraternal nature of scientific effort, combined with squabbling over priorities of discovery and highly partisan attitudes to national schools of natural philosophy.

The first attempt at a history of medicine in the modern sense was made by Daniel Leclerc (1696), whose *Histoire de la médecine* was similar to the parallel pioneering *History of Philosophy* (1685) of Thomas Stanley, and concerned exclusively with ancient medicine. As a concession to later medicine Leclerc added to the second edition (1723) an appendix summarizing the development of medicine from Galen to the sixteenth century, while from the modern period Paracelsus and Paracelsianism were singled out for comment (Roethlisberger 1964). The judgement of Leclerc concerning the importance of Paracelsianism provides an interesting example of the manner in which the older histories run contrary to interpretations prevalent in modern histories of science. Despite dealing only with ancient medicine, Leclerc's work represents the complete fulfilment of his plan, by contrast with modern works of distinction, such as the histories by Neuburger (1906–10) and Sigerist (1951–61), in which the completed sections on ancient medicine represent a torso of much larger projects. These examples indicate the almost insurmountable problems of scale facing a single author attempting to write a history of medicine extending from antiquity to the present day.

A sequel to the work of Leclerc was provided by the Newtonian John Freind (1725–6) whose own project ended with the humanists of the sixteenth century. Freind illustrates the degree to which the 'moderns' attached importance to an appreciation of the lives and works of the 'ancients'. Despite writing in the vernacular, Leclerc and Freind demonstrate the tenacious hold of classical medical culture at the outset of the Enlightenment. Despite their limitation to classical subject matter, these works are pervaded by the idea of progress.

General interest in the history of medicine persisted in France and Britain, being reflected in minor surveys, but the major impetus for the development of the subject shifted to and was to remain in Germany. Even at the end of the nineteenth century the translator of the handbook by Baas (1876) complained of the lack of contribution to the history of medicine of the Anglo-Saxon world. This subject had become 'a peculiarly German department of science' (Baas, trans. Handerson: 657–8).

A few years later William Osler tried to redress the balance, but in 1912 he complained to a disciple at Oxford that 'the Germans are doing so much; it seems a pity we should be so far behind' (Osler to R.T. Gunther, 5 June 1912; Oxford, History of Science Museum, Old Ashmolean Letter Book I). Ironically the full development of the history of medicine in the Anglo-Saxon world was to await the arrival of exiled German scholars during the 1930s.

The flow of German histories of medicine began with works by Johann Conrad Barchusen (1710) and Johann Heinrich Schulze (1728). This movement was given new momentum by the bibliographical labours of Albrecht von Haller (1771–9), and in the last two decades of the century some half-dozen significant general histories of medicine were produced in Germany. By far the most important of these came from Kurt Sprengel (1792–1803). This work, whether in its original five-volume form or in its later greatly expanded editions and French translation, has lost none of its stature, being as thoughtful as any later work, but better digested and more alert to the need to relate to other branches of history. Sprengel's work seems all the more remarkable when it is appreciated that it represents a small part of his literary output, Sprengel's reputation in the field of botany easily matching that in medicine. Sprengel's intellectual debts are only partially revealed and they are not easy to work out, but he felt a particular kinship with the philologist Johann Christoph Adelung, a fellow Pomeranian, whose works included *Pragmatische Staatsgeschichte Europens* (1762–9), *Versuch einer Geschichte der Cultur des Menschlichen Geschlechts* (1782) and *Geschichte der Menschlichen Narrheit* (1785–9), all pertinent to the formation of Sprengel's historical outlook. The characteristic term 'pragmatic' was not discussed by Sprengel, but its use in his title carried two senses – firstly the idea that history has lessons for the present, secondly in the sense developed more fully by Hegel that progress in medicine or other aspects of culture is to be understood as a form of internal necessity. German histories of medicine continued to make free use of the term pragmatic without much attempt to specify which of its range of meanings was implied.

Sprengel saw his work as a contribution to the history of the progress of civilization. He aimed at an exact science of history that would demonstrate that revolutions in medicine were reflections of the general drama of history. Thus, in order to determine the causes of change in medicine it was necessary to pay attention to antecedent factors, among which philosophy was the most relevant. Sprengel used history to demonstrate that medical systems had been dictated by changes of fashion in philosophy, thereby supporting his own view that such systems, which had successively dominated medicine throughout the ancient and modern period, appeared to represent scientific progress but in fact had detracted from the progress of empirical research. Despite his own strong predilections, Sprengel purposely avoided writing his history in a strongly partisan spirit, aiming to arrive at a balanced view of the strengths and weaknesses of the medical doctrines generated during each historical period. His project exhibited significant differences from the earlier histories: the balance was shifted decisively from the ancient to the modern period; the traditional succession of lives of great doctors was replaced by discussion of schools of thought in which there was a more realistic appreciation of the relationship between major and minor figures; finally, this process of subdivision allowed the subject matter to be assembled into sections conforming with major historical periods. It was a subject for note and fierce criticism from later medical historians (e.g. Daremberg 1870: vol. 1, 36–9) that Sprengel pigeon-holed modern medicine into periods coinciding with political history, rather than judging it according to its internal evolution. Despite its seeming perversity, categorization of medical history in terms of the Lutheran Reformation, the Thirty Years' War and the reign of Frederick the Great, as adopted by Sprengel, deserves serious consideration, and it can be defended for certain major purposes in the history of medicine. Sprengel's controversial analysis marked the onset of a long debate concerning the identification of natural 'epochs', as if a natural classification suitable for all purposes, and possessing the veracity of natural classification within the organic kingdom, was within the reach of the taxonomist of the history of science and medicine. In the present century the divisions adopted have taken on a more settled appearance, and are thought to possess scientific validity by virtue of the application of Kuhnian language of stereotypes of scientific revolutions (see chapter 7 on philosophy of science). But there is much in our standard categorization that is contradicted by research, and one suspects that the edifice persists for reasons of deep-seated ideological appeal and didactic usefulness rather than historical validity.

Following Sprengel, the histories of J.F.K. Hecker (1822–9), Damerow (1828–9) and Isensee (1840–4) betray the historiographical influence of Hegel and Schelling (Seemen 1926; Risse 1969). Although Hecker failed to bring his work up to the modern period, it was conducted together with pioneering studies (e.g. 1839) of historical pathology, a subject almost completely ignored in previous histories. Hecker's programme was completed by Heinrich Haeser whose handbook first appeared in 1845 and was drastically revised and expanded on two further occasions, reaching its full three-volume form in the third edition (1875–82). Haeser is the recognizable direct ancestor of all subsequent major handbooks of the history of medicine, and none has effectively supplanted it. The author purposely avoided a popular format, adopting for his work the structure of a scientific treatise, to the extent of using numbered paragraphs and interposed bibliographical summaries and specialized digressions. This was the first history of medicine to be exhaustively documented. Hecker's tendency to reduce the number of historical divisions was extended by amalgamating Hecker's fourth and fifth periods, Paracelsus to Harvey, and from Harvey onwards, into a single modern period. By a further subtle change, Paracelsus was dethroned in favour of Vesalius and the humanists as the major turning point in modern medicine. A further effect of this amalgamation was to bypass the issue of relating medical change to transitions in political history. Haeser shifted the emphasis of his work to the evolution of the modern medical specialisms. Despite the move towards Ranke and *Quellenforschung*, the influence of *Naturphilosophie* was still evident with Haeser, although largely in his judgements regarding medical theory; even in the last edition of his work he showed himself a partisan of Röschlaub, Schönlein, and the natural history and parasitist school of pathology. Accordingly Haeser's conception of history seemed old-fashioned and retrogressive to impatient younger contemporaries, and it was met with running criticism from C.A. Wunderlich whose rival history called for a strong partisan approach in favour of the exact sciences and experimental physiology (Wunderlich 1859; Temkin and Temkin 1958; Temkin 1966). Wunderlich exhibited no patience with historical figures departing from what he regarded as the progressive line. He was thus preparing the way for the highly selective approach of modern works dominated by the history of the biomedical sciences.

Perhaps the most original feature of the Haeser handbook was the substantial section devoted to the history of epidemics. In the final edition this occupied the entire third volume. However, Haeser's jumbling of all diseases into a chronological catalogue was much less satisfactory than Hecker's studies of single diseases. In this field Haeser was overtaken by his contemporary August Hirsch (1881–6), whose handbook of historical and geographical pathology in its final form provided a comprehensive and well-ordered survey of the subjects covered by Haeser (Beck 1961). Undoubtedly, in view of the complexity of the subject matter and lack of a firm empirical basis over much of the field, studies that confined themselves to a single geographical area (Creighton 1894), or preferably to a single disease, as in the case of most of the studies by Hecker, were more satisfactory from both the historical and practical point of view. Historical pathology in the hands of the above authors was not merely or primarily an historical exercise. Following in the tradition of Hippocrates and Sydenham, or the later medical topographers, it was hoped that the exhaustive chronicling of the course of disease would reveal environmental causes and facilitate appropriate remedial action. This point of view was essentially at odds with the bacterial conception of disease. However, regardless of its motives, this school, along with the pioneers of vital statistics, provided a substantial basis for modern historical demography and epidemiology.

In 1865 Charles Daremberg dedicated to Haeser his short review of the history of medicine, thereby producing the first significant general history by a Frenchman since Leclerc. Even strong patriotic sentiment was insufficient to summon up enthusiasm for the work of his predecessors. The little book by the famous Cabanis designed to meet the revolutionary situation was dismissed by Daremberg as 'plus ornés que solides'. Indeed the *Coup d'oeil sur les révolutions et sur la réforme de la médecine* (1804) by Cabanis was primarily a vehicle for promoting the medical ideas of the *idéologues*, the slight historical component being entirely derivative. Apart from the popularization of P.V. Renouard, Daremberg had little competition from his countrymen in the composition of general surveys, although at the more scholarly level the French contribution was considerable (Edelstein 1947). Daremberg's major historical work (1870) was appropriately dedicated to his mentor, Emile Littré, the editor of Hippocrates. Not surprisingly Daremberg's strength was in his exposition of ancient medicine, but his lucid and philosophically acute discussion of physiological ideas of the modern period is unsurpassed, and far more liberal in conception than the widely consulted *Lectures on the History of Physiology* (1901) by Sir Michael Foster.

Daremberg made no attempt to deal exhaustively with all aspects of medicine. His emphasis was firmly on the science of life and the use of history to demonstrate the interrelationships between the constituent parts of the biomedical sciences. The

progress of medicine was thought to be entirely dictated by the
state of development and restraints exercised by its various
scientific 'tributaries'. By contrast with speculators and idealists,
Daremberg described his approach as one of 'brutal materialism'
with respect to evidence and texts. Daremberg nevertheless betrayed the influence of a strong positivist legacy inherited from
Littré. His earlier *Essai sur la détermination et les caractères des
périodes de l'histoire de la médecine* (1850) provided a framework
for the description of progress in medicine in terms of eight
'epochs', akin to the system of Sprengel but with an entirely
different justification, having reference to autonomous developments in the sciences, so avoiding Sprengel's idea of the interrelationship between science and political change.

The 'splitting' tendency evident in Daremberg, developed in
opposition to Haeser, was taken even further by J.L. Pagel (1898).
His short survey was divided into twenty-five lectures. This
retained its position into the 1930s as the most widely used
introductory textbook in the editions edited by Karl Sudhoff (W.
Pagel 1951; Sigerist 1951).

The more exhaustive handbooks reached their zenith at this
time. J.H. Baas, a keen amateur, composed two major surveys
(1876, 1896), the later – untranslated and lesser-known – being
better structured and more fully digested. Both have the merit of
dealing with a variety of more practical aspects of medicine, rather
than concentrating on advanced research in the biomedical sciences. To his contemporaries Baas seemed old-fashioned, or out of
touch, but he had much to say about medical education, the
organization of the profession, minor practitioners, and fringe
medicine, and he was genuinely cosmopolitan in approach. On the
other hand, in the attempt to be encyclopaedic, his work tends to
be excessively synoptic and frequently degenerates into lists of
names and dates.

Theodor Puschmann of Vienna shared many of the interests of
Baas, and was himself a pioneer of the history of medical
education (Lesky 1976: 571–4). Realistically appreciating that an
authoritative history of medicine covering the whole range of
medical specialisms was beyond the reach of a single author, he
drew together a team of authors to produce a major survey
(Puschmann 1902–5). This work retains its value for reference
purposes, but its value as history is severely limited by the
compartmental arrangement. In a remarkable virtuoso effort
designed to restore the philosophical and historical dimension to
this work, Puschmann's pupil Neuburger contributed an introduction to the second volume, attempting to recapitulate the entire
history of modern medicine in some 150 pages. Fortuitously this

essay was to provide his major comment on modern medicine, since his own ambitious handbook of medical history was not carried beyond the Middle Ages (Neuburger 1906–10; Kagan 1943). The last major German history of medicine makes no concessions to twentieth-century historiography (Diepgen 1914–28, 1949–55), despite the adoption of periodization (e.g. Baroque, Enlightenment) suggesting reference to cultural history. Small sections on 'Das ärztliche Leben' provide minimal information on the subjects emphasized by Baas and Puschmann. Otherwise the history runs along predictable lines. Diepgen is solid, detailed and accurate, pro-Paracelsianism, but anti-Romantic. His later and fuller book is still the best summary guide to nineteenth-century German medicine.

The twentieth century has produced many histories of medicine, but it is doubtful whether collectively or individually they are as useful as their nineteenth-century forebears. F.H. Garrison (1913) will retain its reference value on account of its exhaustive coverage of the basic data and its sound indexing. Osler's survey (1921) has no appeal outside the Osler fraternity. The best-known English language history of medicine was produced by Charles Singer (1928), more recently issued in a greatly expanded form by E.A. Underwood (Singer 1962). The original edition is dedicated to E.T. Withington, himself the author of a useful short history of medicine (1894). Singer was a prolific author, his short histories being especially widely consulted. His history of medicine is similar in character to, but not as successful as, his *History of Anatomy and Physiology from the Greeks to Harvey* or the *Short History of Biology*. In the *Short History of Medicine* his characteristic lightness of touch carries the penalties of thinness of content and lack of intellectual depth. The substantial additions made by Underwood leave us with a volume of uneven character, with the added disadvantage of parochialism. Singer's historiographical standpoint reflects the attitudes of the founders of the history of science and medicine in Britain, who saw the two subjects as having a close identity of purpose. Singer's aim was to treat 'medicine as a science' and his text was intended to be read in close juxtaposition with his history of biology. The volume began and ended with a defence of vitalistic biology. As in the case of the superior historical writings of E.S. Russell, the history of biology and medicine was seen as a vehicle for rehearsing the strengths of the vitalist position, at that time coming under increasing pressure from the younger generation of biochemists. For further discussion of their work, see chapters 18 and 19 on medicine and experimental life sciences.

The concern with promoting the values of science and contributing to the philosophy of science led to the history of medicine becoming almost completely identified with the history of biology and the biomedical sciences, and resulted in the formation of that sterile hybrid 'the history and philosophy of science'. So long as the latter provided the institutional and intellectual framework for the history of science, it was very difficult for the history of medicine to achieve an independent identity in the Anglo-Saxon world. The major spur towards a new view of the history of science and medicine in Britain was the publication of *Science at the Cross Roads* (1931), the Soviet contribution to the Second International Congress of the History of Science and Technology organized by Singer in 1931 and centrally designed to promote discussion of the vitalist controversy. Singer's position was not effectively advanced by this conference, but *Science at the Cross Roads* popularized the Marxist conception of the sociology of knowledge, and this experience was instrumental in furthering the interest in the social history of science and medicine of such figures as J.D. Bernal and J. Needham, both of whom had been unsympathetic to Singer's vitalism at the congress.

This meeting marked the beginning of a vigorous debate that has deeply influenced the subsequent course of the study of the history of science and medicine. On the one side a rigorous distinction was drawn between pure and applied science, the progress of the former being regarded as independent of social factors and determined by the free exercise of individual genius and the internal logic of the scientific situation. The other side questioned the validity of this distinction and urged that every aspect of scientific enquiry was influenced by economic and social factors. As Professor Gowing explains in chapter 6, these two views of history were associated with opposing ideas concerning the future planning of science. History was thus drawn into a controversy that affects the entire future of science in Western society. The history of medicine occupied particularly sensitive territory in view of its subsistence at the fringe of the pure and applied. In the light of this controversy, it is possible to detect an incentive towards narrowing the focus of definition of the history of medicine, greater concentration on the history of the biomedical sciences, and consequent elimination or trivialization of all other aspects of the subject. Any movement towards broadening the conception of the history of science or medicine might be seen as a concession to the 'extravagant idea of subordinating science to the planning of welfare' and hence as 'part of a general attack on the status of intellectual and moral life' (Polanyi 1941, 1945).

Effective consolidation of a broader conception of the history of medicine occurred primarily in the USA and was particularly associated with the Johns Hopkins Institute for the History of Medicine. Replying to criticisms from the famous historian of science George Sarton, made in his journal *Isis* (Sarton 1935), Sigerist argued for the independent status of the history of medicine: 'Medicine is not a *branch of science* and will never be. If medicine is a science, then it is a social science', and not an applied science. If any dimension was needed to make the subject more complete, it was integral reference to political history, social history, economic history and the history of religion (Sigerist 1936). He called for social history of medicine, not as a complement or supplement to the history of medical science, but as a substitute for it. He wanted the history of medicine not to 'limit itself to the history of science, institutions, and characters of medicine, but [to] include the history of the patient in society, and that of the physician and the history of the relations between physician and patient. History thus becomes social history' (Sigerist 1940). Following this line of argument, which amounted to an indictment of the history of medicine in both its traditional and modern forms – since neither was consistent with either Marxist historiography or the social sciences – there was need for a general history of medicine conceived according to Sigerist's point of view. This was clearly a major undertaking and only the first two volumes of this history, dealing exclusively with ancient medicine, were completed (Sigerist 1951–61). These volumes are model demonstrations of the application of the Sigerist call for a 'New History of Medicine'.

The most satisfactory survey of modern medicine consistent with the viewpoint of Sigerist, but produced largely independently, came from the scholar who was to become Sigerist's successor at the Johns Hopkins Institute (Shryock 1936). Shryock's work reflected the growing interest among American social historians in the problems of health and medicine. The increasing bias towards American subject matter in the later sections of the book is not detrimental to its qualities as a survey of the problems of health and medicine, especially since 1800. It is interesting to note the degree to which even Shryock's book was dominated by a relatively positivist conception of stages in intellectual progress. He believed that in 1800 the European intellect had reached its 'fourth level' of development (ch. 8). His own survey was concerned with mapping the progress of medicine in its fully mature form.

The scene is now set for the appearance of further collaborative histories of medicine. Various such projects are currently underway, and are announced in somewhat pretentious terms. However, there is no sign that current effort will rise to anything like the stature of the work of Puschmann's associates. And despite claims to the contrary the newer histories of medicine are remarkably conservative in their points of emphasis. Even the more broadly based histories are essentially concerned with the notion of progress and with the identification of major stages in the story of progress; authors have disagreed merely over the degree to which it was necessary to refer to extraneous factors in explaining the major transitions of outlook accomplished by the chief historical figures in medicine. Attempts to depart from this formula have been more persuasive in prescription or programme than in performance. Social history now risks becoming a painlessly absorbed and fashionable panacea, while the discipline out of inertia retains its traditional centre of gravity. There is little sign of historians of medicine abandoning their traditional preoccupation with great doctors and great books. The pressure for a complete change of perspective emanates from outside – from social historians, demographers, historical geographers, who need to enquire into the state of health of communities in the past in connection with their investigations into material life or the dynamics of personal relationships. Histories of pathology by Hecker, Haeser, Hirsch and Creighton provide valuable materials for this exercise, but these authors were not interested in social history. Patients were of interest merely as the passive vehicles of particular diseases. Historians of public health, hygiene or social medicine (e.g. Simon 1890; Fischer 1933; Sand 1952) dwelt on problems of health care in more realistic terms. Fischer, Puschmann and Baas have provided insights into the higher ranks of the medical profession. But we are still at a primary stage of data gathering (see Imhof 1980 for a survey of current work) with respect to compiling a history of medicine that would place its primary emphasis on the changing pattern of health of the population as a whole, and on the mechanisms of health care in proportion to their relevance to the health needs of the major sections of the community.

Bibliography

Baas, J.H. (1876). *Grundriss der Geschichte der Medicin und des heilenden Standes.* Stuttgart; F. Enke. Trans. H.E. Handerson (1889). New York; Vail. Reprinted (1971). New York; R.E. Krieger

Baas, J.H. (1896). *Die geschichtliche Entwicklung des ärztlichen Standes und der medicinischen Wissenschaften.* Berlin; Friedrich Wreden

Beck, E. (1961). Die 'Historisch–Geographische Pathologie' von August Hirsch, *Gesnerus*, Vol. 18, 33–44

Creighton, C. (1894). *A History of Epidemics in Britain*. 2 Vols. London; Cambridge University Press. 2nd edn (1965) with additional material by D.E.C. Eversley, E.A. Underwood and L. Ovenall. 2 Vols. London; Frank Cass

Damerow, H. (1828–9). *Die Elemente der nächsten Zukunft der Medicin, entwickelt aus der Vergangenheit und Gegenwart. Ein Blick*. Berlin; Reimer

Daremberg, C. (1865). *La Médecine. Histoire et doctrines*. Paris; Didier and Baillière

Daremberg, C. (1870). *Histoire des sciences médicales*. 2 Vols. Paris; J.B. Baillière

Diepgen, P. (1914–28). *Geschichte der Medizin*. 5 Vols. Berlin and Leipzig; Sammlung Göschen

Diepgen, P. (1949–55). *Geschichte der Medizin*. 2 Vols in 3 parts. Berlin; Walter de Gruyter

Edelstein, L. (1947). Medical Historiography of 1847, *Bulletin of the History of Medicine*, Vol. 21, 495–511

Fischer, A. (1933). *Geschichte des Deutschen Gesundheitswesens*. 2 Vols. Berlin; Oscar Rothacker. Reprinted (1965). Hildesheim; G. Olms

Freind, J. (1725–6). *The History of Physick; from the Time of Galen, to the Beginning of the Sixteenth Century*. 2 Vols. London; J. Walthoe

Garrison, F.H. (1913). *An Introduction to the History of Medicine*. Philadelphia and London; W.B. Saunders. 4th edn (1929). Philadelphia; W.B. Saunders. Reprinted (1960)

Haeser, H. (1875–82). *Lehrbuch der Geschichte der Medicin und epidemischen Krankheiten*, 3rd edn. Jena; Hermann Dufft and Gustav Fischer

Haller, A. von (1771–2). *Bibliotheca botanica*. 2 Vols. London; prostant apud C. Heydinger

Haller, A. von (1774–5). *Bibliotheca chirurgica*. 2 Vols. Berne; Haller. Basle; Schweighauser

Haller, A. von (1774–7). *Bibliotheca anatomica*. 2 Vols. Zürich; apud Orell, Gessner, etc.

Haller, A. von (1776–9). *Bibliotheca medicinae practicae*. 4 Vols. Berne; Haller

Hecker, J.F.K. (1822–9). *Geschichte der Heilkunde nach den Quellen bearbeitet*. 2 Vols. Berlin; T.C.F. Enslin

Hecker, J.F.K. (1839). *Geschichte der neueren Heilkunde*. Berlin; T.C.F. Enslin

Heischkel, E. (1931). Die Medizinhistoriographie im XVIII Jahrhundert, *Janus*, Vol. 35, 67–105, 125–151

Heischkel, E. (1938). *Die Medizingeschichtsschreibung von ihren Anfängen bis zum Beginn des 16. Jahrhunderts*. Abhandlungen zur Geschichte der Medizin und der Naturwissenschaften, No. 28. Berlin; Emil Eberling

Heischkel, E. (1949). Die Geschichte der Medizingeschichtschreibung, *Einführung in die Medizinhistorik*. Ed. W. Artelt. Stuttgart; F. Enke, 202–237

Hirsch, A. (1881–6). *Handbuch der historisch–geographischen Pathologie*, 2nd edn. 3 Vols. Stuttgart; F. Enke. Trans. C. Creighton (1883–6). 3 Vols. London; New Sydenham Society

Imhof, A.E., Ed. (1980). *Mensch und Gesundheit in der Geschichte*. Abhandlungen zur Geschichte der Medizin und der Naturwissenschaften, No. 39. Husum; Matthiesen Verlag

Isensee, E. (1840–4). *Die Geschichte der Medicin und ihrer Hilfswissenschaften*. 6 Vols. Berlin; Nauck

Kagan, S.R. (1943). Professor Max Neuburger, *Bulletin of the History of Medicine*, Vol. 14, 423–448

Leclerc, D. (1696). *Histoire de la médecine*. Geneva; J.A. Chouët and D. Ritter

42   The historiography of medicine

Leclerc, D. (1723). *Histoire de la médecine ... augmentée d'un plan pour servir à la continuation de cette histoire ... jusques au milieu du XVII*. Amsterdam; Aux dépens de la Compagnie

Lesky, E. (1976). *The Vienna Medical School of the Nineteenth Century*. Trans. L. Williams and I.S. Levij. Baltimore and London; Johns Hopkins University Press. 1st German edn (1965)

Miller, G., Ed. (1966). *A Bibliography of the Writings of Henry E. Sigerist*. Montreal; McGill University Press

Neuburger, M. (1906–10). *Geschichte der Medizin*. 2 Vols. Stuttgart; F. Enke. Trans. E. Playfair (1910–25). London; Oxford University Press

Osler, W. (1921). *The Evolution of Modern Medicine*. New Haven; Yale University Press

Pagel, J.L. (1898). *Einführung in die Geschichte der Medizin*. 2 Vols. Berlin; S. Karger

Pagel, W. (1951). Julius Pagel and the Significance of Medical History for Medicine, *Bulletin of the History of Medicine*, Vol. 25, 207–225

Polanyi, M. (1941). The Growth of Thought in Society, *Economica*, Vol. 8, 428–456

Polanyi, M. (1945). The Planning of Science, *The Political Quarterly*, Vol. 16, 316–328

Puschmann, T. (1902–5). *Handbuch der Geschichte der Medizin*. Ed. M. Neuburger and J.L. Pagel. 3 Vols. Jena; G. Fischer

Risse, G.B. (1969). Historicism in Medical History. Heinrich Damerow's 'Philosophical' Historiography in Romantic Germany, *Bulletin of the History of Medicine*, Vol. 43, 201–211

Roethlisberger, P. (1964). Daniel Le Clerc und seine 'Histoire de la médecine', *Gesnerus*, Vol. 21, 126–141

Sand, R. (1952). *The Advance to Social Medicine*. London; Staples Press. Ist French edn (1948)

Sarton, G. (1935). The History of Science versus the History of Medicine, *Isis*, Vol. 23, 313–320

Science at the Cross Roads (1931). Papers presented to the International Congress of the History of Science and Technology held in London from June 29th to July 3rd 1931 by the Delegates of the USSR. London; Kniga (England). 2nd edn (1971). New foreword by J. Needham and new introduction by P.G. Werskey. London; Cass

Seemen, H. von (1926). *Zur Kenntnis der Medizinhistorie in der deutschen Romantik*. Leipzig Univ. Inst. für Geschichte der Medizin, Beiträge, No. 3. Zürich; O. Füssli

Shryock, R.H. (1936). *The Development of Modern Medicine. An Interpretation of the Social and Scientific Factors Involved*. Philadelphia; University of Pennsylvania Press. 2nd edn (1947). Paperback edn (1979). Madison; University of Wisconsin Press

Sigerist, H.E. (1936). The History of Medicine and the History of Science, *Bulletin of the Institute of the History of Medicine*, Vol. 4, 1–13

Sigerist, H.E. (1940). The Social History of Medicine, *Western Journal of Surgery, Obstetrics and Gynecology*, Vol. 48, 715–722

Sigerist, H.E. (1951). On the 100th Anniversary of Julius Pagel's Birth, *Bulletin of the History of Medicine*, Vol. 25, 203–206

Sigerist, H.E. (1951–61). *A History of Medicine*. 2 Vols. New York; Oxford University Press

Simon, J. (1890). *English Sanitary Institutions, Reviewed in their Course of Development and in some of their Political and Social Relations*. London; Cassell. Reprinted (1970). New York and London; Johnson Reprint Corporation

Singer, C. (1928). *A Short History of Medicine.* Oxford; Clarendon Press
Singer, C. (1962). *A Short History of Medicine.* Ed. E.A.Underwood. Oxford; Clarendon Press
Sprengel, K. (1792–1803). *Versuch einer pragmatischen Geschichte der Arzneykunde.* 5 Vols. Halle; Gebauer
Temkin, O. (1966). Wunderlich, Schelling and the History of Medicine, *Gesnerus,* Vol. 23, 188–195
Temkin, O. and Temkin, L. (1958). Wunderlich versus Haeser. A Controversy over Medical History, *Bulletin of the History of Medicine,* Vol. 32, 97–104
Withington, E.T. (1894). *Medical History from the Earliest Times.* London; Scientific Press
Wunderlich, C.A. (1859). *Geschichte der Medicin. Vorlesungen gehalten zu Leipzig.* Stuttgart; Ebner und Seubert

3

The history of technology

Arnold Pacey

Traditional approaches

There has not always been a sharp distinction between the history of technology in its modern sense and 'histories of trades' of the sort advocated by Francis Bacon in the seventeenth century. Some early accounts of the chronological development of particular types of machine (e.g. Farey 1827) were also intended as guides to current practice. The same is partly true of some writings on the 'history of manufactures', of which there are nineteenth-century examples from Europe (e.g. D'Aubuisson 1802), Britain (Barlow 1836) and, most notably, North America (Bishop 1863; Bolles 1878; Clark 1929). The usefulness of these books as sources for the modern historian is considerable, as one may see from citations of them in recent works (e.g. Rosenberg 1976). But by 1900, the *genre* had become largely the province of economic historians, who produced useful surveys of industry not only in America and Western Europe, but also in India (Dutt 1902) and Russia (Tugan-Baranovskii 1907). Where historians of technology have continued to work along these lines, they have generally concentrated on particular industries, such as automobile manufacture (Rae 1959) or chemicals (Haber 1969; J.G. Smith 1979; Warren 1980).

Two other traditional approaches are those that document the lives of engineers and inventors, and those that describe the evolution of particular types of machine or device. The biographical approach became well established in the last century with

44

popular books portraying the engineer as something of a folk-hero (Smiles 1861; Stuart 1871), and it continues today in carefully researched modern works on 'great engineers' (Goulden 1982). Histories of particular types of device and their invention cover every conceivable kind of hardware: machine tools (Woodbury 1960), bridges (Hopkins 1970), radio (Leinwoll 1979) and dams (N. Smith 1971). Other books deal more generally with electrical and mechanical inventions (Dunsheath 1962; Usher 1954), and with specialized aspects of agriculture (Trow Smith 1959; Rossiter 1975).

These traditional ways of documenting the history of engineering and invention still predominate in the senior British journal, *Transactions of the Newcomen Society* (1920–), despite the many new approaches demonstrated by the principal American journal in the field, *Technology and Culture* (1959–). The traditional style also persists in two useful multi-volume reference works edited by Daumas (1979–80) and by Singer *et al.* (1954–9, updated by T.I. Williams 1978). Short bibliographies in the former work are particularly helpful with leads to French and German literature in the field. These works, of course, deal predominantly with Western technology; Chinese technology (and science) is dealt with in an even more monumental reference book by Needham (1954–80).

There is a certain lack of perspective in much of the writing that follows the traditional pattern, arising partly from a relative neglect of the institutions and social structures that influence (and sometimes restrict) the development of technology. Even so, traditional approaches have produced much good work, particularly on engineering in Antiquity (Camp 1960; Landels 1978) and during the European Renaissance (Parsons 1939; Reti 1972).

Among books that are more innovative in approach, there is a general history of technology edited by Kranzberg and Pursell (1967). There is also Klemm's (1959) stimulating anthology of technical literature and Braudel's (1973) novel synthesis of technological and social history. More specialist works that succeed in looking at technology from a social as well as a technical point of view include two or three dealing with the Middle Ages (White 1962; Gimpel 1958). With regard to studies of Renaissance technology, there are also valuable works by Gille (1966) and Keller (1967, 1976), and there is an important symposium on many aspects of 'pre-modern' technology edited by Hall and West (1976).

One important theme in all these books is the transfer of technological ideas and discoveries from one culture to another.

The well-known examples relate to the way in which medieval
Europe adopted technological ideas from China (often via Arab
intermediary applications) and directly from the Islamic world –
for instance, gunpowder, the magnetic compass, paper-making
and perhaps some clock mechanisms. However, it is still not
adequately recognized to what extent the diffusion of technological ideas quickened during the period of European colonial expansion. Not only were new medicinal herbs and food crops introduced into Europe from newly explored countries, but many
technical ideas were copied also. Travellers noted specific techniques (such as calico printing in India), and they also observed that
apparently primitive hand-production methods in many countries
could turn out better quality goods than were made in Europe.
The most notable examples were paper and porcelain in China and
cotton textiles in India, which Europeans tried hard to equal
throughout the eighteenth century. But around 1800, travellers in
both Africa (Wilson 1969: 144–5) and India (Dharampal 1971)
sent back reports of locally made ironware that equalled or
excelled the quality of British products, and the history of a small
British paper mill reveals that, as late as 1874, considerable
research was needed to equal the quality of special paper imported
from East Asia (Carter 1957).

So important were these processes of technological borrowing
that a major source for the historian of technology is the many
journals, diaries and reports written by the technically minded
travellers most responsible for the transmission of ideas. One of
the best books presenting this kind of material deals with European travellers in India (Dharampal 1971), but travellers in Asia
have in general received much less attention than the journeys of
Europeans visiting other Western countries (Henderson 1966,
1968).

Another topic that has attracted considerable attention is the
relationship between technology, science and academic learning.
A good starting point is to examine the influence of Renaissance
translations of classical texts in stimulating experiment on
machines, pneumatics and hydraulic devices (Keller 1967).
Galileo's achievements could well be included in such studies, for
there is a growing appreciation of the significance of his writings
on three aspects of engineering: machines, scale models and
ballistics. However, most books in English portray Galileo only as
a natural philosopher, and one must turn to Italian scholars for
fuller assessment of his technological background (e.g. Bulferetti
1964). Even when seen in this light, though, his achievements may
seem very limited. In fact, historians have argued that, in general

terms, 'seventeenth century science still lacked the depth of precise, quantitative information that alone is useful to engineers' (Hall 1961).

Some scholars disagree with this assessment, but there is no way of resolving the issue except by paying more attention to the social networks by which new knowledge spread to practising engineers and craftsmen. Such networks included the private teachers of mathematics in France (e.g. Mariotte and Parent), and the activities of instrument makers, educational reformers and popular lecturers in England (documented by Taylor 1954, Brown 1979 and Webster 1975, with pioneer work on the industrial revolution by Musson and Robinson 1969). However, there is scope for more work in this area, perhaps using techniques developed to study literacy (Laqueur 1976) in examining the growth of numeracy among millwrights, masons and other craftsmen. In the absence of such research, one can only draw on impressions – of canal-builders in America in the 1790s hamstrung by poor knowledge of surveying (Morison 1974: 21), of Thomas Telford's advisers using a Galileo theory, and of James Watt's friends baffled by the algebra in French textbooks (Pacey 1976: 225–9).

Some work on the relationships between science and technology has been based on the assumption that influence always proceeds from 'science' to 'technology'. Within the last century that is how things have often worked out, with discoveries in chemistry affecting agriculture (Rossiter 1975), textile industries and the development of plastics, and with discoveries in electromagnetism leading to the invention of radio (Leinwoll 1979). However, interactions of the opposite kind have often been important. The clearest instance is the development of thermodynamics in the first half of the nineteenth century, where Cardwell (1971) has clearly shown that conceptual development grew out of experience with hydraulic machines and steam engines. Further discussion of relations between science and industry is provided in chapter 6.

Technology as practice

Recent discussion of the current state of work in the history of technology has emphasized two main options for future studies – either the further development of specialist researches on 'internalist' lines, or a broadening of perspectives informed by the larger field of social history (Hounshell 1981; compare Cardwell *et al.* 1981). This choice can be put into sharper focus by noting that internalist histories of technology nearly always turn out to be histories of innovation. By contrast, the 'social history' approach is more comprehensive – it offers the prospect of new insights into innovation as a social process, but it can also open up for study aspects of the day-to-day practice of technology that have hitherto been scarcely examined at all. These might include questions about the persistence of traditional technologies and the decline of obsolescent ones as well as the use that is actually made of innovations. It would certainly give due weight to examining how both practice and innovation are affected by professional, educational and industrial institutions, and also by work disciplines.

The great strength of many 'internalist' histories of technology is that their authors have taken great pains to understand in detail the working of the machines or processes that they discuss. But there is danger in overemphasis on the working principles of machines. One can end up with a description of how machines *ought* to have worked that disregards problems encountered in day-to-day practice. Lynn White's (1962) discussion of how the medieval plough revolutionized agriculture is in many ways a brilliant example of how the history of technology and social history can illuminate one another. But White's arguments do sometimes depend on internalist deductions about how the plough ought to have worked that seem overly idealized when confronted with information on the difficult soils in which the plough had to operate and the 'puny' oxen available to pull it (Long 1979).

Similarly, internalist analysis of industrial innovation frequently needs to be amplified by evidence about practice. For example, to understand the 'American system of manufactures', one certainly needs to know what machine tools it depended on and how they worked (Woodbury 1958, 1960). But one also requires evidence of the social attitudes that lay behind the system (Sawyer 1954) and the economic structure of the industries in which it operated (Rosenberg 1963, 1976). Only when these three aspects are pulled together is a full understanding possible – and this has been very largely achieved by Merritt Roe Smith (1977).

This kind of synthesis is difficult to arrive at because of the broad spectrum that must be covered, which includes labour history, business history and institutional change as well as the real nuts and bolts of the engineering. Thus it is perhaps not surprising that much of the best work of this kind has focused on small communities or restricted geographical areas (Trinder 1973; Wallace 1978). On a national or international scale, any similar synthesis is almost entirely lacking, and the nearest one comes to it is in the work of a few outstanding economic historians, especially Landes (1969), who deals with the whole of Europe from 1750 onwards, and Rosenberg (1972) on America. Much related material can be gained by *selective* use of two multi-volume economic histories of Europe (including Russia) – the *Cambridge Economic History* (see especially Habakkuk and Postan 1965), and the more recent work edited by Cipolla (1972–6). For America there is also Boorstin's (1973) account emphasizing the social implications of technological change.

The perspectives of 'technology as practice' that economic historians sometimes offer are also better suited than an internalist approach to the comparative study of technology in different countries. Thus, although readers interested in the early technology of Asian civilizations can approach the subject through the history of science (see chapters 21, 22 and 23 in this book), a more direct introduction is provided by works on economic history by Simkin (1968, on the whole of south Asia) and Elvin (1973, on China), and by some extremely stimulating but more specialist papers (Hartwell 1966, 1967; Okita 1966; Lockwood 1955: 167–235).

Economic history is sometimes very usefully complemented by archaeology, which can confront one very vividly with detail of technology as it was really practised, especially when used to investigate relatively modern industries. Archaeology can also provide new perspectives on technological development as a world-wide process through what it reveals about ancient civilizations, African cultures and pre-Columban America. One's understanding of pre-modern technology is inevitably challenged, for example, by evidence of fourteenth-century mining and metal-refining operations in Zimbabwe, which could support extensive trade with Arab merchants including occasional imports of celadon pottery from China (Summers 1969; Garlake 1973). Norman Smith's (1971) use of archaeological evidence and field observation from various parts of the Middle East and Spain is instructive as to method, and Evenari *et al.* (1971) describe in a striking way how archaeologists rediscovered forgotten water conservation techniques and reapplied them for the benefit of modern communities.

Despite the interest of such work, it is the mutant form known as 'industrial archaeology' that has gained the widest following in recent years, particularly in the United States, Britain, Germany and Sweden. Results from this field have so far been seen mainly in topographical surveys (e.g. Buchanan 1980; Historic American Engineering Record 1974–9), or in the specialist journals listed by Hudson (1979). The growing number of industrial museums that Hudson also mentions mostly illustrate the practice of technology in specific regions, leaving the more traditional science museums to focus on innovation, and often to produce scholarly publications (e.g. Brown 1978; Ferguson 1962). It should not be forgotten either that ever since the publication of Klingender's (1947) book on art and industry, art galleries have occasionally held exhibitions of technological source material documented by useful catalogues (e.g. S. Smith 1979). One of the best of all recent publications on the history of technology is related to a Welsh Arts Council exhibition of engineering drawings (Baynes and Pugh 1978), and shows how drawing as a medium of communication reflects the social and institutional history of engineering design. Important specialist museums have been established, as at Ironbridge and the Museum of English Rural Life at Reading University. Sources for specialist studies of invention include museum catalogues and patents. Bennet Woodcroft (1854–) promoted the printing of nearly all early British patents from 1617 during the 1850s, and searches among more recent patents may be greatly aided by manuals such as Liebesny's (1972).

Over long periods of history, the day-to-day practice of technology was the province of craftsmen who did not leave written records or even drawings to show what they designed and built. This not only underlines the importance of archaeology, but points to the possible role of oral history studies in recording recently obsolete craft processes (Rix 1979) or technical knowledge possessed by illiterate farmers or millwrights (e.g. in India, Gimpel 1979; Howes and Chambers 1979). One problem that inhibits serious study in this area is that the craftsman's specialist knowledge is not only part of an oral tradition, but is organized in categories that are completely alien to modern science. Sturt (1923) illustrates this in relation to twentieth-century wheelwrights, but the problem is even more acute for students of medieval and Renaissance metallurgy, where much craft knowledge was conceived in terms akin to alchemy; only a minority of historians of technology have the inclination and patience to get inside this world view (C.S. Smith, 1960; 1970).

Conceptual agendas and social responsibilities

Although the writings of economic historians can be very useful in their coverage of industry and also of agriculture (Bairoch 1969; Chambers and Mingay 1966), they are by definition limited to economically productive processes, and usually say little about such subjects as military technology and public health engineering.

With a few exceptions (Cipolla 1970; Nef 1950), historians of technology also deal inadequately with military developments. In other areas, too, they appear to work with an agenda or conceptual framework that severely limits the development of their subject. For example, until recently, technology was treated as a purely utilitarian activity, and the strong aesthetic impulse in much innovation was not recognized. Recent writings that develop a perspective on this artistic aspect of technology may therefore indicate the first of several ways in which there is scope for enlarging the conceptual agenda of historical study.

The pioneer work here was done by C.S. Smith (1960, 1970) in his writing about the history of metals and ceramics. More recently, Florman (1976) and Ferguson (1978) have reviewed much other evidence for an aesthetic dimension, while Billington (1979) has made a detailed study of the artistic creativity of one of the engineers involved in developing reinforced concrete as an important structural material. This approach not only offers new insights into the process of innovation, but makes possible a more intelligent treatment of the non-utilitarian application of technology in the building of cathedrals (Gimpel 1958), the Eiffel Tower (Harris 1976) or particle accelerators (Weinberg 1961: 161).

A second way of broadening the agenda of the history of technology may develop from the studies of science policy and institutions that have been used to describe developments during and since the Second World War (Gowing 1964, 1974; Zuckerman 1966). By extending this approach over much longer periods of time, it may be possible to understand better how military requirements influenced the development of technology (Armytage 1965). There are indeed a few isolated works that discuss technology policy and institutions even for the seventeenth and eighteenth centuries (Cole 1964; Artz 1966; Farrar 1971). However, the way in which every nation or other political unit must arrive at a balance between military and industrial technology if it is to survive is not always recognized. The balance may be achieved informally rather than through explicit policies but, either way, an understanding of it can provide a framework for an integrated history of military and industrial developments. This is clearly demonstrated for medieval China in a seminal work by Elvin (1973: 84–110).

A third opportunity for enlarging frames of reference could arise from the concept of 'technology as practice' put forward in the previous section. The point of this idea is to free oneself of the habit of thinking of technology as a self-contained activity in which day-to-day practice and social demands are external and secondary. Styles of management and of work discipline are integral to most technology, affecting even the design of equipment, and are not to be distanced as merely its 'social relations'. But historians rarely discuss these things, despite the call of Marxist writers for a 'critical history of technology' that would pay particular attention to the effect of innovation on human relationships within the labour process (Braverman 1974: 186).

Another aspect of this theme is illustrated by a case study in 'contemporary history' that describes how engineers failed to deal with persistent breakdowns of apparently very simple pumps. The difficulty ultimately transpired to be that the engineers thought of the breakdowns as self-contained technical problems requiring mechanical adjustment of the pumps, whereas the real issue was one of social organization affecting the way pumps were used and maintained (Pacey 1977). Many parallels could be quoted from the history of the steam engine or of the early factory, and, in all these areas, internalist history is in constant danger of mistakenly identifying organizational problems as technical ones, because of the way it concentrates on the scientific logic of innovation largely to the exclusion of its social logic. One should also note how the concepts that historians use to structure their work reflect the ways in which many other people perceive technology; the engineers who failed to understand the social element in the pump problem and the internalist historian are victims of the same misperception.

A fourth aspect of the historian's frame of reference that also has a connection with the way non-historians perceive technology relates to ideas about technical progress. Much writing on the history of technology tends to reinforce conventional wisdom about progress because of the inclination, already noted, to concentrate on advancing and innovative technology rather than technology in everyday use. Historical episodes in which technology did not advance or when skills were lost are ignored, and so are periods when reform movements challenged aspects of their contemporary technology and sought to foster modified patterns of innovation (Webster 1975; Finer 1952: 439–52). Lack of interest in such themes seems to reflect a feeling that they are irrelevant to the central task of the historian, which is to show how early discoveries laid foundations for more recent advances, and to portray technology as developing along a consistent, unvarying, linear path. In histories influenced by this 'linear view' of progress, the relevance of inventions to the problems of their own time is often forgotten, and they are discussed only in terms of what they contributed to the ultimate development of modern technology.

It is only too easy to fall into the trap of looking at history in this way. I have on occasion found myself discussing the eighteenth-century French literature on steam engines like this, assessing it in terms of the much later development of thermodynamics (Talbot and Pacey 1971). What I should have recognized is that much of that literature reflects the institutional and cultural preoccupations of a movement in engineering known as *architecture hydraulique* (Grinevald 1977). This came to an end during the French Revolution, and only a fraction of its discoveries were useful within the new directions of engineering development that followed in the nineteenth century.

A conceptual model of technical progress capable of dealing with such episodes would be one that portrayed progress, not as an unvarying linear advance, but as a series of movements that develop to a certain point and are then abandoned in favour of other approaches. Using this model, one may see how 'history proceeds by changing the subject' (Dahrendorf 1975), and how technology develops by periodic changes of emphasis. These changes come about as new movements grow and others decline, and as new knowledge is discovered in one field while skills are lost elsewhere.

Although this approach has not been much developed, some well-defined movements can be readily identified. Apart from *architecture hydraulique*, they include Smeatonian civil engineering around 1800, 'high farming' in nineteenth-century British agriculture (Orwin and Wetham 1964), and the 'American system of manufactures'. For earlier periods of history, some movements in technology can be identified in terms of the strongly idealistic impulses that motivated them. Among these are the building of cathedrals during the High Middle Ages, the exploration of mathematical relationships in engineering during the Renaissance, and later attempts to create a 'philanthropic' technology devoted to social welfare (Pacey 1976).

Historians of technology have recently commented on their inability to achieve a successful synthetic account of technological history (Hounshell 1981), despite the many insights gained from recent researches. Part of the reason for this is probably the inherent unworkability of the linear view with which so many historians operate, and part of the solution may be to give attention to distinctive movements in technology and the values and institutions that characterized them.

A final aspect of the ideology of progress that may sometimes influence writing on the history of technology is the idea that technological advance is the chief, and perhaps the only, locomotive of social progress. Thus devices such as Arkwright's spinning machine or Baird's invention of television are seen as leading inexorably to the social changes that followed their introduction. This deterministic view is greatly modified if one can show that such inventions were themselves a response to social change, and may simply have reinforced a social process that had already begun. Raymond Williams (1974) makes this point in a brief sketch of the invention of television, and Marglin (1976) does the same with respect to cotton spinning machinery. Indeed, Marglin presents an especially stimulating argument to the effect that the key inventions made during the industrial revolution were the outcome of a social change in industry in which businessmen were seeking and gaining firmer control over craftsmen and work-people. Such interpretations are not yet widely accepted, not least because of their Marxist background, but they perform a great service in showing how it is at least possible to construct a model of technical innovation in which social forces play a credible part.

With new and vigorous studies in 'philosophy of technology' gaining ground in America (Carpenter 1978), we may perhaps expect that some of these issues connected with progress and determinism will shortly receive closer attention. We may also perhaps expect that a better focus will be given to the strong sense of social responsibility evident in much recent writing on the history of technology. Apart from well-known work by established authors in the field (White 1968; Mumford 1934, 1971), there has been an impressive series of works using historical perspectives to illuminate modern problems of resources and of the diffusion of technology to Third World countries; authors who have attempted this include Bairoch (1971), Pacey (1976), Rosenberg (1976), Grinevald (1977) and Gimpel (1979).

Much of this writing is valuable and stimulating, but there is considerable danger that these efforts in 'applied history' (Buchanan 1979) may distract historians from more basic responsibilities. For example, one reason why efforts to transfer technology to Third World countries have often been inept and destructive is an assumption that these countries have no significant technological traditions of their own. Yet recent work has begun to uncover a considerable body of traditional technical knowledge. Such knowledge is often not recognized because it is not organized according to modern scientific categories, but in some subjects (botany, geology, soils) it is in certain respects more detailed and discriminating than corresponding scientific knowledge (Howes and Chambers 1979). The best service that a historian of technology can perform will often be to show that in countries as diverse as India (Dharampal 1971) and Zimbabwe (Summers 1969) such knowledge is part of a long-standing and significant technical and craft tradition. In other words, the historian may often contribute most by doing a straight historical job rather than by trying to 'apply' history in some more indirect way.

Another basic historical task that needs doing relates to the conceptual frameworks about progress and practice in technology that historians use. I have already noted that some of these concepts are not just the property of the historian but may extend into the wider world to influence the work of practising engineers. The way in which politicians and industrialists use these same concepts, supported by historical anecdotes (usually about James Watt), should also be noted. The use of such anecdotes may be fairly casual (as when a new micro-electronics venture in Britain was announced recently), or it may take the form of an extended and serious historical essay (Benn 1971). The responsibility that rests with the historian is clear. The conventional wisdom about technical progress should not be something that he accepts unquestioningly. And the ideas about the history of technology that get into general circulation through school books, popularizations, and engineering education should be a matter of active and serious concern.

Bibliography

Armytage, W.H.G. (1965). *The Rise of the Technocrats*. London; Routledge

Artz, F.B. (1966). *The Development of Technical Education in France, 1500–1800*, Cambridge, Mass.; MIT Press

Bairoch, P. (1969). Agriculture and the Industrial Revolution, in *The Fontana Economic History of Europe*. Ed. C.M. Cipolla. London; Fontana/Collins, Vol. 3: 452–506

Bairoch, P. (1971). *Le Tiers Monde dans l'impasse: le démarrage économique du XVIIIe au XXe siècle*. Paris; Gallimard

Barlow, P. (1836). *A Treatise on the Manufactures and Machinery of Great Britain*. London; Baldwin and Cradock

Baynes, K. and Pugh, F. (1978). *The Art of the Engineer* (exhibition catalogue plus wallet of drawings). Cardiff; Welsh Arts Council. Enlarged edn (1981). London; Butterworth

Benn, A. Wedgwood (1971). Introduction, The Growth of Technology, *The Man-made World*. Milton Keynes; Open University Press

Billington, D.P. (1979). *Robert Maillart's Bridges: The Art of Engineering*. Princeton; Princeton University Press

Bishop, J.L. (1863). *A History of American Manufactures from 1608 to 1860*. 3 Vols. Philadelphia; Young & Co

Bolles, A.S. (1878). *The Industrial History of the United States*. Norwich, Conn.; Henry Bill

Boorstin, D. (1973). *The Americans: the Democratic Experience*. New York; Random House

Braudel, F. (1973). *Capitalism and Material Life, 1400–1800*. London; Weidenfeld and Nicolson. Originally published (1967) as *Civilisation matérielle et capitalisme*. Paris; Librairie Armand Colin

Braverman, H. (1974). *Labour and Monopoly Capital*. New York and London; Monthly Review Press

Brown, J. (1978). *Mathematical Instrument-makers in the Grocers' Company 1688–1830*. London; Science Museum Monographs, HMSO

56   The history of technology

Brown, J. (1979). Guild Organisation and the Instrument-making Trade, 1550–1830, *Annals of Science*, Vol. 36, 1–34

Buchanan, R.A. (1978). History of Technology in the Teaching of History, in *History of Technology 1978*. Ed. A.R. Hall and N. Smith. London; Mansell, 13–28

Buchanan, R.A. (1979). *History and Industrial Civilisation*. London and Basingstoke; Macmillan

Buchanan, R.A. (1980). *Industrial Archaeology in Britain*, revised and enlarged edn. London; Allen Lane

Bulferetti, L. (1964). *Galileo Galilei nella società del suo tempo*. Manduria; Lacaito Editore

Camp, L.S. de (1960). *The Ancient Engineers*. New York; Doubleday. London; Souvenir Press

Cardwell, D.S.L. (1971). *From Watt to Clausius: The Rise of Thermodynamics in the Early Industrial Age*. London; Heinemann

Cardwell, D.S.L. (1972). *The Organisation of Science in England*, revised edn. London; Heinemann. Ist edn (1957)

Cardwell, D.S.L., Marsh, J.O. and Pickstone, J.E. (1981). *British Society for the History of Science. A Workshop on New Perspectives in the History of Technology*. Papers of Conference held at UMIST. Manchester

Carpenter, S.R. (1978). Developments in the Philosophy of Technology in America, *Technology and Culture*, Vol. 19, 93–9

Carter, Harry (1957). *Wolvercote Mill: a Study of Paper-making in Oxford*. Oxford; Oxford University Press

Chambers, J.D. and Mingay, G.E. (1966). *The Agricultural Revolution*. London; Batsford

Cipolla, C.M. (1970). *European Culture and Overseas Expansion*. Harmondsworth; Pelican

Cipolla, C.M., Ed. (1972–6). *The Fontana Economic History of Europe*. 6 Vols. London; Collins/Fontana

Clark, V.S. (1929). *History of Manufactures in the United States*. 3 Vols. New York and Washington; Carnegie Institution of Washington

Cole, C.W. (1964). *Colbert and a Century of French Mercantilism*. 2 Vols. London; Cass

Dahrendorf, R. (1975). *The New Liberty: Survival and Justice in a Changing World*. London; Routledge. Stanford, Calif.; Stanford University Press

D'Aubuisson, J.F. (1802). *Des Mines de Freiberg*. 2 Vols. Leipzig; Pierre Philip Wolf

Daumas, M. (1979–80). *A History of Technology and Invention: Progress through the Ages*. Trans. E.B. Hennessy. 3 Vols. New York; Crown Publishers. London; Murray. Originally published as *Histoire générale des techniques* (1962–8). Paris; Presses Universitaires de France

Dharampal, S. (1971). *Indian Science and Technology in the Eighteenth Century. Some Contemporary European Accounts*. Delhi; Impex India

Dickson, D. (1974). *Alternative Technology and the Politics of Technical Change*. London; Fontana/Collins. New York; Universe Books

Dunsheath, P. (1962). *A History of Electrical Engineering*. London; Faber

Dutt, R. (1902). *The Economic History of India under Early British Rule*. London; Kegan Paul. Reprinted (1950). London; Routledge

Dutt, R. (1904). *The Economic History of India in the Victorian Age*. London; Kegan Paul. Reprinted (1950). London; Routledge

Elvin, M. (1973). *The Pattern of the Chinese Past*. London; Eyre Methuen

Evenari, M., Shanan, L. and Tadmor, N. (1971). *The Negev: The Challenge of a Desert*. Cambridge, Mass.; Harvard University Press

Farey, J. (1827). *A Treatise on the Steam Engine.* London; Longman, Rees, Orme, Brown and Green

Farrar, D.M. (1971). The Royal Hungarian Mining Academy, University of Manchester Institute of Science and Technology MSc Thesis

Ferguson, E.S. (1962). *Kinematics of Mechanism from the Time of Watt*, Washington DC; United States National Museum, Bulletin 228

Ferguson, E.S. (1978). Elegant Inventions: the Artistic Component of Technology, *Technology and Culture*, Vol. 19, 450–460

Finer, S.E. (1952). *The Life and Times of Sir Edwin Chadwick.* London; Methuen

Florman, S.C. (1976). *The Existential Pleasures of Engineering.* New York; St Martin's Press

Garlake, P.S. (1973). *Great Zimbabwe.* London; Thames and Hudson

Gille, B. (1966). *The Renaissance Engineers.* London; Lund Humphries. Originally published (1964) as *Les Ingénieurs de la Renaissance.* Paris; Hermann

Gille, B. (1978). *Histoire des techniques.* Paris; Gallimard, Encyclopédie de la Pléiade

Gimpel, J. (1958). *Les Bâtisseurs de cathédrales.* Paris; Editions du Seuil

Gimpel, J. (1977). *The Medieval Machine.* London; Gollancz. Originally published (1976) as *La Révolution industrielle du Moyen Age.* Paris; Editions du Seuil

Gimpel, J. (1979). La Technologie appropriée: une expérience en Inde, *La Recherche*, Vol. 10, No. 103, 916–925

Goulden, S. (1982). *Great Engineers.* Vol. 1, *From Antiquity through the Industrial Revolution.* New York; St Martin's Press

Gowing M. (1964). *Britain and Atomic Energy, 1939–45.* London; Macmillan

Gowing, M. with L. Arnold (1974). *Independence and Deterrence: Britain and Atomic Energy, 1945–52.* 2 Vols. London and Basingstoke; Macmillan

Grinevald, J. (1977). Révolution industrielle, technologie de la puissance et révolutions scientifiques, *La fin des outils: technologie et domination.* Cahiers de l'IUED Genève, No. 5. Paris; Presses Universitaires de France, 149–201

Habakkuk, H.J. (1962). *American and British Technology in the Nineteenth Century.* Cambridge; Cambridge University Press

Habakkuk, H.J. and Postan, M., Ed. (1965). *The Cambridge Economic History of Europe.* Vol. 6, *The Industrial Revolutions and After.* Cambridge; Cambridge University Press

Haber, L.F. (1969). *The Chemical Industry in the Nineteenth Century.* London; Oxford University Press

Haber, L.F. (1971). *The Chemical Industry 1900–1930.* Oxford; Clarendon Press

Hall, A.R. (1961). Engineering and the Scientific Revolution, *Technology and Culture*, Vol. 2, 333–341

Hall, A.R. and Smith, N., Ed. (1976–). *History of Technology.* Annual volumes. London; Mansell

Hall, B.S. and West, D.C., Ed. (1976). *On Pre-Modern Technology and Science: A Volume of Studies in Honor of Lynn White Jr.* Malibu, Calif.; Undena

Harris, J. (1976). *The Eiffel Tower: Symbol of an Age.* London; Paul Elek

Hartwell, R. (1966). Markets, Technology… and the Eleventh-century Chinese Iron and Steel Industry, *Journal of Economic History*, Vol. 26, 29–58

Hartwell, R. (1967). A Cycle of Economic Change in Imperial China; Coal and Iron in N.E. China, 750–1350, *Journal of the Economic and Social History of the Orient*, Vol. 10, 104–120

Henderson, W.O. (1966). *J.C. Fischer and his Diary of Industrial England 1814–15.* London; Cass

Henderson, W.O. (1968). *Industrial Britain under the Regency: the Diaries of Escher, Bodmer, May and de Gallois.* London; Cass

58   The history of technology

Hills, R.L. (1970). *Power in the Industrial Revolution.* Manchester; Manchester University Press

Historic American Engineering Record (1974–9). *Inventory of Historic Engineering and Industrial Sites, New England.* Ed. T.A. Comp (1974). *The Lower Peninsula of Michigan.* Ed. D.B. Abbott (1976). *Rhode Island.* Ed. G. Kulik (1979). Washington, DC; US Department of the Interior, Heritage Conservation Service

Hopkins, H.J. (1970). *A Span of Bridges.* Newton Abbott; David and Charles

Hounshell, D.A. (1981). On the Discipline of the History of American Technology, *Journal of American History,* Vol. 67, 854–865

Howes, M. and Chambers, R. (1979). Indigenous Technical Knowledge: analysis, implications and issues, *IDS Bulletin* (University of Sussex), Vol. 10, No. 2, 5–23

Hudson, K. (1979). *World Industrial Archaeology.* Cambridge; Cambridge University Press

Keller, A.G. (1967). Pneumatics, Automata and the Vacuum in the Work of Aleotti, *British Journal for the History of Science,* Vol. 3, 338–347

Keller, A.G. (1976). Besson's *Livre des instruments,* in *On Pre-Modern Technology and Science: A Volume of Studies in Honor of Lynn White Jr.* Ed. B.S. Hall and D.C. West. Malibu, Calif.; Undena.

Klemm, F. (1959). *A History of Western Technology.* Trans. D.W. Singer, London; Allen and Unwin. Originally published (1954) as *Technik: eine Geschichte ihrer Probleme.* Freiburg; Verlag Karl Alber

Klingender, F.D. (1947). *Art and the Industrial Revolution.* London. Revised version (1972). Ed. A. Elton. London; Paladin

Kranzberg, M. and Pursell, C.W. (1967). *Technology in Western Civilisation.* 2 Vols. Madison; University of Wisconsin Press

Landels, J.G. (1978). *Engineering in the Ancient World.* Berkeley; University of California Press. London; Chatto and Windus

Landes, D.S. (1969). *The Unbound Prometheus: Technological Change and Industrial Development in Western Europe from 1750 to the Present.* Cambridge; Cambridge University Press

Laqueur, T.S. (1976). The Cultural Origins of Popular Literacy in England 1500–1800, *Oxford Review of Education,* Vol. 2, 255–275

Leinwoll, S. (1979). *From Spark to Satellite: a History of Radio Communications.* New York; Scribner

Liebesny, F., Ed. (1972). *Mainly on Patents.* London; Butterworths

Lockwood, W.W. (1955). *The Economic Development of Japan: Growth and Structural Change, 1868–1938.* London; Oxford University Press

Long, W.H. (1979). The Low Yields of Corn in Medieval England, *Economic History Review,* 2nd ser., Vol. 32, 459–469

Lovell, B. (1973). *The Origins and International Economics of Space Exploration.* Edinburgh; Edinburgh University Press

Marglin, S.A. (1976). What do Bosses do?, in *The Division of Labour.* Ed. A. Gorz. Hassocks; Harvester Press

Morison, E.E. (1974). *From Know-how to Nowhere: the Development of American Technology.* New York; Basic Books

Mumford, L. (1934). *Technics and Civilization.* New York; Harcourt Brace. Reprinted (1946). London; Routledge

Mumford, L. (1971). *The Myth of the Machine.* London; Secker and Warburg

Musson, A.E. and Robinson, E. (1969). *Science and Technology in the Industrial Revolution.* Manchester; Manchester University Press

Needham, J. (1954–). *Science and Civilisation in China.* Cambridge; Cambridge University Press. 5 Vols so far. See especially Vol. 4, *Physics and Physical Technology,* Part II, *Mechanical Engineering* (1965) and Part III, *Civil Engineering and Nautics* (1971)

Nef, J.U. (1950). *War and Human Progress: an Essay on the Rise of Industrial Civilisation*. London; Routledge

Okita, S. (1966). Choice of Technique: Japan's Experience, in *Economic Development with Special Reference to East Asia*. Ed. K. Berrill. London; Macmillan

Orwin, C.S. and Whetham, E.H. (1964). *A History of British Agriculture, 1846–1914*. London; Longmans Green and Co. 2nd edn (1971). Newton Abbot; David and Charles

Pacey, A. (1976). *The Maze of Ingenuity: Ideas and Idealism in the Development of Technology*. Cambridge, Mass.; MIT Press

Pacey, A. (1977). *Hand-pump Maintenance*. London; Intermediate Technology Publications

Parsons, W.B. (1939). *Engineers and Engineering in the Renaissance*. Baltimore; Williams and Wilkins. Reprinted (1967). Cambridge, Mass.; MIT Press.

Rae, J.B. (1959). *American Automobile Manufacturers*. Philadelphia; Temple Press

Reti, L. (1972). Leonardo and Ramelli, *Technology and Culture*, Vol. 13, 577–605

Rix, M. (1979). Oral History Seminar, *Association for Industrial Archaeology Bulletin*, Vol. 6, Part 3, 5–6

Rosenberg, N. (1963). Technological Changes in the Machine Tool Industry, *Journal of Economic History*, Vol. 23, 414–443

Rosenberg, N. (1972). *Technology and American Economic Growth*. New York; Harper

Rosenberg, N. (1976). *Perspectives on Technology*. Cambridge; Cambridge University Press

Rossiter, M. (1975). *The Emergence of Agricultural Science: Justus Liebig and the Americans, 1849–1880*. New Haven and London; Yale University Press

Sawyer, J.E. (1954). The Social Basis of the American System of Manufacturing, *Journal of Economic History*, Vol. 14, 361–379

Simkin, C.G.F. (1968). *The Traditional Trade of Asia*. London; Oxford University Press

Singer, C., Holmyard, E.J., Hall, A.R. and Williams, T.I., Ed. (1954–9). *A History of Technology*. 5 Vols. London; Oxford University Press

Smiles, S. (1861). *Lives of the Engineers*. 3 Vols. Reprinted (1968). Newton Abbott; David and Charles

Smith, C.S. (1960). *A History of Metallography*. Chicago; Chicago University Press

Smith, C.S. (1970). Art, Technology and Science; Notes on their Historical Interaction, *Technology and Culture*, Vol. 11, 493–549

Smith, C.S., and Kranzberg, M. (1979). Materials in History and Society, in *Material Science and Engineering: Evolution, Practice and Prospects*. Ed. M. Cohen. Lausanne; Elsevier Sequoia

Smith, J.G. (1979). *The Origins and Early Development of the Heavy Chemical Industry in France*. Oxford; Clarendon Press

Smith, M.R. (1977). *Harpers Ferry Armory and the New Technology*. Ithaca, NY; Cornell University Press

Smith, N. (1971). *A History of Dams*. London; Peter Davies

Smith, S. (1979). *A View from the Iron Bridge* (catalogue of an exhibition at the Royal Academy, London). Telford, Shropshire; Ironbridge Gorge Museum Trust

Stuart, C.B. (1871). *Lives and Works of Civil and Military Engineers of America*. New York; D. Van Nostrand

Sturt, G. (1923). *The Wheelwright's Shop*. Cambridge; Cambridge University Press

Summers, R. (1969). *Ancient Mines in Rhodesia and Adjacent Areas*. Harare, Zimbabwe; National Museums

Talbot, G.R. and Pacey, A.J. (1971). Antecedents of Thermodynamics in the Work of Guillaume Amontons, *Centaurus*, Vol. 16, 20–40

Taylor, E.G.R. (1954). *The Mathematical Practitioners of Tudor and Stuart England*. Cambridge; Cambridge University Press for the Institute of Navigation

Taylor, E.G.R. (1966). *The Mathematical Practitioners of Hanoverian England 1714–1840*. Cambridge; Cambridge University Press for the Institute of Navigation

Trinder, B. (1973). *The Industrial Revolution in Shropshire*. London and Chichester; Phillimore

Trow Smith, R. (1957). *A History of British Livestock Husbandry to 1700*. London; Routledge

Trow Smith, R. (1959). *A History of British Livestock Husbandry, 1700–1900*. London; Routledge

Tugan-Baranovskii, M.I. (1907). *The Russian Factory in the Nineteenth Century*. English Trans. (1970). Homewood, Ill.; R.D. Irwin

Usher, A.P. (1954). *A History of Mechanical Inventions*. Cambridge, Mass.; Harvard University Press

Wallace, A.F.C. (1978). *Rockdale: the Growth of an American Village in the Early Industrial Revolution*. New York; Knopf

Warren, K. (1980). *Chemical Foundations: The Alkali Industry in Britain to 1926*. Oxford; Clarendon Press

Webster, C. (1975). *The Great Instauration: Science, Medicine and Reform, 1626–1660*. London; Duckworth

Weinberg, A.M. (1961). Impact of Large-scale Science on the United States, *Science*, Vol. 134, 161

White, L. (1962). *Medieval Technology and Social Change*. London; Oxford University Press

White, L. (1968). The Historical Roots of our Ecological Crisis, in *Machina ex Deo: Essays in the Dynamics of Western Culture. Essays by Lynn White*. Cambridge, Mass.; MIT Press

Williams, R. (1974). *Television: Technology and Cultural Form*. London; Fontana/Collins

Williams, T.I., Ed. (1978). *A History of Technology*. Vols 6 and 7, *The Twentieth Century to c. 1950*. Oxford; Clarendon Press. For Vols 1–5, see Singer *et al.* (1954–9)

Wilson, M. (1969). The Sotho, in *The Oxford History of South Africa*. Ed. M. Wilson and L. Thompson. 2 Vols. Oxford; Clarendon Press, Vol. 1: 131–167

Woodbury, R.S. (1958). *History of the Gear-Cutting Machine*. Cambridge, Mass.; MIT Press

Woodbury, R.S. (1960). *History of the Milling Machine*. Cambridge, Mass.; MIT Press

Woodcroft, B. (1854–). *Alphabetical Index of Patentees and Applicants for Patents of Invention*. London; Commissioners of Patents for Inventions. Vol. 1 for 1617–1852, reprinted (1969). New York; Kelley

Woodcroft, B. (1854–). *Chronological Index of Patents Applied for and Patents Granted*. London; Commissioners of Patents for Inventions

Zuckerman, S. (1966). *Scientists and War: the Impact of Science on Military and Civil Affairs*. London; Hamish Hamilton

4

Anthropological perspectives on the history of science and medicine

Michael MacDonald

Anthropology is in vogue among social historians. During the past decade they have plundered the works of French and British anthropologists and enriched their studies with theoretical and comparative booty. Emmanuel Le Roy Ladurie, Keith Thomas and Natalie Davis are rightly celebrated for their sensitive use of anthropological concepts in their reconstructions of popular culture in medieval and early modern France and England. Edward Thompson, Jacques Le Goff and Carlo Ginzburg have displayed their ethnographic prizes less prominently, but they have all profited greatly from the looting. In France it has become chic to speak of historical ethnography, and in England one historian, Alan Macfarlane, has actually undergone the arduous initiation rites and become a social anthropologist.

Historians of science and medicine have not shown much interest in these clamorous raids into alien territory. Apparently the relevance of *la pensée sauvage* to the development of science is not immediately obvious. It was not always so. 'Primitive' beliefs and practices aroused the interest of historians of science early in this century, and three of the most famous medical historians, Henry E. Sigerist, Erwin Ackerknecht and George Rosen, recognized the potential usefulness of anthropological materials to students in their field. Each of these noted polymaths believed that ethnography illuminates the social history of medicine.

Ackerknecht was deeply interested in anthropology and its application to medical history. He studied ethnology in Paris

61

during the 1930s and wrote an important series of papers about primitive medicine after he immigrated to the United States in the 1940s. His aims were to discover the common features of the many different medical practices described by ethnographers and to relate them to the social history of medicine. He drew five broad conclusions from his studies. Primitive medicine is not embryonic modern medicine; it deserves study in its own right, not as a stage in the development of scientific rationalism, but as an aspect of culture. Medicine is part of a total cultural pattern. Diseases are socially defined in primitive cultures, and illness has significant social dimensions even in modern nations. The medical beliefs and practices of primitive peoples encourage conformity to the prevailing values of their culture. Primitive medicine is largely magical but partially empirical; modern medicine is largely empirical but partly magical (Ackerknecht 1971).

Ackerknecht did not integrate these views into his own historical research successfully, but he made a number of striking observations and comparisons to suggest how they might be used by medical historians. In a discussion of autopsies among African peoples, for example, he remarked that the practice of dissection does not necessarily lead to the accumulation of anatomical knowledge. The development of anatomy during the Renaissance cannot therefore simply be ascribed to the increasing frequency of dissections; a reorientation in the cultural context in which dissections were practised was necessary for the birth of an empirically based anatomy: 'To understand the development of modern anatomy our interest should be concentrated rather on the fundamental cultural and spiritual implications and orientations rather than on technical problems' (1971: 94). Theory precedes observation, and theory, in the general sense of a framework within which people make sense of the natural world, is shaped by culture.

Sigerist took up some of the themes sketched by Ackerknecht and elaborated on them. In the first volume of his *History of Medicine*, about primitive and archaic medicine, he echoed Ackerknecht's emphasis on the influence of culture on primitive and historical conceptions of disease: 'The theories of medicine are products of their own time, in their cultural setting' (1951: 11). Even the patterns of symptoms, observations about the signs of particular illnesses, were guided by culturally determined assumptions about the nature of sickness: 'As long as the concept of disease was different than ours, the grouping of symptoms was different' (1951: 29). Society's response to ill people was, like its understanding of illness itself, shaped by culture. A pressing priority in the history of medicine was, in Sigerist's opinion, investigation of the ways in which patients as well as physicians are affected by cultural factors: 'What did disease mean to the individual, how did it affect his life? While there is a good deal of literature on the history of the physician, the history of the patient has been neglected' (1951: 15). Like Ackerknecht, Sigerist was struck by the variations among the beliefs and practices recorded by ethnographers, and he was persuaded that pre-modern medicine in the West had been sensitive to historical change in much the same manner as primitive medicine is shaped by cultural variations.

Neither Ackerknecht nor Sigerist was, I think, entirely comfortable with the general lessons they drew from medical anthropology. They both regarded modern medicine as a system that was relatively free from cultural influences, and they both neglected to examine in detail medical history from an anthropological perspective. Rosen, however, did contribute several examples illustrating how anthropological findings might be used to illuminate the history of particular diseases (1968, 1970). Perhaps the most successful of Rosen's papers integrating anthropology and medical history is his study of psychic epidemics in Europe and America since the Middle Ages (1968). Drawing on the works of anthropologists who have studied ecstatic movements in a wide variety of settings, he concluded that phenomena such as dance frenzies, demonic possession and enthusiastic religious movements cannot be understood simply by applying modern conceptions of psychopathology to them. These episodes, he felt, contained within them a 'rational core', a logically explicable relationship to the social conditions in which they arose. Following Firth and Wallace, he saw behind these epidemics of apparent mass hysteria a pattern of protest against intolerably stressful conditions (1968: 223–5). They served a social function by providing a means to express frustration and to restore the equilibrium of the social system or to change it. To approach such events strictly from the point of view of medical science, he argued, was inadequate: 'It is equally essential to investigate the psychological and the social in relation to each other' (1968: 224).

Despite the suggestions of Ackerknecht and Sigerist and the examples of Rosen, historians of science and medicine must still find it difficult to see how anthropological studies of pre-literate and folk societies may illuminate their own investigations of scientific development in complex historical settings. The problems are manifold. The inconsistencies between the sentiments expressed by Ackerknecht and Sigerist and their own practice as historians demonstrate that they cannot be ignored if anthropological concepts are to be applied successfully to subjects that are nearer to the traditional concerns of the history of science and medicine than exotic psychopathological states. The aim of the rest of this paper will therefore be to describe a few of the most significant issues raised by anthropological studies of traditional thought and of medicine and to demonstrate, with historiographical examples where they are available, their relevance to the history of science and medicine in the West. I shall not discuss the anthropology or history of science and medicine in India and China because these most important societies receive expert attention elsewhere in this volume (chapters 22 and 23).

Science, magic and religion

However great the influence of science has been on modern society, rigorous scientific thought has always been practised by a small intellectual élite. Every historian knows that science developed in cultures dominated by magical and religious beliefs, and many scholars are aware that the interplay of natural philosophy and supernatural beliefs in medieval and early modern Europe was very complex. Contemporaries seldom distinguished sharply between natural and supernatural phenomena as we do. Even the greatest seventeenth-century scientists viewed them as overlapping domains, and they disagreed about the criteria that ought to be employed to map and explore the realms of reason and faith. Many historians of science have recognized that it is anachronistic to view the scientific revolution as a simple triumph of reason over unreason, and they have in recent years devoted a great deal of attention to the religious beliefs of early scientists and the influence of magical and religious traditions on scientific activity. The yearning to depict science, magic and religion simply as rival systems of thought nevertheless persists, and very little attention has been given to the diffusion of scientific ideas and discoveries beyond the small band of virtuosi who understood them. The growth in the prestige and influence of scientific interpretations of our experience of the world around us is the most profound change in the *mentalité* of Western culture since the Middle Ages. The pervasive spread of scientism has received little attention from historians, who have usually assumed that it was the more or less automatic consequence of the theoretical advances of science and the provision of mass education. It is obvious, however, that the upper classes of late seventeenth- and eighteenth-century Europe developed confidence in the theories and methods of science before there had been spectacular improvements in technology (Thomas 1971) and that even today scientific ideas are accepted by laymen as matters of faith and not as fully comprehended matters of fact. The history of science cannot therefore neglect popular beliefs, and it is reasonable to suppose that anthropological studies of science, magic and religion in cultures less fully secularized than our own will illuminate the past.

Keith Thomas's brilliant and richly detailed study of magic and religion in early modern England remains the most ambitious attempt to use anthropological concepts to clarify the history of ideas in the period of the scientific revolution (1971). A consideration of his debts to anthropology and of his failings in the eyes of one critical anthropologist, Hildred Geertz (1975), will illuminate the potentials and the perils of interdisciplinary history. As Geertz rightly observes, Thomas's analysis of the nature and functions of magical beliefs is eclectic, but he borrows heavily from Bronislaw Malinowski's theories about magic (1954: 69–90) and from E.E. Evans-Pritchard's study of Azande witchcraft (1937). Like them he was concerned to discover the social functions of magical beliefs. He rejects the crude determinism of Malinowski's argument that magic is a kind of pseudo-science designed to achieve through mystical means ends that cannot be attained technologically. Nevertheless, like Malinowski he emphasizes that magical rites serve to allay the anxiety of people vulnerable to the forces of nature and that popular magic is a collection of techniques designed to manipulate the physical world, rather than a complex social and intellectual institution like religion. Thomas's debt to Evans-Pritchard is very large. His drafts on the rich intellectual deposits banked in *Witchcraft, Oracles and Magic Among the Azande* are of three types. First, he borrows insights into the logic of specific magical practices: like Azande diviners, for example, cunning men reinforced their clients' own suspicions and inclinations (1971: 216–17). Second, he borrows general propositions about the social functions of magical beliefs: witchcraft provides an explanation of why misfortune befell particular people, not of the causes of accident and disease in general, and witchcraft beliefs function to strengthen social obligations (1971: 535–46, 566–7; Macfarlane 1970, 1977). Third, he borrows Evans-Pritchard's view of the 'closed' character of magical thought: magical beliefs form a self-confirming system that cannot be successfully challenged from within. Once the premises of magical thought are accepted, predictive failures may be explained away (1971: 641–3).

Thomas's judicious use of the ideas of Malinowski, Evans-Pritchard and, it should be noted, many other anthropologists, greatly adds to the explanatory power of his arguments. According to Geertz, however, the book is much less valuable than it seems because it relies on anthropological currency that has been recalled and replaced by a new coinage based on a completely different theory of culture. Repudiating psychological and functional explanations of popular beliefs, she charges that Thomas's reliance on Malinowski and his misunderstanding of Evans-Pritchard result in a kind of historical ethnocentrism. In particular she assails the validity of the distinction between magic and religion formulated by the classical anthropologists of the last century and accepted by Malinowski. Beguiled by these authorities, Thomas has imposed anachronistic conceptual categories on his material. The essence of her argument is that magical practices did not constitute a hodgepodge of intellectually miscellaneous techniques, as the misguided historian assumes. Popular magic must have been based on a view of the world that was coherent and comprehensive from the point of view of its practitioners. Because England was a complex and partially literate society there must have been several different conceptual schemes available to contemporaries, and instead of trying to isolate the social and psychological functions of this or that belief, the historian should busy himself with reconstructing the various cultural codes present in early modern society. This, she argues, is the real burden of Evans-Pritchard's work, whose study of Azande magic and witchcraft was intended to show how those beliefs form a coherent ideational system that was expressed in social behaviour (Evans-Pritchard 1937: 2).

Geertz's objections to Thomas's book emphasize that many anthropologists today are interested primarily in the expressive qualities and structural coherence of belief systems. The alternative approaches they advocate differ greatly, but they share the conviction that the study of ideas and behaviour must attempt to understand them as cultural codes – patterns of thought and action that are meaningful to participants, even if they appear at first illogical from our perspective. As Evans-Pritchard observes in his lucid discussion of classic theories of primitive religion (1965), this methodological orientation is not new, but it has recently prevailed and stimulated brilliant interpretations of symbolism, ritual and systems of classification. I do not have space to describe here all of the literature potentially relevant to the history of science. The notes to Geertz's critique (1975), Firth's survey of symbolism (1973) and the review articles on cognitive anthropology, symbolism, structuralism and semiotics in the *Handbook of Social and*

Cultural Anthropology (Honigmann 1973) and the *Annual Review of Anthropology* (1972–) and its predecessor, the *Biennial Review* (1959–1971), are convenient guides to current scholarship. Margaret Currier (1976) assesses the bibliographic tools available for anthropology usefully, but from a narrowly American perspective. Some influential anthropologists should be mentioned specifically, although my selection is bound to be arbitrary and incomplete.

Historians of science are all aware of the symbolic quality of scientific thinking, but they seldom attempt to relate the specialized symbolism of science to the other kinds of symbolic thought and behaviour found in the societies and periods they study. The nature of symbolism and ritual has been the topic of important works by Evans-Pritchard (1956), Clifford Geertz (1973), Victor Turner (1967, 1968, 1974, 1975), Mary Douglas (1969, 1970, 1975), Edmund Leach (1961, 1976), and Claude Lévi-Strauss (1963). A closely related subject, the classification of knowledge, has also stimulated insightful analyses by Emile Durkheim and Marcel Mauss (1963), the founders of the French sociological school, and by Douglas (1969, 1970, 1975), Leach (1964), Tambiah (1969), Terence Turner (1969) and Lévi-Strauss (1966). A number of American anthropologists have developed a methodologically rigorous approach to classification based on sociolinguistics. Their position is well represented in a collection of papers edited by Stephen A. Tyler (1969) and in articles about medical ideas and practices by Charles O. Frake (1961), Horacio Fabrega Jr. (1970), and Peter K. Manning and Fabrega (1976). The works of all of the anthropologists singled out here should interest historians because they offer fresh discussions of the ways in which knowledge is organized and expressed in speech and action. Some of their concerns are directly relevant to topics in the history of science: for example, animal and plant classifications, ritual healing, ideas about pollution, and conceptions of time. They represent a wide variety of theoretical positions and offer quite different strategies for placing knowledge and beliefs in their social context. Perhaps the most important reason to read them is that they cast familiar concerns in unfamiliar contexts. Stuart Clark, for instance, found that the binary oppositions noticed by many anthropologists in the thought of non-Western peoples (and emphasized by Lévi-Strauss and his followers) inform the writings of early modern demonologists, and he remarks that the language of contraries also played a role 'in individual disciplines like physics, medicine, natural magic, astrology, [and] psychology' (1980: 106). Whether or not such a suggestion lends support to structuralist theories about the nature of thought, it could lead to a clearer understanding of the interconnections between belief systems in the past.

Geertz's complaint is that Thomas overlooks current anthropological theories that stress the interconnections of magical practices and religious beliefs; her suggestion is that there were several webs of discourse and meaning in early modern England. Thomas's thoughtful and enlightening response (1975) grants that he might profitably have devoted more attention to the development of the categories 'magic' and 'religion' in contemporary thought, but he justly emphasizes that they were seventeenth-century concepts, not the inventions of unfashionable anthropologists. Even if Geertz's arguments are correct – and they do embody a valuable methodological suggestion – the historian must still confront the fact that the varieties of meaning and action present in early modern Europe differed not merely in their cultural context in the wider society, they differed in complexity and explanatory power. He cannot, in short, ignore the possibility that scientific thought may not be explicable in the same ways that other cultural codes are interpretable.

Anthropologists disagree about the epistemological status of modern science, but most of them are, like Lévi-Strauss, impressed by its achievements and cosmopolitanism (1978: 288–311). Robin Horton and Jack Goody have written the most perceptive anthropological discussions of the characteristics of Western science and the cultural conditions in which it is practised. Borrowing Karl Popper's terminology, Horton (1967) argues that the unique character of scientific thinking is that it is an 'open' system. Scientists adopt a critical attitude towards theory and continually seek to improve their explanations for observed phenomena. Traditional African cosmologies, on the other hand, are 'closed' systems. Although there are striking similarities between traditional religious thought and scientific theorizing, African peoples have a protective attitude toward theory and seek to explain away its failures to predict events. Goody (1968, 1977) recognizes that Horton's arguments fail to explain why some cultures produce science and others do not. He urges that literacy is the necessary precondition for scientific progress, pointing out that, in literate societies, storing pertinent information, comparing data and ideas, and preserving discoveries may be done more effectively than in oral cultures. Elizabeth Eisenstein (1979) has applied a modified version of Goody's hypothesis to the history of science and medicine, stressing that the proliferation of printed books facilitated scientific progress.

Goody might well have pointed out that literacy permits the formation of cultural traditions and intellectual networks in which the élite of many societies can participate. The problem confronting the historian of science is to trace the development of scientific theorizing within the cosmopolitan tradition of European philosophy and to show how science influenced and was influenced by the cultures of individual nations. Robert Redfield's distinction between great and little traditions is useful in this context: the great tradition is cultivated by scholars and priests; the little tradition 'works itself out and keeps itself going in the lives of the unlettered in their village communities' (1969: 42). Viewed from this perspective Western science was an aspect of the great tradition, practised by a small élite who adopted a critical attitude towards scientific theory and enjoyed access through print to the ideas, data and discoveries necessary to advance it. The mass of their countrymen knew little of the philosophical theories they propounded and lived out their lives entirely within the webs of meaning that formed the little tradition. Great and little traditions were not, however, completely independent. Every scientist participated in both traditions, and his thought and priorities were influenced by the culture in which he lived. Laymen incorporated some scientific ideas into their beliefs and integrated them into the traditions of popular culture. The advantage of this scheme is that it permits one to integrate the approaches of Thomas and Geertz and to clarify the relationships among science, magic and religion. Scientific thinking is not reduced merely to a culturally determined belief system, but it is not detached from culture altogether. The evolution of the pejorative concept 'magic' may be clarified if it is understood as a product of the educated élite's hostility toward beliefs and practices that persisted in the little tradition after they had been repudiated by scientists and theologians.

An example of this general approach is Carlo Ginzburg's wonderful reconstruction of the beliefs of a sixteenth-century Italian miller, condemned by the Inquisition, whose cosmogony was based on an analogy with cheesemaking. The analogy was used by Aristotle to explain human conception and often repeated in medieval texts; it survives among some French Basque shepherds today. Ginzburg (1976) shows how it was woven into the fabric of popular thought, and his exchanges with his critics and the anthropological study of the Basques illuminate the interplay of the great tradition of science and orthodox religion and the little tradition of 'superstition' and 'heresy' (Ott 1979; Elliott 1980). Opportunities to trace the shifting fortunes of a single idea and to see how it was integrated into scientific thinking at one time and popular culture at another are rare. But the relationship between scientific beliefs and practices in great and little traditions can be studied directly in the history of medicine, and in the next section of this chapter I shall review the works of medical anthropology and history relevant to this theme.

Anthropology and the history of medicine

The conflict between the cosmopolitan tradition of Western science and the local traditions of indigenous medical systems has polarized the field of medical anthropology and subjected individual anthropologists to opposing methodological attractions. A useful textbook by George M. Foster and Barbara Gallatin Anderson (1978), the comprehensive review articles by Horacio Fabrega, Jr. (1972), Richard W. Lieban (1973), Anthony C. Colson and Karen E. Selby (1974), and the bibliographies by Ira E. Harrison and Sheila Cosminsky (1976) and Steven Feierman (1979b) all demonstrate that the literature is divided between studies based on Western biomedicine and interpretations of disease and traditional medicine in their cultural context. At one pole are ecological and epidemiological works, which have defined disease strictly in Western scientific terms and investigated the distribution of diseases geographically and socially. At the other pole are studies of 'ethnomedicine', which regard disease and healing from the perspective of sufferers and their healers and explore their social and cultural dimensions. Biomedicine and traditional medical systems identify and treat diseases very differently, and the extent to which they can be reconciled, either by the anthropologist or by the people they study, has been the topic of sharp disagreement.

Anthropologists have made significant contributions to medical ecology and to epidemiology, and their work illuminates the dynamics of illness within societies and the spread of diseases between cultures. The range of approaches employed by anthropologists is illustrated in the excellent collection of important papers assembled by David Landy (1977). Two aspects of this scholarship seem to me to be peculiarly anthropological: its emphasis on the importance of customary behaviour as a factor in promoting health or sickness and its inclination to regard disease and healing as part of the overall pattern of human adaptation to changing environments. Thus, for example, Benjamin D. Paul, John Cassell and R.S. Khare (Landy 1977) have contributed to our understanding of the role of beliefs and customs in public health; Frederick L. Dunn and Arthur J. Rubel (Landy 1977) and René Dubos (Dubos 1965) have discussed the adaptive hypothesis imaginatively. Some of the most important writing about ecology and epidemiology has been explicitly historical. Good examples are Judith Friedlander's study of malaria and historical demography in Mexico, Alfred W. Crosby's well-known examination of the early history of syphilis, and Marc H. Dawson's intriguing reconstruction of smallpox epidemics in Kenya from 1880 to 1920

(Landy 1977; Dawson 1979). Paul Slack's (1972) brilliant doctoral thesis about plague in early modern England shows how anthropological perspectives can add a new dimension to European medical history. Slack remarks that the measures taken by municipal authorities to control the spread of the plague clashed with customary responses to disease and death, and his analysis reveals with striking clarity the interplay of élite notions about health and public order and popular beliefs about sickness and rituals of neighbourliness and death.

Ecological and epidemiological studies of sickness all define disease as a biomedical phenomenon; even psychiatric maladies, which are manifestly different from culture to culture, have frequently been regarded as 'objective' conditions that are found in varying guises and amounts from place to place (Favazza and Oman 1977; Kiev 1972; Honigmann 1973). Many sociologists and anthropologists have, however, rightly observed that, even in modern Western societies, professional and lay definitions of disease differ, and they have stressed that the patients' conceptions of illness are integrated into the larger pattern of beliefs and behaviour that makes events comprehensible and guides people's responses to them (Fabrega 1974). They have therefore turned their attention to studying indigenous classifications of disease and the social and cultural significance of traditional healing practices. Most students of ethnomedicine emphasize the ultimate coherence of beliefs and practices, but they tend to discuss ideas about the nature and causes of disease separately from indigenous forms of medical care. I shall exaggerate the distinction between these topics here, because binary thinking, even perhaps when it is arbitrary, helps to organize disparate concepts and materials clearly.

Ideas about the types of disease and their signs are astonishingly diverse. In some societies, such as the Subanun, studied by Charles O. Frake (1961), the empirical observation of symptoms and classifications of them are very highly developed; in other societies, such as the Gnau, studied by Gilbert Lewis (1975), the observation of symptoms and their classification are of no interest at all. The perception of ill health is profoundly shaped by culture. Working among people who have elaborate notions of human pathology, Frake (1961) and Fabrega and Daniel B. Silver have used the methods of American cognitive anthropology to discover the linguistic categories that identify and describe sicknesses and to show how and when they are used (Fabrega and Silver 1973; Fabrega 1970). Many other anthropologists, relying less on sociolinguistics and statistics, have produced careful analyses of disease classifications and methods of diagnosis in a very wide range of cultures. Some of the most interesting work has been reprinted in Landy (1977) and in a collection of papers edited by J.B. Loudon (1976), and there are useful discussions of the relevant scholarship in the review articles by Fabrega (1972) and Lieban (1973). As Fabrega remarks, a great deal of attention has been given to the recognition and classification of mental disorders, perhaps to the detriment of the field, because the concentration on psychiatric maladies has often led to the assumption that the illnesses laymen and non-Western peoples identify do not have 'real' biological causes (Fabrega 1974; Corin and Bibeau 1975). The literature about the cultural specificity of psychiatric illness is indeed vast and controversial. Convenient guides to it are the survey by Ari Kiev (1972), the selections of papers edited by him (1964) and by Landy (1977), and the bibliography by A.R. Favazza and M. Oman (1977); pertinent articles and reviews appear regularly in the *Transcultural Psychiatric Research Review* (1960–). When the biological aetiologies of diseases are not discernible, as they are not in most psychiatric afflictions, efforts to categorize maladies naturally focus on the patient's symptoms. The signs of illness are interpreted in light of beliefs that are profoundly influenced by the same cultural factors that affect the classifications of other types of knowledge: for example, the symbolic conventions and social structure of the group among which the sufferer lives.

Surprisingly, diseases are often identified not by their symptoms but by their putative causes. Anthropologists have been particularly fascinated by magical beliefs about the origins of disease and misfortune, and they have fostered the impression that supernatural explanations for them are characteristic. The attention lavished on witchcraft, spirit possession and taboo has immensely enriched our understanding of the dynamics of many non-Western societies, for, as Horton observes (1967), such beliefs frequently explain afflictions as the consequences of social disharmony. Sensitive scholars like Lewis (1975), Turner (1968), and Evans-Pritchard (1937) have shown that among diverse peoples disease is regarded as a species of misfortune that may be interpreted in the idiom of supernatural beliefs as the outcome of transgressions against the rules of orderly conduct that govern people's behaviour. Examples might be multiplied indefinitely, and historians already have before them the examples of Thomas (1971) and Macfarlane (1970) to show how beliefs about the supernatural causes of misfortune might be used to understand the past more fully. In addition to the anthropological works cited by Thomas and

Macfarlane, the studies of witchcraft, possession and religious thought by Alan Harwood (1970), Alfred Adler and Andras Zempléni (1972) and Ellen Corin (1979) seem especially suggestive from the perspective of medical history. Despite their interest in supernatural explanations for disease, many scholars have stressed that the peoples they have studied recognize both natural and supernatural causes for diseases, and they have demonstrated that different types of causation are invoked according to the nature of the malady or the circumstances in which it occurs (Evans-Pritchard 1937; Loudon 1976; Landy 1977; Janzen 1978). Historians should attend carefully to this aspect of medical anthropology, because they have been too ready to depict magic and medicine as rival aetiological schemes, employed on the one hand by credulous rustics and on the other by progressive rationalists. The complex interplay of natural and supernatural ideas about disease and misfortune described by Thomas (1971) could profitably be developed further and explored in other historical contexts.

Causal explanations for illnesses are inevitably linked with the methods that are used to relieve them. Healing practices vary widely and even simple societies possess many curing techniques. A regiment of anthropological irregulars has attacked the problem of folk healing on three broad fronts: the conceptual coherence of beliefs about disease and healing, the meaning and function of curative rituals, and the efficacy of traditional medical practices. Almost every work of medical anthropology discusses healing techniques. The most comprehensive treatment is Jerome Frank's (1974) discussion of psychotherapy in Western and non-Western settings. Many of Frank's observations apply to therapies for physical diseases as well, because few peoples make a rigid distinction between psychological and physical afflictions. His arguments about faith healing and the psychodynamics of traditional medical practices are stimulating and perceptive; they should interest historians particularly because he carefully traces the parallels between methods of Western psychiatrists and physicians. But the book also represents the distressing tendency of conventional scholarship to rationalize traditional beliefs and practices in terms of Western theories about psychopathology and the placebo effect that are not much more scientific than the notions they seek to explain. The large and largely useless literature about shamanism achieves the nadir of this approach; madmen, medicine men and psychoanalysts appear interchangeably, like totemistic creatures in the subtler thought of African pastoralists and Asian peasants (Eliade 1974). The best work about traditional therapeutics has been concerned with the logic of medical practices and the expressive qualities of ritual. Victor Turner's (1967, 1968) analysis of Ndembu disease classifications, treatments and healing rituals achieves the zenith of this approach; aetiological ideas, classifications of maladies and remedies, the symbolism and drama of rituals are brilliantly described and placed firmly in their cultural context (Douglas 1975: 142–52). The texts and review articles already mentioned will enable medical historians to locate what is useful in the earlier scholarship. Lévi-Strauss's discussion of sorcery and shamanistic symbolism, and the analyses of hot and cold categories in Latin American folk medicine will help historians to see how attention to symbolism and ritual might illuminate medical systems, like Galen's, that were based on similar concepts (Lévi-Strauss 1963: 167–205; Loudon 1976: 422–99; Foster and Anderson 1978: 56–60).

The distribution of medical knowledge and healing skills within societies obviously influences the ways in which diseases are identified and treated. The types of healers found among non-Western peoples are as various as their notions about the causes and cures of illness. Anthropologists have recently begun to study in detail the dynamics of medical practice, identifying the different kinds of therapies performed by laymen and specialists, clarifying the social organization of the varieties of healers, and discovering the grounds on which laymen select particular therapies and healers. The introduction of Western medicine into traditional societies, either by hiring doctors and building hospitals or by importing medicaments and distributing them through clinics, missions and chemists, has added to the pluralistic character of medicine in Africa, Asia and Latin America. The array of natural and supernatural remedies, biomedical and traditional practitioners that sufferers can turn to in their quest for therapy is very like the profusion of treatments and healers available in early modern Europe. The residents of Lusaka, Zambia, for example, have many healers to choose from, and individual practitioners mingle symbols and remedies from biomedicine and traditional beliefs eclectically; no single set of rituals is prescribed to relieve sickness and patients select treatment in much the same pragmatic manner as seventeenth-century Londoners must have done (Frankenberg and Leeson 1976; Pelling and Webster 1979). Steven Feierman (1979a), in an indispensable review of the literature about medical pluralism in African history, isolates many of the similarities and differences between healing practices in early modern England and in modern Africa, and he incisively demonstrates that the conceptual problems raised by the study of medical history in both cultures are the same. Western medicine and traditional therapeutic systems exist side by side; each of them is effective in the eyes of some people and ineffective in the eyes of others. The central problem is to explain how one medical system achieves hegemony and to show how that change is related to broader transformations in the society and culture. European historians must attempt to assess the attractiveness of all kinds of treatments to laymen if we are ever to understand why the prestige of physicians rose and the reputations (but not the business) of astrologers and empirics fell in eighteenth- and early nineteenth-century Europe. Lola R. Schwartz's (1969) discussion of the 'hierarchy of resort' in Melanesia, historical anthropology by Feierman (1979a), John Janzen (1978), Eva Gilles (1976), and by many Latin Americanists, who have studied the interaction between the changing great tradition of Western medicine and the development of a folk medicine that still includes elements of Galenic humoral pathology, are relevant to this endeavour (Foster and Anderson 1978: 56–60).

Conclusion

The premise of the anthropological works mentioned in this chapter is that the study of culture should be based upon the fullest possible understanding of people's thought and actions from their own perspective. Only when the actors' assumptions about the world have been decoded can the scholar move to a higher level of analysis and assess the significance of social structure and change. This approach to the study of society is appealing to historians because they, too, seek to ground their interpretations on the perceptions of contemporaries, who wrote the documents they use. It is not surprising, therefore, that historians of *mentalité* have produced work that often parallels anthropological research. Michel Foucault's (1972, 1973, 1975) deconstruction of historical taxonomies in medicine and the human sciences; Jean-Pierre Peter's analyses of disease classifications (1971, 1975); my own attempt to discover the logic of popular conceptions of insanity and psychological healing (MacDonald 1981); Marc Bloch (1973) and Ronald Finucane's (1977) discussions of miraculous curing; Margaret Pelling's and Charles Webster's (1979) catalogue of medical practitioners; Paul Slack's (1979) and Natalie Davis's (1975) examinations of popular medical literature; Keith Thomas's (1971) synthetic treatment of the beliefs of early modern Englishmen; and François Lebrun's (1971) portrayal of peasant reactions to sickness and death in Anjou, for example, resemble anthropological studies of science and medicine. The similarities are, of course, deliberate in some instances. And yet in spite of these examples and the work of generations of folklorists, the historical anthropology of science and medicine is still more preached than practised. Some of the conceptual obstacles to its development have been discussed in this chapter. I believe that recognition of the differences between the great traditions of scientific thought and the little traditions of popular culture, and sensitive analysis of the interactions between them, will remove some of those obstacles. Even so, practical difficulties remain. Anthropologists, even when they are interested in History, tend to treat historians with contempt. A recent text for anthropologists about sociocultural change does not cite a single historian in its discussion of historicism (Bee 1974). If my own experiences are representative, historians are as welcome in the gatherings of anthropologists as logical positivists are at Parisian dinner parties. Moreover, E.P. Thompson (1972, 1978) has demonstrated with devastating precision that historians can easily distort and trivialize their own work with irrelevant anthropological comparisons removed from their original context. Nevertheless, as Thompson himself argues, we have much to gain from anthropologists. Each of the three types of ideas Thomas takes from Evans-Pritchard – explicit comparisons, parallels between social processes, and general approaches to the structure of thought and action – can enrich the work of historians of science and medicine if they are used with a proper awareness of their provenance. With the development of anthropological scholarship about belief systems, ritual processes and medical practices, we are in a position at last to realize Sigerist's and Ackerknecht's vision of a history of science and medicine that comprehends the lives of whole peoples, not merely the thought of a small élite. Historians will have to chart difficult passages through very unfamiliar territories to gain the most valuable insights from the anthropological literature. But it is the most daring voyagers who return with the richest prizes.

Acknowledgements

I am grateful to Steven Feierman for help navigating through the relevant anthropological literature and to Carol Dickerman for assistance at the oars during the beginning and the end of the project.

Bibliography

Ackerknecht, E.H. (1971). *Medicine and Ethnology*. Bern; Verlag Hans Huber
Adler, A. and Zempléni, A. (1972). *Le Bâton de l'aveugle: divination, maladie et pouvoir chez les Moundang du Tchad*. Paris; Hermann
Bee, R.L. (1974). *Patterns and Processes: An Introduction to Anthropological Strategies for the Study of Sociocultural Change*. London; Collier Macmillan
Bloch, M. (1973). *The Royal Touch: Sacred Monarchy and Scrofula in England and France*. Trans. J.E. Anderson. London; Routledge and Kegan Paul. Ist edn (1924). *Les Rois thaumaturges*. Strasbourg; Librairie Istra. London; Oxford University Press
Buxton, J. (1973). *Religion and Healing in Mandari*. Oxford; Clarendon Press
Clark, S. (1980). Inversion, Misrule and the Meaning of Witchcraft, *Past and Present*, No. 87, 98–127
Colson, A.C. and Selby, K.E. (1974). Medical Anthropology, *Annual Review of Anthropology*, Vol. 3, 245–263
Corin, E. (1979). A Possession Psychotherapy in an Urban Setting: Zebola in Kinshasa, *Social Science and Medicine*, Vol. 13B, 327–338
Corin, E. and Bibeau, G. (1975). De la forme culturelle au vécu des troubles psychiques en Afrique, *Africa*, Vol. 45, 280–315
Currier, M. (1976). Problems in Anthropological Bibliography, *Annual Review of Anthropology*, Vol. 5, 15–34
Davis, N.Z. (1975). *Society and Culture in Early Modern France*. Stanford; Stanford University Press
Dawson, M.H. (1979). Smallpox in Kenya, 1880–1920, *Social Science and Medicine*, Vol. 13B, 245–250
Douglas, M. (1969). *Purity and Danger*, 2nd edn. London; Routledge and Kegan Paul
Douglas, M. (1970). *Natural Symbols*. New York; Vintage Books
Douglas, M. (1975). *Implicit Meanings*. London; Routledge and Kegan Paul
Dubos, R. (1965). *Man Adapting*. New Haven; Yale University Press
Durkheim, E. and Mauss, M. (1963). *Primitive Classification*. Trans. R. Needham. London; Routledge and Kegan Paul. Originally published (1902)
Eisenstein, E. (1979). *The Printing Press as an Agent of Change*. Cambridge; Cambridge University Press
Eliade, M. (1974). *Shamanism: Archaic Techniques of Ecstasy*. Princeton, NJ; Princeton University Press
Elliott, J.H. (1980). Rats or Cheese?, *New York Review of Books*, Vol. 27, No. 11, 38–39
Evans-Pritchard, E.E. (1937). *Witchcraft, Oracles and Magic Among the Azande*. London; Oxford University Press
Evans-Pritchard, E.E. (1956). *Nuer Religion*. London; Oxford University Press
Evans-Pritchard, E.E. (1965). *Theories of Primitive Religion*. London; Oxford University Press
Fabrega, H., Jr. (1970). On the Specificity of Folk Illnesses, *Southwestern Journal of Anthropology*, Vol. 26, 305–314
Fabrega, H., Jr. (1972). Medical Anthropology, *Biennial Review of Anthropology 1971*, Vol. 7, 167–229
Fabrega, H., Jr. (1974). *Disease and Social Behavior: An Interdisciplinary Perspective*. Cambridge, Mass.; MIT Press
Fabrega, H., Jr. and Silver, D.B. (1973). *Illness and Shamanistic Curing in Zinacantan*. Stanford; Stanford University Press
Favazza, A.R. and Oman, M. (1977). *Anthropological and Cross-Cultural Themes*

in *Mental Health: An Annotated Bibliography 1925–1974*. Columbia, Mo.;
University of Missouri Press

Feierman, S. (1979a). Change in African Therapeutic Systems, *Social Science and Medicine*, Vol. 13B, 277–284

Feierman, S. (1979b). *Health and Society in Africa: A Working Bibliography*. Waltham, Mass.; Crossroads Press

Finucane, R.C. (1977). *Miracles and Pilgrims*. London; J.M. Dent and Sons

Firth, R. (1973). *Symbols: Public and Private*. London; George Allen and Unwin

Foster, G.W. and Anderson, B.G. (1978). *Medical Anthropology*. New York; John Wiley and Sons

Foucault, M. (1972). *Histoire de la folie à l'âge classique*. Paris; Gallimard. 1st French edn (1961). Trans. (1965) as *Madness and Civilisation*. New York; Mentor. 2nd edn (1971). London; Tavistock

Foucault, M. (1973). *The Order of Things*. New York; Vintage Books. 1st French edn (1966). *Les Mots et les choses*. Paris; Gallimard

Foucault, M. (1975). *The Birth of the Clinic*. Trans. A.M. Sheridan Smith. New York; Vintage Books. 1st French edn (1963). *Naissance de la clinique*. Paris; Presses Universitaires de France

Frake, C.O. (1961). The Diagnosis of Disease Among the Subanun of Mindanao, *American Anthropologist*, Vol. 63, 113–132

Frank, J.D. (1974). *Persuasion and Healing*, 2nd edn. New York; Schocken

Frankenberg, R. and Leeson, J. (1976). Disease, Illness and Sickness: Social Aspects of the Choice of Healer in a Lusaka Suburb, in *Social Anthropology and Medicine*. Ed. J.B. Loudon. London, New York and San Francisco; Academic Press, 223–258

Geertz, C. (1973). *The Interpretation of Cultures*. New York; Basic Books

Geertz, H. (1975). An Anthropology of Magic and Religion, I, *Journal of Interdisciplinary History*, Vol. 6, 71–89

Gilles, E. (1976). Causal Criteria in African Classifications of Disease, in *Social Anthropology and Medicine*. Ed. J.B. Loudon. London, New York and San Francisco; Academic Press, 358–395

Ginzburg, C. (1976). *Il Formaggio e i Vermi*. Turin; Giulio Einaudi. Trans. J. and A. Tedeschi (1980) as *The Cheese and the Worms*. Baltimore; Johns Hopkins University Press

Goody, J. (1968). *Literacy in Traditional Societies*. Cambridge; Cambridge University Press

Goody, J. (1977). *The Domestication of the Savage Mind*. Cambridge; Cambridge University Press

Harley, G.W. (1941). *Native African Medicine with Special Reference to its Practice in the Mano Tribe of Liberia*. Cambridge, Mass.; Harvard University Press

Harrison, I.E. and Cosminsky, S. (1976). *Traditional Medicine*. London; Garland Publishing

Harwood, A. (1970). *Witchcraft, Sorcery and Social Categories Among the Safwa*. London; Oxford University Press

Honigmann, J.J., Ed. (1973). *Handbook of Social and Cultural Anthropology*. Chicago; Rand McNally

Horton, R. (1967). African Traditional Thought and Western Science, *Africa*, Vol. 37, 50–71; 155–187

Janzen, J.M. (1978). *The Quest for Therapy in Lower Zaire*. Berkeley, Calif.; University of California Press

Kiev, A., Ed. (1964). *Magic, Faith, and Healing*. New York; Free Press

Kiev, A. (1972). *Transcultural Psychiatry*. Harmondsworth; Penguin

Landy, D., Ed. (1977). *Culture, Disease, and Healing*. New York; Macmillan

Leach, E. (1961). *Rethinking Anthropology*. London; Athlone Press

Leach, E. (1964). Anthropological Aspects of Language: Animal Categories and Verbal Abuse, *New Directions in the Study of Language*. Ed. E.H. Lenneberg. Cambridge, Mass.; MIT Press, 23–63

Leach, E. (1976). *Culture and Communication*. Cambridge; Cambridge University Press

Lebrun, F. (1971). *Les Hommes et la mort en Anjou aux XVIIᵉ et XVIIIᵉ siècles*. The Hague; Mouton

Lévi-Strauss, C. (1963). *Structural Anthropology*. Trans. C. Jacobson and B.G. Schoepf. New York; Basic Books. Ist French edn (1958)

Lévi-Strauss, C. (1966). *The Savage Mind*. London; Weidenfeld and Nicolson. Ist French edn (1962)

Lévi-Strauss, C. (1978). *Structural Anthropology 2*. Trans. M. Layton. Harmondsworth; Penguin. Ist French edn (1973)

Lewis, G. (1975). *Knowledge of Illness in a Sepik Society*. London; Athlone Press

Lieban, R.W. (1973). Medical Anthropology, in *Handbook of Social and Cultural Anthropology*. Ed. J.J. Honigmann. Chicago; Rand McNally, 1031–1072

Loudon, J.D., Ed. (1976). *Social Anthropology and Medicine*. London, New York and San Francisco; Academic Press

MacDonald, M. (1981). *Mystical Bedlam: Madness, Anxiety and Healing in Seventeenth-Century England*. New York and Cambridge; Cambridge University Press

Macfarlane, A.D.J. (1970). *Witchcraft in Tudor and Stuart England*. London; Routledge and Kegan Paul

Macfarlane, A.D.J. (1977). Witchcraft in Tudor and Stuart Essex, in *Crime in England 1550–1800*. Ed. J.S. Cockburn. London; Methuen. Princeton; Princeton University Press, 72–89

Malinowski, B. (1954). *Magic, Science, and Religion and Other Essays*. Garden City; Doubleday Anchor Books. Ist edn (1948)

Manning, P.K. and Fabrega, H., Jr. (1976). Fieldwork and the 'New Ethnography', *Man*, n.s. Vol. 11, 39–52

Ott, S. (1979). Aristotle Among the Basques: The 'Cheese Analogy' of Conception, *Man*, n.s. Vol. 14, 699–711

Pelling, M. and Webster, C. (1979). Medical Practitioners, in *Health, Medicine and Mortality in the Sixteenth Century*. Ed. C. Webster. Cambridge; Cambridge University Press, 165–235

Peter, J.-P. (1971). Les Mots et les objets de la maladie, *Revue historique*, No. 499, 13–38

Peter, J.-P. (1975). Disease and the Sick at the End of the Eighteenth Century, in *Biology of Man in History. Selections from the Annales*. Ed. R. Forster and O. Ranum. Trans. E. Forster and P.M. Ranum. Baltimore and London; Johns Hopkins University Press, 81–124

Redfield, R. (1969). *Peasant Society and Culture*. Chicago; University of Chicago Press

Rosen, G. (1968). *Madness in Society: Chapters in the Historical Sociology of Mental Illness*. Ed. B. Nelson. Chicago; University of Chicago Press

Rosen, G. (1970). Mental Disorder, Social Deviance, and Culture Pattern, *Psychiatry and its History. Methodological Problems in Research*. Ed. G. Mora and J.L. Brand. Springfield, Ill.; Charles C. Thomas, 172–194

Schwartz, L.R. (1969). The Hierarchy of Resort in Curative Practice: The Admiralty Islands, Melanesia, *Journal of Health and Social Behavior*, Vol. 10, 201–209

Sigerist, H.E. (1951). *Primitive and Archaic Medicine*. Vol. 1 of *A History of Medicine*. New York; Oxford University Press

Slack, P.A. (1972). Some Aspects of Epidemics in England, 1485–1640, University of Oxford DPhil Thesis

Slack, P.A. (1979). Mirrors of Health and Treasures of Poor Men: The Uses of the Vernacular Medical Literature of Tudor England, in *Health, Medicine and Mortality in the Sixteenth Century*. Ed. C. Webster. Cambridge; Cambridge University Press, 237–273

Tambiah, S.J. (1969). Animals are Good to Think and Good to Prohibit, *Ethnology*, Vol. 8, 423–459

Thomas, K.V. (1971). *Religion and the Decline of Magic*. London; Weidenfeld and Nicolson. New York; Charles Scribner's Sons. Paperback edn (1973). Revised (1980). Harmondsworth; Penguin

Thomas, K.V. (1975). An Anthropology of Religion and Magic, II, *Journal of Interdisciplinary History*, Vol. 6, 91–109

Thompson, E.P. (1972). Anthropology and the Discipline of Historical Context, *Midland History*, Vol. 1, 41–55

Thompson, E.P. (1978). Folklore, Anthropology and Social History, *Indian Historical Review*, Vol. 3, 247–266

Turner, T. (1969). Oedipus: Time and Structure in Narrative Form, *Proceedings of the American Ethnological Society*, 26–68

Turner, V. (1967). *The Forest of Symbols*. Ithaca; Cornell University Press

Turner, V. (1968). *The Drums of Affliction*. Oxford; Clarendon Press

Turner, V. (1974). *Dramas, Fields, and Metaphors*. Ithaca; Cornell University Press

Turner, V. (1975). Symbolic Studies, *Annual Review of Anthropology*, Vol. 4, 145–162

Tyler, S.A. (1969). *Cognitive Anthropology*. New York; Holt, Rinehart and Winston

5

The social sciences and history of science and medicine

L.J. Jordanova

Introduction

The relationships between the history of science and medicine and the social sciences are many and complex. They are not new either; the recognition that science and medicine are social products in the sense that they represent and express the conflicts, tensions and sources of power within the social structure goes back at least as far as the French Revolution (Gillispie 1959; Pearce Williams 1959). Many nineteenth-century thinkers saw science and medicine as parts of larger transformations of Western capitalist society, while Engels (1940; Carver 1981: ch. 6) attempted to develop a Marxian analysis of systematic understanding of nature.

The development of a distinct discipline that addresses the question of how sociology can be applied to science is a phenomenon of the twentieth century that is generally associated with the work of Robert Merton (1938, 1970, 1973) and his disciples. It was not until the 1970s that the sociology of science grew into a fully fledged field with its own journals, jargon and commonly agreed upon tasks, and with enough practitioners to constitute a field in its own right. The foundation of the journal *Science Studies* (now *Social Studies of Science*) in 1971 marked a point of recognition of the new field, as did publications such as Ben-David's account of 'the emergence and development of the social role of the scientist, and of the organisation of scientific work'

(1971:vii), and the collections of readings in sociology of science prepared by Barber and Hirsch (1962) and Barnes (1972).

The varied disciplinary backgrounds of those who work in the sociology of science suggest its diverse intellectual antecedents in scholarly traditions of the nineteenth and early twentieth centuries. However, the explosion of the 1970s occurred not because of any startlingly new theoretical insights but because of a wide range of social and intellectual circumstances such as anti-psychiatry, feminism, the anti-nuclear and anti-war movements (e.g. Easlea 1973, 1981; Illich 1977). The radical politics of the late 1960s addressed itself to developing a critique of science and medicine and their privileged epistemological and social position. Social theories were an obvious source of inspiration, but so, significantly enough, was the philosophy of science with its insistence, at least in some influential quarters, that facts were theory-laden, that perception, with all the implications of subjectivity that word contains, was a crucial part of scientific activity, and that science could be described in terms of instrumentalism – the idea that scientific theories are merely useful approximations to nature, instruments for knowledge production, rather than true accounts of the physical world (Hesse 1963, 1970; Teich and Young 1973; Hanson 1958). All these factors combined to produce a form of relativism – Western science did not embody any absolute truth in the form of value-free knowledge. Instead, it was a phenomenon to be explained, like any other, in terms that related it to its social context. This relativism had political bite; among many other events, the Vietnam war demonstrated the extraordinary scale of destruction possible in an age of scientific warfare. The claim that science and medicine were activities that directly benefited the mass of the population now seemed like a hollow lie calculated more to deceive than inform. Practising scientists were active in movements that expressed concern at the social impact of science as they had been in the 1930s (Bernal 1939), and, although this did not of itself generate a social analysis of science, it opened the way for science studies being incorporated into scientific curricula, often in the disappointing form of courses designated by the bland juxtaposition 'science *and* society' (Rose and Rose 1970; Mathias 1972). What now goes under the name of 'science studies' varies enormously (Cairncross 1980), but it can act as a convenient umbrella under which social approaches to science can be explored. The establishment of science studies and the analogous foundation of courses in behavioural sciences applied to medicine were thought to be 'humanizing' influences on the sciences; they were never intended to be, and by and large never became, centres for a radical critique of contemporary science and medicine or places where social theory was taught and applied. Institutionally, power remained with scientists and medical practitioners on whom social scientists who wish to study those fields depend not just for jobs or research funds but for access to the laboratory, the hospital and the consulting room in order to pursue their research.

The development of the new sub-disciplines, sociology of science and sociology of medicine, is only one of the ways in which relationships have been forged between history of science and medicine and the social sciences. In this case historical studies serve as classic examples to illustrate a sociological point, but historical research itself may be guided and inspired by a particular social theory. While this is a common approach among sociologists, historians are conventionally reluctant to attach a clear theoretical label to their work. Those who have done so have frequently been severely criticized (Rudwick 1980). Sociological approaches to science and medicine are sometimes part of a broader critique of science, from an ethical and/or political perspective. Much rarer is the sociological theorist who uses material from science or medicine as an integral part of his or her analysis – Parsons' development of the notion of sick role and his approach to motivated deviance based on an examination of medical practice is one of the best known examples (Parsons 1951: ch. 10).

The move towards a social approach to science and medicine has not been without its critics, who frequently reassert the epistemological distinctiveness of science and stress that the special form of knowing involved in the sciences means that, although social factors may affect science, they do not do so in ways that undermine its logic and value-neutrality. It should be noted that this view is also prevalent among those doing social history or sociology of science (Ben-David 1971; Graham 1977).

In the late 1960s it became fashionable to characterize a social approach to science as externalist, a term used to describe work that gave priority to factors deemed extrinsic to the kernel of science, which was taken to be its concepts, theories and methods. The dichotomy thereby posed between an internalist and externalist approach was unhelpful and misguided, and distracted scholars into making elaborate, but somewhat unnecessary, justifications of their positions. This debate, like others mentioned here, must be seen in its historical context. What it betrayed was a deep distrust of the social sciences, and of sociology in particular, which was frequently caricatured as simplistic, reductionist and riddled with jargon. Internalists claimed that externalism was an absurd, extreme doctrine, so preposterous that only a fool, a sociologist or, worst of all, a Marxist would propound it. With hindsight what was significant was the way in which the internal/external debate incorrectly equated social approaches to science with externalism. By contrast I would suggest that methods, concepts and theories from the social sciences can be applied to the study of all aspects of science and medicine. So far, those working in the history of science and medicine have used the social sciences in rather limited ways, drawing surprisingly little from the major traditions of social theory, while employing scientistic methods that bear little relationship to serious attempts to comprehend the individual and society in a theoretically sophisticated, holistic manner.

It is the attempt to explain the manifold relationships between individuals, classes and society as a whole that characterizes the social sciences, a field that subsumes a diversity of approaches and a number of disciplines – history, anthropology, economics and psychology, as well as sociology. The term sociology can easily be misleading, since it suggests a monolithic discipline of deep conceptual and methodological unity – which, of course, is not the case.

It is important to recognize that disciplines rarely act on each other directly but frequently do so by means of intermediates. For example, many of the newer ideas about social history have come to the study of science and medicine from mainstream history, which, in taking up some major sociological themes, addressed the question of how, as a discipline traditionally devoted to questions of politics, diplomacy and foreign policy, history could incorporate social analysis. However, history of science and medicine cannot be understood merely as fields within general history. Although many scholars would argue that they should become so, up to now this has not happened for very good reasons. Until relatively recently, extremely few historians of science and medicine had any historical training; rather they were scientists, mathematicians or medical practitioners who had shifted fields. They, inevitably, were preoccupied with questions related to the distinctiveness of scientific and medical knowledge, which were of relatively little interest to historians as a whole. To a large extent history of science, more so than history of medicine, has remained – institutionally and conceptually – a separate field, although both disciplines have been profoundly influenced by changes within historical scholarship such as the development of quantitative methods and of prosopographical techniques (Pyenson 1977). The point is that insights, ideas and methods from the social sciences have frequently come to the history of science and medicine in a roundabout way.

Although there are several valid intellectual reasons for speaking about 'science' as a phenomenon, it is also important to stress the diversity subsumed under the name of science. Some scholars have explored this variety by describing the distinct characteristics of constituent scientific disciplines and charting their history from a social perspective. Much current work in the sociology of science examines the process of discipline/field formation and growth such as Edge and Mulkay's classic study of radio astronomy (1976) and Mackenzie's recent work on statistics (1981). This method can only be applied to historical periods where the notion of discipline is appropriate. Many other approaches to science as a social phenomenon also stress that a vast array of processes, persons and organizations all come under the heading of science and require study. Thus, the more emphasis is placed on social aspects of science, the more multi-faceted science appears to be. It is therefore appropriate that medicine is no longer treated as if it were merely a scientific discipline and, in fact, sociology of science differs markedly from sociology of medicine. In the case of the former, most attention has been paid to explaining changing theories and practices, especially the processes of discovery, innovation and the communication networks between scientists (Mulkay 1972). In the latter, the dominant emphasis is on the social analysis of interpersonal relationships, such as the professionalization and socialization of medical doctors, 'illness behaviour' and encounters between practitioners and patients, where these are taken as a microcosm of social relations in general (Freidson 1970; Mechanic 1968).

So far, we have noted a number of different relationships between the history of science and medicine and the social sciences that embrace all the possibilities from the deliberate use of social theory in historical studies (Hahn 1971; Peterson 1978) to the incorporation of ideas that have come into common academic use, such as modernization theory (Ehrenreich and English 1979). There is, of course, no consensus as to what a social analysis of science and medicine entails, or, indeed, what we mean by 'science' and 'medicine'. Here it is possible to mention only a few of the most important issues raised by bringing a social perspective to the history of science and of medicine.

Social analyses of science

The answers to the question 'What is science?' determine the content and form of historical and sociological work. Until relatively recently history of science meant the history of scientific *ideas*, which in turn meant the history of the *progress* of scientific theories. It was, quite simply, as a challenge to this hegemony that demands were made for a social history of science (Teich and Young 1973). This entailed challenging two cardinal dogmas: that science was an activity that produced ever more truthful accounts of the natural world, and that it was an autonomous activity that was fostered or impeded by particular social circumstances, but not *determined* by them. In the search for alternatives to Whiggish definitions of science a number of possibilities presented themselves.

The sociology of knowledge has played a central role in the move towards seeing science as a social phenomenon, particularly for those scholars concerned with the philosophical aspects of scientific knowledge. Such work draws on traditions indebted to Durkheim, to the structural anthropology of Mary Douglas (see chapter 4 above) and to such classics in the sociology of knowledge as Berger and Luckmann's *The Social Construction of Reality* (1967). The recent debates have centred both on the theoretical validity of the 'strong programme' in the sociology of knowledge (Bloor 1976: ch.1; Millstone 1978) and on empirical case studies (Mackenzie 1981; Barnes and Shapin 1979).

Although it tends to remain at an abstract, philosophical level, Bloor's demand for a 'strong programme' in the sociology of knowledge expresses two precepts that are of interest. He argued that the sociologist's task is closely akin to that of the scientist in finding regularities and general principles in the data, and then building theories to explain them. The second point follows directly from this, that the sociology of knowledge should be causal and provide naturalistic explanations of science (Bloor 1976: 3–5). Bloor, and others working in closely related perspectives, acknowledge the importance of such factors as intellectual environment and personal commitments and interests, but there is a limit to the extent to which they provide a materialist analysis of science; nor could they be said to have been influenced by or practising within Marxist traditions.

Rather than pursuing a philosophical, causal approach to the social analysis of science, Marxists have sought to decode the social relations implicit in science. For them knowledge is socially constructed in such a way as to conceal social/class interests behind an apparently value-neutral, universal account of nature. As a result, science veils the relations between the natural and the social – indeed it inverts them, so that what we take to be natural phenomena can only be understood as highly mediated forms of relationships and processes in social life. Science can thus be construed as the classic example of ideology in a capitalist society, and it becomes an important project to investigate the precise way in which science functions in a given context, paying particular attention to the power relations between different social groups (Young 1977, 1979; Figlio 1978, 1979; Haraway 1978, 1979).

What sociologists of knowledge and Marxists have in common is their emphasis on scientific knowledge, belief and concepts. They differ, however, in that the former emphasize a philosophically rigorous, naturalistic method applied to detailed, illustrative case studies, while the latter pursue a materialist analysis of power relations. Nevertheless, in both cases the precise content of scientific knowledge is crucial.

There are influential traditions in the sociology of science that see their foothold in the potential for a social analysis of scientific behaviour – what scientists do, rather than how or what they think, becomes the field of study. The social analysis consists in describing the practice of science in particular institutional settings: the laboratory, the university, the school, industry, and scientific societies. Common sense suggests that scientific practices are determined by a whole range of non-scientific factors, such as government policy, traditions of education, economic patterns, business and industry, trade needs, and so on. Furthermore, it is equally clear that how scientists behave is also affected by their personalities, their education and training, their class backgrounds and career aspirations, their age, and their relationships with students, technicians, peers and superiors. Taking science as practice thus opens the way to a vast array of possible topics and methods, from looking at the role of the state as patron to patterns of socialization, and from functionalism to symbolic interactionism (Barnes 1972; Ben-David 1971; Berman 1978; Edge and Mulkay 1976; Hahn 1971). All the by-products of everyday scientific work can become grist to the mill of this type of historical sociology, which uses oral as well as written evidence. Furthermore, there is here a potential for quantitative work, for the study of the biographies and psychological make-up of individual practitioners, and of the conditions most conducive to discovery, innovation and success. Although such methods are built on the premise that science cannot be understood as a purely rational activity, those who use them rarely delve very deeply into the subjective aspects of doing scientific work. They do, of course, make assumptions about human behaviour and consciousness, but these tend to be implicit and are frequently of a mechanistic nature, in that they see people as responding to particular stimuli in predictable ways, given their interests. Their interests impel actors to maximize their individual advantage in career and class terms as defined by rewards of income, status and prestige.

So long as individual scientific practitioners are the main object of study, it makes sense to examine all aspects of individuals, including their creativity and imaginative processes. We know that these are central features of the scientific enterprise and that these aspects of human activity may indeed be analysed from a social perspective (Berger 1972; Williams 1977, 1981). It would be mistaken, however, to allow the application to science of methods and insights from the sociology of culture to perpetuate old-fashioned ideas about the isolation and autonomy of 'exceptional' individuals – be they scientists, writers or painters – from the social fabric. In this sense, the struggles of historians of art, literature and culture to bring to their fields a sociological perspective that does not take the individual as the ultimate unit of explanation can be used by historians of science (McNeil 1979) as models of what can be done.

In addition to the relatively new field of the sociology of culture, other major intellectual traditions also repudiate the emphasis on individual actors as the appropriate unit of social analysis. It is, for example, an important tenet of structuralism, which is clearly seen in the writings of Michel Foucault (1967, 1970, 1972, 1973, 1979) who has had considerable influence on historians and sociologists of science and medicine in the English-speaking world. The value of his approach lies in his delineation of conceptual homologies between diverse aspects of intellectual, social and political life. Science has no privileged status here other than the power it can be shown to wield, which is, for Foucault, of immense significance from the late eighteenth century onwards.

It may be helpful to remind ourselves that each of these approaches to science as a social phenomenon must itself be understood in social terms. Foucault's background in French epistemology, his work with psychiatric patients and his participation in the 'events' of May 1968 in Paris are integral to his intellectual project. For the fields of science studies and science policy (MacLeod 1975), relations with governments and grant-giving bodies have no small effect on the shape of research. One result of the service relationship of much sociology of science to government and other agencies is that history of science is drawn on less than is contemporary science for examples of topical relevance. In certain respects the line between the history and the sociology of science remains a fine one, just as the one between history and sociology is (Burke 1980).

In many ways the relationship between the history and the sociology of science reflects the changing relationship between history as a whole and the social sciences, which has produced the development of 'social history' as a new field (Judt 1979). Social history has spawned two characteristic approaches that illuminate recent, parallel changes in the history of science. These are the use of quantitative methods, and the interpretation of 'social' as everyday, connected with ordinary persons, non-political, 'history with the politics left out'. Many historians have enthusiastically embraced quantitative methods and at the same time turned away from synthetic explanations and theoretical work. To sustain a quantitative approach to science, its exponents will have to show that those features that are susceptible to quantification provide important insights into scientific theory and practice, and that this does indeed constitute a *social* analysis in a non-trivial sense of that term. At the moment the case is not yet proven.

By now it should be clear why the internal/external debate was so obfuscating and unhelpful (Reingold 1980: 487–91). It suggested that science be seen in one of two radically opposed and mutually exclusive ways. On an internal view, sets of ideas changed according to internal logic and either approached ever closer an objective account of nature, or achieved pragmatically an increasingly close fit with observations. For an internalist, social features extrinsic to scientific knowledge might illuminate, though not fundamentally affect, the character of science in a given historical situation. Accordingly, the externalist examined the residuum after the internalist had done his or her job. The classic example of externalism is often taken to be Boris Hessen's article 'The Social and Economic Roots of Newton's "Principia"' from the controversial book *Science at the Cross Roads* (1931; in Basalla 1968: 31–8). No doubt some recent sociology of science could be seen as externalist in its emphasis on career structures, status, citation patterns, reward systems, prestige and so on. But, in fact, these would only be genuine cases of an externalist analysis if the authors argued that factors external to scientific thought determined and explained all other aspects of science as well. Such claims are rarely made. Indeed, those concerned with the historical sociology of science frequently repeat their conviction that the internal/external dualism is meaningless. Neither knowledge nor practice should be taken as an object of study in isolation from the other. Furthermore, it is not, in fact, correct to identify traditional history of science with an internal approach, or sociological perspectives with an externalist one.

Medicine, history and the social sciences

Like science, medicine is frequently defined as a form of know-ledge; unlike science, its conceptual apparatus is both formed through and applied to encounters between practitioners and other people. There have, in fact, been two related openings for a social approach to medicine that were not so readily available for science. First, the relationships between practitioners and patients provided an obvious and concrete object of social analysis. Second, the objects of medical enquiry – health and disease – appear to be inherently social and political in a way that the object of scientific enquiry – the physical world – does not. In the case of medicine, then, the notion of *practice* takes on additional meaning since here it is a directly social relationship. For these reasons it has been relatively easy to bring a sociological element to medical history and to use historical material in medical sociology.

A limited range of sociological concepts and historical themes tends to recur. Relationships between doctors and patients are seen as a microcosm of social relationships in society as a whole, with respect to the differential exercise of power according to class, race and gender (Ehrenreich and English 1979). Thus, the analysis of doctor/patient interactions generally rests on some conventional notion of dominance by professionalized middle-class élites over working-class, vulnerable patients. By logical extension, the striving for privileged status by the medically trained – professionalization – is taken to be the crucial process in medical history. Sociological models of professionalization abound (Freidson 1970; Johnson 1972; Parry and Parry 1976; Larson 1977; Heraud 1979) and are readily incorporated into historical work (Peterson 1978; Woodward and Richards 1977: ch.5). The professions are at the centre of heated dispute with regard both to their social and moral basis (King 1968; Kennedy 1981; Entralgo 1969) and to the characteristics that define professionalization. Some of the most widely used criteria are closure (restricted entry), monopoly, specialization, and esoteric knowledge.

The theories, ideas and concepts of medicine are often treated by sociologists as the *occasion* for upward social mobility, class domination, or sexual exploitation (Holloway 1964; Parry and Parry 1976; Ehrenreich and English 1979). This partly results from a reaction against a traditional approach to medicine that glorified the march of medical progress through scientific research (see chapter 19 below) rather than examining the interaction between theories and practice in a concrete situation (Figlio 1978, 1979). One consequence of recent concern with professional power is a new dualism, with 'proper' scientific medicine on one side and its improper use by scheming, ambitious practitioners on the other. This 'use/abuse' model suggests that scientific-cum-medical knowledge is itself neutral, that in principle it could be used in a morally, politically and socially disinterested way, and that class dominance results from the abuse of doctors in the service of their own self-interests. It is hard to sustain the use/abuse model unless the existence of autonomous knowledge composed of disinterested facts can be demonstrated. This model may also be attacked on intellectual and political grounds (Young 1977; Wright 1980; Figlio 1979). For example, it clearly implies that fault may reasonably be attributed to doctors and scientists as professional groups, and so can easily degenerate into doctor/scientist 'bashing'.

Sociological perspectives on medicine draw heavily on American views of social change and social structure, such as those of Freidson (1970) and Parsons (1951), and particularly those aspects that employ theories of modernization. Change is construed as movement from traditional society to the modern state, from magic and superstition to science and rationality, from static communities to mobile individuals. This image of historical process endows the development of a professional middle class with considerable social significance and enhances the plausibility of considering professionalization and medical power as major social phenomena. Here again, we can note a difference in the way in which modernization has been taken up by students of science and those of medicine. The former have been concerned to trace the development of science as a profession (Ben-David 1971), in the sense of providing a sufficient, secure income and suitable institutional backing, while the latter have paid most attention to control and exclusion of unlicensed practitioners, since it has been possible for many different groups to make a living practising medicine for a long time. The modernization perspective, with its suggestion of continual processes of change and development, appeals to historians and sociologists alike but does not have any real explanatory power (Smith 1973; Judt 1979).

The widespread concern with the social role of the doctor is based on more than a recognition of the rise of the professional middle classes. It derives from the attribution to doctors of power to define health and normality. The potential for social authority and domination by doctors, and those with allied interests like pharmaceutical companies, seemed almost endless (Illich 1977; Foucault 1967, 1973). Such approaches have tended vastly to exaggerate the social impact of the medically trained, although their stress on the power of the medical system as a whole has been a valuable antidote to the 'miracles of modern medicine' view but less relevant to historical studies.

To some extent the problems of bringing together historical and sociological perspectives are equally severe for both science and medicine. In both cases an oversimplistic conceptual framework is frequently relied upon, and nowhere is this more marked than in the current vogue for the concept 'medicalization' (Foucault 1973; Illich 1977). The term refers to the process of making spheres of everyday life into a medical domain and it nicely illustrates current preoccupations with the personal power of doctors and with the use of scientific/medical knowledge as an instrument of oppression. As a term, medicalization alludes to unspecified historical/sociological processes, yet these are hard to pin down; hence the term is of little analytical value.

It is because of these preoccupations with medicine and medical power that relatively little attention has been paid to developing an historical sociology of health. This omission is all the more surprising in view of the recent challenge to the efficacy of medicine and the assertions that health is determined by a large number of social and environmental variables. Certainly some new avenues of research into the social determinants of health are currently being opened up, using methods from the social sciences, particularly demography and epidemiology. In reconstructing family and community structures, demographers have used mortality data, fertility patterns, disease distributions, and information on diet and epidemics, all of which are essential ingredients for an understanding of the historical sociology of health (Laslett 1965; Appleby 1973; Smith 1979). Just as demographers have developed sophisticated quantitative techniques yet found it hard to produce a synthetic history of the family, so there does not yet exist a broadly based account of health in a socio-historical context.

Conclusion

Since the 1960s, there has been extensive discussion of the viability of a social approach to science and medicine without any consensus being reached. Several different frameworks and methods have been employed in the attempts to root science and medicine in their social context. Although some scholars have, with varying degrees of success, synthesized history and the social sciences, their works remain isolated instances without a firm foothold in either set of disciplines.

Historians still have much to learn from the social sciences, although it seems likely that those who study science and medicine will continue to find it difficult to develop a fruitful relationship with traditions of sociological analysis. This is partly because, at some level, they see science and medicine as 'special', a specialness usually linked with their epistemological status. Thus, much social theorizing is simply assumed to be inapplicable to historical studies of science and medicine. It must also be said that, as sub-disciplines, the sociology of science and of medicine stand outside many of the major traditions of social thought, both because their objects of study, as conventionally understood in Western society, encourage a separation between themselves and other phenomena, and because practitioners and institutions from within science and medicine have maintained considerable power over the newly emerging fields of social studies of science and medicine.

The most serious obstacle in the way of an historical sociology of science and medicine is the implicit assumption in many circles that such a discipline should take the form of a science of science. It is arguable that there can be no consensus on developing a social analysis of science or medicine, not least because of the complexity of the objects of study. An historical sociology of science and medicine needs to have a critical orientation towards its subject matter, to go beyond static description, to transcend the internal/external dichotomy and to eschew mechanistic definitions of the kind derived from functionalism. The project of developing these new fields requires a social analysis that is historical, and historical explanation that is informed by social understanding. Furthermore, stereotypical and entrenched definitions of science and medicine have to be superseded. Hence, new insights will come not from within the sciences but from outside them.

Bibliography

Appleby, A.B. (1973). Disease or Famine? Mortality in Cumberland and West-morland, 1580–1640, *Economic History Review*, Second Series, Vol. 26, 403–431
Barber, B. and Hirsch, W., Ed. (1962). *The Sociology of Science*. New York; The Free Press. London; Collier Macmillan
Barnes, B., Ed. (1972). *Sociology of Science*. Harmondsworth; Penguin
Barnes, B. (1974). *Scientific Knowledge and Sociological Theory*. London and Boston; Routledge and Kegan Paul
Barnes, B. (1977). *Interests and the Growth of Knowledge*. London, Henley and Boston; Routledge and Kegan Paul
Barnes, B. and Shapin, S., Ed. (1979). *Natural Order. Historical Studies of Scientific Culture*. Beverly Hills and London; Sage

Basalla, G., Ed. (1968). *The Rise of Modern Science. Internal or External Factors?* Lexington, Mass.; Heath

Ben-David, J. (1971). *The Scientist's Role in Society. A Comparative Study.* Englewood Cliffs, NJ; Prentice-Hall

Berger, J. (1972). *Ways of Seeing.* London; British Broadcasting Corporation. Harmondsworth; Penguin

Berger, P.L. and Luckmann, T. (1967). *The Social Construction of Reality. A Treatise in the Sociology of Knowledge.* Harmondsworth; Penguin

Berman, M. (1978). *Social Change and Scientific Organization. The Royal Institution 1799–1844.* London; Heinemann Educational Books. Ithaca, NY; Cornell University Press

Bernal, J.D. (1939). *The Social Function of Science. Part 1, What Science Does. Part 2, What Science Could Do.* London; George Routledge

Bloor, D. (1976). *Knowledge and Social Imagery.* London, Henley and Boston; Routledge and Kegan Paul

Burke, P. (1980). *Sociology and History.* London; George Allen and Unwin

Cairncross, A. (1980). *Science Studies. A Report to the Nuffield Foundation.* London; The Nuffield Foundation

Carver, T. (1981). *Engels.* Oxford; Oxford University Press

Daniels, G.H. (1967). The Process of Professionalization in American Science: The Emergent Period, 1820–1860, *Isis*, Vol. 58, 151–166

Easlea, B. (1973). *Liberation and the Aims of Science. An Essay on Obstacles to the Building of a Beautiful World.* London; Chatto and Windus for Sussex University Press

Easlea, B. (1981). *Science and Sexual Oppression. Patriarchy's Confrontation with Woman and Nature.* London; Weidenfeld and Nicolson

Edge, D.O. and Mulkay, M.J. (1976). *Astronomy Transformed. The Emergence of Radio Astronomy in Britain.* New York and London; John Wiley

Ehrenreich, B. and English, D. (1979). *For Her Own Good. 150 Years of the Experts' Advice to Women.* London; Pluto

Engels, F. (1940). *Dialectics of Nature.* New York; International Publishers

Entralgo, P.L. (1969). *Doctor and Patient.* Trans. F. Partridge. London; Weidenfeld and Nicolson

Figlio, K. (1978). Chlorosis and Chronic Disease in Nineteenth-Century Britain: The Social Constitution of Somatic Illness in a Capitalist Society, *Social History*, Vol. 3, 167–197. Revised version (1979). *International Journal of Health Services*, Vol. 8, 589–617

Figlio, K.M. (1979). Sinister Medicine? A Critique of Left Approaches to Medicine, *Radical Science Journal*, No. 9, 14–68 and 148–160 (Critical Bibliography I: Medicine)

Foucault, M. (1967). *Madness and Civilisation. A History of Insanity in the Age of Reason.* Trans. R. Howard. London; Tavistock

Foucault, M. (1970). *The Order of Things. An Archaeology of the Human Sciences.* London; Tavistock. 1st French edn (1966). *Les Mots et les choses.* Paris; Gallimard

Foucault, M. (1972). *The Archaeology of Knowledge.* Trans. A.M. Sheridan Smith. London; Tavistock. 1st French edn (1969)

Foucault, M. (1973). *The Birth of the Clinic: An Archaeology of Medical Perception.* Trans..A.M. Sheridan Smith. London; Tavistock. 1st French edn (1963). *Naissance de la clinique.* Paris; Presses Universitaires de France

Foucault, M. (1979). *The History of Sexuality.* Volume I, *An Introduction.* Trans. R. Hurley. London; Allen Lane

Freidson, E. (1970). *Profession of Medicine. A Study of the Sociology of Applied Knowledge.* New York; Dodd, Mead

Gillispie, C.C. (1959). The *Encyclopédie* and the Jacobin Philosophy of Science: A Study in Ideas and Consequences, in *Critical Problems in the History of Science.* Ed. M. Clagett. Madison, Wisconsin and London; University of Wisconsin Press, 255–289

Graham, L. (1977). Science and Values: The Eugenics Movement in Germany and Russia in the 1920s, *American Historical Review*, Vol. 82, 1133–1164

Hahn, R. (1971). *The Anatomy of a Scientific Institution: The Paris Academy of Sciences, 1666–1803.* Berkeley; University of California Press

Hanson, N.R. (1958). *Patterns of Discovery. An Inquiry into the Conceptual Foundations of Science.* Cambridge; Cambridge University Press

Haraway, D. (1978). Animal Sociology and a Natural Economy of the Body Politic, Part I: A Political Physiology of Dominance, Part II: The Past is the Contested Zone: Human Nature and Theories of Production and Reproduction in Primate Studies, *Signs*, Vol. 4, 21–36, 37–60

Haraway, D. (1979). The Biological Enterprise: Sex, Mind, and Profit from Human Engineering to Sociobiology, *Radical History Review*, No. 20, 206–237

Heraud, B. (1979). *Sociology in the Professions.* London; Open Books

Hesse, M.B. (1963). *Models and Analogies in Science.* London; Sheed and Ward

Hesse, M.B. (1970). Is There an Independent Observation Language?, in *The Nature and Function of Scientific Theories.* Ed. R.G. Colodney. Pittsburgh; University of Pittsburgh Press

Holloway, S. (1964). Medical Education in England, 1830–1858: A Sociological Analysis, *History*, Vol. 49, 299–324

Illich, I. (1977). *Limits to Medicine. Medical Nemesis: the Expropriation of Health.* Harmondsworth; Penguin

Johnson, T.J. (1972). *Professions and Power.* London and Basingstoke; Macmillan

Judt, T. (1979). A Clown in Regal Purple: Social History and the Historians, *History Workshop Journal*, No. 7, 66–94

Kennedy, I. (1981). *The Unmasking of Medicine.* London; George Allen and Unwin

King, M.D. (1968). Science and the Professional Dilemma, in *Penguin Social Sciences Survey 1968.* Ed. J. Gould. Harmondsworth; Penguin, 34–73

Larson, M.S. (1977). *The Rise of Professionalism. A Sociological Analysis.* Berkeley, Los Angeles, London; University of California Press

Laslett, P. (1965). *The World We Have Lost.* London; Methuen

Mackenzie, D.A. (1981). *Statistics in Britain 1865–1930. The Social Construction of Scientific Knowledge.* Edinburgh; Edinburgh University Press

MacLeod, R.M. (1975). The Historical Context of the International Council for Science Policy Studies, *Archives Internationales d'Histoire des Sciences*, Vol. 25, 314–323

MacLeod, R.M. (1977). Changing Perspectives in the Social History of Science, in *Science, Technology and Society. A Cross-Disciplinary Perspective.* Ed. I. Spiegel-Rösing and D. Price. Beverly Hills and London; Sage, 149–195

McNeil, M. (1979). A Contextual Study of Erasmus Darwin, Cambridge PhD Thesis

Mathias, P., Ed. (1972). *Science and Society 1600–1900.* Cambridge; Cambridge University Press

Mechanic, D. (1968). *Medical Sociology: A Selective View.* New York; Collier-Macmillan

Merton, R.K. (1938). Science, Technology and Society in Seventeenth Century England, *Osiris*, Vol. 4, part 2, 360–632. Reprinted (1970) with new introduction. New York; H. Fertig. Paperback edn (1978). New York, Humanities Press

Merton, R.K. (1973). *The Sociology of Science; Theoretical and Empirical Investigations.* Chicago; University of Chicago Press

Millstone, E. (1978). A Framework for the Sociology of Knowledge, *Social Studies of Science*, Vol. 8, 111–125
Mulkay, M. (1972). *The Social Process of Innovauon. A Study in the Sociology of Science*. London; Macmillan
Mulkay, M. (1979). *Science and the Sociology of Knowledge*. London; George Allen and Unwin
Parry, N. and Parry, J. (1976). *The Rise of the Medical Profession: A Study of Collective Social Mobility*. London; Croom Helm
Parsons, T. (1951). *The Social System*. London; Routledge and Kegan Paul
Pearce Williams, L. (1959). The Politics of Science in the French Revolution, in *Critical Problems in the History of Science*. Ed. M. Clagett. Madison, Wisconsin and London; University of Wisconsin Press, 291–308
Peterson, M.J. (1978). *The Medical Profession in Mid-Victorian London*. Berkeley; University of California Press
Pyenson, L. (1977). 'Who the Guys Were': Prosopography in the History of Science, *History of Science*, Vol. 15, 155–188
Ravetz, J.R. (1973). *Scientific Knowledge and its Social Problems*. Harmondsworth; Penguin
Reingold, N. (1980). Through Paradigm-Land to a Normal History of Science, *Social Studies of Science*, Vol. 10, 475–496
Rose, H. and Rose, S. (1970). *Science and Society*. Harmondsworth; Penguin
Rudwick, M. (1980). Social Order and the Natural World, *History of Science*, Vol. 18, 269–285
Science at the Cross Roads (1931). Papers presented to the International Congress of the History of Science and Technology held in London from June 29th to July 3rd 1931 by the Delegates of the USSR. London; Kniga (England). 2nd edn (1971). New foreword by J. Needham and new introduction by P.G. Werskey. London; Cass
Smith, A.D. (1973). *The Concept of Social Change. A Critique of the Functionalist Theory of Social Change*. London, Henley and Boston; Routledge and Kegan Paul
Smith, F.B (1979). *The People's Health 1830–1910*. London; Croom Helm
Sociology of the Sciences. A Yearbook (1977–). Dordrecht
Teich, M. and Young, R.M., Ed. (1973). *Changing Perspectives in the History of Science. Essays in Honour of Joseph Needham*. London; Heinemann
Williams, R. (1977). *Marxism and Literature*. Oxford; Oxford University Press
Williams, R. (1981). *Culture*. Glasgow; Fontana
Woodward, J. and Richards, D., Ed. (1977). *Health Care and Popular Medicine in Nineteenth Century England. Essays in the Social History of Medicine*. London; Croom Helm
Wright, P.W.G. (1980). The Radical Sociology of Medicine, *Social Studies of Science*, Vol. 10, 103–120
Young, R.M. (1977). Science *is* Social Relations, *Radical Science Journal*, No. 5, 65–129
Young, R.M. (1979). Interpreting the Production of Science, *New Scientist*, Vol. 81, 1026–1028

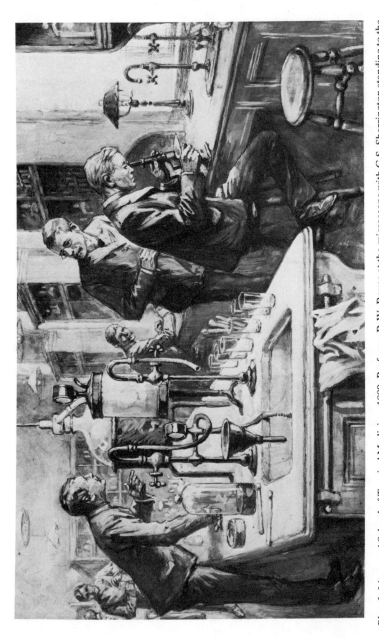

Plate 2. Liverpool School of Tropical Medicine, 1889. Professor R.W. Boyce at the microscope with C.S. Sherrington standing to the left. By courtesy of the Wellcome Trustees

6

The history of science, politics and political economy

Margaret M. Gowing

The history of science as a profession and intellectual discipline in the English-speaking world of the mid-twentieth century developed under the stimulus of George Sarton and Alexandre Koyré. Sarton's background was in philosophy and natural science and Koyré's was in philosophy, religious thought and intellectual history. Both were inspired by a strong, philosophical idealism. Sarton had been interested in the activities of the politically oriented British Fabian Society, and 'his' History of Science Society and *Isis* proclaimed an interest in the social and cultural relations of science. Nevertheless he saw the history of science above all as 'the history of mankind's unity, of its sublime purpose, of its gradual redemption', while Koyré analysed the crucial battles of ideas waged by the great scientists. The history of science profession that developed under their tutelage was inseparable from philosophy of science, as the titles of most of the university departments created in the subject in the 1940s, 1950s and beyond demonstrated. It was primarily 'internalist', concerned with the evolution of ideas.

Thus, with some exceptions (such as A.R. Hall's early work of 1954), historians of science were concerned with 'basic' or 'pure', not applied, research. Nor were they concerned with the complex relationships between the two varieties. The history of technology and of medicine were usually quite separate from the history of science except in the case of an individual such as Charles Singer. The historians of science reflected the scientists' idealistic faith in their own profession and their hierarchy of values, with theoretical mathematically based science at the peak. They believed in the cumulative advance of scientific understanding and thus of mankind towards ever nobler and expanding intellectual realms. The scientists themselves tended to emerge from history as exceptionally high minded, almost ethereal people, whose non-scientific preoccupations disappeared from view.

Most, though not all, of the exceptions among the historians of science were idealists of another philosophical school – Marxism. At the Second International Congress of the History of Science and Technology in London in 1931 (*Science at the Cross Roads* 1931) they heard Boris Hessen explain the history of the physical sciences from the seventeenth to the nineteenth centuries in terms of the rise of capitalism, which created new demands for technology and also deep political and religious divisions within English society. Historical materialism became the faith of Marxist historians of science, including in particular the two eminent scientists J.D. Bernal and Joseph Needham. This led at worst to Bernal's *Science in History* (1954), where vast masses of events and facts were pushed into a ready-made theoretical framework, and at best to his excellent *Science and Industry in the Nineteenth Century* (1953) and to Needham's great multi-volume *Science and Civilisation in China* (1954–; see chapter 23 below). Here, Marxism helped to determine the authors' interests in the relationship between scientific advances and technical needs and processes but they pursued the evidence with the care and respect of true historians. Other Marxists – Farrington, a classicist, and J.G. Crowther, a journalist – wrote at a popular level about the social relations and the statesmen of science (e.g. Farrington 1951; Crowther 1965). The anti-collectivist opposition, led by Polanyi, did not write history of science.

Philosophical questions about science will always be of very great interest to historians. But history and philosophy are two very different disciplines and their combination, whether the philosophy was of the Sarton–Koyré 'internalist' variety or Marxist and 'externalist', had many disadvantages for the infant history of science profession. Philosophically minded historians attached a body of generalizations to science, using historical examples as illustrations, without analysing historical evidence systematically. The internalists gave natural science its own separate lineage through the ages separated from the mainstream historical context of each period. Scientists were too often treated as a race apart and the turmoil of history was lost. The Marxists were usually restricted in their choice of relevant internal and external factors.

Because of its conceptual framework and its struggle for a unique identity from all except its philosophical twin, the history of science developed as a separate discipline and was mostly far removed in educational background, in interests and in contacts from mainstream academic history. Its recruits were more often scientists or philosophers than historians.

Historians of science showed little interest in the relationship of science with politics in its widest sense: how men govern themselves; how they distribute power and resources within a society and between societies; how they choose between different objectives and between different means to any single objective. They were equally uninterested in politics in its narrower formal sense: institutions and administration; parties and pressure groups; diplomacy; laws; political happenings. The major exception was a continuous interest in the foundation and operation of the Royal Society and similar academies, but here again the approach was mostly governed by an idealistic view of high-minded scientists preoccupied in all their activities with objectivity and 'truth'. Bernal (1939: 323–4) expressed the rosy view that

> Science has been at all times a commune of workers, helping one another, sharing their knowledge, not seeking corporately or individually more money or power than is needed for their work. They have at all times been rational and international in outlook and thus fundamentally in harmony with the movements that seek to extend that community of effort and enjoyment to social and economic as well as to intellectual fields.

He concluded that we have 'in the practice of science the prototype for all human common action'. Bernal voiced the opinion, still common among scientists over forty years later, that, while science is pure, party politics are essentially dirty. The scientist may, he wrote (1939: 404),

> become a politician but he will never become a party politician [because] he sees the social, economic and political situation as a problem to which a solution must first be found and then applied, not as a battleground of personalities, careers and vested interests ... Only when the parties can get together on a broad programme of social justice, civil liberty and peace can the full help of the scientist be expected.

If Bernal, with his passionate interest in politics, felt like this, the historians of science might feel justified in recoiling with distaste from the nasty business of politics (Gowing 1977a).

By contrast, mainstream history syllabuses in mid-century remained largely concerned with political history. Intellectual history had little place in it, at least in the English-speaking world, but economic history was flourishing. Few leading English-speaking mainstream historians took any interest in science; Herbert Butterfield and G.N. Clark were rare exceptions. Butterfield's work (1949) was 'internalist' in the prevailing history of science mode despite his contributions to political history, but Clark's short book on *Science and Social Welfare in the Age of Newton* (1937) was – along with Merton's roughly contemporary sociological study of seventeenth-century science (1938) – an early landmark in widening the frame of reference for historical study of scientific developments. In recent years few mainstream seventeenth-century historians would ignore the scientific revolution (Hill 1965), but their nineteenth- and twentieth-century colleagues have continued to omit science almost completely from their politics. For example, a notable biography of Sir Robert Peel (Gash 1972) acknowledges that, of all the leading politicians of the day, Peel was the most sympathetic to science; yet in a book of 716 pages two are devoted to it. A.J.P. Taylor's *English History 1914–1945* (1965) barely mentions science.

The Second World War might well have turned the attention of historians of science to the political dimensions of their subject and the attention of the mainstream political historians to science. In the First World War, science, especially chemistry, had shown that its ancient connections with military matters had been greatly strengthened by modern industrial technology. Indeed, as modern technology had become science-based in the late nineteenth century, science and its infrastructure had become important factors in Anglo-German rivalry. The Second World War was scientific from top to bottom: from major new science-based weapons systems that might dominate strategy and the outcome of the war to, in beleaguered Britain, the nutrition of the whole population, whether munitions workers or expectant mothers. In the belligerent countries, all non-pacifist scientists were mobilized for war work and scientists who had been close colleagues across national frontiers became enemies. The fierce competition for priority in discovery was harnessed to vital political ends. Surprisingly few books have, however, been written on science in the war or the relationships between scientists and politicians. In Britain the official war histories are important (Postan *et al.* 1952; Scott and Hughes 1955). R.V. Jones' book on scientific intelligence (1978) has been deservedly popular as well as valuable. R.W. Clark's *Tizard* (1965) is still the best account of the well-known political rows between Tizard and Cherwell over radar; the biography of Cherwell (Birkenhead 1961) is unsatisfactory as is Snow's work on the subject (1961, 1962). The wartime relationship between scientists and politicians was at its most dramatic in the development of the atomic bomb. Here there are many books and I summarize the political elements of this story to demonstrate the challenge it presented to historians of science. The bomb did not 'win the war' and was less immediately important than the competition in radar. But the famous British Maud report of 1941, which pushed into action the floundering American atomic project, had written: 'the lines on which we are now working are such as would be likely to suggest themselves to any capable physicist' (Gowing 1964). It is conceivable that the very able scientists who had remained in Nazi Germany might have made an atomic bomb before the Allies – if they had concentrated on one route, plutonium, if the great Bothe had not miscalculated the cross-section of graphite, if the scientists had been better at organizing themselves and in securing government support (Goudsmit 1947; Irving 1967). With a different mix of science and politics, Hitler in his bunker might have had an atomic bomb to hurl. Information is now also increasing about the Russian (Holloway 1981) and Japanese work on atomic bombs (Weiner 1978; Hughes 1980).

The British and American decisions to develop an atomic bomb and then to merge the two projects involved all kinds of political decisions about administrative organizations, and about the relative roles of the scientists and the military and of the Allied partners. These international decisions were also to have important consequences, which reverberate to the present day, for France, whose pioneering refugee scientists were part of the British atomic team (Weart 1979) and for Canada whose scientific and power status was greatly raised by her willingness at British behest to establish an atomic project within the small National Research Council (Eggleston 1965).

The scientists – American, British, French and Canadian – were closely involved in these decisions for developing the project, and some of them were involved in the two other big political decisions about the bomb: Should the bomb be used against Japan? What could be done to forestall a postwar nuclear arms race? One of the many misconceptions about the decision to drop the bombs is that it was taken in the face of the opposition of the atomic scientists, that 'the tender consciences of the scientists had little influence on its use' (Ravetz 1971). Scientists were deeply involved in the operational planning (Hewlett and Anderson 1962). Half the members of the American committee under the Secretary of State for War that recommended that the bombs should be dropped on Japanese cities were scientists, and four very eminent physicists comprised the scientific advisory panel. As is well known, a powerful memorandum by six Chicago scientists headed by James Franck urged that hopes of international control of atomic energy would be fatally prejudiced if the United States released this new means of indiscriminate destruction. Nevertheless, the scientific panel saw no acceptable alternative to direct military use but added that as scientific men they had no proprietary rights.

It is true that we are among the few citizens who have had occasion to give thoughtful consideration to these problems during the past few years. We have however no claim to special competence in solving the political, social and military problems which are presented by the advent of atomic power [Stimson 1947: 101].

The political leaders of the United States and Britain were reluctant during the war to ask what could be done to forestall a postwar nuclear arms race, although Niels Bohr did more than anyone else to make them understand the problem (Gowing 1964). When the British brought Bohr from German-occupied Denmark in 1943 and told him of the atomic bomb he at once saw that it would lead to still more horrible weapons, such as the hydrogen bomb, and that it would bring fundamental change in the world. He saw before most others that postwar life would be dominated by tension between Russia and the West and that the only chance of forestalling a nuclear arms race was to tell the Russians about the bomb before it had been used and to attempt to agree on control before there was threat of duress. This belief became Bohr's chief preoccupation for the rest of the war and he spent his time in political antechambers tirelessly advocating it. Churchill was deeply suspicious of Bohr and one clause of an agreement that he and Roosevelt signed implied that Bohr might be a Russian spy. Bohr's efforts failed: if Russia had been consulted about the bomb during the war it might have made no difference but the fact that she was not consulted doomed the early postwar attempts at international control.

Nuclear physics, one of the finest fruits of the human intellect and the epitome of 'pure' science, had produced a weapon that could determine the balance of power, and the life and death of populations and nations. In 1945 the bomb emphasized the world shift in power more than anything else. Its sole possessor was the United States, the supreme world power. In 1949 Russia's first bomb test lifted her to the position of a superpower (Holloway 1981). It was also a shattering moment of truth for Britain, coming three years before her own first test (Gowing 1974). Indeed, Britain's wartime role in the development of the atomic bomb helped to conceal from her the facts of changing power. Would she have come to terms sooner with her status in the postwar world if her own and her refugee scientists had been less clear-sighted in 1940 and 1941, if the Maud report had never been written and if she had played no part in a wartime atomic project?

During the war, the atomic scientists and governments had worked extremely closely together and the first nine postwar years were with some rare exceptions (not only the atomic spies, Fuchs and Nunn May) a period of symbiosis between them. Even Einstein insisted in the early postwar years that the United States should keep control of the bomb until a world government was ready to function. No American scientists complained when, in 1946, the McMahon Act made impossible the collaboration in atomic technology with Britain, their close wartime partner.

The American nuclear physicists however proved to be, in the immediate postwar years, an extraordinarily powerful pressure group on those matters they cared about (Smith 1965). In 1949, the United States had to decide whether or not to proceed with the super or hydrogen bomb (Hewlett and Duncan 1969). The chairman of the United States Atomic Energy Commission (USAEC) described some eminent scientists as 'drooling and blood-thirsty with the prospect' (Lilienthal 1964: 582). But, with one member (Seaborg) absent, the Commission's General Advisory Committee (GAC) of scientists and engineers – Oppenheimer (chairman), Conant, DuBridge, Fermi, Rabi, H. Rowe, Cyril Smith, Buckley of Bell Laboratories – opposed the development, hoping that other countries would refrain. Recent work (York 1976) confirms the wisdom of their view. Nevertheless, after President Truman decided to go ahead, all the members of the GAC did everything they could to hasten the superbomb. The end of the era of scientific solidarity between the government and the scientists was signified by the bitter 1954 hearings, which resulted in the withdrawal of Oppenheimer's security clearance (Major 1971; Stern 1971; USAEC 1954). The nuclear arms race, which may yet obliterate civilization, depends today, as it has done for forty years, on the inventiveness of very clever scientists in all the five nuclear-armed countries.

Since 1940, many of the most eminent scientists in the United States, Britain, France and Russia have been up to their necks in politics, especially military politics. Reflections by the scientific advisers to Presidents Eisenhower, Kennedy and Johnson are most illuminating (Kistiakovsky 1976; Wiesner 1965). Some have loved it, and some have found it profoundly distasteful. Paradoxically, scientists were being submerged in politics in the 1940s and 1950s just as the history of science profession was propagating the idealist version of science and the scientist as essentially international, pure, objective, uninterested in power, so different from the dirt of politics and politicians – the image that the scientists themselves still saw and to some extent still see. The infant history of science profession might well have been excited by the extraordinary profusion of genius gathered in the wartime bomb story and the possibilities of gathering their views and recollections: Bohr, Einstein, Fermi, Chadwick, Joliot-Curie and great physicists galore; chemists including Urey, Seaborg and H.S. Taylor; metallurgists such as Cyril Smith. Yet well into the 1960s the history of science journals contained scarcely any articles about the twentieth century and very little except the internalist, intellectual aspects of science. Of the sixteen papers discussed at the Wisconsin meeting of the Institute for the History of Science in 1957 (Clagett 1962), only one was concerned with politics and that with the French Revolution. The momentous atomic upheaval was not apparently mentioned in the 1961 meeting of the International Union of the History and Philosophy of Science on scientific change (Crombie 1963). There was, and is, equally little concern with these events in mainstream academic history departments in the United Kingdom. This may not be true in the United States, where developments are decribed by Beardsley in chapter 20. The balance of power remains staple fare but most, though not all, historians – staff and students alike – remain scared of the simple technicalities of modern science, which has so profoundly affected political power.

In the 1950s the USAEC and the UK Atomic Energy Authority (UKAEA) both commissioned histories of their atomic projects (including power as well as weapons), appointing authors who were historians not in university posts (Hewlett, a 'mainstream' historian for the USAEC, and myself, an economic historian, for the UKAEA) (Hewlett and Anderson 1962; Hewlett and Duncan 1969, 1974; Gowing 1964, 1974). The histories were scholarly, not 'house' productions, and have been received as such. They have helped to confirm the importance for the history of science of 'federal history' in the US or 'official history' in the UK, which had already been opened up by other war histories. By way of autobiographical detail, I recall that when Oxford appointed me to the new chair in the history of science in 1972, there were official complaints from the history of science profession.

Histories of other countries' early atomic projects have until recently been left to freelance writers – Irving (1967) for Germany, and Kramish (1959) for Russia, though his work is now overtaken by that of Holloway (1981), a political scientist. Eggleston (1965), a journalist, wrote the Canadian story. Weart's history of the French atomic scientists (1979) was the first atomic energy history produced by the history of science profession and it was preceded by that of Scheinman (1965), a political scientist. The recent nuclear power debate is ripe for historical treatment (Williams 1980).

Political scientists in the United States during the last fifteen years have been foremost in using the experience of the Second World War and the succeeding years to analyse the relationship between science, scientists and government. Such interest is still very rare in Britain. After pioneering work by Gilpin (1962), Don Price, Dean of the Graduate School of Public Administration at Harvard, published his profound book *The Scientific Estate* (1965). This was followed by Greenberg's (1967) documented and deeply serious but irreverent polemic on the politics of American pure science. (Though a *Science* journalist, he wrote the book as visitor at the Johns Hopkins History of Science Department.) After these two books the stereotype of the scientist could never be the same again. But even though the history of science profession was now developing twentieth-century interests, these still lay mainly in intellectual or internalist history.

One of the central points in the books of Price and Greenberg was money: the cost of the new big science and the scientists' battles for resources in relation to democratic principles of political control. In the mid-1960s the United States was spending more dollars on research and development than the entire federal budget before Pearl Harbor. The books also showed the dependence of America's pure science in the post-1945 years upon money from the defence departments. British academic research was not similarly funded, but even in 1978 Britain spent more of its public research money on defence than any other European nation: 51.5 per cent compared with 33.3 per cent in France and 12.2 per cent in Germany. The total government research budget and its distribution have been political questions. Non-scientists in other countries besides the United States began to ask what benefits the taxpayer received for his money.

In Britain around 1960 science and technology seemed the talisman that would, through modernization, solve the problems of her relatively slow economic growth and relative industrial decline. At the 1964 general election, science became a main platform and a rallying cry for both political parties but more especially for Labour, which won a majority. Attention had focused on scientific manpower, education, science organization, research priorities and techniques (Vig 1968). By 1970 disillusion with science had returned.

In the late 1960s and 1970s concern concentrated more especially on the relationship between pure and applied research and technology, investment and industrial innovation. It was frequently remarked that Japan, with one of the lowest percentages of gross national product spent on research development, had one of the highest economic growth rates. The economics as well as the politics of research and development had come to the fore. 'Science policy' became a major activity inside and outside governments and on an international scale; in particular, the Organisation for Economic Cooperation and Development (OECD) in Paris proliferated committees and publications on the subject. The book on *Science and Politics* (1973) by the head of its Science Policy Division J.-J. Salomon, a former professor of philosophy, is especially valuable.

Science policy research was endowed in universities and elsewhere. At one stage euphoria produced a discipline called 'the science of science'. This derived partly from new interest in Bernal's *The Social Function of Science* (1939), which believed that planned science could revolutionize the human condition (Werskey 1978). Bernal's book included, far ahead of its time, a remarkable quantitative and qualitative analysis of scientific activity. A historian of science, de Solla Price, gave the subject a further quantitative twist in *Little Science, Big Science* (Price 1963), with graphs of numbers of scientific and abstract journals, scientific papers and their authors and the extent of consultation, scientific manpower (including experimental growth and saturation limits), universities, etc. A later, more sophisticated quantitative approach to the history of science was to be illuminating in the study of physics in 1900 (Forman *et al.* 1975). However, Price's phrase 'the science of science', which was coined for this kind of study and which had a great vogue in the mid and late 1960s (Goldsmith and Mackay 1964), was meaningless and misleading, implying as it did the possibility of discovering laws for the whole activity of science. After a few years the phrase was quietly dropped.

De Solla Price had defined the phrase as a shorthand for a study called 'history, philosophy, sociology, psychology, economics, political science and operations research (etc.) of science, technology, medicine (etc)', which is what many people in recent years have tried to pursue. No longer prepared to take science and the scientists at their own estimation, writers have asked all kinds of new questions drawn from all these disciplines. For a time it was accepted by many, as the acclaim for Ravetz's work showed, that a lot of the problems were new, dating only from 'the bomb'; that right up to the Second World War science was indeed 'pure', and 'industrialized' thereafter; that the former Paradise could be regained. This was absurd, even by reference to elementary histories; Kelvin, after all, owned seventy patents. In the last decade historians of science have become more healthily sceptical.

The frontiers of the history of science widened as its practitioners examined people, projects, phenomena and periods. Scientific activity meant not only ideas, laboratories and experiments but the political activities of scientists, scientific and technological education, and the relationships between science, technology and the economy (Gillispie 1980). Some individuals had already been pioneers in this kind of history of science. Scientific ideas and social progress were so intertwined in the foundation of the American Republic that American historians beginning to write about their native science looked at the evolution of government policy for science. Hunter Dupree, a mainstream historian, published in 1957 an important history of the scientific activity in the US federal government up to 1940. No comparative institutional study exists for Britain, but *The Organisation of Science in England* (1957) by Cardwell, a physicist–engineer turned historian, is still in demand as a textbook. Poole and Andrews (1972) is also helpful. There are articles but no books on the first agitation for a British 'science policy' in the 1830s; Morrell and Thackray's book (1981) on the early years of the British Association partly fills a gap. MacLeod's pioneering studies of mid and late Victorian science are presented in many articles (e.g. 1972 and 1976) and merit a book, while his current work on Science and Empire will be valuable (not yet published). See also Brock (1976) and Turner (1980). There is little on Edwardian, First World War or interwar science, although interest is growing (Moseley 1978). Clearly much remains to be done: there is still, for example, no biography of Lyon Playfair, chemist, politician and civil servant who was active in public life for forty years of the nineteenth century.

A major theme in the history of British science policy is the diffusion of science and technology through education into the culture and economy of a society. Brock's bibliography (1975) is invaluable; see also Gowing (1977b) for the late nineteenth century. This theme is often related in the literature to the relative (not, of course, absolute) decline of British industry from the late nineteenth century up to the present, the 'British disease', and so on. The Royal Commission on Scientific Instruction and the Advancement of Science (the Devonshire Commission) issued eight reports between 1871 and 1875 and the 14 000 questions and answers in the oral evidence provide rich source material.

The relations between science, technology, industry and agriculture in the past are a growing historical theme. Within the history of science profession, Webster's book on the Puritan Revolution (1975; see chapter 1 above) was a landmark. Otherwise the subject has belonged mainly to economic history. Landes (1969) *'The Unbound Prometheus'* has been the major work, and books and articles too numerous to mention have, before and since, studied individual industries. Mathias (1972) surveys the literature for 1600–1800. A review of the nineteenth and twentieth centuries is badly needed. One of the most illuminating industrial studies is Reader's history of Imperial Chemical Industries (1970, 1975). In discussing British and German performance he shows the influence of the chemical industry on the balance of power. He emphasizes in addition another important point of science and politics: how the logic of the new science-based industry led to international arrangements within it that cut clean across the nation state. He stresses the importance of Nobel, a gifted chemist neglected in traditional history of science.

This chapter has concentrated mostly on work in and about the United Kingdom and the United States. Interest in science, politics and government is growing in Australia and Canada. American and British work on other European countries is also developing. Work on French history of science from the seventeenth century onwards has shown much greater interest in political history than most history of science (Fox 1976 gives references for 1800–70). The history of the politics and economics of German science has been neglected – surprisingly since so many comparisons have been made between German and British science for so long. The relationships between German science and Nazism are now being explored (Beyerchen 1977), as are relationships between quantum mechanics and the culture of the Weimar Republic (Forman 1971; Hendry 1980). Work is in progress, but substantial studies have not yet been published, on aspects of biology and politics, on Social Darwinism and on the eugenics movement in Germany.

As the biological sciences have returned to the forefront in the last thirty years or so, the history of contemporary science is increasingly concerned with them. Indeed historians are sometimes joining teams that study crucial debates as they take place. For example, Charles Weiner has been a leader of the MIT team for their Technology, Science and Society programme, which has systematically followed the genetic engineering controversies. The study of the history of science is undoubtedly a far more cheerful prospect than it was fifteen years ago. The profession is no longer exclusive in its search for identity but cooperates with many other disciplines. It is as much concerned with very recent history as with the distant past. At a time of university retrenchment, the study of science and technology policy or liberal studies in science may attract funds much more easily than history of science and technology or than mainstream history, but the name of departments does not matter. What is essential is that careful academic study and evaluation of science and technology in the past (whether ancient or very recent) should continue and that it should be related to the wider life of society – including politics.

Bibliography

Bernal, J.D. (1939). *The Social Function of Science. Part 1, What Science Does. Part 2, What Science Could Do.* London; George Routledge

Bernal, J.D. (1944–1945). Lessons of the War in Science. *Reports in Progress in Physics*, Vol. 10, 418–436. Reprinted (1975) as pp. 439–591 of A Discussion on the Effects of the Two World Wars on the Organization and Development of Science in the United Kingdom. Organized by R.V. Jones. *Proceedings of the Royal Society*, Ser. A, Vol. 342

Bernal, J.D. (1953). *Science and Industry in the Nineteenth Century.* London; Routledge, Kegan Paul. Also (1969). Bloomington; Indiana University Press

Bernal, J.D. (1954). *Science in History.* London; G.A. Watts. 3rd edn revised (1969). 4 Vols. London; G.A. Watts and Penguin

Beyerchen, A.D. (1977). *Scientists under Hitler: Politics and the Physics Community in the Third Reich.* New Haven, Conn.; Yale University Press

Birkenhead, Earl of (1961). *The Prof in Two Worlds.* London; Collins

Brock, W.H. (1975). From Liebig to Nuffield: A Bibliography of the History of Science Education, *Studies in Science Education*, Vol. 2, 67–99

Brock, W.H. (1976). The Spectrum of Science Patronage, *The Patronage of Science in the Nineteenth Century.* Ed. G. L'E. Turner. Leyden; Noordhoff

Butterfield, H. (1949). *The Origins of Modern Science. 1300–1800.* London; G. Bell and Sons. New revised edn (1957). London; Bell

Cardwell, D.S.L. (1957). *The Organisation of Science in England.* London; Heinemann. Revised edn (1972). London; Heinemann

Clagett, M., Ed., (1962). *Critical Problems in the History of Science.* Madison; University of Wisconsin Press

Clark, G.N. (1937). *Science and Social Welfare in the Age of Newton.* Oxford; Clarendon Press

Clark, R.W. (1965). *Tizard.* London; Methuen

Clark, R.W. (1973). *Einstein: The Life and Times.* London; Hodder and Stoughton

Clark, R.W. (1980). *The Greatest Power on Earth: The Story of Nuclear Fission.* London; Sidgwick and Jackson

Crombie, A.C., Ed. (1963). *Scientific Change. Historical Studies in the Intellectual,*

Social and Technical Conditions for Scientific Discovery and Technical Innovation, from Antiquity to the Present. Symposium on the History of Science, University of Oxford, 9–15 July 1961. London; Heinemann

Crowther, J.G. (1965). *Statesmen of Science.* London; Cresset Press

Dupree, A.H. (1957). *Science in the Federal Government: A History of Policies and Activities to 1940.* Cambridge, Mass.; Harvard University Press

Eggleston, W. (1965). *Canada's Nuclear Story.* Toronto; Clarke Irwin

Farrington, B. (1951). *Francis Bacon: Philosopher of Industrial Science.* London; Lawrence and Wishart. 1st edn (1949)

Fleming, D. and Bailyn, B. (1969). *The Intellectual Migration.* Cambridge, Mass.; Harvard University Press

Forman, P. (1971). Weimar Culture, Causality and Quantum Theory, 1918–1927: Adaptation by German Physicists and Mathematicians to a Hostile Intellectual Environment, *Historical Studies in the Physical Sciences*, Vol. 3, 1–115

Forman, P., Heilbron, J. and Weart, S.R. (1975). Physics circa 1900, *Historical Studies in the Physical Sciences*, Vol. 5, 1–185. Princeton; Princeton University Press

Fox, R. (1976). Scientific Enterprise and the Patronage of Research in France 1800–70, in *The Patronage of Science in the Nineteenth Century.* Ed. G.L'E. Turner. Leyden; Noordhoff

Gash, N. (1972). *Sir Robert Peel.* London; Longmans

Gillispie, C.C. (1980). *Science and Polity in France at the End of the Old Regime.* Princeton; Princeton University Press

Gilpin, R. (1962). *American Scientists and Nuclear Weapons Policy.* Princeton; Princeton University Press

Gilpin, R. (1965). *France in the Age of the Scientific State.* Princeton; Princeton University Press

Gilpin, R. and Wright, C., Ed. (1964). *Scientists and National Policy Making.* Princeton; Princeton University Press

Goldschmidt, B. (1980). *Le Complexe atomique. Histoire politique de l'énergie nucléaire.* Paris; Fayard

Goldsmith, M. and Mackay, A., Eds. (1964). *The Science of Science.* Harmondsworth; Penguin. 2nd revised edn (1966)

Goudsmit, S.A. (1947). *Alsos.* New York; Schuman

Gowing, M.M. (1964). *Britain and Atomic Energy 1939–45.* London; Macmillan

Gowing, M.M. with Arnold, L. (1974). *Independence and Deterrence: Britain and Atomic Energy, 1945–52.* Vol. 1. *Policy Making*, Vol. 2. *Policy Execution.* London and Basingstoke; Macmillan

Gowing, M.M. (1977a). *Science and Politics.* Eighth J.D. Bernal Lecture. London; Birkbeck College

Gowing, M.M. (1977b). Science, Technology and Education: England in 1870, *Notes and Records of the Royal Society of London*, Vol. 32, 71–90

Gowing, M.M. (1978). *Reflections on Atomic Energy History.* Cambridge: Cambridge University Press

Greenberg, D. (1967). *The Politics of Pure Science: An Inquiry into the Relationship between Science and Government in the United States.* New York; New American Library. Also (1969) as *The Politics of American Science.* London; Penguin Books

Gummett, P. (1980). *Scientists in Whitehall.* Manchester; Manchester University Press

Hall, A.R. (1954). *The Scientific Revolution 1500–1800.* London; Longmans

Hendry, J. (1980). Weimar Culture and Quantum Causality, *History of Science*, Vol. 18, 155–180

Hewlett, R.G. and Anderson, O.E. (1962). *The New World, 1939–1946*. Vol. 1 of *A History of the United States Atomic Energy Commission*. University Park, Pa.; Pennsylvania State University Press

Hewlett, R.G. and Duncan, F. (1969). *Atomic Shield, 1947–1952*. Vol. 2 of *A History of the United States Atomic Energy Commission*. University Park, Pa.; Pennsylvania State University Press

Hewlett, R.G. and Duncan, F. (1974). *Nuclear Navy, 1947–1962*. Chicago; Chicago University Press

Hill, J.E.C. (1965). *Intellectual Origins of the English Revolution*. Oxford; Clarendon Press

Holloway, D. (1979). Research Note: Soviet Thermonuclear Development, *International Security*, Vol. 4, 192–197

Holloway, D. (1981). Entering the Nuclear Arms Race: the Soviet Decision to Build the Atomic Bomb, 1939–45, *Social Studies in Science*, Vol. 11, 159–197

Hughes, P.S. (1980). Wartime Fission Research in Japan, Notes and Letters, Abstract. *Social Studies in Science*, Vol. 10, 345–349

Irving, D. (1967). *The Virus House*. London; Kimber

Jones, R.V. (1978). *Most Secret War*. London; H. Hamilton

Jungk, R. (1958). *Brighter than a Thousand Suns: The Moral and Political History of the Atomic Scientists*. London; Gollancz and Hart-Davis

Kevles, D.J. (1978). *The Physicists: The History of a Scientific Community in Modern America*. New York; Knopf

Kistiakovsky, G.B. with introduction by Maier, C.S. (1976). *A Scientist at the White House; The Private Diary of President Eisenhower's Special Assistant for Science and Technology*. Cambridge, Mass.; Harvard University Press

Kramish, A. (1959). *Atomic Energy in the Soviet Union*. Stanford; Stanford University Press

Landes, D.S. (1969). *The Unbound Prometheus: Technological Change and Industrial Development in Western Europe from 1750 to the Present*. Cambridge; Cambridge University Press

Lilienthal, D.E. (1964). *The Atomic Energy Years, 1945–1950*. Vol. 2 of *The Journals of David E. Lilienthal*. New York; Harper and Row

MacLeod, R.M. (1972). Resources of Science in Victorian England, 1868–1900, in *Science and Society 1600–1900*. Ed. P. Mathias, Cambridge; Cambridge University Press

MacLeod, R.M. (1976). Science and the Treasury: Principles, Personalities and Policies, 1870–85, in *The Patronage of Science in the Nineteenth Century*. Ed. G.L'E. Turner. Leyden; Noordhoff

Major, J. (1971). *The Oppenheimer Hearing*. London; Batsford

Mathias, P. (1972). Who Unbound Prometheus? Science and Technical Change 1600–1800, in *Science and Society 1600–1900*. Ed. P. Mathias. Cambridge; Cambridge University Press

Melville, H. (1962). *The Department of Scientific and Industrial Research*. London; Allen and Unwin

Merton, R.K. (1938). Science, Technology and Society in Seventeenth Century England, *Osiris*, Vol. 4, Part 2, 360–362. Reprinted (1970) with new introduction. New York; H. Fertig. (1978). New York; Humanities Press

Moorehead, A. (1952). *The Traitors*. London; H. Hamilton

Morrell, J.B. and Thackray, A. (1981). *Gentlemen of Science: The Early Years of the British Association for the Advancement of Science*. Oxford; Oxford University Press

Moseley, R. (1978). The Origins and Early Years of the National Physical

Laboratory: A Chapter in the Pre-History of British Science Policy, *Minerva*, Vol. 16, 222–250
Needham, J. (1954–). *Science and Civilisation in China.* Cambridge; Cambridge University Press
Nieburg, H.L. (1964). *Nuclear Secrecy and Foreign Policy.* Washington DC; Public Affairs Press
Pierre, A.J. (1972). *Nuclear Politics : The British Experience with an Independent Strategic Force, 1939–1970.* London; Oxford University Press
Poole, J.B. and Andrews, K. (1972). *The Government of Science in Britain.* London; Weidenfeld and Nicolson
Postan, M.M., Hay, D. and Scott, J.D. (1952). *Design and Development of Weapons. History of the Second World War: United Kingdom Civil Series.* London; HMSO and Longmans
Price, D. J. de Solla (1963). *Little Science, Big Science.* New York; Columbia University Press
Price, D.K. (1965). *The Scientific Estate.* Harvard; Belknapp Press
Ravetz, J.R. (1971). *Scientific Knowledge and its Social Problems.* Oxford; Oxford University Press. Paperback edn (1973). Harmondsworth; Penguin
Reader, W.J. (1970–75). *Imperial Chemical Industries : A History.* Vol. 1, *The Forerunners 1870–1926.* Vol. 2, *The First Quarter of the Century 1926–1952.* London; Oxford University Press
Royal Commission on Scientific Instruction and the Advancement of Science (Devonshire Commission) (1871–75). *Parliamentary Papers* (1871), Vol. 24; (1872), Vol. 25; (1873), Vol. 28; (1874), Vol. 22; (1875), Vol. 28
Royal Society (1975). Discussion on the Effects of the Two World Wars on the Organisation and Development of Science in the United Kingdom, *Proceedings of the Royal Society*, ser. A, Vol. 342, 441–586
Salomon, J.-J. (1973). *Science and Politics.* London; Macmillan
Scheinman, L. (1965). *Atomic Energy Policy in France under the Fourth Republic.* Princeton; Princeton University Press
Science at the Cross Roads (1931). Papers presented to the International Congress of the History of Science and Technology held in London from 29th June to 3rd July 1931 by the Delegates of the USSR. London; Kniga (England). 2nd edn (1971). New foreword by J. Needham and new introduction by P.G. Werskey. London; Cass
Scott, J.D. and Hughes, R. (1955). *The Administration of War Production. History of the Second World War: United Kingdom Civil Series.* London; HMSO and Longmans
Sherwin, M.J. (1975). *A World Destroyed: The Atomic Bomb and the Grand Alliance.* New York; Knopf
Smith, A.K. (1965). *A Peril and a Hope: The Scientists' Movement in America, 1945–47.* Chicago; Chicago University Press
Snow, C.P. (1961). *Science and Government.* London; Oxford University Press
Snow, C.P. (1962). *A Postscript to Science and Government.* London; Oxford University Press
Stern, P.M. with Green, H.P. (1971). *The Oppenheimer Case: Security on Trial.* New York; Harper and Row
Stimson, H.L. (1947). The Decision to Use the Atomic Bomb, *Harper's Magazine*, Vol. 194, No. 1161, 97–107
Taylor, A.J.P. (1965). *English History 1914–1945.* Oxford; Clarendon Press
Turner, F.M. (1980). Public Science in Britain 1880–1919, *Isis*, Vol. 71, 589–608
United States Atomic Energy Commission (1954). *In the Matter of J. Robert Oppenheimer.* Washington DC; Government Printing Office. Reprinted (1971). Cambridge, Mass.; MIT Press

Varcoe, I.M. (1974). *Organising for Science in Britain: a Case-Study*. London; Oxford University Press

Vig, N. (1968). *Science and Technology in British Politics*. Oxford; Pergamon Press

Weart, S.R. (1975). Scientists with a Secret, *Physics Today*, Vol. 29, No. 2, 23–30

Weart, S.R. (1979). *Scientists in Power*. Cambridge, Mass; Harvard University Press

Weart, S.R. and Szilard, G.W., Ed. (1978). *Leo Szilard: His Version of the Facts*. Cambridge, Mass; MIT Press

Webster, C. (1975). *The Great Instauration: Science, Medicine and Reform, 1626–1660*. London; Duckworth

Weinberg, A.M. (1967). *Reflections on Big Science*. Oxford; Pergamon Press

Weiner, C. (1978). Retroactive Saber Rattling?, *Bulletin of the Atomic Scientists*, Vol. 34, 10–12

Wersey, G. (1978). *The Visible College*. London; Allen Lane

Wiesner, J.B. (1965) *Where Science and Politics Meet*. New York; McGraw Hill

Williams, R. (1980). *The Nuclear Power Decisions: British Policies 1953–78*. London; Croom Helm

York, H. (1976). *The Advisors: Oppenheimer, Teller and the Superbomb*. San Francisco; W.H. Freeman

Zuckerman, S. (1966). *Scientists and War: The Impact of Science on Military and Civil Affairs*. London; Hamish Hamilton

Zuckerman, S. (1980). Science Advisers and Scientific Advisers, in *Proceedings of the American Philosophical Society*, Vol. 124, No. 4, 241–255. Also London; Menard Press

7

Philosophy of science in relation to history of science

Paul Wood

During the past twenty years the philosophy of science has undergone a profound reorientation, due in part to developments internal to the discipline, and, perhaps more importantly, to renewed contact and confrontation with the history of science. The first section surveys this philosophical reorientation, and outlines its historical background. The remainder of the chapter then reviews major themes in the recent literature of the philosophy of science related to methodological and historiographical problems that face the practising historian of science or medicine. This review is necessarily selective, and ignores the technical and often highly formalized literature on scientific explanation, probability and confirmation. It is my firm conviction that the bulk of this literature is irrelevant to the historian, since it largely deals with problems remote from actual scientific practice. The reader wishing to explore these topics should consult Michalos (1980) or Asquith and Kyburg (1979) for bibliographical guidance.

Historical developments in the philosophy of science, 1750 to the present

During the eighteenth and nineteenth centuries, the history of science and the philosophy of science were complementary fields. Perhaps the dominant historiographical tradition in the history of

116

science throughout this period was that of *histoire raisonné*, or conjectural history. In the works of Jean D'Alembert, Joseph Priestley and Adam Smith, for example, we find the development of a genre of history in which historical narrative and explanation are structured by an antecedent epistemological theory (D'Alembert 1963; McEvoy 1979; Smith 1980). History was used in this tradition to exemplify the abstract epistemic principles governing the progress of the human mind and to further various ideological ends.

Philosophical studies of science often integrated logical and historical modes of analysis. The most influential exponents of this approach during the nineteenth century were William Whewell, Ernst Mach and Pierre Duhem. In their philosophical works, history was used both to illustrate and to justify their epistemological and methodological principles (Whewell 1847; Hiebert 1970; Duhem 1954). These principles, in turn, provided the analytical categories for their historical studies, all of which were written in the style of conjectural history (Whewell 1857; Mach 1902, 1926; Duhem 1969). The historical and philosophical investigations of Whewell, Mach and Duhem were, moreover, intended to inform and legitimate their own scientific practice. Whewell, for example, was concerned to defend the wave-theory of light and the use of analytical mathematics in physics, while Mach and Duhem employed history and philosophy in the service of thermodynamics, in opposition to kinetic theories of heat.

In the early decades of the twentieth century, however, the history and the philosophy of science began to be pursued relatively independently. With the rise of the Vienna Circle and logical positivism in the 1920s, the philosophy of science rapidly became ahistorical in character. Inspired by Whitehead and Russell's *Principia Mathematica*, the positivists attempted to transform philosophical method through the use of the techniques of formal logic. They turned away from traditional problems of scientific method to analyse the meaning of scientific terms, the structure of scientific explanation, and the logical status of scientific laws. While leading figures such as Rudolf Carnap and Hans Reichenbach were interested in contemporary physical science, specifically Einstein's theory of relativity and the quantum theory, unlike their philosophical predecessors they did not turn to history for analytical insights. Moreover, it is arguable that the philosophical issues related to contemporary science raised by the Vienna Circle were purely academic, and that the positivists showed no inclination to contribute to the improvement of actual scientific practice. Although the history of science written during this period was premissed on positivistic assumptions, leading historians such as George Sarton owed more to Comte than to Carnap, and no major work integrating the history and the philosophy of science comparable to that of Whewell, Mach and Duhem was produced.

Through the 1930s and 1940s logical positivism evolved into what became known as logical empiricism, and it was this philosophy that dominated the discipline for the next two decades. Beginning in the late 1950s, however, the logical empiricist consensus came under increasingly concerted attack. As the influence of Ludwig Wittgenstein grew in Anglo-American philosophical circles, a number of philosophers inspired by his work began to reassess a range of problems in the philosophy of science, most notably Stephen Toulmin (1953, 1963) and N.R. Hanson (1958, 1963). Toulmin and Hanson began to undermine the sharp distinction that had been drawn by the logical empiricists between theory and observation through subtle analyses of how theories function as ways of seeing and ordering natural phenomena, and they questioned the empiricists' account of how theoretical terms acquire their meaning. Hanson also challenged another central distinction of logical empiricism, that between the contexts of discovery and justification. He argued for the existence of a logic of discovery, whereas the logical empiricists had previously denied the possibility of reconstructing the discovery of scientific theories in logical terms. Significantly, the argumentative strategies of Toulmin and Hanson harken back to the tradition overthrown by the logical positivists earlier in the century, for they combined historical and logical modes of analysis in their writings.

Undoubtedly the most influential philosophical alternative to logical empiricism to emerge since the 1950s has been that advocated by Sir Karl Popper. Although he was in contact with members of the Vienna Circle from 1929 until 1936, Popper has long been critical of their philosophical methods, their obsession with questions of meaning, their dismissal of metaphysics, and their inductivism. Popper has countered the logical positivists and empiricists by arguing that metaphysics is a cognitively significant form of discourse, and that scientific theories have their origins in metaphysical ideas. Like Toulmin and Hanson, Popper rejects any distinction between theory and observation, believing that all observations are theory-laden. His rejection of inductivism, and his falsificationist solution to the problem of demarcating science from pseudo-science, has led Popper to re-emphasize the importance of a number of issues relating to scientific method and the nature of progress that the positivists systematically ignored.

Apart from occasional experiments in conjectural history (1958–9), Popper has made little appeal to the evidence of history to justify his position, since he believes that methodology cannot be based on empirical study (1972a: 50–3).

Unlike Popper, his followers have repeatedly appealed to the historical record to show that their falsificationist methodology accurately represents the manner in which science progresses. Paul Feyerabend first adopted an historical style of argument when he was allied with the Popperians early in his career (Feyerabend 1962, 1964, 1965a,b,c), and he later turned it to devastating effect against them in his Brechtian study of Galileo (Feyerabend 1970, 1975). Joseph Agassi also made extensive use of history to illustrate his Popperian philosophy, and in an innovative work he criticized the inductivist historiographical assumptions adopted by the majority of historians of science from a Popperian perspective (Agassi 1963, 1964, 1966, 1971). The figure who took this trend to its extreme was the late Imre Lakatos, who proposed an analysis of the interrelationships of the history and the philosophy of science, which will be discussed below (Lakatos 1971).

The most controversial challenge to logical empiricism came in the early 1960s from the philosophically inclined historian T.S. Kuhn, whose *The Structure of Scientific Revolutions* (Kuhn 1970a; first published in 1962) is in the tradition of Whewell, Mach and Duhem, combining as it does philosophical analysis with historical exposition. Kuhn's research in the history of science, initially inspired by the works of Alexandre Koyré, Anneliese Maier, Hélène Metzger and Émile Meyerson, eventually led him to question the logical empiricists' model of scientific progress and, like Popper, he began to be interested primarily in the dynamics of scientific growth. Like Toulmin and Hanson, Kuhn rejected the logical empiricists' distinction between theory and observation and their account of the meaning of scientific terms. The distinctive feature of Kuhn's approach is his use of sociological factors to explain the development of science, in particular his appeal to the nature of scientific communities to elucidate the mechanisms governing theoretical change. The intrinsically sociological character of Kuhn's approach was at odds with the assumptions of both logical empiricists and Popperians, and it has since inspired the Edinburgh school of sociologists of knowledge who are currently challenging the presuppositions of philosophically oriented history of science (Barnes 1974; Bloor 1976). However, Kuhn has explicitly disowned the use made of his work by the Edinburgh school, and his recent emphasis on the intellectual autonomy of mature scientific communities would seem to preclude the kinds of social influences on theory-choice that the Edinburgh programme seeks to reveal.

During the past decade the achievements of the historical approach to the philosophy of science have been consolidated by the work of a number of figures, of whom Buchdahl (1969, 1973), Hesse (1974, 1980), and Laudan (1977) deserve particular mention. Drawing on post-positivist philosophy of science, Ravetz (1971), Feyerabend (1978) and others have begun to analyse the ethical and social dimensions of scientific activity. The period has also seen the beginnings of a cross-fertilization between Anglo-American and Continental traditions in the philosophy of science. Stegmüller (1976), for example, has been heavily influenced by Kuhn, while Hesse (1980), Gaukroger (1976, 1978) and Hacking (1975) have taken up the works of Bachelard (1927, 1972), Foucault (1970, 1972) and Habermas (1972). Historians too have recently begun to utilize the works of Bachelard and Foucault (Albury and Oldroyd 1977; Schaffer 1980).

Laudan (1969) provides an indispensable bibliographical guide to both the primary and secondary sources for the history of scientific method up to the early years of this century. Losee (1980) is a brief but useful introductory history of the philosophy of science, which can be supplemented by the collections of articles in Madden (1966), Butts and Davis (1970), Giere and Westfall (1973), and the readings in Kockelmans (1968). A reliable summary of logical empiricism and subsequent developments in the philosophy of science is given by Brown (1977). Contemporary Continental philosophies of science are discussed in Heelan (1979), Gutting (1979) and Michalos (1980), who also provide further bibliographical guidance.

The units of appraisal in science

With the shift towards historical analysis, a number of philosophers of science have come to reject the logical positivists' and empiricists' view that individual theories are the units of scientific appraisal. Reflecting his awareness of the metaphysical origins of scientific theories, Popper has drawn attention to the importance of what he calls 'metaphysical research programmes' in the history of science (1974: 118–21). For Popper, Darwinism is just such a research programme; although he maintains that Darwinism is untestable, and hence metaphysical, Popper argues that a number of testable theories have been derived from it and subjected to empirical criticism (1974: 133–43). Furthermore, Popper sees the metaphysical ideas at the heart of these programmes as undergoing development in response to logical and conceptual criticism. Unfortunately Popper has yet to publish a systematic exposition of his theory of metaphysical research programmes, but some of his earlier papers suggest the lines along which such an exposition would run (Popper 1949, 1958).

Kuhn has also identified larger units of appraisal, which he first called 'paradigms', and now refers to as 'disciplinary matrices' (1970a: 181–91). These consist of four elements: first, symbolic generalizations like $f=ma$, which function either as laws or definitions; secondly, models that specify the theoretical entities to be employed, suggest the general structural features of acceptable theories, and identify the important problems to be solved; thirdly, values such as methodological standards; and fourthly, the most important element, the exemplars, which are concrete problem-solutions that scientists use as patterns in their puzzle-solving activities. Disciplinary matrices do not, according to Kuhn, undergo change. During periods of what he calls 'normal science', change occurs at the level of individual theories, which are designed to solve empirical problems within the constraints imposed by the disciplinary matrix. In a scientific revolution, one disciplinary matrix is relinquished for a rival. Despite the suggestiveness of Kuhn's conception of disciplinary matrices, it has not received the attention it deserves from either philosophers or historians of science. The same can be said for Toulmin's (1972) discussion of what he calls 'intellectual disciplines', which has so far been virtually ignored in the literature.

Various aspects of Kuhn's and Popper's ideas have been amalgamated by Imre Lakatos, whose 'methodology of scientific research programmes' is based on the explicit realization that the unit of appraisal in science is a succession of closely related theories, rather than an isolated single theory. Lakatos' research programmes consist of a 'hard core', a 'protective belt', a 'positive heuristic' and a 'negative heuristic'. The hard core is either a metaphysical world-view such as Cartesian mechanism, or an empirical theory such as Newton's theory of gravitation, which is protected from refutation by methodological *fiat*. Like the basic assumptions contained in a Kuhnian disciplinary matrix, the hard core of a research programme does not change through time. The negative heuristic of a programme is a set of methodological rules that specify how to protect the hard core by diverting potential refutations into the protective belt of auxiliary theories, which are revised and replaced according to the specifications of the rules of the positive heuristic (Lakatos 1970: 47–52). As compared with Kuhn and Toulmin, the drawback of Lakatos's conception of scientific research programmes is that it is highly schematic. Moreover certain aspects of his discussion of hard cores are very problematic. First, Lakatos contradicts his otherwise static picture of hard cores by suggesting that in fact they take time to emerge, thereby raising the question of how research programmes are to be individuated in their initial stages. Secondly, more precision is needed in specifying what can function as the hard core of a research programme. It is reasonable to assume that a research programme based on a metaphysical world-view would exhibit a number of significant differences from one based on an empirical theory such as Newton's law of gravitation, and it is a critical weakness of Lakatos' discussion that he does not sufficiently differentiate between these two cases.

Laudan has identified a number of faults in the analyses of Kuhn and Lakatos, and has offered an alternative theory of what he calls 'research traditions' (Laudan 1977: ch. 3). Following his predecessors, Laudan specifies the constituents of research traditions as being a set of metaphysical and methodological commitments that define a tradition, along with a series of specific empirical theories that exemplify those commitments. Unlike Kuhn and Lakatos, Laudan believes that the core assumptions of a tradition are either reformulated or replaced over time. More importantly, whereas Kuhn and Lakatos believe that disciplinary matrices and research programmes are assessed in terms of their empirical success alone, Laudan emphasizes the importance of conceptual problems in the assessment of competing research traditions. Thus, to take an obvious example, Newton's theory of gravitation was attacked in the early eighteenth century because it employed the problematic concept of forces acting at a distance. Laudan also provides a more refined taxonomy of the various relationships that exist between the core assumptions of a tradition and the specific theories that exemplify it.

Patterns of scientific change

Bearing in mind the alternative descriptions of the units of appraisal in science reviewed in the preceding section, I shall now turn to examine the various models of scientific change that have been advanced. Popper has portrayed science as being in a perpetual state of revolution. Drawing an analogy with the Darwinian theory of evolution, he sees continual competition between rival theories and, presumably, rival metaphysical research pro-grammes. Similarly, Lakatos conceives of the history of science as a chronicle of the rivalry between successive scientific research programmes, and Feyerabend has emphasized the catalytic effect of inter-theoretical criticism in science, going so far as to argue that rationality can only be ensured by the proliferation of incompatible theories and world-views (Feyerabend 1975: chs. 3–4). Toulmin (1972) has explored the evolutionary analogy at greater length, and has pictured science as progressing through a process of conceptual variation and selection.

A very different model of scientific change has been proposed by Kuhn (1970a), who discerns in the historical record a pattern of alternating periods of 'normal' and 'revolutionary' science. During periods of normal science, *one* paradigm or disciplinary matrix is adhered to by a scientific community. Those who do not accept the dominant paradigm are, according to Kuhn, often labelled as cranks and excluded from the scientific community. Using the theoretical and methodological assumptions of the disciplinary matrix, scientists engage in what Kuhn calls 'puzzle-solving'; that is, they are primarily concerned with improving the fit between paradigmatic theories and experimental data, and the failure to produce an improved fit is taken to reflect on the competence of the individual scientist rather than on the validity of the para-digmatic theories. However, anomalies inevitably arise and accumulate, eventually (Kuhn does not say when) provoking a crisis, which causes the community to suspend its absolute alle-giance to the hitherto dominant disciplinary matrix. (Although Kuhn denies that crises are the necessary preliminary to revolu-tion, he suggests no other mechanism by which the hold of a disciplinary matrix over a community can be loosened.) A period of revolutionary science then ensues, during which a number of alternative matrices compete for the allegiance of the community. After an interregnum, one of these alternatives emerges as the victor, the revolution is resolved, and another period of normal science begins.

Hence unlike Popper, Lakatos, Feyerabend and Toulmin, Kuhn believes that there are long periods during which a particular disciplinary matrix exerts hegemonic control over a community of scientists. Kuhn also questions the traditional view that science progresses in a cumulative manner. Popper and Lakatos, for example, hold that a theory T′ is progressive if and only if T′ can explain all of the phenomena accounted for by a preceding theory T, and T′ can explain some further phenomenon or phenomena unaccounted for by T. Kuhn allows that cumulative progress occurs within periods of normal science, but insists that some previously explained phenomena are usually left unaccounted for after a scientific revolution. Indeed Kuhn and Feyerabend have argued that the competing theoretical systems in scientific revolutions are incommensurable, because of profound differences in methodological standards and metaphysical presuppositions, and the changed meanings of key theoretical and observational terms (Kuhn 1970a: chs 10, 12; Feyerabend 1962). The incommensurability thesis has proved extremely controversial, its critics including Shapere (1966) and Kordig (1971). Kuhn has since reformulated his original position, and has argued that there are shared standards by which competing disciplinary matrices can be judged, and that partial translation of the theoretical languages of competing matrices can be achieved (Kuhn 1970b, 1977a). Feyerabend has attempted to specify more precisely the conditions under which rival theoretical systems may be said to be incommensurable (Feyerabend 1975: ch. 17).

Following Kuhn's lead, Laudan (1977) has proposed an interesting non-cumulative model of scientific progress, based on the assessment of the problem-solving capacities of rival research traditions. Yet Laudan rejects the incommensurability thesis, and the pattern of scientific change that he describes differs from that of Kuhn, since Laudan underlines both the existence and importance of competition between research traditions in the history of science.

Rationality

The problem of scientific change, as discussed in the literature surveyed in the last section, has highlighted a number of issues concerning the rationality of science. Traditionally, empirical criteria of confirmation or corroboration, along with logical criteria like consistency, have been considered to be the rational parameters of theory assessment and choice in science. Other criteria such as simplicity have, at least by empiricists, either been dismissed as non-rational or reinterpreted in empirical terms (Popper 1972a: ch. vii). Many of the critics of logical empiricism, like Popper (1972d), Lakatos (1970) and Feyerabend, continue to restrict the parameters of theory assessment to criteria such as consistency, empirical content and predictive success, a restriction that allows Feyerabend (1975: ch. 17) to conclude that the choice between rival cosmological systems is based largely on aesthetic, religious and other 'irrational' factors.

Alternatives to the traditional theory of rationality have been canvassed by a number of writers in response to a growing awareness, based on historical inquiry, of the complexity of theory assessment and choice in science. Although Kuhn offers an uncontroversial list of methodological criteria by which scientists appraise rival theories or disciplinary matrices, he challenges the traditional theory of rationality by arguing that an individual scientist's application of these criteria is mediated by an array of factors ranging from aspirations and beliefs drawn from the scientist's culture, to previous research experience, career prospects and personal psychological idiosyncrasies (Kuhn 1977a). Thus methodological criteria do not, on Kuhn's view, unequivocally determine the choice of one particular theory or matrix in preference to another, as the traditional account of rationality assumes. Rather, methodological criteria function as values, which are variously applied according to the differing interpretations of each member of a scientific community.

As noted above in the second section, Laudan has convincingly argued that theories and research traditions are assessed in terms of their empirical and conceptual problem-solving capacities. An important theme of his argument concerning conceptual problems is that theories and research traditions are often assessed in terms of metaphysical, theological, and political or ideological beliefs (Laudan 1977: 61–4). Moreover Laudan suggests that rational belief has a social dimension, and hence denies the traditional assumption that social factors are intrinsically arational or irrational. However, this suggestion is left undeveloped, and, unlike Kuhn, Laudan does not explore the social and institutional structures that he thinks underlie research traditions.

The most radical critique of previous theories of rationality has come from Toulmin (1972), who has attacked the view, which he traces back to the Greeks, that rationality presupposes absolute, atemporal standards, analogous to formal systems of mathematics and logic. Toulmin wishes to replace this static picture of rationality with one in which the standards of rationality evolve historically, and this leads him to analyse rationality in terms of its intellectual and social dimensions. Thus for Toulmin the assessment of conceptual variation and change involves the interaction of the explanatory ideals and standards of a given scientific discipline with cultural and institutional factors. Consequently he denies any absolute historiographical distinction between internal (intellectual) and external (institutional and social) factors affecting conceptual change, as this distinction rests on the basic assumptions of the traditional theory of rationality that he rejects.

Finally, brief mention should be made of Maxwell's (1972, 1974, 1976) criticisms of the theory of rationality of standard empiricism, and his alternative theory of 'aim-oriented empiricism'. Although Maxwell does not develop his position historically, his emphasis on the rational importance of aims and values and on 'metaphysical blueprints' in science has suggestive implications for historical analysis.

The relationships between the history and philosophy of science

In this concluding section, I shall confront the problematic nature of the relationships between the history and philosophy of science. Despite the professionalization of history and philosophy of science as a joint discipline, manifested in the establishment of academic departments and the publication of the journal *Studies in History and Philosophy of Science* (1970–), a consensus concerning the interrelationships of the two uneasy partners has yet to emerge. Indeed, in practice most philosophers of science continue to ignore history, while historians of science on the whole react negatively to the occasional historical forays by philosophers.

As we have seen in the first section, leading critics of logical empiricism like Hanson believed that 'profitable philosophical discussion of any science depends on a thorough familiarity with its history and its present state' (Hanson 1958: 3). Hanson himself argued that though there was no *logical* relationship between the history and philosophy of science, philosophical analysis had to begin with the raw materials provided by history. A much stronger thesis was developed by Lakatos (1971), who claimed that rival methodologies of science should be tested against the historical record. However Kuhn (1971) and McMullin (1970) argue that Lakatos' account of testing methodologies against history is circular, since Lakatos claims that all historical evidence is 'theory-laden', that is, already interpreted in terms of some methodology. Worrall (1976) has attempted to salvage Lakatos' position by admitting that much of the historical record is not theory-laden, and hence that it can be used to test methodologies in the way in which Lakatos had originally suggested.

Giere (1973) has criticized these attempts to justify philosophical positions historically, on the grounds that methodological norms cannot be derived from the way in which science has happened to be practised in the past. In reply to Giere, Laudan (1977: ch. 5) has argued that Giere's appeal to contemporary scientific practice is in principle the same as an appeal to the past, and has outlined a solution to the problem of deriving methodological norms from descriptions of scientific practice. Like Lakatos, Laudan believes that the history of science should be used to adjudicate between rival methodologies of science. Burian (1977) has responded to Giere by arguing that, because theories develop and undergo structural change through time, history is needed both to identify particular lines of development and to evaluate the progress of a given theory, concluding that the normative task of philosophy cannot be accomplished without the aid of historical analysis. Burian makes the further point that history can and should be used to criticize the normative standards of assessment proposed by philosophers of science.

The relevance of the philosophy of science to the history of science has been argued for in a number of ways. Hanson (1971) has made the weak claim that the historian of science must be acquainted with the philosophy of science in order to be able to give a proper logical reconstruction of the theories and arguments that he studies. Grünbaum (1963) has argued that the historian must first understand the philosophical or conceptual foundations of a theory, like that of special relativity, before he can ask illuminating historical questions about the development of that theory and assess the contributions of those scientists who developed it. But these arguments are inconclusive, for they do not show that a historian must *necessarily* turn to the philosophical literature on the structure of scientific theories or on special relativity in order to display the logical acumen that Hanson desires or the understanding of fundamental theoretical concepts that Grünbaum demands.

A stronger thesis has been developed by Agassi (1963), Lakatos (1971), Worrall (1976) and Laudan (1977), which purports to show that for epistemological and logical reasons the historian must necessarily rely on a philosophical view of science for his narrative and explanatory concepts. However, this thesis rests on two questionable assumptions. First it is assumed that the type of theory required by the historian to record and interpret the science of the past will be that offered by philosophers of science. This assumption is gratuitous since historians might equally well turn to sociology or social anthropology for their analytical frameworks, as indeed they have recently begun to do. Secondly, it is generally assumed that historical explanations are deductive in structure, and can be analysed in terms of Hempel's 'covering-law' model. Yet Hempel's model has been widely, and trenchantly, criticized by a number of philosophers of history (Gardiner 1974). Consequently this 'strong' thesis, as it has been argued so far, is less than persuasive.

Historians of science have generally resisted the often patronising arguments of philosophers of science concerning the interrelatedness of their subjects, much as their colleagues in general history have resisted the arguments of social scientists urging greater integration of the two disciplines. But as the social sciences provide the general historian with valuable theoretical resources, so the philosophy of science can provide the historian of science with analytical tools that can be refined through historical practice.

Acknowledgements

I wish to thank J.R.R. Christie for a number of discussions concerning the historical relationships between the history and the philosophy of science, and Dr G.N. Cantor for his helpful criticisms of an earlier draft of this chapter.

Bibliography

The major journals for the philosophy of science are *Philosophy of Science*, *The British Journal for the Philosophy of Science* and *Studies in History and Philosophy of Science*. The main bibliographical guide to the periodical literature is *The Philosopher's Index: An International Index to Philosophical Periodicals* (1967–), Bowling Green Ohio: Philosophy Documentation Center, Bowling Green University. The *Isis Critical Bibliography* (1912–) also lists books and articles in the philosophy of science.

Agassi, J. (1963). *Towards an Historiography of Science*. History and Theory Studies in the Philosophy of History, Vol. 2. The Hague; Mouton and Co
Agassi, J. (1964). Scientific Problems and Their Roots in Metaphysics, in *The Critical Approach to Science and Philosophy*. Ed. M. Bunge. New York; The Free Press, 189–211
Agassi, J. (1966). Sensationalism, *Mind*, Vol. 75, 1–24
Agassi, J. (1971). *Faraday as a Natural Philosopher*. Chicago and London; University of Chicago Press
Albury, W.R. and Oldroyd, D.R. (1977). From Renaissance Mineral Studies to Historical Geology, in the Light of Michel Foucault's *The Order of Things*, *The British Journal for the History of Science*, Vol. 10, 187–215
Asquith, P.D. and Kyburg, H.E., Jr. (1979). *Current Research in Philosophy of*

Science. *Proceedings of the P.S.A. Critical Research Problems Conference*. East Lansing, Pa.; Philosophy of Science Association

Bachelard, G. (1927). *Étude sur l'évolution d'un problème de physique: La propagation thermique dans les solides*. Paris; Vrin

Bachelard, G. (1972). *La Formation de l'esprit scientifique. Contribution à une psychanalyse de la connaissance objective*, 4th edn. Paris; Vrin. Ist edn (1938)

Barnes, B. (1974). *Scientific Knowledge and Sociological Theory*. London and Boston; Routledge and Kegan Paul

Bloor, D. (1976). *Knowledge and Social Imagery*. London, Henley, and Boston; Routledge and Kegan Paul

Brown, H.I. (1977). *Perception, Theory and Commitment. The New Philosophy of Science*. Chicago; Precedent Pub. 2nd edn, Chicago and London; University of Chicago Press

Buchdahl, G. (1969). *Metaphysics and the Philosophy of Science. The Classical Origins. Descartes to Kant*. Oxford; Basil Blackwell

Buchdahl, G. (1973). Explanation and Gravity, in *Changing Perspectives in the History of Science. Essays in Honour of Joseph Needham*. Ed. M. Teich and R.M. Young. London; Heinemann, 167–203

Bunge, M., Ed. (1964). *The Critical Approach to Science and Philosophy*. New York; The Free Press

Burian, R.M. (1977). More Than a Marriage of Convenience: On the Inextricability of History and Philosophy of Science, *Philosophy of Science*, Vol. 44, 1–42

Butts, R.E. and Davis, J.W., Ed. (1970). *The Methodological Heritage of Newton*. Oxford; Basil Blackwell

Cohen, I.B. (1974). History and the Philosopher of Science, in *The Structure of Scientific Theories*. Ed. F. Suppe. Urbana, Chicago and London; University of Illinois Press, 308–349

Cohen, R.S., Feyerabend, P.K. and Wartofsky, M.W., Ed. (1976). *Essays in Memory of Imre Lakatos*. Boston Studies in the Philosophy of Science, Vol. 39. Dordrecht and Boston; D. Reidel

D'Alembert, J. (1963). *Preliminary Discourse to the Encyclopedia of Diderot*. Trans. R.N. Schwab and W.E. Rex. Indianapolis and New York; Bobbs-Merrill

Duhem, P. (1954). *The Aim and Structure of Physical Theory*. Trans. P.P. Wiener. Princeton; Princeton University Press. Ist French edn (1906)

Duhem, P. (1969). *To Save the Phenomena: An Essay on the Idea of Physical Theory from Plato to Galileo*. Trans. E. Doland and C. Maschler. Chicago and London; University of Chicago Press. Ist French edn (1908)

Feyerabend, P.K. (1962). Explanation, Reduction, and Empiricism, in *Scientific Explanation, Space, and Time*. Ed. H. Feigl and G. Maxwell. Minnesota Studies in the Philosophy of Science, Vol. 3. Minneapolis; University of Minnesota Press, 28–97

Feyerabend, P.K. (1964). Realism and Instrumentalism: Comments on the Logic of Factual Support, in *The Critical Approach to Science and Philosophy*. Ed. M. Bunge. New York; The Free Press, 280–308

Feyerabend, P.K. (1965a). Problems of Empiricism, in *Beyond the Edge of Certainty. Essays in Contemporary Science and Philosophy*. Ed. R.G. Colodny. University of Pittsburgh Series in the Philosophy of Science, Vol. 2. Englewood Cliffs, NJ; Prentice-Hall, 145–260

Feyerabend, P.K. (1965b). On the 'Meaning' of Scientific Terms, *The Journal of Philosophy*, Vol. 62, 266–274

Feyerabend, P.K. (1965c). Reply to Criticism, in *Boston Studies in the Philosophy of Science*. Ed. R.S. Cohen and M. Wartofsky. Boston Studies in the Philosophy of Science, Vol. 2. Dordrecht; D. Reidel, 223–261

Feyerabend, P.K. (1970). Problems of Empiricism, Part II, in *The Nature and Function of Scientific Theories. Essays in Contemporary Science and Philosophy.* Ed. R.G. Colodny. University of Pittsburgh Series in the Philosophy of Science, Vol. 4. Pittsburgh; University of Pittsburgh Press, 275–353

Feyerabend, P.K. (1975). *Against Method.* London; New Left Books

Feyerabend, P.K. (1978). *Science in a Free Society.* London; New Left Books

Finocchiaro, M.A. (1973). *History of Science as Explanation.* Detroit; Wayne State University Press

Foucault, M. (1970). *The Order of Things. An Archaeology of the Human Sciences.* London; Tavistock Publications. Ist French edn (1966). *Les Mots et les choses.* Paris; Gallimard

Foucault, M. (1972). *The Archaeology of Knowledge.* Trans. A.M. Sheridan Smith. London; Tavistock Publications. Ist French edn (1969)

Gardiner, P. (1974). *The Philosophy of History.* Oxford; Oxford University Press

Gaukroger, S.W. (1976). Bachelard and the Problem of Epistemological Analysis, *Studies in History and Philosophy of Science,* Vol. 7, 189–244

Gaukroger, S.W. (1978). *Explanatory Structures: A Study of Concepts of Explanation in Early Physics and Philosophy.* Hassocks; Harvester Press

Giere, R.N. (1973). History and Philosophy of Science: Intimate Relationship or Marriage of Convenience, *The British Journal for the Philosophy of Science,* Vol. 24, 282–297

Giere, R.N. and Westfall, R.S., Ed. (1973). *Foundations of Scientific Method: The Nineteenth Century.* Bloomington and London; Indiana University Press

Grünbaum, A. (1963). The Special Theory of Relativity as a Case Study of the Importance of Philosophy of Science for the History of Science, in *Philosophy of Science: The Delaware Seminar.* Ed. B. Baumrin. New York; Interscience Publishers, Vol. 2: 171–204

Gutting, G. (1979). Continental Philosophy of Science, in *Current Research in Philosophy of Science. Proceedings of the P.S.A. Critical Research Problems Conference.* Ed. P.D. Asquith and H.E. Kyburg Jr. East Lansing, Pa.; Philosophy of Science Association, 94–117

Habermas, J. (1972). *Knowledge and Human Interests.* London; Heinemann. Also (1971). Boston; Beacon Press

Hacking, I. (1975). *The Emergence of Probability: A Philosophical Study of Early Ideas about Probability, Induction and Statistical Inference.* Cambridge, London, New York and Melbourne; Cambridge University Press

Hanson, N.R. (1958). *Patterns of Discovery. An Inquiry into the Conceptual Foundations of Science.* Cambridge; Cambridge University Press

Hanson, N.R. (1963). *The Concept of the Positron. A Philosophical Analysis.* Cambridge; Cambridge University Press

Hanson, N.R. (1971). The Irrelevance of History of Science to Philosophy of Science, in N.R. Hanson. *What I Do Not Believe, and Other Essays.* Ed. S. Toulmin and H. Woolf. Dordrecht; D. Reidel, 274–287

Hanson, N.R. (1973). *Constellations and Conjectures.* Ed. W.C. Humphreys. Dordrecht and Boston; D. Reidel

Heelan, P.A. (1979). Continental Philosophy and the Philosophy of Science, in *Current Research in Philosophy of Science. Proceedings of the P.S.A. Critical Research Problems Conference.* Ed. P.D. Asquith and H.E. Kyburg Jr. East Lansing, Pa.; Philosophy of Science Association, 84–93

Hesse, M.B. (1961). *Forces and Fields. The Concept of Action at a Distance in the History of Physics.* London; Nelson

Hesse, M.B. (1963). *Models and Analogies in Science.* London; Sheed and Ward

Hesse, M.B. (1974). *The Structure of Scientific Inference.* London and Basingstoke; Macmillan

Hesse, M.B. (1980). *Revolutions and Reconstructions in the Philosophy of Science.* Brighton; Harvester Press

Hiebert, E.N. (1970). Mach's Philosophical Use of the History of Science, in *Historical and Philosophical Perspectives of Science.* Ed. R.H. Stuewer. Minnesota Studies in the Philosophy of Science, Vol. 5. Minneapolis; University of Minnesota Press, 184–203

Howson, C., Ed. (1976). *Method and Appraisal in the Physical Sciences. The Critical Background to Modern Science, 1800–1905.* Cambridge, London, New York and Melbourne; Cambridge University Press

Kockelmans, J.J., Ed. (1968). *Philosophy of Science: The Historical Background.* New York; The Free Press

Kordig, C. (1971). *The Justification of Scientific Change.* Dordrecht; D. Reidel

Kuhn, T.S. (1970a). *The Structure of Scientific Revolutions*, 2nd edn. Chicago and London; University of Chicago Press. Ist edn (1962)

Kuhn, T.S. (1970b). Reflections on My Critics, in *Criticism and the Growth of Knowledge.* Ed. I. Lakatos and A. Musgrave. Cambridge; Cambridge University Press, 231–278

Kuhn, T.S. (1971). Notes on Lakatos, in *PSA 1970: In Memory of Rudolf Carnap.* Ed. R.C. Buck and R.S. Cohen. Boston Studies in the Philosophy of Science, Vol. 8. Dordrecht and Boston; D. Reidel, 137–146

Kuhn, T.S. (1977a). Objectivity, Value Judgment, and Theory Choice, in Kuhn (1977c), 320–339

Kuhn, T.S. (1977b). The Relations between the History and the Philosophy of Science, in Kuhn (1977c), 3–20

Kuhn, T.S. (1977c). *The Essential Tension. Selected Studies in Scientific Tradition and Change.* Chicago and London; University of Chicago Press

Kuhn, T.S. (1980). The Halt and the Blind: Philosophy and History of Science, *The British Journal for the Philosophy of Science*, Vol. 31, 181–192

Lakatos, I. (1970). Falsification and the Methodology of Scientific Research Programmes, in Lakatos and Musgrave (1970), 91–195

Lakatos, I. (1971). History of Science and Its Rational Reconstructions, in *Boston Studies in the Philosophy of Science*, Vol. 8, 91–135

Lakatos, I. (1976). *Proofs and Refutations. The Logic of Mathematical Discovery.* Ed. J. Worrall and E. Zahar. Cambridge, London, New York and Melbourne; Cambridge University Press

Lakatos, I. (1978). *Philosophical Papers.* 2 Vols. Ed. J. Worrall and G. Currie. Vol. 1, *The Methodology of Scientific Research Programmes.* Vol. 2, *Mathematics, Science and Epistemology.* Cambridge, London, New York and Melbourne; Cambridge University Press

Lakatos, I. and Musgrave, A., Ed. (1970). *Criticism and the Growth of Knowledge.* Proceedings of the International Colloquium in the Philosophy of Science, London, 1965, Vol. 4. Cambridge; Cambridge University Press

Laudan, L. (1969). Theories of Scientific Method From Plato to Mach, *History of Science*, Vol. 7, 1–63

Laudan, L. (1977). *Progress and Its Problems. Towards a Theory of Scientific Growth.* London and Henley; Routledge and Kegan Paul

Losee, J. (1980). *A Historical Introduction to the Philosophy of Science*, 2nd edn. Oxford, New York, Toronto and Melbourne; Oxford University Press

McEvoy, J. (1979). Electricity, Knowledge, and the Nature of Progress in Priestley's Thought, *The British Journal for the History of Science*, Vol. 12, 1–30

Mach, E. (1902). *The Science of Mechanics: A Critical and Historical Account of its Development*, 2nd revised and enlarged edn. Trans. T.J. McCormack. Chicago; Open Court. 1st edn (1883). Leipzig; F.A. Brockhaus

Mach, E. (1926). *The Principles of Physical Optics: An Historical and Philosophical*

Treatment. Trans. J.S. Anderson and A.F.A. Young. London; Methuen. Reprinted (1953). New York; Dover Books

Machamer, P.K. (1973). Feyerabend and Galileo: The Interaction of Theories, and the Reinterpretation of Experience, *Studies in History and Philosophy of Science*, Vol. 4, 1–46

McMullin, E. (1970). The History and Philosophy of Science: A Taxonomy, in *Historical and Philosophical Perspectives of Science*. Ed. R.H. Stuewer. Minnesota Studies in the Philosophy of Science, Vol. 5. Minneapolis; University of Minnesota Press, 12–67

Madden, E.H., Ed. (1966). *Theories of Scientific Method: The Renaissance Through the Nineteenth Century*. Seattle and London; University of Washington Press

Manier, E. (1980). History, Philosophy and Sociology of Biology: A Family Romance, *Studies in History and Philosophy of Science*, Vol. 11, 1–24

Maxwell, N. (1972). A Critique of Popper's Views on Scientific Method, *Philosophy of Science*, Vol. 39, 131–152

Maxwell, N. (1974). The Rationality of Scientific Discovery, *Philosophy of Science*, Vol. 41, 123–153, 247–295

Maxwell, N. (1976). *What's Wrong with Science? Towards a People's Rational Science of Delight and Compassion*. London; Bran's Head Books

Michalos, A.C. (1980). Philosophy of Science: Historical, Social, and Value Aspects, in *A Guide to the Culture of Science, Technology, and Medicine*. Ed. P.T. Durbin. New York; The Free Press. London; Collier Macmillan, 197–281

Popper, K.R. (1949). Towards a Rational Theory of Tradition, *The Rationalist Annual*, 36–55. In Popper (1972b), 120–135

Popper, K.R. (1958). On the Status of Science and Metaphysics, *Ratio*, Vol. 1, 97–115. In Popper (1972b), 184–200

Popper, K.R. (1958–9). Back to the Presocratics, in *Proceedings of the Aristotelian Society*, N.S., Vol. 59, 1–24. In Popper (1972b), 136–165

Popper, K.R. (1972a). *The Logic of Scientific Discovery*, revised edn. London; Hutchinson. Ist edn (1935)

Popper, K.R. (1972b). *Conjectures and Refutations. The Growth of Scientific Knowledge*, 4th revised edn. London; Routledge and Kegan Paul. Ist edn (1963)

Popper, K.R. (1972c). *Objective Knowledge. An Evolutionary Approach*. Oxford; Oxford University Press

Popper, K.R. (1972d). Truth, Rationality, and the Growth of Scientific Knowledge, in Popper (1972b), 215–250

Popper, K.R. (1974). Autobiography, in *The Philosophy of Karl Popper*. 2 Vols. Ed. P.A. Schilpp. LaSalle; Open Court, Vol. 1: 3–181

Popper, K.R. (1975). The Rationality of Scientific Revolutions, in *Problems of Scientific Revolution. Progress and Obstacles to Progress in the Sciences*. Ed. R. Harré. Oxford; Oxford University Press, 72–101

Radnitzky, G. (1970). *Contemporary Schools of Metascience*, 2nd edn. Göteborg; Akademiförlaget

Ravetz, J.R. (1971). *Scientific Knowledge and its Social Problems*. Oxford; Oxford University Press. Paperback edn (1973). Harmondsworth; Penguin

Schaffer, S. (1980). Natural Philosophy, in *The Ferment of Knowledge. Studies in the Historiography of Eighteenth-Century Science*. Ed. G.S. Rousseau and R.S. Porter. Cambridge, London, New York, New Rochelle, Melbourne and Sydney; Cambridge University Press, 55–91

Shapere, D. (1964). The Structure of Scientific Revolutions, *Philosophical Review*, Vol. 73, 383–394

Shapere, D. (1966). Meaning and Scientific Change, in *Mind and Cosmos. Essays in Contemporary Science and Philosophy.* Ed. R.G. Colodny. University of Pittsburgh Series in the Philosophy of Science, Vol. 3. Pittsburgh; University of Pittsburgh Press, 41–85

Shapere, D. (1974). *Galileo: A Philosophical Study.* Chicago and London; University of Chicago Press

Smith, A. (1980). *Essays on Philosophical Subjects.* Ed. W.P.D. Wightman, J.C. Bryce and I.S. Ross. Oxford; Oxford University Press

Stegmüller, W. (1976). *The Structure and Dynamics of Theories.* New York, Heidelberg and Berlin; Springer-Verlag

Stuewer, R.H., Ed. (1970). *Historical and Philosophical Perspectives of Science.* Minnesota Studies in the Philosophy of Science, Vol. 5. Minneapolis; University of Minnesota Press

Suppe, F., Ed. (1974). *The Structure of Scientific Theories.* Urbana, Chicago and London; University of Illinois Press

Temkin, O. (1977). On the Interrelationship of the History and the Philosophy of Medicine, in *The Double Face of Janus and other Essays in the History of Medicine.* Baltimore and London; Johns Hopkins University Press, 101–109

Toulmin, S. (1953). *The Philosophy of Science: An Introduction.* London; Hutchinson

Toulmin, S. (1963). *Foresight and Understanding. An Enquiry into the Aims of Science.* New York and Evanston; Harper and Row

Toulmin, S. (1972). *Human Understanding.* Oxford; Oxford University Press

Wallace, W.A. (1972–4). *Causality and Scientific Explanation.* 2 Vols. Ann Arbor; University of Michigan Press

Watkins, J.W.N. (1958). Confirmable and Influential Metaphysics, *Mind*, Vol. 67, 344–365

Watkins, J.W.N. (1975). Metaphysics and the Advancement of Science, *The British Journal for the Philosophy of Science*, Vol. 26, 91–121

Whewell, W. (1847). *The Philosophy of the Inductive Sciences, Founded upon their History*, new edn. 2 Vols. London; J.W. Parker. Reprinted (1967). London; Frank Cass

Whewell, W. (1857). *History of the Inductive Sciences, from the Earliest to the Present Time*, 3rd edn. 3 Vols. London; J.W. Parker. Reprinted (1967). London; Frank Cass. Ist edn (1837)

Worrall, J. (1976). Thomas Young and the 'Refutation' of Newtonian Optics: a Case-study in the Interaction of Philosophy of Science and History of Science, in *Method and Appraisal in the Physical Sciences. The Critical Background to Modern Science, 1800–1905.* Ed. C. Howson. Cambridge, London, New York and Melbourne; Cambridge University Press, 107–179

Part II

8

Guide to bibliographical sources

Pietro Corsi

This chapter provides basic information on reference material relating to the history of science and medicine. Any listing of bibliographies, reference books, dictionaries and historical works can only indicate the *type* of sources a historian is likely to find useful. It is therefore appropriate to discuss publications providing a wide range of information on research in the history of science and medicine, as well as literature on libraries, collections and museums, which contain a broad spectrum of sources. Bibliographies appended to subsequent chapters dealing with specialized topics will integrate and add to the information provided below.

Bibliographical aids

History of science and history of medicine in the English-speaking world have already been objects of surveys and general bibliographies (Sarton 1952, 1953; Neu 1967; Canguilhem 1970). Probably the most successful and satisfactory presentation of publications and research is the survey by Thornton and Tully of scientific books, libraries and collectors (1971; Supplement 1978). The authors consider in some detail a wide range of bibliographical sources and studies, with particular emphasis on the physical and life sciences. More selective and discursive is the book on sources of the history of science by Knight (1975b; see Jayawardene 1977). The author provides critical assessment of research publications, with particular emphasis on nineteenth-century physical and life sciences. Lastly, a French publication is worth mentioning, even though critics (Black and Thomson 1973: 25) have pointed out slight inaccuracies in the citation of works. This is the bibliography of the history of science and technology by Russo, first published in 1954, and reissued with considerable change and improvement in 1969. From 1958 to 1968 Russo was the editor of the history of science and technology section of the *Bulletin Signalétique* (which is examined below) and benefited from the powerful resources and expertise of the Centre National de la Recherche Scientifique (CNRS) bibliographic team. Russo's listings, subdivided topically and chronologically, can still be of use to readers wishing to acquire basic bibliography on major topics and figures in the history of science and technology. General bibliographies relating to the history of medicine are not to be found in the works quoted above.

Useful representative examples of a new interest in area studies are works edited by Jarrell and Ball (1980) on the development of the history of science and technology in Canada, and by Shortt (1981) on medicine in Canadian society. These contain selective bibliographical appendices, including a list of museums of Canadian science and technology.

Growing public and scholarly interest in history of science and medicine is also testified to by the *Dictionary of the History of Science* (Bynum, Browne and Porter, 1981). This is organized by subjects, thus providing brief historical accounts of themes, concepts and discoveries, primarily in Western science. Furthermore there is a substantial single-volume survey of the history of science and medicine: *A Guide to the Culture of Science, Technology and Medicine* (Durbin 1980). Jayawardene (1982) has compiled a *Handlist* of 1000 major reference works for the historian of science, based on the resources of the Science Museum Library, as the principal library in Britain for history of science and technology.

All these general surveys provide selective guides to publications and sources relevant to the history of science. Detailed bibliographical information requires use of more specialized sources. Many bibliographies differ in organization, however, by applying divergent criteria. It is therefore appropriate to remind the reader that bibliographies are not neutral instruments or aids, but often embody particular convictions about the field surveyed, and about significant conceptual or historical priorities. It is advisable to consult, when possible, more than one bibliography relating to the same or a closely related subject. A particularly useful guide to bibliographical services throughout the world is provided by a series of handbooks compiled under the auspices of UNESCO (1969, 1972, 1977). As far as bibliographies of bibliographies are concerned, Collison (1968) is an easy to use and selective guide to the contents, organization and purpose of bibliographies, arranged by topics and geography. A more comprehensive survey of bibliographies that includes diverse aspects of the history of science and medicine is the classic five-volume *World Bibliography of Bibliographies* edited by the late Theodore Besterman (1965–6). This undoubtedly represents one of the most ambitious enterprises in information science. A two-volume supplement has appeared (Toomey 1977). Equally useful is the scholarly work edited by Malclès (1950–8), of which Part 3, Vol. 4 is devoted to specialized bibliographies relevant to the history of the exact sciences and technology.

Information on currently published bibliographies, and on various aspects of the history of science is provided by *Isis*, one of the longest-running journals of the history of science. The *Isis* Critical Bibliographies appear as a separate issue of each volume of the journal. Yearly bibliographies from 1913 to 1965 have been collated and published in a three-volume work compiled by Whitrow; volumes 4 and 5 are awaited. The *Isis Cumulative Bibliography* is undoubtedly the most useful specialized listing of works in the history of science (Whitrow 1972–6). Jayawardene (1979) has critically evaluated the criteria that guided the selection of the *Isis* bibliography entries in the early phases of the life of the journal. This bibliographical aid should be complemented by use of the quarterly issues of the *Bulletin Signalétique* (Centre National de la Recherche Scientifique 1947–), which systematically surveys hundreds of journals and magazines in all languages. Only articles and reviews of books are listed, not books or other publications. The *Bulletin Signalétique* is a source not often mentioned or used in English-speaking countries, so its usefulness should be stressed. Information provided by the *Bulletin* is of particular value for coverage of articles in the history of science and technology published in Eastern European and Soviet journals. However, while the *Bulletin* constitutes the delight of the scholar, it also represents a bibliographer's nightmare. Its original title, *Bulletin Analytique. Philosophie,* changed in 1956 to *Bulletin Signalétique.* The titles, arrangement and subheading of its various sections have altered almost every two years, owing to a constant search for a more efficient arrangement, and the very titles and divisions of the history of science section portray the conceptual reorientation of the field. Thus, the 'Histoire des sciences' section originated as a subsection of the *Bulletin Analytique. Philosophie.* In Vol. 9, 1955, the section was headed 'Histoire des sciences et des techniques', and in 1957, Vol. 11, a separate paragraph 'Technologie' appeared. Moreover, from 1956 to 1960 the *Bulletin* was headed *Bulletin Signalétique. Philosophie Sciences Humaines,* and was changed in 1961 to *Bulletin Signalétique. 19 Sciences Humaines Philosophie.* The 'Histoire des sciences et des techniques' subsection was given the number 22. In 1964 the section numbers appeared in the title (*19–23*), and in 1966 one more section, 'Sciences du langage', was added (*19–24*). In 1968 the title was yet again revised, and became *Bulletin Signalétique (19–24) Sciences Humaines.* In 1969 the various sections were printed in separate volumes, and the *Bulletin Signalétique. 522 Histoire des Sciences et des Techniques* appeared. In many respects, the *Bulletin* can be regarded as complementary to the *Isis Critical Bibliography.* It appears quarterly, and has monthly indexes, whereas *Isis* lists books, reviews and articles published in the course of the entire year. It should also be pointed out that, since the history of science is becoming characterized by a variety of approaches and historiographical priorities, many historians of science and medicine are increasingly aware that research in allied disciplines such as the history of philosophical or religious thought, economic history, social history, historical anthropology, etc. is indispensable to the investigation of past scientific cultures. Thus, the sections of the *Bulletin Signalétique* provide valuable information on papers published in many types of journals by experts in a variety of topics that cannot be *a priori* excluded as irrelevant to historians of science and medicine. Sections *519 Philosophie, 520 Sciences de l'Education, 521 Sociologie Éthnologie, 527 Sciences Religieuses* are of particular interest to the historian of scientific cultures and their historical development. Useful basic bibliographies are also to be found in the *New Cambridge Bibliography of English Literature* (Watson 1974–7).

The bibliographies for the history of medicine deserve separate consideration, and will be discussed in detail in chapter 19 and with relation to the publications of the National Library of Medicine and the Wellcome Institute. It is however appropriate to mention here a standard work, *A Medical Bibliography* by Garrison and Morton (Morton 1970), and the brief survey of historical sources for medicine by Gaskell, in a volume of the Butterworths Use of Literature series (Morton 1977). A useful historical work on medical bibliographies by Brodman (1954) listed 300 medical bibliographies published between 1500 and 1950. This book is also of some historical interest, since it contains a discussion of the working of the Larkey Committee, set up in 1948 to inquire into the possibility of a computerized bibliography for the Army Medical Library of the United States (afterwards the National Library of Medicine). The American Medical Library Association, which published Brodman's book, has recently published a work by Adams, *Medical Bibliography in an Age of Discontinuity* (1981). This reflects on the new and often dramatic developments of information techniques and the conceptual and cultural challenges they provide.

A last type of general bibliographical source relevant to investigation of the historical development of scientific theories, institutions and practices is reference books and directories (Walford 1973–7). Two general guides have recently been edited by Sheey and Burkett. Sheey has written an informed survey of reference books, while Burkett has compiled a directory of scientific directories (Sheey 1976, 1980; Burkett 1979a). Both kinds of source are particularly relevant to students of contemporary science and medicine – tracing the activities of a modern scientist might involve requesting information and sources from relevant institutions and organizations.

Biographies

The biographical approach to the history of science is and has been an almost natural, if at times misleading, way of dealing with the development of scientific theories or of social and cultural practices based on the exploitation of natural and medical sciences. A wide range of biographical dictionaries – national, chronological, topical, professional or otherwise – is available to students. Slocum (1967) is a bibliography and guide to biographical dictionaries, and lists various kinds of sources likely to contain biographical information. Current publications such as the *American Men and Women of Science* edited by Cattell Press (1978b, 1979) or the *McGraw-Hill Modern Men of Science* (1966–8) provide information on leading scientists currently or recently active. Such sources are obviously complemented by various types of *Who's Who* and similar publications (see, e.g., Debus 1968).

A major source of biographical and bibliographical information is the classic *Biographisch-Literarisches Handwörterbuch zur Geschichte der exacten Naturwissenschaften*, started by the German physicist and scholar Johann Christian Poggendorff (1858–). The Poggendorff volumes provide skeleton biographical information and bibliographies, with particular emphasis on articles published in journals. Poggendorff listed naturalists and men of science in general and avoided selective criteria based on acknowledged eminence or discoveries. Many of the entries are thus concerned with scientists otherwise not mentioned in specialized biographies or national dictionaries of biography. The volumes are particularly important for natural and life sciences of countries like Italy, which have started their comprehensive national biographies only in the last few years. Poggendorff often remains the only source of information on scores of naturalists, collectors or taxonomists who substantially contributed to their disciplines without achieving fame or academic eminence. However, specialized biographical enterprises like the *Dictionary of British and Irish Botanists* (Desmond 1977) show that the listing provided by Poggendorff can be further expanded, and emphasize the limits of the German work as far as botanical practitioners are concerned. (See also Mayerhöfer 1959–70.)

A useful index of biographical fragments in unspecialized scientific journals has been compiled by Scott Barr (1973). The book is the result of a survey of a few major scientific journals like *Nature*, the *Philosophical Magazine* and the *Proceedings* of classic institutions like the London or the Edinburgh Royal Societies. The tracing of 15 000 citations relating to 7700 scientists gives an idea of the reward brought by this kind of biographical investigation. It is hoped that historians of science and information experts will use the facilities offered by computerized systems to produce further inventories on a larger scale, using a greater variety of journals and sources.

An important enterprise in the field of scientific biography has been undertaken and completed in the last decade – the *Dictionary of Scientific Biography* (Gillispie 1970–80). Sixteen volumes have been published, including a Supplement (Vol. 15) and an excellent Index (Vol. 16). The *Dictionary* is divided into biographical entries of various length and value. Critics have pointed out the lack of uniformity in criteria adopted for different disciplines and epochs, and the under-representation of medical practitioners and theoreticians. Serious gaps have been indicated, and better bibliographical citations suggested. The enterprise inevitably encountered serious obstacles regarding criteria of selection of authors and the state of the profession in various fields of the history of science. The *Dictionary* is very much a reflection of the history of science as a collective academic and scholarly undertaking, as it is of the decisions taken by the editors. Furthermore, the debate aroused by this publication and the proposal mooted from various quarters that the *Dictionary* should continue with additional volumes covering gaps and redressing imbalances represent a positive element of critical evaluation of the requirements and needs of research and researchers in the history of science and the history of medicine (Fleming *et al.* 1980).

Biographical information and articles surveying the general cultural relevance of scientific debates in the past can also be obtained from general dictionaries and encyclopaedias. Several general bibliographies of these sources are available, whether surveying the history of encyclopaedias (Collison 1966) or providing a critical listing of major modern Anglo-American encyclopaedias (Walsh 1968). The *International Bibliography of Dictionaries* (1972) is also useful for ferreting out multi-volume enterprises of general or specific relevance to the history of scientific cultures, as well as biographies of eminent personalities in various fields of natural and social investigation. The Larousse *Grand Dictionnaire Universel* (1866–90) represents a particularly significant instance of a general dictionary with many valuable entries on European naturalists, physicists and medical practitioners or agronomists and agriculturists, mainly of the eighteenth and nineteenth centuries. For example, entries on philosophical and scientific French authorities were compiled by the outstanding historian F. Picavet. The *Dictionary of National Biography* (1882–1900), conceived by Leslie Stephen, contains many useful entries on early seventeenth-century to nineteenth-century naturalists and physicians.

It is appropriate to close this section on biographies by referring to biobibliographies of historians of science themselves. It is self-evident, or it should be, that histories of science are the product of historians, and not the recording of universally acknowledged contributions to human knowledge. The prestige, authority and power of science in the modern world should not make scholars less alert to the role of contemporary assumptions about the concept and role of science in the historical reconstructions of scientific activities and programmes of the past. It is therefore important to refer in this context to the checklist of biographical notices of historians of science by Jayawardene and Lawes (1979). Their list absorbs and supersedes previous work by Sarton and Mieli.

Museums and libraries: collections and catalogues

Museums are probably the aristocrats among sources for the history of science and the history of medicine. The collection of natural wonders and minerals, fossils, plants and flowers was often the preliminary and at times amateurish stage of studies in the natural world. It is sufficient to recollect the importance of the Tradescant–Ashmolean collection, or the impact of the centralization in Paris of natural scientific collections during the Napoleonic era on the development of modern taxonomy and biology, to realize the relevance of museum collections to the history of science. There are numerous and excellent bibliographies listing museums in the world and their collections. *Museums of the World* (1975), which lists 17500 museums in 150 countries, provides general reference to collections. More specialized are the listings of British museums by Hudson and Nicholls (1975) and the *Official Museum Directory 1981* (1980) for the United States and Canada. Of historical value is the survey by Markham (1948) of British museums, sadly indicating in an appendix the museums and the collections lost in the years of war. A selective survey of museums in Great Britain with scientific and technological collections is also available in an improved second edition that corrected some omissions in the first issue of the volume (Smart 1978). Museums frequently publish series of pamphlets, indexes of their collections, and even periodicals. This provides the reader with a wide range of sources tracing the whereabouts or stressing the importance of collections of natural objects or human artefacts, current information on exhibitions and bibliographical references. A selective listing of such publications is available, though it needs integration with more recent works mentioned above (Clapp 1962).

Museums were also primary centres for collections of scientific books and periodicals. Curiosity, the pursuit of rarity by the *virtuosi*, research interests and the need for books complementing the objects collected have made museum libraries important centres for the history of science and the history of medicine (Harvard University 1976; Wellcome 1927, 1960). The Science Museum in London issued catalogues of *Book Exhibitions* (Science Museum 1952–60). A bibliography of the Science Museum's publications (catalogues, guides to the galleries, exhibitions, administrative publications and monographs) is in preparation. The American Museum of Natural History (1977–8) has recently produced an extremely useful author and classified *Research Catalog* of its library, which holds 325000 books and more than 17000 periodicals and serials. The British Museum (Natural History) (1955–64) issues a periodical list of accessions to the Museum Library. The Smithsonian Institution – the United States' national museum – publishes a range of periodicals and catalogues illustrating the collections and holdings of its library and research department in the history of science and technology (Smithsonian Institution 1959–, 1978, 1979).

Specialized and general libraries provide important sources of bibliographical information through their catalogues, which are often published. Regional and local libraries should not be overlooked, since they are likely to contain special collections relating to particular scientists and institutions. Their catalogues may therefore provide leads to the compilation of more complete bibliographies and studies. There are several surveys of European and American libraries, specifying their locations, holdings, and collections preserved (Cattell Press 1978a; Bowns 1972; Lewanski 1978; Burkett 1979b). In 1977, Young, Young and Kruzas compiled a five-volume directory of special libraries and collections. Volume 3 was devoted to health sciences, volume 4 to social sciences and humanities, volume 5 to natural sciences and technology. Equally important is the *World Guide to Libraries*, edited by Legenfelder (1980). Volume 8 lists a wide range of libraries providing specialized information and documentation, including more than 70 history of medicine and 63 history of science and technology libraries.

Accurate descriptions of library collections are also to be found in a subject collection guide published by a team of information experts led by Ash (1978). The guide, like almost all recent important directories, was compiled using computer techniques and facilities. It lists collections of medical books up to the year 1800, history of science collections, etc. (Ash 1978: 655, 978–9). Guides to more restricted geographical areas are also available (Roberts *et al.* 1978; Tait and Tait 1976). Wasserman and Herman (1975) have published a list of library bibliographies and indexes, which is a useful guide to resources available from libraries and information centres in the United States and Canada. It is also appropriate to reiterate that scientific societies and research departments usually hold small or large specialized libraries, many of which are catalogued. The reader may find useful information about scientific societies and learned societies in general by consulting available guides and directories (*Scientific and Learned Societies* 1964; Gribbin 1961; Macreavy 1971).

Major catalogues of leading world libraries are a means of providing bibliographical information and data on the diffusion and editions of a particular text. The *National Union Catalog*, the *British Museum Catalogue* (now *British Library*), or the *Union Catalogue of Scientific Libraries in the University of Cambridge* (University of Cambridge, 1975) are standard authorities, which are usually readily available. American Library of Congress information experts have prepared a series of bibliographical aids and guides for which there also exists a useful handbook (Library of Congress 1977).

Series of catalogues of specialized libraries should also be mentioned, to indicate the importance of their holdings to the history of specific issues and periods. Here may be cited the catalogue of the Warburg Institute Library (University of London 1967), one of the leading centres for the study of Renaissance culture. Volumes 3, 4 and 5 list its holdings of subjects like religion, magic and science, and philosophy. The *Author Catalogue* of the Royal Botanic Gardens Library at Kew, transferred from the royal family to the nation in 1841, makes information available from one of the largest botanical libraries in the world (Royal Botanic Gardens 1974). Some catalogues of scientific societies and academies have both intrinsic and historical use, insofar as they provide information on subjects and literature valued by the naturalists who established the library. The *Catalog of the Library of the Academy of Natural Sciences of Philadelphia* (Academy of Natural Sciences of Philadelphia 1972) is worth mentioning as an instance of this type of library holding. The library contains more than 150 000 books on taxonomic biology, palaeontology and stratigraphical geology. In 1936 it absorbed the library of the American Entomological Society. The catalogues of books and libraries associated with major collective scientific enterprises also deserve consideration. An outstanding example is the *Catalog of the United States Geological Survey Library* (Department of Interior 1964–76). The library, as the title suggests, originated from collections of sources acquired by the geological survey of the United States, and it is the largest geological library in the world.

Catalogues of libraries collected by private individuals often represent important sources of information on specialized subjects. Private collections donated to academic, private or national libraries frequently constituted the core of extremely important libraries devoted to the history of science and the history of medicine (Crerar Library 1967; Countway Library 1973; *Bibliotheca Osleriana*, Osler 1969). It is possible to reconstruct the list of the books possessed by individual naturalists or groups of naturalists from descriptions of individual libraries of the past. Key sources of information are sale catalogues of collectors and libraries. General information on sale catalogues can be obtained from the recently published *Index to British Literary Bibliography* edited by Howard Hill (1969–1979, iv: 296–7; i: 147–8). A volume on sale catalogues of eminent scientists, reproducing examples of important catalogues, has been compiled by Feisenberger (1975).

Particular mention must be made of the two leading libraries for the history of medicine and the medical sciences, namely the National Library of Medicine (NLM) of the United States and the Library of the Wellcome Institute for the History of Medicine in London. The National Library of Medicine was established in October 1956. It incorporated the Armed Forces Medical Library and other holdings of significant historical value. The NLM is now the largest medical library in the world and the major world centre for medical bibliography; it operates sophisticated computerized information systems and publishes bibliographical aids. Indeed, as mentioned above, the NLM was the first major library to evaluate the possibility of large-scale use of modern technology in librarianship and information science. MEDLARS, the computerized system devised by NLM and IBM experts, is today connected with 900 libraries and research centres throughout the world (Rogers 1982). One programme, HISTLINE, is particularly designed to meet the requirements of the historian of medicine and of medical sciences. It contains 35 000 references to articles, monographs, symposia and general publications relating to the history of medicine. It has however to be pointed out that the data available refer to publications appearing after 1970, though there are selective references for the period 1964–1970. The related library catalogues, from the *Index Catalogue of the Library of the Surgeon-General's Office* to the modern *Current Catalog*, still represent the major reference source for historians. Particularly relevant are the *Index of NLM Serial Titles*, and the short-title catalogues of eighteenth- and sixteenth-century printed books. *Index Medicus* and the *Bibliography of the History of Medicine* are compiled by the staff and information experts at the NLM. For further information on the great variety of editorial initiatives and bibliographical services offered by the NLM it is possible to address queries directly to the Office of Inquiries and Publications Management at the NLM, Rockville Pike, Bethesda, Maryland. (For full citations of NLM references, see the bibliography of chapter 19 below.)

The Wellcome Institute in London and the attached library are probably the largest specialized institution for the history of medicine in the world, certainly in Europe. Though established comparatively recently – the library was opened to the public in 1949 – the scholarship of its librarians has made it a centre for rare medical books, incunabula and historical medical publications, not to mention rich manuscript collections covering all aspects of medical systems and practices. There are catalogues of the incunabula preserved in the library, as well as of books published before

1641 and between 1641 and 1850, reaching letter L in volume three. A multi-volume reprint of its subject, biographical and topographical catalogues of the history of medicine and related sciences appeared in 1980. The Wellcome Institute also publishes a useful international bibliography, *Current Work in the History of Medicine*, since 1974 compiled partly on the basis of computer print-outs from the MEDLARS station in Boston Spa. (For full citations of Wellcome references see the bibliography of chapter 19 below.)

Histories of science and its teaching

Various studies of particular areas of scientific investigation and practice are mentioned in other chapters in this book. The general bibliographies mentioned above, and the *Isis Critical Bibliography* in particular, provide information on recent attempts systematically to survey specific or general problems in the history of science. It is however to be pointed out that new trends of research in the history of science and the history of medicine often do not appear to have produced any significant change in the books and topics selected or advised for history of science courses. Teachers or readers are also advised to take the precaution of reading book reviews cited by the *Isis Critical Bibliography* and the *Bulletin Signalétique*. The different and at times opposite reactions of other historians of science can alert a reader to problems or debatable features of any work.

A number of bibliographies of major studies in the history of science for the use of students are also available. Rider (1970) has prepared a select bibliography listing major works in every department of the history of science. He paid only incidental attention to the history of medicine, since he rightly regarded the subject as 'an extensive field' in its own right. A selective and competent bibliographical guide to the history and philosophy of science for students at Oxford was compiled by Black and Thomson (1973). Of a more systematic nature are the publications of the Library of Congress designed to provide students and teachers with basic bibliographies. The *L.C. Tracer Bullet* has already covered specialized topics like the history of technology, science and education in America, science and society and women in the sciences (1973, 1975, 1976, 1977).

The history of science and the history of medicine have rapidly expanded in the past few years and become part of curricula in the sciences and the humanities. The plurality of approaches is reflected by different priorities stressed by scholars engaged in the teaching of the subject. *Annals of Science* has recently followed the example of *Isis*, and introduced a section devoted to discussion of the teaching of history of science and technology. Of particular interest was the publication of the Interim Report by the Committee on Undergraduate Education of the History of Science Society of the United States. The Committee, chaired by Sharlin, surveyed the methodological and institutional problems facing history of science as an academic discipline, and was particularly alert to the consequences of changes of historiographical priorities in the history of science (Sharlin 1975). Knight (1975a) reported in the same issue of *Annals of Science* on educational programmes and facilities in the history of science in British universities and polytechnics. *Isis* publishes a News of the Profession section, surveying debates, organization, opinion and curricula of the history of science as an academic and scholarly discipline (Price 1967). The *Revue d'Histoire des Sciences* and the *Archives Internationales d'Histoire des Sciences* perform similar functions.

Lists of theses in the history of science, in progress or recently completed, give the impression that the history of science in British universities is increasingly concerned with topics in contemporary and late nineteenth-century Anglo-American history of science and technology. There appears to be a significant shift away from classic, early modern European-oriented history of science (Morrell 1980). For a general survey of history of science courses in the American universities, the directory of interdisciplinary studies in the humanities published by Bayrel (1979) offers a list of the major history of science, technology and medicine departments in the USA. Burns (1979) compiled a survey of teaching of medical history to college undergraduates in the USA and Canada, a study undertaken by the Educational Committee of the American Association for the History of Medicine. Isis (1980) has produced a *Directory of Members and Guide to Graduate Studies*. Dissertation abstracts also provide information on trends in research in American, English, Canadian and European universities (Reynolds 1975).

It is appropriate to conclude with some consideration of new computerized systems of bibliography. Techniques of information and systems of retrieval of data have undergone considerable qualitative and quantitative change in the past few years. There are a number of publications providing bibliographical information on studies and developments of what are called 'on-line systems'. (By 'on-line' is meant direct communication from the main information centre to a terminal in the user's library, as opposed to 'off-line', when a computer print-out is sent to the user.) I have already pointed out that on-line systems are operative for the history of medical sciences. These also offer the possibility of eliciting information on a question and answer basis, but this demands considerable skill and understanding of the system on the part of the scholar. Hall has published an on-line information retrieval sourcebook (1977), and a bibliographical directory (1979). In 1977 a magazine was also started, *Online Review. The International Journal of Online and Videotex Information Systems* (1977–). Developments in information science will undoubtedly facilitate the work of historians, even though it is clear that the critical judgement of librarians in preparing the data systems and of historians in evaluating complex problems and interdisciplinary features of the history of science, technology and the history of medicine will remain the cornerstone of scholarly enterprise.

Bibliography

Academy of Natural Sciences of Philadelphia (1972). *Catalog of the Library of the Academy of Natural Sciences of Philadelphia.* 16 Vols. Boston, Mass; G.K. Hall

Adams, S. (1981). *Medical Bibliography in an Age of Discontinuity.* Chicago; The Medical Library Association

American Museum of Natural History (1977–8). *Research Catalog of the Library of the American Museum of Natural History. Authors*, 13 Vols (1977); *Classed*, 12 Vols (1978). Boston, Mass.; G.K. Hall

Ash, L. (1978). *Subject Collections. A Guide to Special Book Collections and Subject Emphases as Reported by University, College, Public, and Special Libraries and Museums in the United States and Canada*, 5th edn. New York and London; R.R. Bowker Co.

Bayrel, E. (1977). *Interdisciplinary Studies in the Humanities. A Directory.* Metuchen, NJ, and London; The Scarecrow Press

Besterman, T. (1965–6). *A World Bibliography of Bibliographies, and of Bibliographical Catalogues, Calendars, Abstracts, Digests, and the Like*, 4th edn. 5 Vols. Lausanne; Societas Bibliographica, 1 rue de Genève

Bibliographic Index (1945–). *A Cumulative Bibliography of Bibliographies.* New York; H.W. Wilson Co.

Black, S. and Thomson, R.B. (1973). *History and Philosophy of Science. A Guide to Study and Research at Oxford University*, 2nd edn. Oxford; Oxford University Press

Bowns, R.B. (1972). *American Library Resources. A Bibliographical Guide.* Chicago; American Library Association

British Museum. *British Museum Catalogue of Printed Books. Photolithographic Edition to 1955* (1966). Replaces previous catalogues. 263 Vols. (1968). Ten Years Supplement, 1956–65. 50 Vols. (1971–2). Five Years Supplement, 1966 –70. 26 Vols. London; The Trustees of the British Museum

The British Library. General Catalogue of Printed Books. Five Years Supplement 1971–5 (1978–9). 13 Vols. London; The British Library, British Museum Publications Ltd.

The British Library General Catalogue of Printed Books to 1975 (1979–). London, London and Munich, New York, Paris; Clive Bingley and K.G. Saur

British Museum (Natural History) (1955–74). *List of Accessions to the Museum Library.* London; British Museum (Natural History)

Brodman, E. (1954). *The Development of Medical Bibliography.* Chicago; The Medical Library Association

Burkett, J. (1979a). *Directory of Scientific Directories. A World Guide to Scientific Directories Including Medicine, Agriculture, Engineering, Manufacturing and Industrial Directories*, 3rd edn. London; Francis Hodgson, Longman Group Ltd.

Burkett, J. (1979b). *Library and Information Networks in the United Kingdom.* London; ASLIB

Burns, C.R. (1979). *1977 Survey of the Teaching of Medical History to College Undergraduates in the United States and Canada.* The Educational Committee of the American Association for the History of Medicine

Bynum, W.F., Browne, E.J. and Porter, R.S. (1981). *Dictionary of the History of Science.* London; Macmillan

Canguilhem, G. (1970). *Introduction à l'histoire des sciences.* Paris; Hachette

Cattell Press, J. (1978a). *American Library Directory*, 31st edn. New York and London; R.R. Bowker

Cattell Press, J., Ed. (1978b). *American Men and Women of Science. Social and Behavioral Sciences*, 13th edn. New York and London; R.R. Bowker

Cattell Press, J. (1979). *American Men and Women of Science. Physical Science and Biological Sciences*, 14th edn. 8 Vols. New York and London; R.R. Bowker

Centre National de la Recherche Scientifique (1947–). *Bulletin Analytique. Philosophie* (1947–55); then *Bulletin Signalétique. Philosophie Sciences Humaines* (1956–60); then *Bulletin Signalétique. 19 Sciences Humaines Philosophie* (1961–3); then *Bulletin Signalétique. 19–23 Sciences Humaines Philosophie* (1964); then *Bulletin Signalétique. 19–24 Sciences Humaines Philosophie* (1965–7); then *Bulletin Signalétique (19–24) Sciences Humaines* (1969); then *Bulletin Signalétique. 522 Histoire des Sciences et des Techniques* (1969–); *519 Philosophie Sciences Religieuses* (1969), then *519 Philosophie* (1970–) and *527 Sciences Religieuses* (1970–); *520 Pédagogie* (1969), then *520 Sciences de l'Éducation* (1970–); *521 Sociologie Éthnologie Préhistoire Archéologie* (1969), then *521 Sociologie Éthnologie* (1970–). Paris; Centre de Documentation du CNRS.

Clapp, J. (1962). *Museum Publications. A Classified List and Index of Books, Pamphlets, and Other Monographs, and of Serial Reprints.* Part II, *Publications in Biological and Earth Sciences.* New York; The Scarecrow Press

Collison, R.L. (1966). *Encyclopaedias : Their History throughout the Ages. A Bibliographical Guide with Extensive Historical Notes to the General Encyclopaedias Issued throughout the World from 350 BC to the Present Day*, 2nd edn. New York and London; Hafner

Collison, R.L. (1968). *Bibliographies. Subject and National. A Guide to their Contents, Arrangement and Use.* London; Crosby Lockwood and Son

Countway Library (1973). *Author–Title Catalog of the Francis A. Countway Library of Medicine. For Imprints through 1959 Harvard Medical Library – Boston Medical Library.* 10 Vols. Boston, Mass.; G.K. Hall

Crerar Library (1967). *The John Crerar Library Author Catalog.* 35 Vols. Boston, Mass.; G.K. Hall

Debus, A.G. (1968). *World Who's Who in Science: a Biographical Dictionary of Notable Scientists from Antiquity to the Present.* Chicago; Marquis and Who's Who

Department of Interior, US Government (1964–76). *Catalog of the United States Geological Survey Library. Department of Interior, Washington D.C.* 25 Vols

(1964); 1st Supplement, 10 Vols (1972); 2nd Supplement, 4 Vols (1974); 3rd Supplement, 6 Vols (1976). Washington DC; US Government Printing Office

Desmond, R. (1977). *Dictionary of British and Irish Botanists and Horticulturists, Including Plant Collectors and Botanical Artists.* London; Taylor and Francis. 1st edn (1893). Ed. J. Britten and J.E.S. Boulger. London; West, Newman and Co. 2nd edn (1931). London; Taylor and Francis

Dictionary of National Biography, The (1882–1900). Ed. L. Stephen and S. Lee. 63 Vols. London; Smith, Elder and Co. *Supplement* (1901). 3 Vols. Reprinted in 22 Vols (1908–9). *Index and Epitome* [i.e. Concise D.N.B. to 1900] (1903). Thereafter in 5 decennial vols, from 1901 (1920–71). London; Oxford University Press. See also Institute of Historical Research, London, *Corrections and Additions to the Dictionary of National Biography Cumulated from the Bulletin...1923–1963* (1966). Boston, Mass.; G.K. Hall

Durbin, P.T., Ed. (1980). *A Guide to the Culture of Science, Technology and Medicine.* New York; Free Press. London; Macmillan

Feisenberger, H.A. (1975). *Scientists.* Vol. 11 of *Sale Catalogues of Libraries of Eminent Persons.* Ed. A.N.L. Munby. 12 Vols. (1971–5). London; Mansell

Ferguson, E.S., Ed. (1968). *Bibliography of the History of Technology.* Society for the History of Technology, Monograph 5. London; Society for the History of Technology. Cambridge, Mass.; MIT Press

Fleming, D., Needham, J., Grant, E., Roger, J. (1980). The Dictionary of Scientific Biography. A Review Symposium, *Isis*, Vol. 71, 633–652

Gillispie, C.C., Ed. (1970–80). *Dictionary of Scientific Biography.* 16 Vols. New York; American Council of Learned Societies, Charles Scribner's Sons

Gribbin, J.H. (1961). *Scientific and Technical Societies of the United States and Canada,* 7th edn. Washington DC; National Academy of Sciences, National Research Council

Hall, J.L. (1977). *On-Line Information Retrieval Sourcebook.* London; ASLIB

Hall, J.L. (1979). *On-Line Bibliographic Data Bases.* London; ASLIB

Harvard University (1968, 1976). *Catalog of the Library of the Museum of Comparative Zoology. Harvard University.* 8 Vols (1968). 1st Supplement (1976). Boston, Mass.; G.K. Hall

Houghton, B. and Convey, J. (1977). *On-Line Information Retrieval Systems: An Introductory Manual to Principles and Practice.* London; Bingley

Howard Hill, T.H. (1969–79). *Index to British Literary Bibliography.* 5 Vols. Oxford; Oxford University Press

Hudson, K. and Nicholls, A. (1975). *The Directory of Museums.* London; Macmillan

International Bibliography of Dictionaries (1972), 5th edn. New York and London; R.R. Bowker. Berlin; Verlag Dokumentation

Index Medicus (1970–). *Cumulative Abridged Index Medicus.* Bethesda and Washington; National Library of Medicine and US Government Printing Office

Isis (1980). *Directory of Members and Guide to Graduate Studies.* Philadelphia; History of Science Society

Jarrell, R.A. and Ball, N.R. (1980). *Science, Technology and Canadian History.* Waterloo, Ontario; Wilfrid Laurier University Press

Jayawardene, S.A. (1977). Review of D. Knight (1975b), *Isis*, Vol. 68, 299–302

Jayawardene, S.A. (1979). Isis Cumulative Bibliography, *Isis*, Vol. 70, 160–163

Jayawardene, S.A. (1982). *Handlist of Reference Books for the Historian of Science.* Science Museum Library Occasional Publications, 2. London; Science Museum

Jayawardene, S.A. and Lawes, J. (1979). Biographical Notices of Historians of Science : A Checklist. For Kurt Vogel on his 90th Birthday (30 September 1978), *Annals of Science*, Vol. 36, 315–394

Karp, W. (1965). *The Smithsonian Institution: an Establishment for the Increase and Diffusion of Knowledge Among Men*. Washington DC; Smithsonian Institution and American Heritage Magazine

Knight, D.M. (1975a). Teaching the History of Science in Some British Universities and Polytechnics, *Annals of Science*, Vol. 32, 163–173

Knight, D.M. (1975b). *Sources for the History of Science*. London; The Sources of History Ltd, Hodder and Stoughton. Now distributed by the Cambridge University Press

Kyed, J.M. and Matarazzo, J.M. (1979). *Scientific, Engineering and Medical Societies Publications in Print 1978–1979*. New York and London; R.R. Bowker

Larousse, P. (1866–90). *Grand dictionnaire universel du XIXe siècle*. Vols 1–15 (1866–76); Vol. 16, 1st Supplement (1878); Vol. 17, 2nd Supplement (1890). Paris; Administration du Grand Dictionnaire Universel

Legenfelder, H. (1980). *Handbook of International Documentation and Information*. Vol. 8 of *World Guide to Libraries*. Munich, New York, London and Paris; G. Saun

Lewanski, R.C. (1978). *Subject Collections in European Libraries*, 2nd edn. London and New York; R.R. Bowker

Library of Congress (1977). *Publications Prepared by the Science and Technology Division 1940–1975*. Washington DC; Library of Congress

Library of Congress Tracer Bullet. T.B. 72.5 *Science Policy*. Comp. S.B. Dresmer, May (1972); T.B. 73.18 *The History of Technology*. Comp. D. Niskern, Nov. (1973); T.B. 74.4 *Science and Technology in 18th Century America*. Comp. C. Carter, June (1974); T.B. 75.12 *Science Education in America*. Comp. C. Carter, Sept. (1975); T.B. 76.2 *Women in the Sciences*. Comp. C. Carter, March (1976); T.B. 77.6 *Science and Society*. Comp. S.B. Dresmer, Feb. (1977). Washington DC; Science and Technology Division

McGraw-Hill Modern Men of Science (1966–8). 2 Vols. New York and London; McGraw-Hill Book Co.

Macreavy, S.E. (1971). *Guide to Science and Technology in the United Kingdom. A Reference Guide to Science and Technology in Great Britain and Northern Ireland*. Guernsey; Francis Hodgson

Malclès, L.-N. (1950–8). *Les Sources du travail bibliographique*. 3 parts in 4 Vols. Geneva; Droz. Lille; Giard. Reimpression (1965). Vol. 4, *Bibliographies specialisées (Sciences exactes et techniques)*

Markham, S.F. (1948). *Directory of Museums and Art Galleries in the British Isles*. London; The Museum Association

Mayerhöfer, J. (1959–70). *Lexicon des Geschichte der Naturwissenschaften. Biographien, Sachwörter und Bibliographien*. Vienna; Verlag Brüder Hollinek

Morrell, J.B. (1980). *A List of Theses in History of Science in British Universities in Progress or Recently Completed*. N.11, 1980–1. Halfpenny Furze, Chalfont St. Giles; The British Society for the History of Science

Morton, L.T. (1970). *A Medical Bibliography (Garrison and Morton): An Annotated Check-List of Texts Illustrating the History of Medicine*, 3rd edn. London; A. Deutsch

Morton, L.J. (1977). *Use of Medical Literature*, 2nd edn. London; Butterworths

Museums of the World. A Directory to 17 500 Museums in 150 Countries Including a Subject Index (1975), 2nd edn enlarged. Munich; Verlag Dokumentation

National Union Catalog. Library of Congress: *The National Union Catalog. Pre-1956 Imprints* (1968–80). Replaces previous catalogues of pre-1956 imprints. 685 Vols. *Supplement* (1980–1). Vols 686–754. London and Chicago; the Library of Congress, with American Library Association, Mansell

The National Union Catalog. A Cumulative Author List Representing Library of

154   Guide to bibliographical sources

Congress Printed Cards and Titles Reported by Other American Libraries (1963). Covers the years 1958–62. 50 Vols. New York; The Library of Congress, with the cooperation of the American Library Association, Rowman and Littlefield Inc. (1969). Covering the years 1963–7. 59 Vols. Ann Arbor; The Library of Congress and the American Library Association, J.W. Edwards Publisher (1973). Covering the years 1968–72. 104 Vols. Ibidem; idem (1978). Covering the years 1973–77. 135 Vols. Totowa; The Library of Congress and the American Library Association, Rowman and Littlefield (1978). Covering the year 1978. 16 Vols. Washington; The Library of Congress, Catalog Publication Division Yearly volumes are published, which will be cumulated in five-year Catalogs.

Neu, J. (1967). The History of Science, *Library Trends*, Vol. 15, 776–792

Official Museum Directory 1981. United States and Canada (1980). Washington DC and Stokie, Ill.; The American Association of Museums and National Register Publishing Co.

Online Review (1977–). *The International Journal of Online and Videotex Systems.* Oxford and New York; Learned Information

Osler, W. (1969). *Bibliotheca Osleriana: A Catalogue of Books Illustrating the History of Medicine and Science, Collected, Arranged and Annotated by Sir William Osler, Bt., and Bequeathed to McGill University.* Montreal and London; McGill University Press. 1st edn (1929)

Poggendorff, J.C. (1858–). *Biographisch–literarisches Handwörterbuch [zur Geschichte] der exakten Naturwissenschaften.* Vol. I, First Issue, Columns 1–576, Jan. 1858; Vol. I, Second Issue, Columns 577–1152, Dec. 1858; Vol. I, Third Issue, Columns 1153–1524, Sept. 1859; Vol. II, Fourth Issue, Columns 1–576, Oct. 1860; Vol. II, Fifth Issue, Columns 577–1152, Jan. 1863; Vol. II, Sixth Issue, Columns 1153–1468, Aug. 1863; Vols. I and II, First Complete Edn., with additions (1863). Vol. III, covering the years 1858–83 (1893). Vol. IV, 1883–1904 (1904). Leipzig; Verlag von Johan Ambrosius. Vol. V, 1904–22 (1926). Leipzig and Berlin; Verlag Chemie. Vol. VI, 1923–31 (1936–40). 6 Vols. Berlin; Verlag Chemie. Vol. VII A, 1932–53 (1956–62). 4 Vols. Supplement (1971). Vol. VII B, 1932–62, letters A–Q, (1967–). 6 Vols. [Vol. 6, N–Q] (1980). Berlin; Akademie Verlag

Pollard, A.W. and Redgrave, G.R. (1950). *A Short-Title Catalogue of Books Printed in England, Scotland and Ireland, and English Books Printed Abroad, 1475–1640.* London; Bibliographical Society

Price, D.J. de Solla (1967). A Guide to Graduate Study and Research in the History of Science and Medicine, *Isis*, Vol. 58, 385–395

Reynolds, M.R. (1975). *A Guide to Theses and Dissertations. An Annotated International Bibliography of Bibliographies.* Detroit; Gale Research Co., The Book Tower

Rider, K.J. (1970). *History of Science and Technology: a Select Bibliography for Students*, 2nd edn. London; The Library Association

Roberts, S., Cooper, A. and Gilder, L. (1978). *Research Libraries and Collections in the United Kingdom: A Selective Inventory and Guide.* London; Clive Bingley. Hamden, Conn.; Linnet Books

Rogers, F.B. (1982). The Origins of MEDLARS, in L.G. Stevenson, Ed., *A Celebration of Medical History, The Fiftieth Anniversary of the Johns Hopkins Institute of the History of Medicine and the Welch Medical Library.* Baltimore and London; The Johns Hopkins University Press, 85–106

Royal Botanic Gardens (1974). *Author Catalogue of the Royal Botanic Gardens Library Kew.* 5 Vols. Boston, Mass.; G.K. Hall

Russo, F. (1969). *Éléments de bibliographie de l'histoire des sciences et des techniques*, 2nd revised edn. Paris; Hermann. 1st edn (1954). *Histoire des sciences et des techniques: bibliographie*

Sarton, G. (1952). *Horus. A Guide to the History of Science. A First Guide for the Study of the History of Science, with Introductory Essays on Science and Tradition*. New York; Ronald Press

Sarton, G. (1953). La bibliographie de l'histoire des sciences, *Archives Internationales d'Histoire des Sciences*, Vol. 32, 395–419

Science Museum (1952–60). *Book Exhibitions. Catalogue*. London; HMSO

Scientific and Learned Societies of Great Britain. A Handbook Compiled from Official Sources (1964). London; G. Allen and Unwin

Scott Barr, E. (1973). *An Index to Biographical Fragments in Unspecialized Scientific Journals*. Alabama; University of Alabama Press

Sharlin, H.I., *et al.* (1975). A Study and Critique of the Teaching of the History of Science and Technology. Interim Report by the Committee on Undergraduate Education of the History of Science Society (USA), *Annals of Science*, Vol. 32, 55–70

Sheehy, E.P. (1976). *Guide to Reference Books*. Chicago; The American Library Association. Supplement (1980)

Shortt, S.E.D. (1981). *Medicine in Canadian Society. Historical Perspectives*. Montreal; McGill-Queen's University Press

Slocum, R. (1967). *Biographical Dictionaries and Related Works*. Detroit; Gale Research Co., The Book Tower

Smart, J.E. (1978). *Museums in Great Britain with Scientific and Technological Collections*, 2nd edn. London; Science Museum

Smithsonian Institution (1959–). *Museum of History and Technology. Contributions from the Museum of History and Technology Papers*. Washington DC; Smithsonian Institution

Smithsonian Institution (1978). *Guide to the Smithsonian Archives*. Washington DC; Smithsonian Institution Press

Smithsonian Institution (1979). *Smithsonian Institution Press. Complete Catalogue 1970–80*. London; Smithsonian Institution

Tait, J.A. and Tait, H.F.C. (1976). *Library Resources in Scotland 1976–1977*. Glasgow; Scottish Library Association

Thornton, J.L. (1966). *Medical Books, Libraries and Collectors: A Study of Bibliography and the Book Trade in Relation to the Medical Sciences*, 2nd edn. London; André Deutsch

Thornton, J.L. and Tully, R.I.J. (1971). *Scientific Books, Libraries and Collectors, A Study of Bibliography and the Book Trade in Relation to Science*, 3rd edn. London; The Library Association. Reprinted (1975). Supplement to 3rd edn covering 1969–75 (1978)

Toomey, A.F. (1977). *A World Bibliography of Bibliographies 1964–1974. A List of Works Represented by Library of Congress Printed Cards, a Decennial Supplement to Theodore Besterman, A World Bibliography of Bibliographies*. 2 Vols. Totowa, NJ; Rowman and Littlefield

UNESCO (1969–77). *Bibliographical Services throughout the World. 1960–1964*, Comp. P. Avicenna (1969); *1965–1969* (1972); *1970–1974*, comp. M. Beaudiquez (1977). Paris; UNESCO Bibliographical Handbooks

University of Cambridge (1975). *Union Catalogue of Scientific Libraries in the University of Cambridge. Scientific Conference Proceedings 1644–1972*. 2 Vols. London; Mansell

University of London (1967). *Catalog of the Warburg Institute Library. University of London*. 5 Vols. Boston, Mass.; G.K. Hall

Walford, A.J. (1973–7). *Guide to Reference Material*, 3rd edn. 3 Vols. 4th edn, Vol. 1 (1980). London; The Library Association

Walsh, S.P. (1968). *Anglo–American General Encyclopaedias. A Historical Bibliography 1703–1967.* New York and London; R.R. Bowker

Wasserman, P. and Herman, E., Ed. (1975). *Library Bibliographies and Indexes. A Subject Guide to Resource Material Available from Libraries, Information Centers, Library Schools and Library Associations in the United States and Canada.* Detroit; Gale Research Co., The Book Tower

Watson, G. (1974–7). *The New Cambridge Bibliography of English Literature.* 5 Vols. Cambridge; Cambridge University Press

Wellcome (1927). *The Wellcome Historical Medical Museum.* London; The Wellcome Foundation Ltd.

Wellcome (1960). *The Wellcome Museum of Medical Science.* London; The Wellcome Foundation

Whitrow, M., Ed. (1972–6). *Isis Cumulative Bibliography: A Bibliography of the History of Science formed from Isis Critical Bibliographies, 1–90 1913–65.* 3 Vols. London; Mansell

Wing, D. (1972). *Short-title Catalogue, 1641–1700*, 2nd edn. New York; Modern Language Association

Young, M.L. and Young, H.C. (1979). *Directory of Special Libraries and Information Centers*, 5th edn. 3 Vols. Detroit; Gale Research Co., The Book Tower

Young, M.L., Young, H.C. and Kruzas, A.T. (1977). *Subject Directory of Special Libraries and Information Centers*, 4th edn. 5 Vols. Detroit; Gale Research Co., The Book Tower

9

Periodical literature and societies

Paul Weindling

In many respects the specialized periodical literature of the history of science and medicine provides an acid test of the effectiveness of the many organizations promoting these studies. A survey of periodicals and societies is timely, because of new titles and the shift away from the conception of the discipline as a branch of the natural sciences. The problems that journals must now confront arise partly from the very different styles of journals in the humanities and sciences, partly from the excessive number of history of science journals in comparison with the paucity of publishing outlets in the history of medicine, and partly because major articles often appear in a wide range of journals beyond those claiming to represent history of science and medicine. The scene is one of many cinderella publications, an occasional ugly sister attempting to hog the stage, and untimely economic pressures that may price journals out of existence unless they adapt themselves to current needs of researchers in their disciplines.

If one takes a step out of the all too closed worlds of the history of science and medicine, the size of the problem may be gauged. Between 1950 and 1970 there were an estimated 220 000 new journals, of which a third were geared to science and medicine. In the same period there arose new abstracting services, citation indexes and innovations like microfiche and camera-ready copy. In 1981, there were approximately 300 current serials for history of science and medicine, nearly half using English as their primary language. The comparatively large number of such publications is

due to long-standing amateur interest and recent professionalization, both of which have their strong and weak points. Factors like
remoteness of country of origin and the obscurity of many societies
could be overcome by greater international cooperation between
the societies themselves and libraries. But a sign of the malaise is
that there is not even a list of current journals in the history of
science and medicine, or a world directory of appropriate
societies. Most defy abstracting services and general directories.
Quality of content is at worst abysmal and in general tends to be
restricted so that the potential of history of science and medicine
remains largely unrealized. If journals are slow to publish, poorly
abstracted and inefficiently circulated they are doing contributors
a disservice, as well as jeopardizing their existence in the face of
competition from publications in related areas. If journals fail to
maintain scholarly standards and to be informative and genuinely
open to worthwhile contributions they are doing a disservice to
subscribers, to society members and to the studies they purport to
represent.

Historical factors

It is to stress the extent to which journals and societies are
cooperative and mutually dependent enterprises that these are
treated together here. Not only have many societies been formed
primarily to establish journals, but societies generate publications
like proceedings, newsletters, bibliographies and editions of standard works. Thus in Britain, some of the earliest societies for the
history of science were formed as publishing ventures. A pioneering but short-lived organization was Halliwell-Phillipps' Historical
Society of Science of 1841. Notable historical contributions were
made by other contemporary groupings: the Sydenham Society
from 1843 and its successor, the New Sydenham Society, under-
took translations of medical classics; the Ray Society, founded in
1844, has continued to publish many classic biological works
(Curle 1954); and the Hakluyt Society dating from 1846 publishes
accounts by early explorers.

Historical forays into the development of medical and scientific
periodicals provide not only bibliographical information, but also
understanding of factors affecting the structuring and diffusion of
knowledge. Kronick suggests, in his well-documented study of the
scientific and technical press between 1665 and 1790, that historical analysis can also be helpful in revaluation of library organization

and of systems of communication (1976, vii). Examples of historical studies are Manzer (1977) on the development of the abstract journal and *Publications in Historical Biobibliography* (1980). Studies have also been encouraged by the Society for the Bibliography of Natural History. Many factors like criteria for selection of papers and publishing history remain under-exploited. However, there are some useful research tools: examples are the cumulative author index, 1802–1906, to Poole's *Index to Periodical Literature* (Wall 1971), *The Wellesley Index* (1966–) and *Waterloo Directory* (1976) of Victorian periodicals.

Periodicals may seem striking evidence of the continuity of a cumulative scientific search for truth, as some publications have lasted for over three centuries. But such publications provide more evidence for viewing science as a discontinuous enterprise everdestructive of once-cherished truths as biased prejudices. Past definitions of history, philosophy and science have so varied that the pioneering *Journal des Sçavans* (1665–) arguably contained little that a modern scientist would recognize and the *Philosophical Transactions* (1665–) of the Royal Society included many credulous anecdotes and items on monsters, beverages and the history of trades.

General journals for the history of science, medicine and technology, adopting long time-spans, tend to give a false even if not altogether intentional image of the continuity of sciences. Whether there is and ought to be a common readership for articles on thirteenth-century mathematics and twentieth-century infant mortality is debatable. But as views on the continuity of scientific endeavour fade, new interests appear in the comparative study of cultures, so posing the challenge to editors of opening their pages to new modes of historical analysis.

Bridging the two cultures?

Further problems relating to the fields of history of science and medicine arise from journals attempting to reconcile divisions between the arts and sciences. There is great inconsistency in the treatment of these pursuits by abstracting services, bibliographical services and libraries. For example, *Annals of Science* is included in the *British Humanities Index* and *Social Science Citation Index*, but *Medical History* and *History of Science* are omitted. Whether journals themselves are open to contributions from neighbouring fields varies: thus the editor of the *Journal of the History of*

Medicine and Allied Sciences has recently attacked the contribution of social historians as history of medicine without medicine (Wilson 1980a). Others indeed hope for a broad audience, yet limitations on style and content show this to be unrealistic, so that even when an item appears that merits wide attention it is liable to be overlooked.

Potential contributors should bear in mind varying circulation figures, price and the degree of specialization of a journal. *Isis* has the largest circulation (2500), is reasonably priced and offers a useful annual bibliographical volume, as well as many reviews. However, the quality of articles has been competent rather than outstanding, although recently there have been signs of rising standards. The number of foreign-language articles has declined since the 1930s, when many contributions were in French. Although 'an international review', as organ of the History of Science Society located in the USA it inevitably has a high proportion of papers and reviews by US scholars. Similarly as medical historians increasingly – and not unjustifiably – work on local and regional topics, so the *Bulletin of the History of Medicine* carries a very high proportion of articles on American subjects.

High circulation figures are in themselves no guarantee of academic excellence. Yet one attraction of publication in a general historical or scientific journal is that these may reach a far larger or more appropriate audience. Many general scientific and medical journals will include occasional historical articles. In 1979 the *Scientific American* had a circulation of 665 395 and *Nature* of about 21 000. A popular historical journal like *Past and Present* has a circulation of 4500. Alternatively an article may merit publication only in a specialized journal. Circulation figures of other leading journals in history of science and medicine are *Ambix* (500), *Archives Internationales d'Histoire des Sciences* (800), *Bulletin of the History of Medicine* (1700), *Centaurus* (700), *Clio Medica* (350), *Gesnerus* (650), *History of Science* (1000), *Journal of the History of Medicine* (1000), *Journal of the History of the Behavioral Sciences* (1000), *Revue d'Histoire des Sciences* (800), Royal Society of London *Notes and Records* (1300), and *Sudhoffs Archiv* (500) (*Ulrich's International Periodicals Directory* 1980).

Criteria for selection are also of importance. Those journals with a fair and expert refereeing system can attract and maintain higher scholarly standards. The editor of *Annals of Science* has provided statistics of papers submitted and outlined criteria of selection – which helps readers as well as potential contributors (Grattan-Guinness 1977). Speedy publication is desirable, so that constructive debate may be conducted, although journals vary greatly in the degree to which they permit or encourage controversy. While it is by no means easy to maintain a balance between providing a permanent repository for research and communicating latest research, and while many academics plan work schedules in terms of weeks and months rather than hours and days, it is important for editors to prevent needless delays and backlogs.

Guides to periodicals

There is a general review journal, *History of Science*, which also carries occasional articles on the literature of history of medicine and technology. This journal has adopted the flexible format of essay reviews dealing either with a series of books, conceptual problems or whole periods, rather than providing systematic coverage of current literature in the tradition of the *Zentralblatt*. The individualistic format has certain advantages, as well as running the risk of disadvantages, such as essay reviews being of uneven length and quality, ranging from perfunctory comment to fully fledged articles by selected contributors. What is needed is more systematic critical bibliography striking a balance between comprehensiveness and critical comment, and also for journals in related areas to cite and comment on new literature. The *Isis Critical Bibliography*, and consequently Whitrow's *Isis Cumulative Bibliography* (1972–6) and Neu's *Cumulative Bibliography* (1979) contain many more journals in specializations other than history of science. Historical journals are beginning to give greater prominence to history of science and medicine. For example, the *Journal of Social History* devoted an issue (Vol. 10, No. 4) to the history of medicine in 1977. Historical journals are also reviewing books on history of medicine and science more frequently, although whether reviewers are always judiciously selected may be questioned. The *Historical Journal* and *American Historical Review* have published a number of articles, mostly disappointing, on the history of science.

On balance the *Isis Critical Bibliography* and *Current Work in the History of Medicine* (now alas no longer gratis) are still the most convenient and economical means for keeping up with periodical literature. The chapter on general bibliographies in this volume (chapter 8) discusses other items relating to periodicals. Comprehensive listings of journals giving locations are the *British Union Catalogue of Periodicals* (BUCOP), now replaced by *Serials in the British Library* (1981–), the *World List of Scientific Periodic-*

als (1963–5), and the *Union List of Serials in the United States and Canada* (1965). For information on publishers and subscription costs, *Ulrich's* directory of serials should be consulted; this has the merit of being subject-indexed. Useful information on new titles may be gleaned from the British Library's *New Periodical Titles* (1964–80) and Library of Congress *New Serial Titles* (1975–).

An attempt to integrate history of medicine and science periodicals into mainstream history is made by *Historical Abstracts*. This contains a topic heading 'Science and Technology, Including Geography and Exploration'. Medicine is unsatisfactorily subsumed in this. These abstracts, begun in 1955, now appear in three sections: Part A, Modern History Abstracts (1450–1914); Part B, Twentieth Century Abstracts (1914–1979); and entries on Canadian and US history in *America: History and Life*. As well as surveying many general science and social science journals, thirty-six history of medicine and science periodicals were covered from varying dates since 1955 (see Bibliography of Journals, p. 501). This is particularly useful for foreign-language journals, and for more obscure publications as from Cuba and Japan; however, most are English-language and readily available.

Citation indexes are a useful means of assessing which authors are most frequently referred to in periodicals, certain monographs series and multi-authored volumes. History of science is a subject category in the well-established *Science Citation Index (SCI)* and *Social Science Citation Index (SSCI)*, and in the newer *Arts and Humanities Citation Index (A&HCI)* (1977–). In 1980 the *SSCI* fully covered twenty-two titles among which were *Cambridge Monographs on the History of Medicine*, *Social Studies of Science* and the *Radical Science Journal*. In 1979 *SCI* covered only fifteen titles in history and philosophy of science, including certain journals like *Medical History* not in *SSCI*. Such indexes raise the interesting problem of adapting citation practices in the sciences to the humanities. Garfield, an information scientist with a long-standing interest in the history of science, has argued (1980) that such problems as citation of works of art and musical compositions have been overcome. Yet the computer finds it difficult to handle features of the citation of older printed books and unpublished sources – problems hardly existing in the natural sciences.

The distinction between what is and is not a scientific paper has long been problematic. For nineteenth-century scientific papers, the Royal Society *Catalogue of Scientific Papers* is an important research tool. But it has important limitations. The first six volumes for 1800–1863 excluded those medical and surgical papers not regarded as adequately scientific, and 'such papers as were merely literary, technical or professional', which today's historian of science would value (i: vii). Its policy then changed to include 'inaugural addresses, biographies and papers on the history of science' (vii: iii). Although the rest of the nineteenth century was covered, index volumes only for mathematics, mechanics and physics were published (1908–13). In 1901 an index of obituaries published in the *Proceedings* from 1860 to 1899 was issued (*Obituary Notices of Fellows of the Royal Society* 1901). For the twentieth century, see the *International Index* (1907–65), becoming the *Social Sciences and Humanities Index* (1965–74) and then the *Humanities Index* (1974–). The *British Humanities Index* (1962–) has the great merit of indexing newspaper articles and general 'weeklies', in which often substantial articles by experts appear. However, it only indexes three history of science journals, the *British Journal for the History of Science*, *Annals of Science* and *Studies in History and Philosophy of Science*.

Bibliographies of past medical journals have been compiled by Garrison (1934; amended by Kronick 1958), and also by LeFanu (1937–8). For locations the appropriate union catalogues should be consulted. For source lists of scientific journals, Kronick (1974) warns that certain items have only been copied from other lists and are in fact 'ghosts'. Thornton and Tully (1971) provide a useful introduction to problems of historical bibliography of science. Sarton (1952: 194–258), aided by Mayer, compiled a comprehensive list of journals relevant to the history (and philosophy) of science. The bibliography of journals at the end of this book is intended to update Sarton's list for English-language publications, as well as providing a select list of foreign journals. It should be noted that journals relating to philosophy and sociology have been excluded, apart from those mentioned in this chapter, and only a few relating to folk medicine and medical anthropology are cited.

Certain journals like *Social Studies of Science* have been included in the appended bibliography because of the consistently high proportion of historical articles on history of science and medicine published. Given the interdisciplinary nature of history of science and medicine, articles relevant to any topic may appear in a very wide range of journals. The cross-cultural approach of a journal concentrating on a particular region or period can be beneficial in promoting awareness of the dependence of science and medicine on particular contexts and circumstances. Investigative techniques of other fields like folklore and anthropology can also have a refreshing effect. Specialized journals in related disciplines provide the opportunity for publishing material of high quality that will attract attention of experts in related fields. In addition to journals mentioned elsewhere, one may cite *Journal of the Courtauld and Warburg Institutes* for the history of the classical tradition, *Minerva* and *History of Education* for educational questions, and *Fabula* for folklore.

Certain journals have not only consistently provided space to history of science and medicine, but have raised standards by encouraging innovation and more rigorous treatment of evidence. A pioneering role was taken by the *Journal of the History of Ideas* resulting in an anthology on the roots of scientific thought (Wiener and Noland 1957). However, such an approach to cultural history has been much criticized, and important new methodologies have been developed by contributors to the French historical journal *Annales*. There have been a series of translations from this edited by Forster and Ranum (e.g. 1975). *Past and Present* has issued a collection of articles on the intellectual revolution of the seventeenth century (Webster 1974), and its conferences have resulted in volumes on the patronage of science (Turner 1976) and on socio-biology (Webster 1981). The *Oxford Review of Education* (Webster 1976–7) included several articles on history of science. General series like the *Transactions* and *Proceedings of the American Philosophical Society* have included important contributions to the history of science and medicine, as well as stimulating specialized newsletters for genetics and biochemistry.

History of science journals

The establishment in 1901 of a section for the history of science and medicine by the Gesellschaft Deutscher Naturforscher und Aerzte gave renewed impetus to history of science journals. In Imperial Germany vigorous scholarly activity was the outcome of the cooperation of historians of medicine in established academic posts and widespread interest among amateurs in national scientific achievements, resulting also in the establishment of major historical institutions like the Deutsches Museum in Munich. The German drive to dominate international scientific circles meant that international meetings demanded appropriate national committees.

This has meant that history of science journals were first general publications fostered on an international or national level. Specialized journals for particular disciplines developed much more slowly, and subject journals were a vogue of the 1960s. The effect of this change was to create a narrower outlook among historians of science, many of whom insisted that scientific training was a prerequisite for holding one of the new academic posts. Of the general journals, *Osiris* ceased publication and the *Archives Internationales* suffered interruptions.

Isis has its roots in the earlier cosmopolitan period: it was established in Belgium by Sarton, before being transplanted to the USA when the History of Science Society was founded in 1924, partly to secure the journal's existence. Mieli was another indefatigable promoter of history of science on an international scale. In 1928 he played a leading part in the establishment of the International Academy of the History of Science. This adopted Mieli's *Archivo di Storia delle Scienze*, founded in 1919 and assuming the title *Archeion* in 1927. It was the predecessor of *Archives Internationales d'Histoire des Sciences* now supported by UNESCO. Mieli also promoted history of science at the Centre de Synthèse in Paris together with Metzger and Rey. The Centre launched the *Revue d'Histoire des Sciences* in 1947, but also had the *Revue de synthèse* (1931–), the successor to Henri Berr's *Revue de synthèse historique* (1900–30).

The cosmopolitan spirit between the wars also resulted in the establishment of *Annals of Science* by Singer in 1936. Although originally limited to post-Renaissance science, owing to the constraints of Singer's positivistic views, it now extends back to the thirteenth century. This is one of the oldest commercially published journals. Some specialized journals are also commercially published, such as the *Journal of the History of Biology*, which reflects the strong American interest in nineteenth-century English and European precursors of the growth of the life sciences in early twentieth-century America. Among the most costly journals is the *Archive for History of Exact Sciences*, which has managed to maintain high standards of technical expertise. Particular countries have general journals of sound quality that are also open to contributors from abroad or review foreign literature. *Janus* is a well-established Dutch journal, *Centaurus* originates in Denmark, and *Gesnerus* is the organ of the Swiss society for the history of science and medicine; *NTM* derives from the German Democratic Republic, originally numbered Bernal among its collaborators and in 1980 devoted an issue to science and industrialization, drawing on studies by British-based academics like Porter and Shapin. Many foreign periodicals publish contributions in English, and occasionally French, German and Russian.

The *Transactions* of the Newcomen Society (1920–) should be regarded as the longest-running British journal for the history of science and technology. *Ambix* (1937–), the Journal of the Society for the History of Alchemy and Chemistry has consistently maintained a high quality. In 1947 the British Society for the History of Science was established. From its *Bulletin* (1949–58) developed *The British Journal for the Philosophy of Science* (1951–) and the *British Journal for the History of Science* (1962–). The largest society with a history of science orientation is the Society for the Bibliography of Natural History, which has a journal (see *Archives of Natural History*) and newsletter with lively discussion of historical problems and sources. The Royal Society (*Notes and Records of the Royal Society* 1938–) and the British Museum (Natural History) (*Bulletin of the British Museum (Natural History), Historical Series* 1953–) also publish serials, broadly relating to their histories and thus including major sources like the Darwin notebooks.

History of medicine journals

Until 1933, German-language history of medicine periodicals were pre-eminent both in quantity and quality. *Sudhoffs Archiv* (1907–) maintains high standards. It also publishes in English and has an interesting series of *Beihefte* as supplements. Although there were a number of American history of medicine periodicals, and prior initiatives by William Osler and his circle, a new impetus was given by German scholarship, overcoming anti-German feelings after the 1914–18 war with the establishment of the American Association for the History of Medicine in 1924–5. This originated in the American delegation to Singer's International Society for the History of Medicine (Krumbhaar 1949; Miller 1976). An institute for the history of medicine, established at Johns Hopkins by William Welch, then attracted the Leipzig-trained Swiss scholar Sigerist. The *Bulletin of the History of Medicine* is now jointly published by the Johns Hopkins Institute and the Association. The *Journal of the History of Medicine* was established in 1946 but has in recent years adopted a controversial stance, criticizing social history and equal opportunities employment in editorials (Wilson 1980a,b). A similar but more sophisticated controversy has been conducted in the *Bulletin* (Fox 1980; Stephenson 1980).

The medical profession has taken particular pride in its achievements and there have been societies for the history of medicine in many countries. These fall into two categories – those with open access, and those with restricted membership. The latter tends to favour the development of exclusive and self-perpetuating élites. There is an International Academy of the History of Medicine, founded in 1962 with a membership limited to fifty fellows and fifty associates. Its journal is *Clio Medica*, although on occasions there have been tensions between the editor and the Academy (King 1976; Lesky 1976). The open and closed models for societies also have their respective supporters, thus giving rise to competition and furthering debate.

Although there has been a long tradition of medical societies in Britain, the development of diverse specialized organizations for the history of medicine did not occur until the twentieth century. The Royal Society of Medicine established a separate section for the history of medicine in 1912 with papers published in its *Proceedings*. The major society is the Society for the Social History of Medicine. There is a Scottish Society of the History of Medicine, and an Osler Club of London since 1928; the Society of Apothecaries has a faculty for the history and philosophy of medicine; and there are societies for pathological, veterinary and pharmaceutical history.

Although Henry Wellcome's plans for a museum of mankind were not realized, the establishment of the Wellcome Library and Medical Museum (which became the Wellcome Institute for the History of Medicine in 1968) has provided an institutional basis for serious study of medical history along with the establishment of units in the universities of London, Cambridge, Oxford and later Edinburgh. *Medical History* was begun in 1957 and from 1965 passed into the ownership of the Wellcome Trust. From 1965 until 1973 it also served as the organ of the British Society for the History of Medicine. This has been moribund since 1973, and only British subjects were eligible as members. There was a Wellcome Historical Monograph series from 1962 to 1973. The Wellcome Unit in Oxford has a series of *Research Publications* (1979–).

The Society for the Social History of Medicine has the largest membership of any medical history organization in Britain, and is an international society. It was established in 1970 and has consistently promoted a broad basis of interest among medical practitioners, historians and social scientists. It issues a *Bulletin*, including summaries of conference papers (of which there were 180 from 1970 to 1980) and details of research in progress.

From this survey it emerges that the history of science and medicine are multi-centred activities, thus encouraging diverse points of view. As a species of literature, periodicals in the history of science and medicine are an interesting hybrid between the clipped style of scientific communications and the more literary format of journals in the humanities. As an interdisciplinary approach to the history of science and medicine prevails, inconsistencies would be removed if abstracting services and bibliographies of the arts, social and natural sciences would include more coverage of history of science and medicine journals. It would also be helpful if there were more extensive bibliographies of relevant articles in non-specialized journals. But libraries and scholars in related areas will not give more attention to history of science and medicine journals unless high standards are maintained while greater breadth of approaches and depth of research are encouraged.

An important discrepancy is the comparatively large number of history of science journals with similar contents, in contrast to the very few journals for history of medicine. Whereas existing journals for the history of medicine cater for the scientific basis of medicine, there is a need for a historical journal concentrating on social rather than scientific aspects of medicine. Journals like *Social Science and Medicine* (now divided into sections for anthropology and medical sociology) have responded to this need. Coverage given to historical literature by the *British Medical Journal*, among other professional journals, is also symptomatic of the openness of the medical profession to historical causes of current concern. Journals for the history of medicine and science must therefore rise to a unique challenge of broadening perspectives in the humanities and bringing new historical and social concerns to medicine and the sciences. Only adoption of broader rather than restricted policies can achieve this.

Bibliography

America. History and Life. Vol. 1, No. 1–, 1964–. Santa Barbara, California; Clio Press

British Humanities Index. Vol. 1–, 1962. London; Library Association

British Union Catalogue of Periodicals (1955–8). 4 Vols. London; Butterworths Scientific Publications. *Supplement to 1960* (1962)

Cambridge Monographs on the History of Medicine, Vol. 1–, 1979–; Cambridge; Cambridge University Press

Curle, R.H.P. (1954). *The Ray Society. A Bibliographical History*. London; The Ray Society

Current Work in the History of Medicine. An International Bibliography (1954–). London; Wellcome Institute for the History of Medicine

Forster, R. and Ranum, O., Ed. (1975). *Biology of Man in History: Selections from the Annales, économies, sociétés, civilisations*. Baltimore and London; Johns Hopkins University Press

Fox, D.M. (1980). Rockefeller Medicine Men Again: Ideology vs. Methodology. An Essay Review, *Bulletin of the History of Medicine*, Vol. 54, 591–593

Garfield, E. (1980). Is Information Retrieval in the Arts and Humanities Inherently Different from that in Science? The Effect that ISI's Citation Index for the Arts and Humanities is Expected to have on Future Scholarship, *Library Quarterly*, Vol. 50, 40–57

Garrison, F.H. (1934). The Medical and Scientific Periodicals of the 17th and 18th Centuries, with a Revised Catalogue and Checklist, *Bulletin of the History of Medicine*, Vol. 2, 285–343

Grattan-Guinness, I. (1977). History of Science Journals: 'to be useful, and to the living'?, *Annals of Science*, Vol. 34, 193–202

Historical Abstracts. Vol. 1–, 1955–. Santa Barbara, Calif.; Clio Press

Humanities Index. Vol. 1–, 1974. New York; The H.W. Wilson Company

International Catalogue of Scientific Literature 1901–1904 (1902–18). 28 Vols. London; The Royal Society for the International Council

International Index to Periodicals (1907–1965). Vols. 1–18. New York; The H.W. Wilson Company. Originally published as *Readers' Guide to Periodical Literature Supplement*. Reprinted (n.d.)

Isis Critical Bibliography (1912–). Originally entitled: 'Bibliographie analytique des publications relatives à l'histoire de la science depuis le 1ier janvier 1912', *Isis*, Vol. 1, 136–192. Issued irregularly in *Isis* with changes of title as follows: No. 2 as (Bibliographie analytique', Vol. 1, 293–326. No. 4 as 'Bibliographie analytique de toutes les publications relatives à l'Histoire et à l'Organisation de la Science', Vol. 1, 757–824. No. 5 as 'Bibliographie analytique de toutes les publications relatives à l'Histoire, à la Philosophie et à l'Organisation de la Science', Vol. 2 (1914) 248–310. No. 7 as 'Critical Bibliography of the History, Philosophy and Organization of Science and of the History of Civilization', Vol. 3 (1920–1921) 90–154. No. 11 as 'Critical Bibliography of the History and Philosophy of Science and of the History of Civilization', Vol. 4 (1922) 390–453. No. 80 as 'Critical Bibliography of the History of Science and Its Cultural Influence', Vol. 49 (1955) 111–220. From Bibliography No. 92, Vol. 58 (1967) appears as Issue No. 5 of each annual volume. Note: *Isis* included in Vol. 2 (1914) 125–161, Sarton's *Bibliographie Synthétique des Revues et des Livres*

King, L.S. (1976). Clio Medica and the International Academy, *Clio Medica*, Vol. 11, 73–75

Kronick, D.A. (1958). The Fielding H. Garrison List of Medical and Scientific Periodicals in the 17th and 18th centuries; Addenda et Corrigenda, *Bulletin of the History of Medicine*, Vol. 32, 456–474

Kronick, D.A. (1974). Studies of the Early Scientific Journal. I. The Basic Source Lists, *Texas Reports on Biology and Medicine*, Vol. 32, 61–74

Kronick, D.A. (1976). *A History of Scientific and Technical Periodicals. The Origins and Development of the Scientific and Technical Press*, 2nd edn. Metuchen, NJ; The Scarecrow Press

Krumbhaar, E.B. (1949). Notes on the Early Days of the American Association of the History of Medicine, *Bulletin of the History of Medicine*, Vol. 23, 577–582

LeFanu, W.R. (1937–8). British Periodicals of Medicine: A Chronological List, *Bulletin of the Institute of the History of Medicine*, Vol. 5, 735–761, 827–846; Vol. 6, 614–648. Publ. sep. (1938). Baltimore; Johns Hopkins Press. Supplemented by A.M. Sheldrake (1963). British Medical Periodicals, 1938–61, *Bulletin of the Medical Library Association*, Vol. 51, 181–196

Lesky, E. (1976). Letter, *Clio Medica*, Vol. 11, 213

Manzer, B.M. (1977). *The Abstract Journal, 1790–1920: Origin, Development and Diffusion*. Metuchen, NJ and London; The Scarecrow Press

Miller, G. (1976). The Missing Seal, or Highlights of the First Half Century of the American Association for the History of Medicine, *Bulletin of the History of Medicine*, Vol. 50, 93–121

Neu, J. (1979). *Isis Cumulative Bibliography 1966–75. A Bibliography of the History of Science formed from Isis Critical Bibliographies 91–100.* Vol. 1, *Personalities and Institutions.* London; Mansell

New Periodical Titles (1964–80). London; Butterworths Scientific Publications

New Serial Titles 1950–1970. Subject Guide (1975). New York and London; Library of Congress

Obituary Notices of Fellows of the Royal Society (1901). Reprinted from the Yearbook of the Society, 1900, 1901. With an Index to the Obituaries published in the *Proceedings* from 1860–1899. London; Harrison and Sons

Publications in Historical Biobibliography (HIBB) (1980). No. 215. Newcastle upon Tyne

Research Publications. Vol. 1–, 1979–. Oxford; Wellcome Unit for the History of Medicine

Royal Society of London (1867–1925). *Catalogue of Scientific Papers, 1800–1900.* 19 Vols. London; HMSO and (from Vol. 9) Cambridge University Press

Sarton, G. (1952). Horus. A Guide to the History of Science. A First Guide for the Study of the History of Science, with Introductory Essays on Science and Tradition. New York; Ronald Press

Science Citation Index. Vol. 1, No. 1–, 1961–. Philadelphia; Institute for Scientific Information

Serials in the British Library. No. 1–, 1981–. London; British Library

Social Science Citation Index. Vol. 1, No. 1–, 1973–. Philadelphia; Institute for Scientific Information

Social Sciences and Humanities Index. Vols. 19–27, 1965–1974. New York; The H.W. Wilson Company

Stephenson, L.G. (1980). A Second Opinion, *Bulletin of the History of Medicine*, Vol. 54, 134–140

Thornton, J.L. and Tully, R.J. (1971). *Scientific Books, Libraries and Collectors. A Study of Bibliography and the Book Trade in Relation to Science*, 3rd edn. London; The Library Association. Reprinted (1975). Supplement to 3rd edn covering 1969–75 (1978)

Turner, G.L'E., Ed. (1976). *The Patronage of Science in the Nineteenth Century.* Leyden; Noordhoff International Publishing

Ulrich's International Periodicals Directory (1980), 19th edn. New York and London; Bowker

Union List of Serials in the United States and Canada (1965), 3rd edn. 5 Vols. New York; The H.W. Wilson Company

Wall, C.E., Ed. (1971). *Poole's Index to Periodical Literature. Cumulative Author Index, 1802–1906.* Ann Arbor; Piernan Press

The Waterloo Directory of Victorian Periodicals 1824–1900. Phase 1 (1976). By M. Wolff, J.S. North and D. Deering. Waterloo, Ontario; Wilfred Laurier Press for the University of Waterloo

Webster, C., Ed. (1974). *The Intellectual Revolution of the Seventeenth Century.* London; Routledge and Kegan Paul for Past and Present Publications

Webster, C., Ed. (1976–77). History and Education, *Oxford Review of Education*, Vol. 2, No. 3 and Vol. 3, No. 1

Webster, C., Ed. (1981). *Biology, Medicine and Society, 1840–1940.* Cambridge; Cambridge University Press for Past and Present Publications

The Wellesley Index to Victorian Periodicals, 1824–1900 (1966–). Ed. W.E. Houghton. London; Routledge (In progress: 3 Vols published)

Whitrow, M. (1972–76). *Isis Cumulative Bibliography: A Bibliography of the History of Science formed from Isis Critical Bibliographies, 1–90, 1913–65.* 3 Vols. London; Mansell

Wiener, P.P. and Noland, A. (1957). *Roots of Scientific Thought, a Cultural Perspective.* New York; Basic Books

Wilson, L.G. (1980a). Medical History Without Medicine, *Journal of the History of Medicine and Allied Sciences*, Vol. 35, 5–7

Wilson, L.G. (1980b). Inequality before the Law: Affirmative Action, *Journal of the History of Medicine and Allied Sciences*, Vol. 34, 377–379

Wilson, L.G. (1981). Schizophrenia in Learned Societies: Professionalism vs. Scholarship, *Journal of the History of Medicine and Allied Sciences*, Vol. 36, 5–8

World List of Scientific Periodicals Published in the Years 1900–1960 (1963–5), 4th edn. Ed. P. Brown and G.B. Stratton. 3 Vols. London; Butterworths

The Diseases and Casualties this Week.

Abortive	6	Kingsevil	10
Aged	54	Lethargy	1
Apoplexie	1	Murthered at Stepney	1
Bedridden	1	Palsie	2
Cancer	2	Plague	3880
Childbed	23	Plurisie	1
Chrisomes	15	Quinsie	6
Collick	1	Rickets	23
Consumption	174	Rising of the Lights	19
Convulsion	88	Rupture	2
Dropsie	40	Sciatica	1
Drowned 2, one at St. Kath- Tower, and one at Lambeth	2	Scowring	13
		Scurvy	1
Feaver	353	Sore legge	1
Fistula	1	Spotted Feaver and Purples	190
Flox and Small-pox	10	Starved at Nurse	1
Flux	2	Stilborn	8
Found dead in the Street at St. Bartholomew the Less	1	Stone	2
		Stopping of the stomach	16
Frighted	1	Strangury	1
Gangrene	1	Suddenly	1
Gowt	1	Surfeit	87
Grief	1	Teeth	113
Griping in the Guts	74	Thrush	3
Jaundies	3	Tissick	6
Imposthume	18	Ulcer	2
Infants	21	Vomiting	7
Kild by a fall down stairs at St. Thomas Apostle	1	Winde	8
		Wormes	18

```
           ⎧ Males──── 83 ⎫         ⎧ Males──── 2656 ⎫
Christned ⎨ Females── 83 ⎬ Buried ⎨ Females── 2663 ⎬ Plague──3880
           ⎩ In all───166 ⎭         ⎩ In all───5319 ⎭
```

Increased in the Burial this Week ──────── 1289
Parishes clear of the Plague ──── 34. Parishes Infected ──── 96

The Assize of Bread set forth by Order of the Lord Maior and Court of Aldermen,
A penny Wheaten Loaf to contain Nine Ounces and a half, and three
half-penny White Loaves the like weight.

Plate 3. London's dreadful visitation: or a collection of all the bills of
mortality for this present year. London; E. Cotes, 1665, fol.K2v,
deaths for 15–22 August 1665. By courtesy of the Wellcome Trustees

10

Research methods and sources

Paul Weindling

New research methods and priorities adopted by historians in recent years pose many challenges to historians of science and medicine. For example, debates are now raging over the application of quantitative methods of evidence, and over the extent to which science and medicine can be interpreted as ideologies. Yet traditional scholarly virtues, such as those relating to textual criticism, to the re-creation of past intellectual and religious systems of belief, or to the provision of basic narrative accounts, have frequently gone unheeded. Accusations of unhistorical procedures of historians of science were often levelled (as by Butterfield in 1950, Briggs in 1963 and Gowing in 1975), making it difficult for general historians to recognize history of science as fully historical. At the same time, apart from economic historians with narrow interests in technical change, general historians were by and large preoccupied with a restricted view of history, often confined to the securing of constitutional and religious liberties. This outlook was comparable to similarly 'whiggish' concerns of historians of science with scientific progress.

The aim of this chapter is to summarize recent historiographical developments for anyone embarking on research in the history of science and medicine. Historical procedures are not self-evident and there is considerable choice of methods and sources available. Comments are offered here on types of sources, on initiatives to ensure preservation of records, and on certain methods of analysis and interpretation. For although a rich variety of little-known and unused sources is available, lack of awareness of their historical importance results in further neglect, deterioration and – all too frequently – their destruction.

For those general historians interested in intellectual history, history of medicine and science have much to offer: But as historians have ventured into new areas of social history, such as demography, popular culture and class formation, a dilemma has developed for history of medicine and science. At worst, a new intolerance has arisen condemning medicine and science as insignificant and obscure aspects of élite culture, irrelevant to the understanding of the lives of the masses or of fundamental social processes like industrialization. Yet, at best, historians of medicine and science, along with the more enlightened social historians, are realizing that the shift of historical concerns greatly increases the historical relevance of health and science. Examples of the reversal of priorities underway are firstly study of medicine as concerned not just with great scientific discoveries but with the health of peoples, and secondly appreciation of science as a reflection of broader social conditions and values.

To some extent new aims mean reinterpretation and more effective use of readily available evidence. Historians of medicine and science may also benefit from or contribute to the work of general historians. For example, John Thelwall, a leading radical of the 1790s, looming large in Thompson's *Making of the English Working Class* (1968), also pioneered speech therapy (Rockey 1980). Rarely exploited material on health conditions poses immense challenges. Such additional sources must be located, and then efficient tools for their investigation have to be fashioned from the wide range of available concepts and analytical techniques, a few of which are discussed here.

It is part of the intrinsic fascination and general importance of history of medicine and science that they straddle the humanities, natural sciences and social sciences, drawing on and recruiting from a wide array of disciplines. There are, however, compelling arguments why history of science should be regarded methodologically as part of history and the social sciences. No amount of scientific knowledge or medical expertise can make a scientist or doctor an expert on the history of his discipline. But when scientists and doctors begin to view evidence historically – that is, in line with criteria of the past rather than the present – then they can be in an advantageous position to make effective contributions. Those trained in the humanities may have other advantages such as conceptual and historical knowledge and linguistic skills. The professions' aim should be maximum cooperation between and contributions from both humanities and sciences, preserving historical priorities.

In the decade since publication of the science-oriented volume *Modern Methods in the History of Medicine* (Clarke 1971), historians of medicine and science have responded to a variety of social and sociological approaches including structuralism and Foucault, anthropology, and historical geography (Young 1979). The argument has become increasingly untenable that the history of medicine is a branch of the history of science, itself an independent technical discipline, now that interest is no longer confined to those scientific innovations most relevant to modern theories.

Broadened perspectives raise new problems. For example, highly abstract conceptual superstructures may be imposed on sources that have been insufficiently mastered when judged by more traditional scholarly criteria. But such dangers are far outweighed by the gains from certain more rigorous historical procedures. For more sustained and historically sensitive methods are essential if the immense potentials of history of medicine and science are to be realized. Whatever conceptual breakthroughs there may be, the historian's craft will remain labour-intensive, requiring broad awareness of the conventions and dynamics of particular periods, mastery of local, personal and technical minutiae, together with scholarly accuracy and precision. Persistence in dealing with sources and imaginative sympathy with the very different priorities of past cultures will always be essential. Scholarly consensus emerges not from a single correct method, but from critical discussions and diversity of methods.

Social history itself requires a more complex multi-factoral approach than most historians of medicine and science have employed. Social history at its best thus increases the conceptual and factual burden, even if the rewards are ultimately greater. The trend away from synoptic histories of particular disciplines to smaller-scale investigations of particular social contexts increases the complexity of problems with the convergence of many different types of evidence (Macfarlane, Harrison and Jardine 1977: 36–7). For history of medicine and science should not be viewed as discrete entities with necessarily distinct sources. This is reflected in discussion of concepts that has reached a consensus of plurality (MacLeod 1977: 150). In practice, however, lack of historical acumen and craftsmanship in the working of source materials has hampered the efforts of historians of science.

Types of sources

Proof of the lack of uniform aims and methods in the history of medicine and science is provided by the wide range of sources used. For some, the starting point is scientific instruments and published papers; for others it is official state papers; and for others again it may be religious sermons and tracts. Some examples of the immense variety of sources employed are considered here.

Systematic cataloguing of previous experiments, of papers published on particular scientific problems or of surviving manuscripts can be of immense value to historical research. Such basic studies may also be of direct relevance to the practising scientist, who may wish to know of prior work on a topic or to clarify the meaning of terms. For example, scientists work historically, albeit in a limited sense, when considering certain questions like taxonomic classification or when criticizing past theories; doctors' case histories are also a type of history. Historians require basic bibliographical compilations to solve further problems with regard to chronology, influence of ideas and people, and institutions. More comprehensive information on scientific societies than in Hume (1847), and on medical practitioners and such institutions as dispensaries and hospitals, is also required.

Another point of departure may be the study of artefacts. This requires a combination of historical and technical skill. While scientific understanding is required for evaluation and preservation of instruments and machinery, it is also necessary to take account of human factors about makers and users. Artefacts may require varied techniques – for example physical anthropology applied to bone finds in order to establish past diseases (Armegelos, Mielke, Winter 1971); archaeological techniques for the remains of buildings; or chemistry and botany to evaluate agricultural improvements, manufacturing processes, drugs and herbal remedies. Extant written sources, such as recipe books, patents, plans, trade cards of instrument makers, should be taken into account. Visual representations such as maps and drawings, which may also rank as works of art, are also fundamental. Appreciation of scientific, medical or cosmological dimensions of works of art may often reveal meanings concealed from the modern eye. In the twentieth century, films and posters require preservation and study as striking features of scientific and health education.

Manuscript sources, which include personal papers such as diaries and letters, working materials like laboratory notebooks, and institutional and administrative documents, are still under-used. Laborious problems may be encountered at the basic level of deciphering handwriting or dating an item. Further difficulties abound at the conceptual level in evaluating medical or scientific procedures and the relations of sources with other printed materials and historical accounts. Historians of medicine and science vary greatly in their use of manuscripts: while failure to look for manuscripts may result in serious errors of interpretation, others become so embroiled in technical problems that they never evaluate their findings. Pioneering study of scientific manuscripts gathered momentum in the nineteenth century with, for example, Libri (1838–41), the historian of mathematics, and Halliwell-Phillipps (see Winsor 1881). But there is still a dearth of collected editions of papers, calendars of letters, or even skeleton checklists of correspondence and other types of private papers. Personal archives are on deposit in a wide range of locations ranging from university libraries, learned societies and record offices to descendants' attics and company warehouses. University College London provides an example of a rich and well-ordered collection of papers of such as Chadwick, Brougham, Galton and Pearson. The Department of Manuscripts at the British Library contains much material (for example, the Prosser collection and Alexander Fleming's papers) of medical, scientific and technological interest, and publishes catalogues of its holdings. In the course of this chapter, finding aids will be discussed.

Printed sources, like manuscripts, are extremely diverse. There are many gaps even in major national collections. At a basic bibliographical level many tasks remain. For example, although many printers and publishers had scientific interests, bibliographies of the works produced by particular printers and publishers are rare, let alone details of the number of copies in an edition. Library and sale catalogues have attracted more attention (Chalmers-Hunt 1976; Thornton and Tully 1971). Periodicals, abstract journals, encyclopaedias and handbooks also raise many bibliographical and historical problems.

Official archives and government records provide rich material about government policies towards science, medicine and education, and about scientists and their activities. They are also important in establishing the context of scientific and medical endeavour. Indeed the under-use of official source material shows that as yet few historians of science and medicine work as fully fledged historians. Some of this material – parliamentary debates and official, published reports and papers – lies in published records available in public and university libraries. Other official sources are either available in Britain in the Public Record Office or are still retained by government departments. Such material may lie in general series of government papers and committees from the Cabinet downwards, in the records of the establishments for scientific, medical and technological research and development, or in the records of government departments that sponsor scientific research or are responsible for scientific education at all levels.

In Britain, historians' use of such records has been erratic. Among the research establishments a few have received systematic attention – for example, the National Physics Laboratory, the Department of Science and Industrial Research, the botanical gardens at Kew, and the Greenwich Observatory. 'Official' – government-sponsored – history has used a variety of documents for histories of the design and development of radar and of the atomic energy project. A multi-volume history of the British medical services in the Second World War (MacNalty 1952–66) was written by doctors not historians, but Richard Titmuss's (1950) history of wartime social policy illuminated the history of the hospital services. The history of the National Health Service from 1947 to 1955 is being prepared by Charles Webster, a historian. There is still much work to be done on sources relating to medicine and science as used for military purposes.

Central government archives vary greatly in their finding aids. Thus the Public Record Office has lists of individual files but no indexes, so it is necessary to use the official guides and develop detective abilities. In the USA the National Archives and Records Service performs a function analogous to the Public Record Office, and the Library of Congress also holds important collections of documents. The National Archives has established two major centres. The holdings of the Center for Polar and Scientific Archives include the records of the Second World War scientific organization. The Center for Cartographic and Architectural Archives has a large variety of scientific and engineering graphs of the federal government from 1785 to the present.

The scope of central government archives clearly varies between countries according to government activities. Thus, where the central or state government has directly controlled academic funding and appointments, government records provide a rich source of information on scientific and medical education and research. In Germany, the records of individual states, rather than the central imperial administration, reveal much about the selection of candidates for appointments, funding, policy, numbers and background of students. In Britain and the USA, by way of further contrast, such information for universities would be available only in the records of individual educational institutions. Paradoxically, most, though not all, universities have been very lax in keeping their own archives.

Thus, particularly in countries with a strong federal system of government, state and local archives may be as or more important for medicine and science than central government archives. In Britain, local archives may include records of individual parishes, places of worship, poor law, schools and police, or manorial or borough records of corporations, courts and guilds (Martin and McIntyre 1972). County records may yield details of industries and public health. Ecclesiastical records may be important, for example in the episcopal licensing of medical practitioners. There are on deposit in local archives many records of scientific societies, schools, industries and hospitals. Many record offices in Britain have good indexes, have published certain types of records and hold specialist libraries. The Church of Jesus Christ of Latter-day Saints are compiling a computer file index to surviving English parish registers currently covering approximately 40 per cent of registers, and 90–95 per cent of London registers. Microfiches are also available at the Society of Genealogists and the Guildhall Library in the City of London. The activities of genealogists, sometimes wrongly despised, have acted as a check on the increasing inaccessibility of some important classes of record (such as wills) and have led to the availability of others in printed form (Camp 1974). The proceedings of archaeological, antiquarian, natural history and record societies have performed similar valuable functions.

Preserving the past

Museums are themselves a feature of the rise of science. They encompass many historical dimensions, such as collections and individual items with particularly interesting histories, and act as centres of historical research (Hudson 1975). There exist many specialist collections and museums for the history of crafts, industrial techniques, medicine and science. It will be to the great benefit of the history of medicine, science and technology as more museums make historical contributions by orienting policies relating to accessions, conservation and display to thorough historical understanding of the past priorities.

As a result of new historical approaches and the need for sources from hitherto neglected areas, several initiatives have combined the energies of archivists, curators, historians and librarians. There exist central directories of archival information such as the National Register of Archives in Britain and the National Historical Publications and Records Commission in the USA (1978b), and central catalogues of manuscripts for France at the Archives Nationales in Paris and for the Federal Republic of Germany at the Staatsbibliothek Preussischer Kulturbesitz in West Berlin. But effective preservation and use of resources require coordinated efforts by actively concerned groups.

The bulk of government and institutional modern records is so great that policies and procedures for the selection of records for preservation are essential. Questions of access may be difficult because of privacy and security requirements, although, if misapplied, these can result in restrictions on legitimate academic inquiries. In Britain, an inquiry into the public records system by the Public Records Committee has examined these issues (Wilson 1981). It includes a chapter on the massive problems of National Health Service records. The initiative in this area was most commendably taken by the Society for the Social History of Medicine. Currently, records prior to 1856 may not be destroyed. It would be simplest if this date were brought forward to 1918. Subsequent records should be treated as 'ancient monuments' of national importance: there should be surveys of surviving materials, public notification of impending destruction, and the right of appeal allowed. It must be stressed that both clinical and administrative records are of great interest to historians and social scientists. Non-government institutions and appropriate private individuals must equally be encouraged to arrange for the selection of documents for preservation, with advice from the historical profession, and to permit access where possible.

More care has been given to records of the history of science than to the more voluminous medical records. Greater pride is taken in scientific collections than in the records of state and private welfare organizations, hospitals, health insurance schemes and pharmaceutical manufacturers. Both in Britain and the USA pioneering initiatives were taken for scientific records in the 1960s, but preservation schemes for medical records have lagged behind in Britain and have hardly started in the USA.

The Contemporary Scientific Archives Centre in Oxford is a model of how a cost-effective scheme may achieve substantial results. The Centre grew out of concern in the 1960s that the records of individual scientists, medical researchers and engineers were being destroyed or dispersed for lack of any interest in their preservation. The combined initiative of Nicholas Kurti, the physicist, and Margaret Gowing, the historian, led to the establishment in 1973 of the Centre, which operates under the aegis of the

Royal Society. With a total staff of two, it locates papers of leading scientists as they die or retire, sorts and catalogues them. The collections – about eighty so far – are deposited in existing archives; the catalogues are kept centrally though are available in microfiche (Alton 1973–8) and are annually updated. The decentralization preserves long-standing connections and has avoided the need for a costly new repository. The Centre has adopted a wide definition of contemporary archives, emphasizing that personal letters and diaries, as well as professional and technical documents merit inclusion. Following the initiatives of the American Institute of Physics (AIP), a recent guide to scientists for organizing and preserving their own papers represents an important step in furthering historical awareness among scientists.

US efforts to preserve manuscript collections arose in the post-Sputnik period of international scientific competition (Weiner 1978). In 1960 a Conference on Scientific Manuscripts was held (*Conference on Science Manuscripts* 1962), and the issue was kept alive by Nathan Reingold of the Library of Congress. In 1961 a project on the archives for the history of quantum physics was launched with Thomas Kuhn as director and the American Physical Society and American Philosophical Society as sponsors; the American Institute of Physics also began a project on recent physics (Kuhn *et al.* 1967). Documents and photographs have been located, catalogued, micro-filmed and deposited, as well as transcripts of oral history interviews. A permanent Center for the History of Physics was established in the AIP. Subsequent projects have been on the development of the electronics industry by the Bancroft Library of the University of California and the Smithsonian, on the history of nuclear physics and chemistry at Berkeley, and the Berkeley Survey of Physics Sources. The American Philosophical Society has sponsored initiatives for the history of genetics with the *Mendel Newsletter*, and housed an international survey of sources for biochemistry with a newsletter (1973–8) leading to final publication of a report and a microfiche index of collections (Bearman and Edsall 1980).

The Charles Babbage Institute has a project underway for archives and history of computing, the US Geological Survey furthers research on the history of American geology, and the American Psychological Association sponsors a centre for the history of psychology at the University of Akron. The American Chemical Society, the Laser Institute and the American Genetics Society are following suit. These American initiatives are important and also heartening because they show the commitment of practising scientists and engineers to the history of their disciplines. Their emphasis on professionally conducted oral history as well as on documents is of value to posterity and in stimulating awareness of the historical dimensions to contemporary problems. It is unfortunate that no professional societies in Britain or other countries are following this lead, although a number of individual researchers and schools of librarianship have embarked on projects. In West Berlin there is the model institution of the archives of the Max-Planck-Gesellschaft and more dispersed initiatives exist in other countries. An interesting series of papers on archives was presented to the Fifteenth International Congress on the History of Science (Forbes 1978: 369–440).

Sources for the history of medicine are poorly served in contrast to the pure sciences. The National Library of Medicine (Bethesda, Maryland) preserves certain papers of modern physicians. Social welfare organizations have been surveyed for the State of Minnesota, and Margaret Dunn's survey of medical records in Ontario is one of several Canadian initiatives ('Archives and Medicine' 1980). Although during the national programme of the New Deal's Works Progress Administration, medical practitioners like midwives left testimonies, there is currently nothing comparable. In Britain, at a time when amalgamation and reorganization in the National Health Service jeopardized many collections and when the Public Records Committee was launched, the relevance of medical records to social history is being increasingly grasped (*Preservation of Medical and Public Health Records* 1979; Jordanova 1980), and efforts to preserve medical records have recently been made. Municipal and state medical activities have only fragmentary records, and destruction has continued. A few historians and archivists have pressed for measures and resources to preserve material, but even medical research has been hampered by destruction of records. A Contemporary Medical Archives Centre was established in 1979 on the pattern of the Contemporary Scientific Archives Centre at the Wellcome Institute to locate records, disseminate information about the value of medical records, and to house a selection of records of a wide range of medical practitioners. Significant regional initiatives have been mounted: in the South East with a Health Records Study Group; in the North Western Health Region based at the Department of History of Science and Technology, University of Manchester Institute of Science and Technology; by the Greater Glasgow Health Authority; and by the archives committee of the Liverpool Area Health Authority (Jordanova 1980).

For general historical purposes, the National Register of Archives (14 Quality Court, Chancery Lane, London) is an efficient means for locating collections through its reports and computer-collated lists of correspondence. The Register also houses reports on archives of hospitals and scientific societies. The handlist of sources for the historian of science, currently available for consultation, has now been published (Royal Commission on Historical Manuscripts 1982). MacLeod and Friday (1972) compiled a microfiche index to archives of British men of science, mainly for the period 1870–1950. A.C. Foskett (1970) has a useful guide to personal indexes. There are also helpful guides to certain types of sources: an example is Batts (1976) on manuscript diaries.

On the whole, the archives situation remains bleak. The US National Historical Publications and Records Commission complains of the paucity of readily available information about even those documents already in repositories (1978a: 22–3). Since 1974 it has established a records programme to identify and salvage sources. A Joint Committee on Archives of Science and Technology established in 1978 has come to the conclusion (Joint Committee of Archives of Science and Technology 1980) that the vast majority of records are destroyed without consideration of their historical value before they come to the attention of records managers and archivists. The Committee found that the US government research and development since the Second World War is virtually undocumented in official archives and that there is an immense backlog in federal record centres. It also established that the records of industrial research, professional associations and journals are particularly quickly destroyed.

Satisfactory decisions on selection of records are thus extremely difficult. For example, exclusive concern with the pre-eminent scientific and medical figures of today or with crucial experiments would be mistaken, and posterity will probably require information about a broad spectrum of activities and people in medicine and science. Historians must also bear this in mind when formulating research topics. No simple solutions exist; historians, archivists and records managers can and must work together to produce procedures and policies that are practicable and well thought out.

Research methods

There is the same rich variety of research methods and organizing concepts in the history of medicine and science as in all history. This survey shows something of this variety, and indicates some of the pitfalls.

At no stage has history of science been free from controversy over methods and concepts. For example, historians in the 1930s could choose between repetition of experiments, Marxist analyses of the effects of methods of production, or idealistic accounts of scientific progress according to an inherent and autonomous development of prevailing scientific knowledge.

Ironically, methods that might seem the most accurate and precise are open to serious objection and require judicious caution. Repetition of experiments is of particular interest in assessing factors limiting observational accuracy. However, history is rife with myths of crucial experiments, which can be misleading. An example is Galileo's law of falling bodies. Koyré (1937) pointed out that Galileo never performed and never mentioned the experiment at the Leaning Tower of Pisa, and further stressed that many of Galileo's experiments were only thought experiments, and that imagination and theory are essential to experimentation (1968). However, if contemporary conditions are strictly observed, the historian can make a practical contribution; Drake (1975) demonstrated that musical technique could provide the means for measuring time in experiments on falling bodies, although here too both accuracy and the narrowness of this approach have been questioned (e.g. Drake 1981).

The relations between observation, systematic experiments and intellectual commitments are the subject of much debate. Harvey's demonstration of cardiovascular circulation has been discussed in relation to questions of metaphysical and political belief, and the Darwin 'industry' has concentrated on relations between Darwin's observations and the principle of natural selection. Evaluation of experiment and observations requires broad consideration of technical, institutional, intellectual and psychological factors. Baker (1943, 1958) and Bradbury (1967) have conducted investigations on accuracy and aberrations in microscopy. Once it is established that certain observations were only artefacts, Koyré's theories on ideas and imagination in experiments are again relevant, and historians have spoken of the fantasy world of microscopy.

Institutional factors can affect equipment and research facilities as well as the social milieu in which investigations are conducted. Indeed, the dramatist Brecht suggested that there is an element of vulgar showmanship in certain of Galileo's experiments (1974). For experiments and mechanical contrivances have since the Renaissance been sources of entertainment and spectacle, into which economic applications may enter. There has been a long tradition of scientific showmen, ranging in the early nineteenth century from quack doctors using Mesmer's magnetism and phrenology to Humphry Davy's fashionable lectures (Altick 1978; Cooter forthcoming). These are echoed today by the Royal

Institution Christmas Lectures for children, and television series as by Jonathan Miller on the body and Robert Young on science and society. Similarly the wonders of the Renaissance *Kunst- und Wunderkammer* developed via the much maligned collector's cabinet into the modern public museum (Balsiger 1970). Another creative but neglected tradition is the literature on scientific and technological utopias, ranging from Bacon's *Solomon's House* to modern science fiction.

In the history of medicine, it is impossible to separate specialized expertise from broader cultural concerns. Technical knowledge, clinical experience and understanding of past social conditions are necessary for the fundamental task of reconstructing past morbidity. Diseases themselves and terminology can vary greatly according to time and place, and thus modern classifications may be inappropriate. Moreover, the incidence of diseases has changed: for example, in earlier ages leg ulcers were a major disabling factor (Loudon 1981) and diagnoses like 'chlorosis' or 'green sickness' once prevalent in young women have disappeared (Figlio 1978; Loudon 1980).

These examples suggest that neither medical scientists nor general historians can provide ready answers without systematic investigation requiring both social and technical understanding. A judicious and historically convincing balance between different aspects of the complexity of past cultural systems is by no means easy to attain. There have been recurrent discussions between adherents of mechanistic, vitalistic and other models of organization. Thus doctrinaire adherence to the mechanistic and corpuscularian theories in seventeenth-century science has obscured the continuing fruitfulness of Aristotelianism, vitalism and natural magic. Excessive emphasis on intellectual traditions may lead to failure to detect contemporary political or religious concerns. There are cases when the anxiety of historians to attribute developments to humanist scholarship has obscured the basis of some ideas in folklore and popular culture. Scientific concepts may change greatly in time, or may mean different things to different practitioners, or may have been translated in a variety of ways.

The relevance of contemporary psychology and sociology depends on the extent to which human nature and social processes are considered as constant or changing through time. Examples of psycho-historical analyses are provided by Manuel on Newton (1968) and Gruber on Darwin (1974). Writings of leading sociologists like Mannheim, Weber and the Frankfurt School have been applied to sciences and medicine by Merton (1938), Zilsel (1942) and Habermas (1971). Their concepts, as Jordanova suggests in chapter 5, have considerably enriched history of science, as when tracing the connections between the Puritan work ethic and the manual labour of experiments or the links between technology and socioeconomic needs. In recent years the motivation of social status has moved to the fore, along with concerns with the relativism of scientific truths. Much confusion has arisen due to differing definitions of current and past concepts. It is therefore valuable to maintain a personal index of definitions of terms in any specific area of interest.

Biography, collective biography and institutional analysis have all come into conflict at times (Holton 1970). Although historians are moving beyond praise of great experiments and selected geniuses, individual biography remains important. A helpful guide to individuals' bibliographies is proved by Arnim (1944–53). Detailed micro-studies can analyse how particular interests were formed and pursued, and how these related to cultural, economic, political, psychological and other social factors. Key figures such as Newton (Westfall 1980) and Darwin (Manier 1978) have been much scrutinized, and this process will go further as their neglected contemporaries are also studied.

Biography, autobiography and oral history all provide data for many purposes. The contribution of autobiography to history is revealing of both past circumstances and prejudices. This can also be a means of gathering and preserving sources. Besides the testimony of celebrities, accounts are much needed of day-to-day medical and scientific activities. These factors are also relevant to oral history. It is a technique of particular value – for non-literate cultures, patients' experiences and revealing the subjective side of scientific achievement. Interviewing and processing require considerable skill. One estimate is that it takes forty hours to process an hour's interview. Less has been done on oral history for medicine and sciences in the UK than the USA, but there is a lot of experience with social oral history (Thompson 1978). Oral history now has a journal, *Oral History*, the journal of the Oral History Society, and there is also an *International Journal of Oral History*. Oral history combined with anthropological concepts and techniques can be of use in the history of medicine. Anthropological and folkloric studies of customs, proverbs, recipes, songs and stories represent important but under-used methods, as Mac-Donald indicates in chapter 4.

In recent years historians of science have enthusiastically embraced prosopography. Pyenson (1977) has noted the important contributions at the turn of the century of classicists, eugenicists, genealogists, empirical sociologists and others who adopted a scientific approach to history. The term prosopography was used in the late sixteenth century to denote biography or personal appearance and has since come to mean systematically analysed collective biographies. Merton produced indices of intellectual achievement from the works of Sarton (1927–48) and of Darmstaedter (1908), and from the *Philosophical Transactions* (1665–1702) and the *Dictionary of National Biography* (1882–1900). After a generation of neglect, the approach was resumed by Shapin and Thackray (1974) in the wake of the social historian Stone (1971). Collective biography provides a means of analysing social movements in terms of component individuals. However, while age, career appointments, income and honours may be readily quantified, details relating to religion, occupation and political affiliations are liable to qualitative changes. Besides such obvious risks as confusion of individuals with the same name, prosopography may be too static and schematic. I would contend that it is important to present conclusions not just as statistics, but retaining individual biographical data, so that others may check on or use the information.

Biographical dictionaries have thus become much-used research aids. Of the specialist libraries, invaluable for study of particular groupings, excellent facilities are provided by Friends House in London for Quaker biography and by Dr Williams's Library, London, for other nonconformist sectarian intellectuals. In dictionaries, it is particularly helpful if comprehensive and uniform information is provided as in the *Neue Deutsche Biographie* (1953–), which systematically cites religion and parental and children's occupations; statistics of social mobility may readily be compiled from such information. But records of many doctors and scientists are difficult to obtain, presenting a challenge to historians who may use anything from registration of births to wills and gravestones.

Biographical information is often required for institutional analyses. There has been a long tradition of house histories of medical and scientific institutions. In recent years determined efforts have been made to study the origins and initial composition of major institutions like the Royal Society (Webster 1975; Hunter 1981), the Royal Institution (Berman 1978) and the British Association for the Advancement of Science (Morrell and Thackray 1981), but little has appeared on their subsequent history. Voyages of exploration have received due attention, and there has been renewed interest in the many minor scientific societies and mechanics' institutes (Ornstein 1928; Schofield 1963). These can be analysed using such criteria as patronage, levels of scientific expertise and other common cultural and economic interests. It is also necessary to take into account the extent of research facilities, financial arrangements and associated publications. Attendance registers provide a readily quantifiable source to gauge participation of individuals or factions. However, sheer longevity of certain institutions may be misleading, as the real centre of activities may have been elsewhere. Institutionalization is often defusing or defensive rather than innovating; movements can be half-dead or uninteresting by the time institutionalization occurs. Informal networks of patronage, friendships, family connections and apprenticeships should all be recognized as being of possible importance. Ian Inkster (1977) has stressed the impact of itinerant lecturers and short-lived scientific schools in the early nineteenth century. Medical institutions like hospitals, dispensaries and colleges pose similar problems. Besides traditional house histories, historians have recently tended to look 'out of doors' to unlicensed practitioners, dissident medical groups or rural practitioners who, in earlier centuries as in the Third World today, came from a wide range of occupations and offered diverse skills.

Historical accuracy does not necessarily depend on a restricted, technical approach to medicine and science. It is essential, however, to maintain standards of scholarly precision, whether biographical, chronological or terminological. For example, in references to botany, standard works like the *Flora Europaea* (1964–80) should be used; in geology, grid references would avoid ambiguity when discussing sites; in cytology, the works by Baker (1933) and Lee (1885) on staining, and editions of *Nomina Anatomica* (Warwick 1977) are useful. The study of reference works like encyclopaedias, handbooks, disease classifications and pharmacopaeias can be of considerable interest. Precision may be assisted by quantification (Hahn 1980), although many phenomena like morbidity may also require expression in qualitative terms. As Edge (1979) argued, quantification should not be a substitute for historical judgement. Pioneering uses of quantification were undertaken by Merton (1938), and by Ellegård (1958) on the diffusion of Darwinism. Ellegard assessed levels of scientific understanding of natural selection in general interest journals by a numerically quantified content analysis. Yet such methods tend to do injustice to concepts, especially when the material quantified may itself be oversimplified. Ben-David's statistics of discoveries in the medical sciences (1971: 189) are shakily based on Garrison's synoptic history (1929), which itself is highly selective. Attempts have been made to quantify citations, co-authorship, conference lists, visitors' books and acknowledgments as providing measurable indexes of scientific communication. As Edge suggests, these lead to distorted and overformalized explanations of the scientific community, and ignore cognitive factors (1979: 15). Caution must be exercised in deducing statistics; problems of making estimates when data are missing for one or more variables cannot be overcome unless there is certainty of a logical or statistical relationship between known and missing variables (Floud 1973: 178–82).

Quantification has immense potential in history of medicine, as basic data on many aspects are lacking. For example, in studying routine medical practice, patients' case histories can be analysed by occurrence of illnesses, prescribed treatments, patients' occupations and numbers of visits. Geographical distribution and types of medical practitioners are also readily shown in diagrammatic or quantified terms. Quantification is an established method in epidemiological and demographic studies, and arguments over the defects of earlier analyses are full of useful lessons: local conditions and differentiating factors relating to age, class and sex have often been overlooked (Imhof and Larsen 1975).

Some technical detail may be useful. In the systematic organization of data, card indexes are increasingly used. Most historians keep basic indexes of authors, biographies and subjects. More elaborate systems can reduce the evidence itself to cards. The more analytical a system is, the more important are the techniques for reconstituting information: for example, cross-referencing cards and carbon copies of evidence so that one copy is kept intact or broken down in a different way. Macfarlane *et al.* provide a good description of methods and problems of indexing in relation to analyses of village communities (1977: 89–98), and these methods are adaptable for medical and scientific communities. Manual analysis of data can be done by transferring data to punch cards, which can be sorted by machine or manually by using a knitting needle. It is imperative to sort out categories and order the data before transferral for computer analysis.

Broader perspectives of social history can thus demand more vigorous analysis, higher historical standards and a variety of techniques. Other questions and dimensions arise: past attitudes to medicine and science are assuming great current importance – as with hostility to vivisection, nuclear power or racism, for example, or with demands for alternatives to scientific medicine, and with feminism. Medicine and science may thus emerge historically not as catalogues of progress but as activities fraught by tensions between practitioners and researchers, and related to broader sociocultural issues. Indeed, the histories of particular disciplines and institutions already often include power struggles, but are frequently intended to enhance the stature of the victorious and diminish the role of the vanquished.

Given the challenge of new methods and sources, the problems of maintaining sound historical standards are great. Although the trend has been away from general histories of science to detailed research on limited areas, historians of science often betray lack of competence outside their areas of immediate expertise. Even in their chosen areas, concepts may be ineptly used: for example, 'radical' in politics, 'secularization' obscuring complex shifts in belief, or 'marginal' as a definition of social status. There is a tendency to erect polarities and attribute 'right' or 'wrong', 'progressive' or 'backward' theories, 'static' or 'dynamic' cosmologies. Greater authenticity demands more attention to sources and their context, as well as conceptual refinements.

To conclude: current practices are increasingly an amalgam of the sources, methods and concepts outlined here and by other contributors. The hope must be that a constructive synthesis will ultimately emergé between history, the social sciences and the history of medicine and science.

Acknowledgements

I am particularly indebted to Professor Margaret Gowing, Margaret Pelling and Roger Cooter for helpful comments.

Bibliography

Altick, R.D. (1978). *The Shows of London*. Cambridge, Mass.; Harvard University Press
Alton, J., Ed. (1973–8). *The Catalogues of Archives of Scientists Compiled by the Contemporary Scientific Archives Centre*. Oxford; Oxford Microform Publications
Archives and Medicine (1980). *Archivaria*, No. 10
Armegelos, G.J., Mielke, J.H. and Winter, J. (1971). *Bibliography of Human Paleopathology*. Amherst; University of Massachusetts
Arnim, M. (1944–53). *Internationale Personal Bibliographie. 1800–1943*, 2nd enlarged edn. 2 Vols. Stuttgart; Hiersemann. Continued by G. Bock and F. Hodes (1963). Vol. 3, *1944–1959*. Continued by F. Hodes (1978–). Vols 3/4, *1944–1975*. 8 Parts published so far
Baker, J.R. (1933). *Cytological Technique. The Principles and Practice of Methods Used to Determine the Structure of the Metazoan Cell*. London; Methuen

Baker, J.R. (1943). The Discovery of the Uses of Colouring Agents in Biological Micro-Technique, *Journal of the Queckett Microscopical Club*, ser. 4, Vol. 1, 256–327

Baker, J.R. (1958). *Principles of Biological Microtechnique. A Study of Fixation and Dyeing.* London; Methuen. New York; John Wiley and Sons

Balsiger, B.J. (1970). The Kunst und Wunderkammern: a Catalogue Raisonné of Collecting in Germany, France and England. 1565–1750, University of Pittsburgh PhD Dissertation. Also Ann Arbor; University Microfilms

Batts, J.S. (1976). *British Manuscript Diaries of the Nineteenth Century. An Annotated Listing.* Totowa, NJ; Rowman and Littlefield

Bearman, D. and Edsall, J.T., Ed. (1980). *Archival Sources for the History of Biochemistry and Molecular Biology. A Reference Guide and Report.* 1 Vol. and Microfiche Supplement. Boston, Mass.; American Academy of Arts and Sciences. Philadelphia; The American Philosophical Society

Ben-David, J. (1971). *The Scientist's Role in Society. A Comparative Study.* Englewood Cliffs, NJ; Prentice-Hall

Berman, M. (1978). *Social Change and Scientific Organization: the Royal Institution 1799–1844.* Ithaca, NY; Cornell University Press. London; Heinemann Educational Books

Bradbury, S. (1967). *The Evolution of the Microscope.* Oxford; Pergamon Press

Brecht, B. (1974). *Life of Galileo.* London; Eyre Methuen

Briggs, A. (1963). Discussion of A.C. Crombie and M. Hoskin, A Note on the History of Science as an Academic Discipline, in *Scientific Change.* Ed. A.C. Crombie. London; Heinemann, 765–769

Butterfield, H. (1950). The Historian and the History of Science, *Bulletin of the British Society of the History of Science*, Vol. 1, No. 3, 49–58

Camp, A.J. (1974). *Wills and their Whereabouts.* London; A.J. Camp

Chalmers-Hunt, J.M. (1976). *Natural History Auctions 1700–1972. A Register of Sales in the British Isles.* London; Sotherby Parke Bernet

Clarke, E., Ed. (1971). *Modern Methods in the History of Medicine.* London; Athlone Press

Collingwood, R.G. (1945). *The Idea of Nature.* Oxford; Clarendon Press

Conference on Science Manuscripts, The (1962). *Isis*, Vol. 53, No. 171, 1–157

Cooter, R.J. (forthcoming). *The Cultural Meaning of Popular Science. Phrenology and the Organization of Consent in Nineteenth-century Britain.* Cambridge; Cambridge University Press

Darmstaedter, L. (1908). *Handbuch zur Geschichte der Natur und der Technik. In chronologischer Darstellung*, 2nd edn. Berlin; Julius Springer

Dictionary of National Biography, The (1882–1900). Ed. L. Stephen and S. Lee. 63 Vols. London; Smith, Elder and Co. *Supplement.* (1901). 3 Vols. Reprinted in 22 Vols (1908–9). *Index and Epitome* [i.e. *Concise D.N.B. to 1900*] (1903). Thereafter in 5 decennial vols, from 1901 (1920–71). London; Oxford University Press. See also Institute of Historical Research, London, *Corrections and Additions to the Dictionary of National Biography Cumulated from the Bulletin...1923–1963* (1966). Boston, Mass.; G.K. Hall

Drake, S. (1975). The Role of Music in Galileo's Experiments, *Scientific American*, Vol. 232, 98–104

Drake, S. (1981). Alleged Departures from Galileo's Law of Descent, *Annals of Science*, Vol. 38, 339–342

Edge, D. (1979). Quantitative Measures of Communication in Science: a Critical Review, *History of Science*, Vol. 17, 102–134

Ellegård, A. (1958). Darwin and the General Reader. The Reception of Darwin's Theory of Evolution in the British Periodical Press, 1859–1872, *Göteborgs*

Universitets Årsskrift, Vol. 64, No. 7. Also published as Gothenburg Studies in English, Vol. 8

Figlio, K. (1978). Chlorosis and Chronic Disease in Nineteenth-Century Britain: The Social Constitution of Somatic Illness in a Capitalist Society, *Social History*, Vol. 3, 167–197. Revised version (1979). *International Journal of Health Services*, Vol. 8, 589–617

Flora Europaea (1964–1980). 5 Vols. Cambridge; Cambridge University Press

Floud, R. (1973). *An Introduction to Quantitative Methods for Historians*. London; Methuen

Forbes, E.G., Ed. (1978). *Human Implications of Scientific Advance. Proceedings of the XVth International Congress of the History of Science*. Edinburgh; Edinburgh University Press

Foskett, A.C. (1970). *A Guide to Personal Indexes Using Edge-notched, Uniterm and Peek-a-boo Cards*, 2nd edn. London; Clive Bingley

Garrison, F.H. (1929). *An Introduction to the History of Medicine*, 4th edn. Philadelphia and London; W.B. Saunders. Reprinted (1960)

Gowing, M. (1975). *What's Science to History or History to Science?* Oxford; Clarendon Press

Gruber, H.E. (1974). *Darwin on Man. A Psychological Study of Scientific Creativity. Together with Darwin's Early and Unpublished Notebooks*. Transcribed and annotated P.H. Barrett. New York; E.P. Dutton. London; Wildwood House

Habermas, J. (1971). *Knowledge and Human Interests*. Boston; Beacon Press. Also (1972). London; Heinemann

Hahn, R. (1980). *A Bibliography of Quantitative Studies on Science and its History*. Berkeley Papers in History of Science, 3. Berkeley; University of California

Holton, G., Ed. (1970). The Making of Modern Science Biographical Studies, *Daedalus*, Fall 1970, 723–1130. Issued as *Proceedings of the American Academy of Arts and Sciences*, Vol. 99, No. 4

Hudson, K. (1975). *A Social History of Museums: What the Visitors Thought*. Atlantic Highlands, NJ; Humanities Press

Hume, A. (1847). *The Learned Societies and Printing Clubs of the United Kingdom*. London; Longman, Brown, Green and Longmans. 2nd edn (1853) with Supplement by A.I. Evans. London; G. Willis

Hunter, M. (1981). *Science and Society in Restoration England*. Cambridge; Cambridge University Press

Imhof, A.E. and Larsen, Ø. (1975). *Sozialgeschichte und Medizin. Probleme der quantifizierenden Quellenbearbeitung in der Sozial- und Medizingeschichte*. Oslo; Universitetsforlaget. Stuttgart; Gustav Fischer Verlag

Inkster, I. (1977). Science and Society in the Metropolis: a Preliminary Examination of the Social and Institutional Context of the Askesian Society of London, 1796–1807, *Annals of Science*, Vol. 34, 1–32

Jayawardene, S.A. (1978). Western Scientific Manuscripts before 1600: a Checklist of Published Catalogues, *Annals of Science*, Vol. 35, 143–172

Jayawardene, S.A. (1982). *Handlist of Reference Books for the Historian of Science*. Science Museum Library Occasional Publications, 2. London; Science Museum

Joint Committee of Archives of Science and Technology (1980). *The Documentation of Science and Technology in America: Needs and Opportunities. Preliminary Report of the Joint Committee of Archives of Science and Technology. History of Science Society, Society of American Archivists, Society for the History of Technology*. [Typescript]

Jordanova, L.J., Ed. (1980). *Medical Records Newsletter*. Oxford; Wellcome Unit for the History of Medicine

Koyré, A. (1937). Galilée et l'expérience de Pise, *Annales de l'Université de Paris*, 441–453

Koyré, A. (1968). *Metaphysics and Measurement. Essays in Scientific Revolution.* London; Chapman and Hall

Kuhn, T.S., Heilbron, J.L. and Forman, P., Ed. (1967). *Sources for History of Quantum Physics.* Philadelphia; American Philosophical Society

Lee, A.B. (1885). *The Microtomist's Vade-Mecum. A Handbook of the Methods of Microscopic Anatomy.* London; J. & A. Churchill. 11th edn (1950)

Libri, G. (1838–41). *Histoire des sciences mathématiques en Italie, depuis la Renaissance des Lettres jusqu'à la fin du dix-septième siècle.* 4 Vols. Paris; J. Renouard et Cie

Loudon, I.S.L. (1980). Chlorosis, anaemia, and anorexia nervosa, *British Medical Journal*, Vol. 281, 1669–1675

Loudon, I.S.L. (1981). Leg Ulcers in the Eighteenth and Early Nineteenth Centuries, *The Journal of the Royal College of General Practitioners*, Vol. 31, 263–273

Macfarlane, A., Harrison, S. and Jardine, C. (1977). *Reconstructing Historical Communities.* Cambridge; Cambridge University Press

MacLeod, R.M. (1977). Changing Perspectives in the Social History of Science, in *Science, Technology and Society: A Cross-Disciplinary Perspective.* Ed. I. Spiegel–Rösing and D. Price. Beverly Hills and London; Sage, 149–195

MacLeod, R.M. and Friday, J.R. (1972). *Archives of British Men of Science.* London; Mansell

MacNalty, A.S., Ed.-in-Chief. (1952–66). *History of the Second World War. United Kingdom Medical Series.* 21 Vols. London; HMSO

Manier, E. (1978). *The Young Darwin and His Cultural Circle. A Study of the Influences which Helped Shape the Language and Logic of the First Drafts of the Theory of Natural Selection.* Boston; D. Reidel

Manuel, F. (1968). *A Portrait of Isaac Newton.* Cambridge, Mass.; Harvard University Press. Reprinted (1980). London; Frederick Mulder

Martin, G.H. and McIntyre, S. (1972). *A Bibliography of British and Irish Municipal History.* Vol. 1, *General Works.* Leicester; Leicester University Press

Merton, R.K. (1938). Science, Technology and Society in Seventeenth-Century England, *Osiris*, Vol. 4, 360–632. Reprinted with new introduction (1970). New York; Howard Fertig. (1978). New York; Humanities Press

Morrell, J.B. and Thackray, A. (1981). *Gentlemen of Science : The Early Years of the British Association for the Advancement of Science.* Oxford; Oxford University Press

National Historical Publications and Records Commission (1978a). *A Report to the President*, Washington DC; National Historical Publications and Records Commission

National Historical Publications and Records Commission (1978b). *Directory of Archives and Manuscripts Repositories in the United States.* Washington DC; National Archives and Records Service

Neue Deutsche Biographie (1953–). Berlin; Duncker & Humblot

Ornstein, M. (1928). *The Role of Scientific Societies in the Seventeenth Century.* Chicago; Chicago University Press

Preservation of Medical and Public Health Records, The (1979). Oxford; Wellcome Unit for the History of Medicine

Pyenson, L. (1977). 'Who the Guys were': Prosopography in the History of Science, *History of Science*, Vol. 15, 155–188

Rockey, D. (1980). *Speech Disorder in Nineteenth Century Britain. The History of Stuttering.* London; Croom Helm

Royal Commission on Historical Manuscripts (1982). *The Manuscript Papers of British Scientists 1600–1940*. London; HMSO

Sarton, G. (1927–48). *An Introduction to the History of Science*. 3 Vols. Baltimore; Williams and Wilkins

Schofield, R.E. (1963). Histories of Scientific Societies. Needs and Opportunities, *History of Science*, Vol. 2, 70–83

Shapin, S. and Thackray, A. (1974). Prosopography as a Research Tool in History of Science: the British Scientific Community 1700–1900, *History of Science*, Vol. 12, 1–28

Stone, L. (1971). Prosopography, *Daedalus*, Vol. 100, No. 4, 46–79

Stone, L. (1979). The Revival of Narrative: Reflections on a New Old History, *Past and Present*, No. 85, 3–24

Thackray, A. (1980). History of Science, in *A Guide to the Culture of Science, Technology and Medicine*. Ed. P.T. Durbin. New York; The Free Press. London; Collier Macmillan, 3–69

Thompson, E.P. (1968). *The Making of the English Working Class*. Harmondsworth; Penguin Books. 1st edn (1963). London; Victor Gollancz

Thompson, P. (1978). *Voice of the Past : Oral History*. Oxford; Oxford University Press

Thornton, J.L. and Tully, R.I.J. (1971). *Scientific Books, Libraries and Collectors. A Study of Bibliography and the Book Trade in Relation to Science*, 3rd edn. London; The Library Association. Reprinted (1975). Supplement to 3rd edn covering 1969–75 (1978)

Titmuss, R.M. (1950). *Problems of Social Policy. History of the Second World War. United Kingdom Civil Series*. London; HMSO

Warwick, R., Ed. (1977). *Nomina Anatomica*, 4th edn. Amsterdam and New York; Elsevier and North Holland

Webster, C. (1975). *The Great Instauration. Science, Medicine and Reform, 1626–1660*. London; Duckworth

Weiner, C. (1978). Sources for History of 20th-Century Science: Progress and Problems, in *Human Implications of Scientific Advance. Proceedings of the XVth International Congress of the History of Science*. Ed. E.G. Forbes. Edinburgh; Edinburgh University Press, 417–429

Westfall, R.S. (1980). *Never at Rest. A Biography of Isaac Newton*. Cambridge; Cambridge University Press

Wilson, D., Chairman (1981). *Modern Public Records. Selection and Access. Report of a Committee appointed by the Lord Chancellor*. London; HMSO

Winsor, J. (1881). *Halliwelliana: a Bibliography of the Publications of J.O. Halliwell-Phillipps*. Cambridge, Mass.; Harvard University Library

Young, R.M. (1979). Interpreting the Production of Science, *New Scientist*, Vol. 81, 1026–1028

Zilsel, E. (1942). The Sociological Roots of Science, *American Journal of Sociology*, Vol. 47, 544–562

Part III

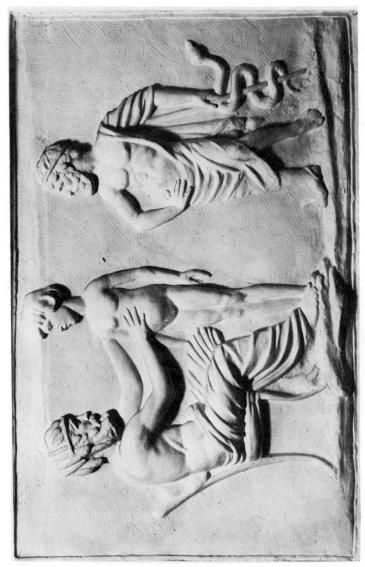

Plate 4. A physician palpating a boy with Aesculapius on the right. Plaque based on an intaglio gem of c. 350 BC. By courtesy of the Wellcome Trustees

11

Science, technology and medicine in the classical tradition

Gian Arturo Ferrari
Mario Vegetti

A view of the field

In the early 1950s Ludwig Edelstein published an important essay review of contributions to the study of classical science (1952). Edelstein was particularly well equipped to survey the literature critically . He was a historian of classical medicine with expertise in the technical and philological issues of the discipline; he was also a historian of ideas, fully aware of the historiographical implications of the categories to be used in dealing with classical science. The two studies he singled out for discussion represented differing historiographical and cultural approaches, though both works shared the assumption that it was possible to offer an emphatically one-dimensional view of Greek science, capable of explaining all its aspects. Moreover, the books reviewed by Edelstein constituted a synthesis and a summary of the historiography of classical science of the previous two decades.

The first of the two books was the massive anthology of primary sources of Greek science edited with critical commentary by M.R. Cohen and I.E. Drabkin (1948). This collection was designed to survey major contributions of the Greek classical tradition to a wide spectrum of disciplines and topics that later became part of the classical heritage of the Western world. The authors used the primary sources in order to reinforce their view that certain methodological features of Greek science were identical with those of modern science. Their selection of texts was thus guided by contemporary scientific priorities and theories. Cohen and Drabkin emphasized the modern distinction between scientific and philosophical or speculative theories, and stressed that Greek science was typified by quantitative approaches to the investigation of nature, by the experimental method, by concepts of mathematization of observational and experimental results, and by the idea of scientific progress. However selective, their criteria undoubtedly brought to light an important collection of texts; yet their emphasis on anachronistic priorities showed the limitation of their study and produced a severely reductive picture of Greek science.

The second book discussed by Edelstein was the history of Greek science by Benjamin Farrington (1944–9), who stressed the relationship between science and political or social ideologies in Greece. Farrington favoured a broad concept of science, inclusive of philosophy and characterized by the dialectical tension between social and political categories, such as 'democratic–oligarchic', or 'progressive–reactionary'. According to Farrington, Greek science had to be seen as divided into two main traditions: the manual, technical, experimentalist, materialist and inductive approach on the one hand, and the abstract, speculative, idealistic and deductive one on the other. The conflict between the two traditions ended with the victory – political and religious at first, and then also cultural – of the conservative and reactionary 'idealist' approach. This victory, the author maintained, was only apparent, since it marked the end, or at least the beginning of the decline, of the Greek scientific tradition, which had lost the vital support of technology and practice. Farrington's thesis was clearly ideologically motivated, although its merit was to emphasize tensions and contradictions within Greek science.

Edelstein was severely critical of Farrington, and sympathized with Cohen and Drabkin. The approach he favoured was, however, opposed to both of their positions. Edelstein was deeply suspicious of great historical syntheses, which to him reduced Greek science to a few selective features and constantly projected modern values into the study of the classical scientific tradition. He objected to Cohen and Drabkin's positivistic leanings, claiming that the modern demarcation between science and pseudo-science, or between science and philosophy, had either different meanings or indeed no meaning at all for the ancient world and the naturalists of the classical tradition. Cohen and Drabkin detached 'Baconian' elements from the mosaic of Greek science, and produced a reconstruction that had little historical credibility. Against Farrington, Edelstein pointed out that the great monuments of Greek science, the works by Ptolemy, Galen and Diophantus, were the product not of the Ionic democratic towns, but of the aristocratic Roman Empire. The heliocentric hypothesis invented by Aristarchus, which Farrington regarded as progressive and revolutionary, and therefore fated to be defeated with the victory of the aristocracy, was never opposed on political grounds. The Epicureans, progressives according to Farrington, were actually little concerned with science.

Edelstein's main contention was that every attempt at providing a comprehensive and consistent picture of Greek science failed to account for its most important feature, which made its study historically and epistemologically important: the Greek concept and practice of science fundamentally differed from those distinguishing modern science. Moreover, the most puzzling feature of this discrepancy was the fact that it characterized the early expressions of Greek science, as well as its more mature stage – the period of the great discoveries and syntheses of the Hellenistic and Imperial eras. Ptolemy was the author of treatises in which mathematical astronomy not only achieved superb mastery of calculus and a sophisticated capacity of prediction, but also represented a summa of ancient astrology.

Edelstein was receptive to ideas on science and the scientific profession elaborated by the German sociologist Max Weber, and consequently stressed that the main peculiarity of Greek science was the lack of integration of scientists and scientific disciplines within the broader social context. This view has been evaluated by Africa (1968), but not conclusively resolved. It could be argued that the sociological approach cannot provide a satisfactory explanation for the diversity of Greek science, for the simple reason that relevant documents and quantifiable data are extremely sparse. It is, however, to be noted that the historians of classical science have accepted Edelstein's main contention. Historians in the past twenty years have shown increasing reluctance to put forward unifying explanatory models for the development and decline of Greek science. Many of the certainties cherished by historians of previous decades now appear as problematic rather than one-sided or positively mistaken, and require critical evaluation on the available evidence.

It could therefore be said that the time for comprehensive

explanatory syntheses is over. Those historians who have approached the issue of Greek science with synthetic ambitions have tended to stress problems rather than certainties (Clagett 1957; Lloyd 1970, 1973). Others have concentrated their investigations on well-defined problems, such as the question of Roman science (Stahl 1962). Current research concentrates on the issue of evaluating the historical role of scientific traditions within the spectrum of disciplines that characterized mature Greek science. This choice has been favoured for various important reasons. Firstly, the study of internal developments within single disciplines like astronomy, mathematics or mechanics requires sophisticated technical expertise. Secondly, even when the name of an author of a scientific corpus was transmitted to posterity – like Hippocrates, Euclid or Hero – it is clear that the treatises were more likely to belong to a tradition than to be the product of a single author. Thirdly, historians have stressed that classical science was characterized by a plurality of rival theories that often flourished independently from each other and rarely interacted. Historians appear inclined to regard Greek science as a plurality of scientific traditions, occasionally in conflict but with none ever achieving final victory over its rivals. The scientific tradition is therefore the historical and epistemological category to be investigated by the historian of classical science. Modern epistemological doctrines concentrating on the transition from a particular theory to a more powerful and more comprehensive one hardly apply in the investigation of Greek science. Historians have directed their efforts to reconstructing the formation and development of particular scientific traditions, the 'mentality' and the ideological contexts that favoured their appearance, and the historically specific epistemological presuppositions and theories that distinguished them.

Techne

In ancient Greek, 'science' and 'technology' were represented by the words *'episteme'* and *'techne'*. However, it should be pointed out that the intellectual practices and the epistemological connotations denoted by these two words were subject to fundamental transformations. The decision about which discipline or type of knowledge belonged to the *techne* and which to the *episteme*, and the systematization of the 'sciences' into an epistemological hierarchy, were the result of a long and complex historical process and of deeply rooted cultural conflicts. The definition of *techne* that emerged from this process referred to any practical activity that required intellectual competence as well as manual dexterity, was based on scientific knowledge, produced results that it was possible to verify, and was governed by well-defined rules that could be transmitted through teaching. This epistemological model was established in the second half of the fifth century BC. It expressed the professional and methodological awareness of practitioners of Hippocratic medicine (Kudlien 1967). The model was then incorporated by Plato into his system, where it referred to all kinds of practical knowledge.

The origins of this model for *techne* were rooted in the mythical tradition. In the tragedy *Prometheus Bound*, written at the beginning of the fifth century, Aeschylus narrated that the hero had stolen the *technai* from the gods, to give them to man. The gift included techniques for the control and the exploitation of nature, such as agriculture and animal husbandry, but also advanced technologies such as metallurgy and navigation, or specific forms of knowledge such as medicine, calculus, writing and divination (Vernant 1965). Some technological activities included by Aeschylus in the definition of *techne* clearly represented long family and communal traditions of skilled craftsmanship. Blacksmiths, doctors and soothsayers were already described by Homer and Hesiod. However, it was within the *polis*, and within the context of the basically egalitarian political atmosphere of the city states, that craftsmen and practitioners of a variety of techniques attained social esteem; and here they elaborated sophisticated intellectual rationalizations of their practices. The transformation was characterized by two major features. Firstly, there was a transition from the mere practice of a craft to the explicit awareness that it implied a rigorous method that guaranteed the rationality and efficacy of the technique deployed. Secondly, the view of a cultural system consisting of a plurality of *technai* emerged within the *polis* (Vernant 1962; Kahn 1960). The *technai* were not seen as controlled by gods; indeed medical practitioners or astronomers and meteorologists were competing against religious personnel providing similar services. The *technai* were described as supported by the autonomous rationality of their method, their efficacy and their proven utility to the society of the *polis*. This was the case with medicine, historiography, architecture, town planning, geography and meteorology. Practitioners of meteorology succeeded in taking control of the calendar away from the Lords of the Time, the figures representing the religious tradition and responsible for the division of the seasons and years (Levêque and Vidal Naquet 1964).

It should be pointed out that the legend of the transmission of the *technai* to men by Prometheus, narrated by Aeschylus, indicated the existence of a rift between gods and men. The gap was further widened as the practitioners of the *technai* attempted to invade fields of activity traditionally monopolized by priests. The success of these attempts contributed to the final decline of the view of human history put forward by Hesiod, who maintained that in the 'age of iron' following the Promethean gift mankind reached the peak of decadence and of estrangement from the gods. The new conception of human history stressed instead that the *technai* freed men from their dependence on the gods and nature. The *technai* were also responsible for the growth of man's power and knowledge, and for the building of a civilization made by men and based on dominion over nature. The fifth century BC thus witnessed the appearance of an ideology of *techne*. The idea of the *homo faber* formulated by Democritus became the key concept of a tradition extending to the Latin poet and philosopher Lucretius, and to the Roman architect Vitruvius (Cole 1967).

It is, however, also to be pointed out that the development of a professional and methodological awareness by practitioners of the *technai* did not imply a complete and radical break with the original dimensions of technological activities. Thus, for instance, the therapeutic success of a medical practitioner was still seen as depending on magical elements, notwithstanding the marked professional difference between doctors and magicians. The figure of Empedocles, shaman and medical practitioner at the same time, well illustrates this point (Temkin 1953; Bollack 1965; Lloyd 1979). Political ideologies and mythical priorities still influenced the articulation of the new forms of knowledge. At the same time, the professional milieu of the *technai* showed little concern for technological innovation and practical applications. There were no institutional structures such as schools devoted to a systematic training of craftsmen. There was no established curriculum of studies that commanded approval and recognition from political or social bodies (Lloyd 1970). Thus, the practitioners of the *technai* were constantly under pressure to defend and justify their claim to be the true *technitai* (technologists) against rival claims by so-called quacks. This defensive exercise was particularly necessary in medicine, as shown by treatises produced by 'Hippocratic' practitioners and Galen himself. The situation of practitioners of the *technai* was thus precarious and vulnerable to changing political and cultural moods or to social developments. The privileged position that practitioners of the *technai* achieved during the fifth century BC appeared as an anachronistic chimera in the changed political situation of the next century (Edelstein 1967a).

Episteme

The form of knowledge at the basis of the *technai* was sometimes described as *episteme*, 'science'. The term did, however, come to refer to a distinctive cultural tradition. At the beginning of the fourth century BC, Plato pointed out that *episteme* was self-evident and certain knowledge, removed from the uncertainty of experience and from the practice of crafts. *Episteme* was concerned with a particular class of objects not subjected to change and deterioration. Plato identified these objects with 'ideas', which were seen as real entities, the only 'objects' in the proper sense of the term. The ensuing Platonic tradition classified the objects with which *episteme* concerned itself into two primary categories: the forms of language, capable of expressing rational contents, and the mathematical forms, arithmetic and above all geometry.

The individuation of a specific and particular class of objects for *episteme* was the key element of a cultural tradition different from, and to some extent opposed to, the culture of the *technai*. The definition of *episteme* emerged from sacred and shamanic traditions. It was elaborated by the 'masters of truth', a category of individuals connected with political rulers, the temple and the exercise of religious rituals (Detienne 1967). They maintained that knowledge was primarily initiation and revelation. Even though the formulation of this concept became increasingly more circumscribed, the 'masters of truth' maintained that the source and the object of knowledge was the divine, and that the divinely inspired word was the best means of propagating it. The sacred context for the production of this kind of knowledge represented the guarantee of its purity and certainty. It should be stressed that the transition (especially by Parmenides and the Pythagoreans) from the ancient holy wisdom of the 'masters of truth' to the new forms of abstract and rational knowledge took place within the sacred tradition. Investigations by Burkert (1972) emphasized the religious and cult-like features of the early Pythagorean movement. Representatives of this tradition expressed the conviction that the astronomical order was the visible image of the divine order, and that mathematics represented the indispensable key to understanding it. This idea was central to the writings of Philolaus and of the Pythagoreans of the fifth century BC. It was from them that Plato and representatives of the astronomical school at the Academy borrowed crucial elements of their philosophical system. Von Fritz (1971) has also pointed out the relevance of Parmenides' powerful analytical thought for the development of forms of abstract logic and mathematical reasoning.

The idea of *episteme* underlying these traditions of thought was therefore deeply rooted in sacred forms and sought to be regarded as the only true form of knowledge, in contrast to other beliefs, which were condemned as ill-founded, impure and contradictory. This was the context that favoured the development of the Platonic epistemological and ontological opposition between 'truth' and 'opinion'. However, Plato himself attempted a conciliation between the two conflicting forms of knowledge. His solution was a hierarchical scheme that put *episteme*, represented by mathematics and astronomy, at the top of man's intellectual activities. The *theoria* was seen as extending the borders of human rationality, and bringing the world to the contemplation of the divine order. The *technai*, concerned with objects subjected to perpetual change through space and time, were seen as inferior to *episteme*. The hierarchy was therefore determined by the nature of the objects investigated, even though Plato acknowledged that both *episteme* and *techne* represented important epistemological values. *Episteme* was characterized by theoretical purity, and by the permanence and truth of its result, which gave it pre-eminence and authority. Practitioners of the *technai*, on the other hand, could boast of the practical efficacy of their methods. Indeed the Platonic dialogue *Timaeus* told of a divine craftsman who ordered the world. The practical relevance of the *technai* was indispensable to the dialectical process through which the philosopher was to transform the existing ethical and political system. Thus the *techne* was seen as the paradigm of productive and efficient knowledge, as important to the activities of the Platonic philosopher-king as was pure theory (Cambiano 1971).

The dream of a dialectical transformation of society faded away, but the intellectual tradition of the Academy and of Platonism stressed the primacy of mathematical knowledge – its superior epistemological dignity and moral value. Aristotle himself accepted the Platonic hierarchy of knowledge, and stressed with even greater emphasis the superiority of *episteme* over *techne*. He did nevertheless considerably expand the sphere of pure theory, since he included within *episteme* objects subjected to change in space and time which Plato and the Platonic tradition had rejected. Natural sciences, from physics to meteorology and zoology, were no longer seen as inferior to mathematics, provided the epistemological requirements of *episteme* were followed. The hierarchy of knowledge was therefore seen as introducing demarcations not between the objects to be investigated, but between two different approaches to research. Thus, for instance, anatomical and physiological features of the medical *techne* were seen as belonging to the section of *episteme* dealing with natural products, and medical *techne* was reduced to therapeutic practice. *Episteme* was thus seen as pure theoretical knowledge, and *techne* as the activity directed to produce and transform objects and natural processes. The new epistemological hierarchy had clear sociological implications. It justified the creation of the Lyceum, the first scientific institution of the Greek world, which was designed to house personnel engaged in theoretical investigation. The Lyceum provided them with adequate instruments for research, and in particular with a library organized by disciplines. In contrast, the practitioners of the *technai* – from doctors to architects and engineers – exercised their skills outside institutional frameworks. Some did of course gain wealth and prestige, but their social position prevented them from attaining the intellectual leadership that had been sought during the fifth century BC.

The sacred tradition

Historical investigations have shown how various forms of *episteme* and *techne* did not represent a clear-cut break from the pre-scientific tradition. Their mature epistemological organization and their growth were influenced by the 'mentality' as well as by the social, ideological and professional conflicts that characterized the early phases of their development. Various examples can be offered of the close links between ancient sacred traditions and the organization of new forms of knowledge. Thus, for instance, astronomers of the fourth century BC severed their connections with meteorologists on the one hand, and with compilers of calendars on the other. Both moves were motivated by the desire to dispense with empirical observation and prediction. Astronomers stressed the value of their investigations in terms of pure knowledge and in the religious terms of the Pythagorean and Platonic traditions, which emphasized the sacredness of the heavens. The consequence of this development was further mathematization of astronomy, a move that could be described as 'rational' in modern terms but was deeply rooted in the religious tradition. Moreover, astronomers pointed out that anomalies of observational data had to be eliminated, since the movements of heavenly bodies were perfect by definition. They therefore multiplied their efforts to devise mathematical models capable of reducing anomalies to order. The Platonic problem of 'saving the appearance' stressed interpreting irregularities of planetary motions as mistakes of observation: truth lay in the 'real' regularity of the heavens, which was to be expressed in mathematical terms. The reduction to mathematical regularity of planetary motions represented one of the major problems of ancient astronomy (Mittelstrass 1962).

Lloyd (1966) has shown that various Pythagorean polarities, based on opposites such as light–darkness, hot–cold, male–female, etc., typical of more ancient mentalities, did in fact influence the organization of disciplines despite apparent 'purification' from pre-scientific elements. Thus, for instance, the Aristotelian biological theory that represented the female as the cold, humid, material element, opposed to the male principle of heat and form, was reminiscent of ancient polarities. Even more influenced by traditional beliefs were the domains of the life sciences, such as anatomy, zoology, botany and medicine. The Aristotelian anatomical map, which could be seen as an epistemological break with traditional conceptions, was in fact evocative of the topology typical of sacrificial practices and of the sacred division of parts of animal bodies between men and gods (Detienne 1972; Detienne and Vernant 1979).

Botanical and zoological taxonomies produced during the fourth century BC by Aristotle, Theophrastus and their disciples were still organized according to mythical preconceptions, which accorded plants and animals an intermediate sphere in the cosmos between men and the gods (Detienne 1972; Detienne and Vernant 1974; Dierauer 1977). As far as medicine was concerned, practitioners of the fifth century BC stressed the rationality of their methods. Yet this did not imply the abandonment of magic and superstitious presuppositions regarding therapeutic practices. Female sterility was cured with fumigation of the uterus by sexual organs of stags, and the flesh of various animals was credited with different dietetic virtues (Joly 1966). Medical treatises, as well as texts of the Aristotelian corpus, often showed the influence of mystical number theories. The number seven was thought to be relevant to the psychological and physiological development of man: for example, female fertility started at the age of 14, male fertility at 21 (Mansfeld 1971).

Psychological and anthropological theories were deeply influenced by extra-scientific traditions. Sources from Empedocles to Aristotle and the Stoics stressed that blood and the heart were the principles of life, both organic and psychic. The primacy of blood is easily explained by primitive linking of blood to life, and to magical interpretations of the role of the blood in vital functions. Moreover, the connection of blood with organic heat made it possible to interpret this principle according to the Pythagorean polarities described above. The shift of the principle of life from the blood to the heart was stressed by medical theoreticians and biologists of the fourth century BC, and was determined by anatomical considerations. However, the supremacy of the heart over the brain and the sense organs was also maintained. With Aristotle and the Stoics, the primacy of the heart reflected the widespread monarchical ideologies of the time, and purported to offer a view of man centred on a single principle, at both the physiological and political levels. In contrast, medical thought of the fifth century BC emphasized the primacy of the brain, at both anthropological and psychological levels. This conviction probably reflected the fading of beliefs in magical connections between man and nature. Human intelligence was seen as capable of control and transformation of nature through the *technai*.

Plato made use of the polarity in his system. He saw the human soul as divided into three parts: the brain was the seat of reason, the heart of passions, and the viscera of greed. It is clear that Plato's divisions did not derive from explanatory needs of biology, but were instead motivated by the intention of establishing a political relationship between the body, the soul and the city state. It is perhaps surprising to note that Plato's psychological and political explanatory model was found to agree with the conclusions of the far more advanced Alexandrian school of anatomy and physiology. Galen reinterpreted the Platonic model in terms of the relationships linking the nervous system to the brain, the arterial system to the heart, and the venous system to the liver. Thus, the Platonic model was preserved without losing its political and anthropological connotations, and became the dominant paradigm for biological investigation. The Galenic division represented the last development of ancient physiology. As a consequence, the cardiocentric tradition of Empedocles, Aristotle and the Stoics, as well as the Hippocratic brain-centred scheme, were finally abandoned (Manuli and Vegetti 1977; Harris 1973).

Scientific treatises and teaching

The fourth century BC witnessed deep changes in the concept of rationality and the institutional organization of scientific knowledge. As far as the criteria of rationality were concerned, recent historiography has stressed the influence of the diffusion of writing on the scientific 'mentality' as well as on the actual production and circulation of knowledge (Havelock 1963). The alphabet provided the model for the constitution of systems open to infinite variation of combinations although based on a limited number of components (*stoicheia*). Moreover, the system was interpreted by reducing it to its components. The atomistic physics of Democritus was evocative of the *stoicheia* (Ferrari 1980; Wissman 1980). The model of rationality suggested by the alphabet reached the peak of its influence in the fourth century BC, as witnessed by Euclid's *Elements* in mathematics and by developments in anatomy. Traditional anatomical doctrines looked on living beings as containers. The surface only was known, as well as the input – food, air – and the output – excrement, cathartic products etc. Aristotle introduced a comparative anatomical approach. The organism was now analysed in terms of its primary elements, i.e. of internal organs and tissues, and interpreted as a system endowed with various levels of complexity (Preus 1975; Vegetti 1979).

The concept of rationality embodied in the *stoicheia* had a further point of contact with the development of writing. The fourth century BC saw the composition of scientific treatises. This development favoured the relative independence of various forms of knowledge from their earlier sacred, social and professional contexts. The scientific treatise promoted disciplinary competence; indeed, the writing of treatises and the division of knowledge into various disciplines were parallel processes. The composition of treatises also favoured the compilation of bibliographies for each discipline. Aristotle and his school introduced the practice of doxography, the compiling of opinions and ideas on a subject by various authors of the past. The treatise was moreover open to further developments of disciplinary knowledge, expressed in the form of commentaries on texts. The literary context of the text and the commentaries provided the basis for the development of the concept of the linear and cumulative progress of scientific knowledge. This idea was explicitly formulated in late classical science by Galen and Ptolomy, but was already implicit in the writings of Aristotle (Edelstein 1967b; Dodds 1973).

Aristotle's contribution to the development of new forms of scientific rationality can hardly be overemphasized. Many studies have stressed his importance for the classical scientific tradition (Düring 1966). The traditional image of Aristotle as the metaphysician, who deduced scientific knowledge from the first principles of theology and ontology, has been subjected to fundamental revision. Historians have analysed the actual research methods employed by Aristotle. The analysis of language and the study of the learning handed down by tradition and of the knowledge embodied in the *technai* were important features of the Aristotelian methodology, as was the approach to scientific investigation that selected specific problems for thorough research.

Aristotle was responsible for the foundation of a variety of autonomous scientific disciplines from zoology to meteorology. He provided these disciplines with a conceptual framework that made them part of a comprehensive encyclopaedia of knowledge. Concepts such as teleology, the four modes of causation, or the pairs form–matter or act–power, provided the unified scheme of reference for all disciplines, whose autonomy was guaranteed by the epistemological presupposition that each single science was organized according to a set of principles, inductively derived from observation of phenomena.

Aristotle also provided the newly developed disciplines with an appropriate institutional basis. The Aristotelian Lyceum or Peripatos was the first Greek 'school' to organize relatively continuous scientific investigation. The Lyceum was provided with a library preserving material relevant to each discipline, and promoted a series of specialized investigations supervised by the philosopher at the head of the school. In contrast to the Platonic Academy, the Lyceum served no immediate political purpose: research and teaching were its primary functions (Lynch 1972).

The Museum of Alexandria

The Museum of Alexandria was established at the beginning of the third century BC under the patronage of King Ptolomaeus I. A group of advisers formerly linked with the Lyceum, including Demetrius of Phalerum and Straton, were the actual initiators of the institution, which implemented the teaching and the organizational structure of the institution established by Aristotle. Fraser (1972) conducted thorough investigations of the institutional features and the teaching at the Museum. It was endowed with a library designed to collect all literary productions up to the present. It has been noted that the problem posed by the classification of the library material reinforced the tendency to use specialized treatises as the favoured means of scientific communication: books had to have an author, a title, and a disciplinary concern. This kind of classificatory preoccupation was at the basis of the formation of the *Corpus Hippocraticum*. The entire medical literature of the fifth and fourth centuries BC, including lectures, professional textbooks, notes for teaching purposes, etc., was organized according to 'works' on single features of medical science and practice. Titles were given and the name of Hippocrates was furnished as the author of all treatises. The fame of Hippocrates guaranteed the success of the collection. The Museum also housed men of science for various disciplines and from every corner of Greece. The Museum was organized according to disciplinary specialities, and there was no place for the philosopher–leader unifying the sciences in an encyclopaedia of knowledge; though under the king's patronage, the scientists did not appear to have lost their intellectual independence. It has however been noted that the organization of the Museum favoured the detachment of the scientist from the society he lived in. The Museum also became the centre of an embryonic scientific community. Scientists, such as Archimedes of Syracuse, living in other regions were connected with the group established in Alexandria (Lloyd 1979). The Museum also favoured the division between theoretical sciences and professional practices. The doctors who took part in the activities of the Museum were biologists rather than practitioners, and their influence on the medical profession was slight.

Mathematics

From the third century BC to the second century AD the Museum was the focus for major developments of classical science. A survey of disciplines studied there, and of studies concerned with the work of the Museum, must start with consideration of mathematical doctrines and teaching. This sector of studies has witnessed important historiographical reassessment. Historians of mathematics active at the end of the nineteenth century and at the beginning of the twentieth century assumed that Greek mathematics constituted a monolithic body of knowledge from Thales to the commentaries of Proclus. This view was shared by historians of idealistic leanings and by philosophers inspired by the Platonist tradition, who stressed the continuity of philosophical developments from Pythagoras and Plato up to Plotinus. This line of thought was construed as the dominant feature of classical philosophy. The rational structure of mathematical theorems and the logico-deductive structure of axiomatic procedures were seen as the distinguishing features of the intellectual 'purity' of Greek mathematics, the dimension that emphasized its 'classical' nature. Further investigation has substantially questioned the lineality and 'purity' of this interpretation. Firstly, thorough analysis of non-Greek mathematical systems, the Babylonian ones in particular, has shown their highly sophisticated technical capacity. These non-Greek mathematical systems were not oriented towards geometrical treatment of mathematical problems and favoured a numerical and algebraic approach, characterized by a strong emphasis on calculus. It was further noted that Hellenistic mathematics reached the peak of its development only after being exposed to foreign influence (van der Waerden 1954; Neugebauer 1957). Secondly, various authors (Becker 1957; Lasserre 1964; Szabo 1969) have pointed out that the axiomatic method was introduced into Greek mathematics only in the fourth century BC. This led to the sophisticated system of Euclid's *Elements*, but signified at the same time the abandonment of previous and to some extent more flexible methods for solving certain types of problems. Lasserre (1966) concentrated his investigation on the work of Eudoxus, one of the figures responsible for the introduction of the axiomatic method. Moreover, historians have analysed Euclid's work searching for traces of systems of traditional and pre-axiomatic mathematical thought embodied in the *Elements* (Cambiano 1967; Knorr 1975). Thirdly, Dijksterhuis (1956) has conducted innovative investigations of the work of Archimedes, and Clagett (1964–80) has shown the persistence of the Archimedean tradition through the Middle Ages. Both authors agreed that Archimedes' thought cannot be described in terms of neo-Platonic philosophy as proposed by Proclus and a long tradition of historians of mathematics. Indeed, Archimedes' mathematical preoccupations were varied, ranging from systems of numbers and obsession with infinity to practical and theoretical mechanical concerns, and the combined use of heuristic and demonstrative methods.

Astronomy

According to the author of the pseudo-Platonic treatise *Epinomides* (probably Philippus of Opunte), numbers were donated to man by the heavens, in the sense that the diurnal sequence of astronomical phenomena, phases of the moon, months and years were divinely pre-ordained to teach numbers and calculus to mortals. The Greek scientific tradition was indeed characterized by the constant relationship between mathematics and astronomy. The close links between the two sciences dated from the beginning of astronomy (van der Waerden 1965), and were expressed by the geometrical model of the universe as composed of two spheres (Kuhn 1957). Historians have recently expanded upon earlier investigations of the astronomico-geometrical model. Pioneering research by the Italian astronomer and historian Schiaparelli (1925–7) on the homocentric planetary spheres invented by Eudoxus has been reassessed by Maula (1974), who has stressed the importance of this model as the first systematic attempt to come to terms with observational anomalies, and its relevance to the development of Aristotelian cosmology. The model also represented the harmonious combination of geometrical concepts with the theory of proportions.

Historians have however devoted more attention to 'mature' Greek astronomy, to the Ptolemaic tradition in particular. Pedersen (1974) has provided a general survey of the historical development of Ptolemaic astronomy, and Newton (1977) has discussed the accuracy and reliability of astronomical observations recorded by Ptolemy. In 1975, Otto Neugebauer published three massive volumes on Greek astronomy, which will long stand as a classic in the field. He strongly emphasized the limited applicability of the history of ideas and the history of philosophy approach to the history of science. His arguments are supported by an impressive display of technical details and accurate reconstructions and interpretations of contemporary astronomical calculations and maps. According to Neugebauer, ancient astronomy reached its peak in the late Hellenistic and Imperial age. He dismisses claims that significant developments occurred in the philosophical, pre-Socratic period, or in the early Hellenistic and Classical periods. Ancient astronomy reached its maturity in the Imperial age, when astronomers combined the spherical geometry of Menelaus with the Babylonian tradition of calculus. The result of the marriage between the two traditions was a theoretical system of great sophistication and complexity, characterized by considerable precision and highly refined technical procedures. Mature Greek astronomy cannot be understood in qualitative or purely philosophical terms, but only in terms of the sophisticated mathematical features of its procedures.

Astrological study of the heavens complemented astronomy. Neugebauer and Hoesen (1959) have contributed interesting perspectives on the relationship between the two disciplines. Gundel and Gundel (1966) have surveyed ancient astrological literature, and Gundel (1968) investigated the connection of astrological ideas with magic and occult practices.

Physics

As is well known, the modern classification of sciences is basically the one put forward by Comte in the mid nineteenth century. Historians of Greek science have become increasingly aware that the modern classification is insufficient if not positively misleading for ancient science. It is true that by the fourth century BC disciplines such as mathematics and astronomy were characterized by conceptual features that can be analysed in terms of modern epistemological theories. However, it would be more difficult to defend this thesis when dealing with ancient physics. Firstly, our modern concept of physics corresponds to what the Greeks called mechanics, i.e. the theory of machinery (Jaouiche 1976). Secondly, various approaches to physics were intimately interwoven with often mutually exclusive philosophical traditions. Thus, Peripatetic physics prospered alongside the rival Stoic physics, or Epicurean and atomistic physics. There were indeed points of contact and mutual influences between these various traditions, but the fact remains that different conceptual and scientific traditions developed along basically separate lines.

Historians active in the last two decades have acknowledged the variety of approaches that characterized ancient physics. They have become reluctant to put forward comprehensive unified views of disciplines anachronistically defined according to modern criteria of demarcation. However, the investigation of ancient scientific traditions has produced results of uneven value. The task of rewriting the history of a particular scientific tradition outside the context set by widely accepted historiographical and philosophical frameworks is a difficult one, and at times open to interpretative risks. Thus Serres (1977) has produced a fascinating account of Epicurean physics interpreted exclusively in terms of fluid mechanics and Archimedean mathematics. His reconstruction was suggestive rather than fully convincing. Sambursky (1956, 1959, 1962) has more persuasively argued that the chief feature of the Stoic physical tradition was its stress on a 'physics of continuum'.

Particularly important results have been obtained by historians investigating the original physical system devised in particular by Aristotle and the Peripatetic tradition. At the beginning of the 1960s, three books put forward new views of Aristotelian physics. Solmsen (1960) proposed a more sophisticated interpretation of the *Physics* of Aristotle. He rejected the pyramidal image traditionally used by historians to describe the strongly hierarchical features of the system. Solmsen pointed out that the various issues Aristotle dwelt upon did not follow each other as parts of a deductive process. Instead, single issues reflected specific interests and were connected with or opposed to analogous topics discussed within the tradition of the Academy. The essays collected by Mansion (1961) concentrated on Aristotelian method; they discerned a dialectical structure within the physical system, and emphasized the key role played by the concept of *phainomenon*. Wieland (1962) analysed the core of Aristotelian physics, i.e. the theory of principles. He argued that principles did not represent the metaphysical *primum* from which the entire body of the theory was then deduced, but were instead seen by Aristotle as 'functional concepts'. These were regarded as specific analytical points of view, deployed for analysing and interpreting physical phenomena at every stage of the inquiry.

The fundamental reassessment of traditional interpretations of Aristotelian physics which characterized the early 1960s has left an important legacy of suggestions. Düring (1969) considered further investigations of the Aristotelian philosophy of nature. Steinmetz (1964) studied the physical system proposed by Theophrastus, and Gatzemeier (1970) devoted attention to the little-known activity of Straton of Lampsacus. Two major results are to be singled out from research conducted since the early 1960s. Firstly, a new image of Aristotelian physics has been produced. Historians now regard it as a succession of attempts to investigate, with the help of a plurality of methods (like linguistic analysis and analogies with techniques), the central theme of mutation and change. Motion, a particular case of change, was eventually singled out for special investigation. Secondly, historians have drawn a sharp distinction between Aristotle and Aristotelianism.

Mechanics

It has been pointed out above that in classical science today's concept of physics corresponds with mechanics. The science of mechanics represented a crucial tradition in ancient science. It incorporated pneumatics, i.e. the science of fluids, and was seen as relevant to theories of the construction of buildings and machinery. This body of knowledge was systematized in important 'encyclopaedias of mechanics'. Those by Philon of Byzantium, Vitruvius and Hero can be singled out for their influence and sophistication. This area of Greek science has not been adequately studied, even though various contributions have pointed out possible approaches to the subject. Drachmann (1963) produced a meticulous commentary on the major treatise composed by Hero, the *Mechanics*, of which the Arabic version only has been transmitted. Marsden (1969–71) contributed a comprehensive study of the theory and practice of military artillery, particularly the construction of catapults. This part of the mechanical tradition is of great historical and scientific interest, since it was characterized by concepts like 'technical improvement', and 'model'. Landels (1978) has verified the actual potential, capacity and achievements of ancient engineering with the help of experimental verifications of ancient descriptions. On the other hand, the lack of systematic investigation of this dimension of ancient science has induced some historians to offer limited and partial views of the subject (Gille 1980). Problems of interpretation are made more difficult by the economic factors related to the mechanical and technological dimensions of ancient mechanics. These require reference to social and cultural factors, as well as investigation of areas hitherto neglected by historians. It is also to be noted that historians active between the two world wars stressed that Greek technology was rarely either sophisticated or significant, thereby preventing even the discussion of the topic. However, studies by Vernant (1965) on archaic and classical craftsmanship, and by Frontisi-Ducroux (1975) on the mythical dimensions of the Greek craftsman's mentality, are available.

Ancient medicine

The essays of Edelstein, collected in the volume *Ancient Medicine* (1967a), represented an important contribution to the study of Greek medicine and biology, and promoted a fruitful line of historical investigation. Recently published studies have questioned the image of Greek medicine put forward by Galen. The latter stressed the continuity and unity of Greek medicine, which was seen as developing from the Hippocratic school of the fifth and fourth centuries BC through Alexandrian anatomy and the dogmatic school up to Galen himself. Historians are not convinced that ancient medicine was characterized by the existence and activities of well-defined schools, such as the ones at Cos and Cnidos. It is instead stressed that there were probably several traditions of medical theory and practice. The only unifying criterion was perhaps their archaic nature, i.e. lack of institutionalization and of anatomical knowledge (Jouanna 1974; Grensemann 1975; Grmek 1980). This tradition remained active in the Hellenistic world, and was represented by a plurality of medical centres at Rhodes, Alexandria and Rome as well as Cos and Cnidos (Kudlien 1979; Scarborough 1969). The anatomical and physiological investigations of the Alexandrian Museum were elements added to the tradition.

One of the issues at the centre of the historiographical debate is the extent and actual diffusion of vivisection and human dissection. There is little doubt that anatomical practices that developed from Aristotelian teaching deeply influenced ancient biology up to Galen, who systematized but hardly added to prior knowledge. It was at the Museum, during the third century, that Herophilus discovered the nervous system and its relationship to the brain, and that Herasistratus distinguished between arteries and veins, and developed the theory of pulsations. These developments were based on the accurate study of the human body, as unanimous testimonies confirm. However, historians have argued that the practice of human dissection only characterized the first period of the Museum. Traditional religious beliefs opposed the practice in the Roman world, and anatomical dissections were abandoned at Alexandria as well. Galen himself probably did establish his anatomy on animal dissections and on the dissection of monkeys in particular, as well as on the occasional observation of human bodies (Kudlien 1969).

Further investigations focused on the medical schools of the Roman and Hellenistic periods. Recent studies have concentrated on pneumatic medicine and its relation to the Stoic philosophy professed by Posidonius, and have investigated practices of the Empirics and of the Methodics and their connection with philosophical scepticism and materialism. Roman medicine was characterized by the conflict between various medical schools. The building of a tradition unifying Hippocratic clinical methods and Alexandrian anatomy, and opposed to empirics and dogmatic 'factions', was the work of Galen. The latter has been subjected to careful scrutiny in the 1970s, and a lively debate developed from Temkin's comprehensive study (1973). Several features of Galenic biological and medical thought have been investigated, including his anatomy and physiology, his theory of the pneuma and the denial of the existence of arterial blood. Historians have stressed two major influences operating within Galenic thought. Firstly, the Aristotelian and Stoic teleology, which emphasized the primacy of anatomy and physiology, and secondly, the theory of temperaments and the traditional Hippocratic clinical approach (Isnardi 1961; Nutton 1981). Much work is still to be done on critical editions and adequate commentaries on the Galenic texts. DeLacy's edition (1980) of the *De Placitis Hippocratis et Platonis* and editions of Arabic versions of Galenic texts represent a positive step in that direction. A satisfactory index to the Galenic corpus, comparable to the one recently prepared by Maloney for the *Corpus Hippocraticum* (to be published), is still a desideratum. Thus, it could be argued that the interpretation of Galenic thought and of its historical and scientific context is far from achieving a satisfactory critical stage and solidity. The state of studies on the history of post-Galenic biology and medicine is less than satisfactory (Kudlien 1968). Suggestions put forward by Temkin (1973) are worth exploring. It will be the task of the next decade to establish the role of the various medical traditions in the encyclopaedias of late antiquity, and to investigate the transmission of the Hippocratic and Galenic tradition to the Middle Ages.

Bibliography

Africa, T.W. (1968). *Science and State in Greece and Rome.* New York, London and Sidney; Wiley

Becker, O. (1957). *Das mathematische Denken der Antike.* Göttingen; Vandenhoeck and Ruprecht

Becker, O., Ed. (1965). *Zur Geschichte der griechischen Mathematik.* Darmstadt; Wissenschaftliche Buchgesellschaft

Bollack, J. (1965). *Empédocle. Introduction à l'ancienne physique.* Paris; Minuit

Burkert, W. (1972). *Lore and Science in Ancient Pythagoreanism.* Cambridge, Mass.; Harvard University Press

Cambiano, G. (1967). Il Metodo ipotetico e le origini della sistemazione euclidea della geometria, *Rivista di Filosofia*, Vol. 58, 116–149

Cambiano, G. (1971). *Platone e le tecniche.* Turin; Einaudi

Clagett, M. (1957). *Greek Science in Antiquity.* London; Abelard-Schuman

Clagett, M. (1964–80). *Archimedes in the Middle Ages.* 4 Vols. Vol. 1, Madison; University of Wisconsin Publications in Medieval Science. Vols 2–4, Philadelphia; American Philosophical Society

Cohen, M.R. and Drabkin, I.E. (1948). *A Source Book in Greek Science.* New York; McGraw-Hill

Cole, T. (1967). *Democritus and the Sources of Greek Anthropology.* American Philological Association, Philological Monographs No. 25. Ann Arbor; Western Reserve University

DeLacy, P. (1980). Galen's De Placitis Hippocratis et Platonis, in *Corpus Medicorum Graecorum*, Vol. 4. Berlin; Akademie Verlag

Detienne, M. (1967). *Les Maîtres de vérité dans la Grèce archaïque.* Paris; Maspéro

Detienne, M. (1972). *Les Jardins d'Adonis.* Paris; Gallimard

Detienne, M. and Vernant, J.-P. (1974). *Les Ruses de l'intelligence. La mêtis des Grecs.* Paris; Flammarion

Detienne, M. and Vernant, J.-P., Ed. (1979). *La Cuisine du sacrifice en pays grec.* Paris; Gallimard

Dierauer, U. (1977). *Tier und Mensch im Denken der Antike. Studien zur Tierpsychologie, Anthropologie und Ethik.* Amsterdam; Hakkert

Dijksterhuis, E.J. (1956). *Archimedes.* Copenhagen; Munksgaard

Dodds, E.R. (1973). *The Ancient Concept of Progress.* Oxford; Clarendon Press

Drachmann, A.G. (1963). *The Mechanical Technology of Greek and Roman Antiquity.* Copenhagen; Munksgaard

Düring, I. (1966). *Aristoteles. Darstellung and Interpretation seines Denkens.* Heidelberg; Winter

218   Science, technology and medicine in the classical tradition

Düring, I., Ed. (1969). *Naturphilosophie bei Aristoteles und Theophrast.* Heidelberg; Stiehm

Edelstein, L. (1952). Recent Trends in the Interpretation of Ancient Science, *Journal of the History of Ideas*, Vol. 13, 573–604. Reprinted (1957) in *Roots of Scientific Thought.* Ed. P.P. Wiener and A. Noland. New York; Basic Books, 90–121

Edelstein, L. (1967a). *Ancient Medicine.* Baltimore; The Johns Hopkins Press

Edelstein, L. (1967b). *The Idea of Progress in Classical Antiquity.* Baltimore; The Johns Hopkins Press

Farrington, B. (1944–9). *Greek Science.* 2 Vols. London; Pelican Books

Ferrari, G.A. (1980). La Scrittura fine della realtà, in *Democrito e l'atomismo antico.* Ed. F. Romano. Catania; Università di Catania, 75–90

Fraser, P.M. (1972). *Ptolemaic Alexandria.* Oxford; Oxford University Press

Fritz, K. von (1971). *Grundprobleme der Geschichte der Antiken Wissenschaft.* Berlin and New York; De Gruyter

Frontisi-Ducroux, F. (1975). *Dédale. Mythologie de l'artisan en Grèce ancienne.* Paris; Maspéro

Garcia Ballester, L. (1972). *Galeno.* Madrid; Guadarrama

Gatzemeier, M. (1970). *Die Naturphilosophie des Straton von Lampsakos.* Meisenheim; Hain

Gille, B. (1980). *Les Mécaniciens grecs.* Paris; Seuil

Grensemann, H. (1975). *Knidische Medizin.* Berlin and New York; De Gruyter

Grmek, M.D., Ed. (1980). *Hippocratica.* Paris; CNRS

Gundel, H.G. (1968). *Weltbild und Astrologie in den griechischen Zauberpapyri.* Munich; Beck

Gundel, W. and Gundel, H.G. (1966). *Astrologumena. Die astrologische Literatur in der Antike und ihre Geschichte.* Sudhoffs Archiv Beiheft 6. Wiesbaden; Steiner

Harris, G.R.S. (1973). *The Heart and the Vascular System in Ancient Greek Medicine from Alcmaeon to Galen.* Oxford; Clarendon Press

Havelock, E.A. (1963). *Preface to Plato.* Cambridge, Mass.; Harvard University Press

Isnardi, M. (1961). Techne, *La Parola del Passato*, Vol. 79, 257–296

Jaouiche, K. (1976). *Le Livre du garastūn de Tābit ibn Qurra. Etudes sur l'origine de la notion de travail et du calcul du moment statique d'une barre homogène.* Leyden; Brill

Joly, R. (1966). *Le Niveau de la science hippocratique. Contribution à la psychologie de l'histoire des sciences.* Paris; Les Belles Lettres

Jouanna, J. (1974). *Hippocrate et l'école de Cnide.* Paris; Les Belles Lettres

Kahn, C.H. (1960). *Anaximander and the Origin of Greek Cosmology.* New York; Columbia University Press

Knorr, W.R. (1975). *The Evolution of the Euclidean Elements. A Study of the Theory of Incommensurable Magnitudes and its Significance for early Greek Geometry.* Dordrecht and Boston, Mass.; Reidel

Kudlien, F. (1967). *Der Beginn des medizinisches Denkens bei den Griechen.* Zurich; Artemis

Kudlien, F. (1968). The Third Century A.D., a Blank Spot in the History of Medicine?, in *Medicine, Science, Culture, Historical Essays in Honor of O. Temkin.* Baltimore; The Johns Hopkins Press

Kudlien, F. (1969). Antike Anatomie und menschlicher Leichnam, *Hermes*, Vol. 97, 78–94

Kudlien, F. (1979). *Der griechischen Arzt im Zeitalter des Hellenismus: seine Stellung in Staat und Gesellschaft.* Wiesbaden; Steiner

Kuhn, T. (1957). *The Copernican Revolution. Planetary Astronomy in the Development of Western Thought.* Cambridge, Mass.; Harvard University Press

Landels, J.C. (1978). *Engineering in the Ancient World.* London; Chatto and Windus. Berkeley; University of California Press

Lasserre, F. (1964). *The Birth of Mathematics in the Age of Plato.* London; Hutchinson

Lasserre, F. (1966). *Die Fragmente des Eudoxos von Knidos.* Texte und Kommentare 4. Berlin; De Gruyter

Levêque, P. and Vidal Naquet, P. (1964). *Clisthène l'Athénien.* Paris; Les Belles Lettres

Lloyd, G.E.R. (1966). *Polarity and Analogy. Two Types of Argumentation in Early Greek Thought.* Cambridge; Cambridge University Press

Lloyd, G.E.R. (1970). *Early Greek Science. Thales to Aristotle.* London; Chatto and Windus

Lloyd, G.E.R. (1973). *Greek Science after Aristotle.* London; Chatto and Windus

Lloyd, G.E.R. (1979). *Magic, Reason and Experience. Studies in the Origins and Development of Greek Science.* Cambridge; Cambridge University Press

Lynch, J.P. (1972). *Aristotle's School. A Study of a Greek Educational Institution.* Berkeley, Los Angeles and London; University of California Press

Mansfeld, J. (1971). *The Pseudo-Hippocratic Tract peri hebdomadon ch. 1–11 and Greek Philosophy.* Assen; Van Gorcum

Mansion, S., Ed. (1961). *Aristote et les problèmes de méthode.* Louvain, Paris; Nauwelaerts

Manuli, P. and Vegetti, M. (1977). *Cuore, sangue e cervello. Biologia e antropologia nel pensiero antico.* Milano; Episteme

Marsden, E.W. (1969–71). *Greek and Roman Artillery.* 2 Vols. Oxford; Clarendon Press

Maula, E. (1974). *Studies in Eudoxus' Homocentric Spheres.* Helsinki; Societas Scientiarum Fennica

Mittelstrass, J. (1962). *Die Rettung der Phänomene.* Berlin; De Gruyter

Neugebauer, O. (1957). *The Exact Sciences in Antiquity,* 2nd edn. Providence; Brown University Press

Neugebauer, O. (1975). *A History of Ancient Mathematical Astronomy.* 3 Vols. Berlin, Heidelberg, New York; Springer

Neugebauer, O. and Van Hoesen, H.B. (1959). *Greek Horoscopes.* American Philosophical Society Memoirs 48. Philadelphia

Newton, R.R. (1977). *The Crime of Claudius Ptolemy.* Baltimore; The Johns Hopkins Press

Nutton, V., Ed. (1981). *Galen. Problem and Prospects.* London; The Wellcome Institute for the History of Medicine

Pedersen, O. (1974). *A Survey of the Almagest.* Odense; Odense University Press

Phillips, E.D. (1973). *Aspects of Greek Medicine.* New York; St Martin's Press

Preus, A. (1975). *Science and Philosophy in Aristotle's Biological Works.* Hildesheim and New York; G. Olms

Sambursky, S. (1956). *The Physical World of the Greeks.* London; Routledge and Kegan Paul

Sambursky, S. (1959). *The Physics of the Stoics.* London; Routledge and Kegan Paul

Sambursky, S. (1962). *The Physical World of Late Antiquity.* London; Routledge and Kegan Paul

Scarborough, J. (1969). *Roman Medicine.* Ithaca and New York; Cornell University Press

Schiaparelli, G.U. (1925–7). *Scritti sulla storia della astronomia antica.* 3 Vols. Bologna; Zanichelli

Serres, M. (1977). *La Naissance de la physique dans le texte de Lucrèce. Fleuves et turbolences.* Paris; Minuit

Smith, W.D. (1979). *The Hippocratic Tradition.* Ithaca and London; Cornell University Press

Solmsen, F. (1960). *Aristotle's System of Physical World.* New York; Cornell University Press

Stahl, W.H. (1962). *Roman Science.* Madison; University of Wisconsin Press

Steinmetz, P. (1964). *Die Physik des Theophrastos von Eresos.* Bad Homburg; Gehlen

Szabo, A. (1969). *Anfänge der griechischen Mathematik.* Munich and Vienna; Oldenbourg

Temkin, O. (1953). Greek Medicine as Science and Craft, *Isis*, Vol. 44, 213–225

Temkin, O. (1973). *Galenism. Rise and Decline of a Medical Philosophy.* Ithaca and London; Cornell University Press

Vegetti, M. (1979). *Il Coltello e lo stilo.* Milan; Il Saggiatore

Vernant, J.-P. (1962). *Les Origines de la pensée grecque.* Paris; Presses Universitaires de France

Vernant, J.-P. (1965). *Mythe et pensée chez les Grecs. Etudes de psychologie historique.* Paris; Maspéro

Waerden, B.L. van der (1954). *Science Awakening.* Groningen; Noordhoff

Waerden, B.L. van der (1965). *Anfänge der Astronomie.* Groningen; Noordhoff

Wieland, W. (1962). *Die aristotelische Physik. Untersuchungen über die Grundlegung der Naturwissenschaft und die sprachlichen Bedingungen der Prinzipienforschung bei Aristoteles.* Göttingen; Vandenhoeck und Ruprecht

Wissman, H. (1980). Réalité et matière dans l'atomisme démocritéen, in *Democrito e l'atomismo antico.* Ed. F. Romano. Catania; Università di Catania

12

Recent trends in the study of medieval and Renaissance science

C.B. Schmitt

Pre-seventeenth century science was a blend of dependence on tradition and of innovation. This is certainly a truism that cannot be contested, but it is important to keep it in mind, since many interpreters have unduly emphasized the slavish adherence to tradition and the degenerate nature of pre-modern science after antiquity. The Middle Ages and Renaissance embraced a wide variation of scientific competence on the part of different individuals in different localities; it was quite at odds with the unified 'scientific world view' of more recent times. It was also different insofar as much of its science was based, directly or indirectly, upon written texts transmitted from an age long past. At its worst, medieval science could be no more than a system of ideas constantly degenerating from the deficient handbooks and *compendia* based on already derivative Roman sources. At its best, it could produce a degree of sophistication that went far beyond the best Greek science and that has properly been adjudged 'precursor' to some of the greatest achievements of seventeenth-century science. Throughout the period in question and, indeed, into the seventeenth century the resources of classical antiquity were held in particular esteem and served as the starting point for scientific, as well as other, studies.

Texts and traditions surviving from classical times not only exerted a remarkable positive influence on the scientific consciousness, but also contributed to the progress of the individual sciences (Lindberg 1978: 1–51). The writings of leading Greek thinkers such as Euclid and Archimedes, Aristotle and Theophrastus, Ptolemy and Galen remained favoured sources of enlightenment and inspiration for many generations of Western Europeans, as well as for men of Jewish and Muslim culture. Indeed, in many specialized fields the technical level of ancient science was more accomplished than anything achieved independently by European science before the sixteenth or seventeenth centuries. Medieval and Renaissance thinkers not only added to the ancient sources a good deal of original material of their own devising, but also drew freely upon non-classical sources that came their way. Thus the scientific fruits of the flourishing Muslim culture, many of whose major contributions were quickly translated into Latin, were assimilated and built upon especially during the twelfth and thirteenth centuries. (For discussion of Islamic science and medicine, see chapter 21.) Medieval science in Western Europe was a mixture of classical, non-Western and post-classical elements, often intimately blended in such a way that the original source of the different strands was all but lost sight of. As time progressed many non-classical elements were abandoned in favour of a 'classical revival' (i.e. Renaissance), but even then numerous 'medieval' characteristics – from both East and West – remained.

In view of the decisive impact of classical texts on later developments, it is rather surprising how few genuine ancient writings were available for much of the Middle Ages and, indeed, how little of the total output of the scientific literature of Greece actually survived the ravages of time. Aristotle, Theophrastus and Galen, for example, are known to have written many more works than have come down to us. Nonetheless, after the low point of Western culture, lasting from about the late ninth to the late eleventh century, when few Greek writings were available in Latin Europe, there was a revival both of interest and of the availability of material. Especially from the twelfth-century Renaissance to the fifteenth-century one, new classical material progressively became available for assimilation within the developing sciences of the day. What survived to play a central role in later science was often the result of pure accident, as with Aristotle, whose unpublished works remained extant to exert a decisive role on later science, while those works generally known in antiquity perished with the fall of the ancient world.

Before moving on to a more detailed discussion of some of these points, it might be worthwhile to say a few words about the meaning of 'science' as the term is used in the present context. (Ancient Greek and Roman definitions are discussed in chapter 11.) In general, 'science' (*episteme, scientia*) meant for those of antiquity, the Middle Ages and Renaissance a theoretical discipline involving certain and unchangeable knowledge desirable for its own sake. It was distinguished from 'art' (*techne, ars*), which had a practical end product such as health (for medicine), a statue (for sculpture), or a table (for carpentry). 'Science' and 'technology' (to use a term coined only in modern times) were also quite separate, and science was not thought of as having a practical or useful end. The clear distinction between art and science was not always upheld, however, and there is in fact a good deal of variation in terminology and practice. For example, among theologians of the thirteenth century, theology was spoken of as the archetypal science. On the other hand, disciplines such as medicine and mathematics, which imply 'science' to many modern ears, were frequently called 'arts', as in Girolamo Cardano's *Great Art* (*Ars magna* 1545), essentially a treatise on algebra.

Another important point to keep in mind is that until the seventeenth century (and even later in certain disciplines and in certain contexts), there was not always a clear differentiation between 'science' and 'pseudo-science' (Thorndike 1923–58). Astrology and astronomy were frequently inextricably intertwined, as for example in Kepler; the mystical and magical content of alchemy was not distinguished – or always distinguishable – from empirical, scientific chemistry. While recent science has established fairly clear-cut criteria for the inclusion or exclusion of material as 'scientific' or 'non-scientific', this was not always the case.

The problem of evaluating ancient, medieval and early modern texts in this light is most difficult for the present-day interpreter. Though recent work has shown the failings of an overly positivistic approach in which contemporary criteria are employed to evaluate the 'scientific' texts of earlier periods, by the same token one must not abandon all critical judgement to put things in 'historical context'.

Beginning with some of the major figures of the so-called 'scientific revolution' itself, e.g. Galileo, Bacon, and Descartes, there was a very strong deprecation of the value of the scientific thought of the Middle Ages. These three, and others, looked upon themselves as reviving true valid science, after various medieval perversions. Such a historiographical interpretation persisted until quite recently. To put matters simply, the history of science could be viewed as an ancient flowering, a medieval interval followed by a new dawn that led on directly to the major accomplishments of seventeenth-century science. Such an interpretation, often in only a slightly modified form, can still be found in many of the textbooks and general surveys in current use.

Though some earlier interpreters had pointed to isolated scientific accomplishments during the Middle Ages (notably Ernst Mach), it was really Pierre Duhem (1906–13, 1913–59; Rosen 1961; Martin 1976) who first put forward a coherent and comprehensive 'continuity thesis' connecting ancient, medieval and early modern science. During the first years of the twentieth century, Duhem turned his attention increasingly from scientific research to the study of the primary sources of pre-seventeenth-century physical science. The first to consider seriously the extensive manuscript sources for the history of medieval science, Duhem was able to show their importance in the development of scientific thought. His 'continuity thesis' stressed, counter to previous interpretations, two main points. First, there was an unbroken tradition of a creative physical science, centred at Paris, from the early thirteenth century to the early sixteenth century. Second, the major scientific results of this tradition were known and built upon by Leonardo da Vinci and Galileo, thus forming the basis for the major developments of early modern science. Duhem stressed the innovating aspects of medieval science, pointing out clearly the ways in which it marked a genuine progress over ancient science, e.g. in the development of methods of quantitative description (intension and remission of forms) and improved laws of kinematics and dynamics (impetus theory, etc.). Though utilizing classical sources, medieval science was marked by a significant positive advance, which was built upon in turn by the major figures of the scientific revolution. (For further discussion of Duhem, see chapter 1.)

Duhem's pioneering work in the manuscript sources of medieval science has been extended by numerous later scholars such as Maier (1949–58), Clagett (1959, 1979), Grant (1974, 1981a,b), Murdoch (1974) and others, who have refined and clarified his theses. Much new material has been brought to light, and many of the key texts have been edited and subjected to intense scrutiny. It can no longer be held that the Middle Ages was a low point in the development of science, though certain problems do remain. Several fourteenth-century thinkers (for example, Jean Buridan, Nicole Oresme, Thomas Bradwardine, Richard Swineshead) came very close to making some of the conceptual breakthroughs that marked the seventeenth century, but it is clear that they failed to take a final step (Clagett 1959; Murdoch 1974). Though discussions of *impetus* came very close to what was later the 'law of inertia' (a seventeenth-century formulation that became a foundation stone for later physics), the breakthrough was not quite managed. In spite of medieval attempts to approach physical science in a quantitative way (Aristotelian physics was wholly qualitative), there was no coherent and systematic application of mathematics to the study of physics.

The extensive and highly competent research that has gone into the study of medieval science, especially during the past fifty years, has thus far failed to establish in a definitive way a genuine continuity between medieval and modern science. There can be no doubt that Duhem's work transformed the study of pre-seventeenth-century science; much of the research still being carried on today stems from the impetus that he initiated. On the other hand, several severe and valid criticisms can be brought against his work. It might be well to mention some of these, since they are still very much at the forefront of present-day discussions. First, there is too much emphasis on the precursors of important scientific discoveries. This often led to a *post hoc, ergo propter hoc* type of reasoning on Duhem's part. This is crucial in the case of Galileo, whose formulations cannot always be linked directly to similar theories of those who pre-dated him.

Second, throughout Duhem's work there is a very strong pro-French bias. It cannot be denied, certainly, that thirteenth- and fourteenth-century Paris was the centre of much important intellectual activity, but the relative contributions of Oxford and the Italian and German universities, as has become apparent in recent research, were severely underestimated.

Third, Duhem essentially paid no attention whatever to the place of the biological sciences in his story, nor did he claim to. Nonetheless, for a more balanced account it will be necessary to consider the very large body of extant material covering the other side of science. This is particularly true in view of the importance of the medical faculties in many universities in Italy and elsewhere.

Fourth, the intensive research of recent years on the recovery of ancient sources during the Renaissance shows that Duhem did not place enough emphasis on this factor as a contributing element to scientific development. Sources such as Archimedes, Hero of Alexandria, Pappus, Theophrastus, (pseudo-)Aristotle's *Mechanics*, and various Greek commentators on Aristotle that were recovered during the Renaissance played an important role in the development of the 'new science'.

The crucial factor, however, which has plagued the study of medieval and Renaissance science in recent decades, is the problem of continuity or discontinuity between medieval and modern science. Put in other terms it is the problem of Renaissance science. Medieval science – at least in broad outline, and in some areas of detail as well – is now fairly well understood, as is the seventeenth-century scientific revolution. A problem remains however: how does the accomplishment of the fourteenth century link up with that of the seventeenth? More precisely, little is known of the continuity of medieval science between the late fourteenth and the late sixteenth centuries. How can Buridan and Oresme be linked to Galileo?

The general view, based upon a very superficial – even trivial – knowledge of the extant sources, holds that the development of humanism marked a turning away from scientific studies and, hence, an interruption in the development of science. Thus the Renaissance, for all of its accomplishments in painting, sculpture, architecture and literature, had a deleterious effect upon the development of the science that had flourished during the Middle Ages. Precise documentation for such an interpretation has been singularly lacking. In fact, the decline of medieval science in such centres as Oxford and Paris was already well under way when humanism entered the picture (Clagett 1959: 628–71; Schmitt 1981: sect. VI). Moreover, the attitude of the humanists as regards science was by no means uniform: some humanists rejected all medieval science; others accepted some parts of science, rejecting others; while still other humanists, partially critical of some aspects of science, contributed to particular sciences in a very positive way. Petrarch rejected much of the scholastic science and logic of his day, which included some of the high-level fourteenth-century contributions. Yet a number of humanists of note – including Coluccio Salutati, Giovanni Pico and Ermolao Barbaro – were clearly influenced by, and not wholly opposed to, so characteristic a doctrine as 'intension and remission of forms' (Dionisotti 1955; Garin 1969: 139–77; Witt 1977). The humanists' role in recovering, editing, translating and explicating some of the key ancient works of science scarcely needs comment (*Catalogus translationum et commentariorum* 1960–; Rose 1975). In fifteenth-century Italy, medieval science continued to exist and even to dominate the arts faculties of the universities while humanism was in full flower. The interaction between these two major intellectual traditions – fourteenth-century Paris and Oxford natural philosophy and logic, on the one hand, and humanism, on the other – has not been fully investigated and is very imperfectly understood. It must be studied in detail before an accurate evaluation of the fifteenth century as a whole and its place in the history of science can be formulated.

This leads us to what is the major problem in the whole historiography of pre-seventeenth-century science, viz. the place of the fifteenth century. Though much studied from the point of view of art history and humanism, the scientific activity of the century has been almost wholly neglected. Thus far we lack even basic biobibliographies for the major figures and, with few exceptions, the major lines of development are not clear (Vasoli 1974: 405–75). We know, for example, that the important contributions of fourteenth-century science were still studied during the fifteenth-century in Central and Eastern Europe, as well as in Paris and various Italian universities. Yet the precise details of this continued interest and what developments it promoted have been investigated in only a few cases. The continuity of the tradition at Paris and Oxford, where it originated the century before, is still very imperfectly understood. From the indications of previous research it appears that, for the most part, the fifteenth century merely transmitted the accomplishment of the previous century in various branches of natural philosophy without contributing very substantially to its further development (Federici Vescovini 1979).

What does seem clear at this point is that some of the most characteristic aspects of late medieval science and philosophy were still current at major centres only until about 1525 or 1530, thereafter surviving, if at all, in a severely diluted form. Therefore, the differences between the natural philosophy taught in Italian universities during the fifteenth century and that taught in the sixteenth are noticeable and manifold. In 1450, say, medieval doctrines such as intension and remission, reaction, first and last instants were being widely discussed, the appropriate texts were still being copied, new commentaries and expositions being written. By 1550 the vestiges of all this were few and there was much more discussion of the Greek commentators on Aristotle and of the other ancient scientific traditions, the sources for which had been recovered by the humanists. On the other hand, certain aspects of the medieval tradition, e.g. the strong influence of Averroes, were still present and, if anything, expanded during the sixteenth century. Nonetheless, the sixteenth century does mark a qualitative change over the fifteenth, though the many regional variations – for example Spain presents a very different picture from Poland, and Italy from England – make generalizations unsafe (Schmitt 1981: sect. VI).

As already suggested, it is at present difficult to specify precisely the role of humanism in the development of science. One thing is sure: the development of scientific thought was significantly influenced by humanistic techniques and aspirations (Garin 1969: 449–500). Many humanists were certainly intensely critical of traditional science with all of its genuine and pretended accomplishments, but the humanists also contributed significantly to later scientific achievements. First, they were responsible for the recovery of many ancient scientific texts unknown to the Middle Ages. Key writings of Theophrastus, Galen, Archimedes, Pappus, Diogenes Laertius (where much information on various ancient traditions of science is contained) and several others were brought to Western Europe from Byzantium by a handful of humanists about the turn of the fifteenth century. Secondly, these and other texts, including many known to the Middle Ages, were newly edited, additional manuscript copies were provided, and new and improved translations were prepared. After the invention of printing, it was the humanists who prepared new editions for the press, thus establishing a firm basis for the later transmission of scientific knowledge (Eisenstein 1979: 453–682). Third, the humanists, including such figures as Lorenzo Valla (1407–57), Angelo Poliziano (1454–94) and Ermolao Barbaro (1454–93), developed refined approaches to the study of classical texts that made possible a more accurate evaluation of the legitimacy of scientific and other texts. Thus, for example, many works that had been attributed to Aristotle during the Middle Ages were shown to be later forgeries and were removed from the canon.

In spite of the new influence of humanism, remnants of medieval science continued to flourish throughout Europe, albeit in a diluted form and with the admixture of new tendencies such as humanism. Sixteenth-century natural philosophy shows a peculiar blend of rather traditional medievalism coupled with new thrusts (e.g. empirical observation, the application of mathematical methods, the consideration of a range of ancient traditions in science other than Aristotelian). It was obviously a time in which traditional scholastic science was being found somewhat deficient, but a single clear-cut and viable alternative had not won general approval.

One decisive fact that must be kept in mind when evaluating the science of the Middle Ages and Renaissance is that 'science' as such was not yet a clearly defined and independent group of disciplines. In university contexts – and many others as well, it should not be forgotten – what we call 'science' was actually a part of natural philosophy. Such a categorization continued down to Newton (*Mathematical Principles of Natural Philosophy*) and beyond. The positivistic tradition in history of science has tended to forget this decisive fact and to evaluate the accomplishment of earlier ages nearly wholly in terms of the criteria of recent times. Buridan, Oresme, Paul of Venice, Blasius of Parma, Pietro Pomponazzi, Iacopo Zabarella and Cesare Cremonini, along with many others, fall into this category. Yet others, for example Cardano, worked in a medical context, which also had strong links with philosophy.

Previously, I pointed out that one of the deficiencies of Duhem's work was his total neglect of the biological sciences. This same neglect has, in fact, been true of most later research on the history of early science. The important accomplishments of the physical sciences during the early modern period had obscured the import-ance of the biological sciences. Yet the extant source material is, if anything, more abundant than for the physical sciences. This abundance is attributable to two facts: (1) much of Aristotelian science is concerned with biological subjects, and (2) the position of the medical faculties in universities fostered a primary concern for those subjects related to medical studies. Indeed, one of the major growth points for scientific studies during the sixteenth and early seventeenth centuries lay in developments within biological science. Botany, for example, emerged in the sixteenth century as an independent discipline largely within university medical facul-ties (Schmitt 1979: 378–9). With the exception of anatomy and a few other disciplines related directly to medical history, the study of the biological sciences during the Middle Ages and Renaissance is in a very primitive state indeed. While key figures such as Vesalius and Harvey have been studied in some detail, disciplines such as botany, zoology and many others have scarcely been considered as subjects worthy of consideration over a long period. Here, as in most other fields of study, the vast commentary literature that has survived – for example on the works of Hippocrates, Galen, Aristotle and Theophrastus – has not even been fully catalogued, let alone evaluated and studied.

At the other end of the spectrum, the most mathematical of the sciences, astronomy, has been subjected to intense study, especial-ly the work of Copernicus and Kepler, both subjects for the scholarly flourishes accompanying their centenaries (1973 and 1971 respectively). With regard to Copernicus, a new critical edition is in progress (Copernicus 1972–), as well as continuing series of publications (*Studia Copernicana*). Among the many things that have turned up in the new research is a realization that Copernicus was closer to the Middle Ages than previously realized (Swerdlow in *Symposium on Copernicus* 1973: 423–512). Also important, from various points of view, is the work that has been done on his reception during the century after his death (Westman, 1975a, 1980). The complexities of Kepler's personality and his intricate scientific work have been unravelled to some degree and his accomplishment interpreted more in its historical context.

Another branch of study, which is somewhat peripheral to history of science during the period in question, but which has forged increasingly close links in more modern times, is history of technology. While Francis Bacon is generally thought to have been the first to connect directly the practice of science with technological productivity, there are earlier roots, some of which involve the traditions of philosophy and mythography (Rossi 1970, 1974). Precedents in the earlier Tuscan tradition have also been uncovered for Galileo's contributions to the practical (technological) aspects of scientific enquiry (Settle 1966, 1971). On the other hand, recent work has tended to diminish the supposed contribution of Leonardo da Vinci to the history of science and technology (Truesdell 1968: 1–83). Duhem's pioneering work on uncovering Leonardo's sources has been extended, so that at present little of the enthusiastic view of Leonardo as a genius to top all geniuses remains untarnished. As a concomitant to this, much new light has been shed on the development of technology during the Middle Ages (White 1962, 1978).

The case of Leonardo is not unique, and there has been a general tendency in recent years to play down the contributions of the 'great men', while re-establishing the importance of various secondary figures previously largely neglected. Thus the contributions of Copernicus, Vesalius and Harvey are seen more as rather long-term developments, than as the work of a single genius appearing unheralded upon the scene (Lesky 1957; Pagel 1967, 1969–70; Plochmann 1963). Moreover, at least in the cases of Copernicus and Harvey, it has also been demonstrated that the acceptance of their novel work did not come so quickly in all quarters as one might expect.

Galileo requires particular comment, since he has long been considered a key figure in the transition from medieval to modern sciences. After several decades of a rather tired approach to Galilean studies, much new work has been done to illuminate him and his context. The roots of his early work in the scholastic, university tradition have been demonstrated with studies of his relations to Padua, Pisa and the Collegio Romano (Schmitt 1981: sect XI; Wallace 1981; Lewis 1980). On the other side, his ties with contemporary Tuscan culture – in such fields as literature, music and non-university science – have been illustrated (Cochrane in

McMullin 1967: 118–39; Walker 1978; Settle 1971; Goldthwaite 1972; van Egmond 1977). Studies on his methodology have gone far beyond the pioneering but out-dated study of Randall (1961), and several suggestive studies situating him within other earlier traditions are now available (Jardine 1976; Wisan 1978). Much attention has been focused upon Galileo's experimental work, with a number of ingenious studies of some rather miscellaneous notes of his preserved in manuscript but not printed in the standard edition of his *Opere*. The interpretation of this material is controversial to say the least, but it shows clearly that the Florentine's experimental approach to the study of motion of bodies was more highly developed and more sophisticated than had previously been demonstrable (Drake 1970, 1978; Wisan 1974; Naylor 1976).

Another important aspect of the development of science that has drawn much interest in recent decades is the pseudo-scientific and occult aspect, which was a very evident concomitant of scientific endeavour during the Middle Ages and Renaissance. The most comprehensive study of this to date is to be found in the work of Lynn Thorndike (1923–58). His massive study brought to light many manuscript sources and built up a strong case for an occultist tradition being intimately interwoven with 'science' as the more positivistic historians view the subject. Later studies pushed the analysis further, almost claiming at times a more central position for pseudo-science than for genuine science (e.g. Yates 1964, and in Singleton 1967: 255–74). A more balanced reaction has set in against these claims, sometimes inspired by traditional positivism and other times by a new attempt to evaluate the history within 'its own context of time and place' (Westman and McGuire 1977; Schmitt 1981: sect. IX). Many questions still remain unanswered on this subject and many of the categories are not yet clear. Further and more balanced research is needed in this area, taking account of the vast range of unstudied materials rather than relying upon a few well-known but unrepresentative sources.

If much, perhaps too much, undisciplined study has been expended on the occult connections of science, too little has been directed towards the study of science in the universities. Not only during the Middle Ages, but during the Renaissance as well, the universities of Europe were the centres of much of the most significant scientific activity. This is particularly true in fields connected with the medical sciences (Siraisi 1973, 1981). Aristotle continued to dominate, but it has been suggested that this was not always as deleterious as previously assumed (Grant 1981b, sect. XVI; Schmitt 1981, sect. VI). Subjects such as anatomy, botany and embryology developed within university contexts to a marked degree and there is reason to believe that other subjects did as well. Even major figures who turned against traditional sciences, e.g. Copernicus, Galileo, Bacon and Kepler, were university trained and in several cases themselves taught in universities.

The continuity of university sciences, along with the use of Latin as the functional language of science and the common core of source materials, problems and aspirations, leads one to question the chronological structure of much of the previous historiography in this field. Almost all writers on the intellectual history of the period have followed the chronological divisions of the general historiography into medieval and Renaissance (or medieval and modern). Yet there are compelling reasons for treating the period from the twelfth to the seventeenth century as a unit, as I have tended to do here. The twelfth century marks a watershed between darkness and enlightenment in Western culture in a more real sense than does the Italian Renaissance. This is not to diminish the importance of the Renaissance, but merely to note the degree to which it was building on the achievements of the twelfth and thirteenth centuries: the rise of universities, the beginning of the assimilation of classical culture and learning, the re-establishment of an intellectual structure (Aristotelian scholasticism) within which a regenerated science could flourish. I believe that the main characteristics of such a culture persisted as long as Latin persisted as the language of science and learning, that is until the end of the seventeenth century, with continuities lasting even longer in a number of contexts. Whether such a hypothesis be accepted or not, it is clear that the term 'Renaissance' as normally used (i.e. applying principally to the fifteenth and sixteenth centuries) has little application to the history of science or philosophy. Rather than being a high point in the history of science, as it is in the arts and letters, the fifteenth century – insofar as one can now understand it on the basis of a defective appreciation of source materials – remains a trough between crests.

Those familiar with the recent historiography of science for post-seventeenth-century developments will find a number of differences when they come to study earlier science. Sources are more meagre (though not so meagre as the surveys suggest) and their interpretation fraught with a number of peculiar problems (the language of expression, the philosophical and theological context, the admixture of many elements extraneous to science as today understood). Most important of all, however, for those brought up on the current (not always admirable or luminiferous) trends, is the fact that the so-called 'sociology of science' is not directly applicable in the terms normally thought. Scientific work was nearly always by a single individual, not by groups; the scientific journal was not yet established and communication was through other means; patronage of science *per se* was rudimentary, if present at all; the structure of learning was such that a clearly defined scientific group, in modern terms, had not yet come to the fore. Moreover, 'national styles' had not evolved, if they were ever to evolve in the terms often supposed. In short, though the social backgrounds of intellectuals and groups of intellectuals (e.g. professors of medicine) can be uncovered in some instances, the general structure of the whole endeavour was so different from that of more modern science that the models used thus far by sociologists of science do not apply.

The reader by this stage should be aware that there are still more problems than answers with regard to the study of science for the period (especially for the Renaissance). It has certainly been bedevilled by inadequate and misleading general surveys and textbooks (here unnamed) based on accidental and cliché-ridden evidence. The plain fact is that, allowing for few exceptions, medieval science has been studied from the roots up through valid methods by competent individuals, while Renaissance science has been little studied, but wildly generalized about by interpreters unfamiliar with the sources and fundamental structure of the subject.

Bibliography

This bibliography is very selective. In compiling it an attempt has been made to assemble a representative selection of the research done in this field during the period 1955–81. Only very few earlier works have been included, while general reference works, e.g. the *Dictionary of Scientific Biography*, as well as translations and editions have generally been excluded. Moreover, an attempt has been made to include representative examples of the work of as wide a range of scholars as possible. Consequently, frequently only two or three publications of even the most active and prolific writers are included. I am also very aware of many exclusions, even of articles and books that I personally admire and of which I have made abundant use in my own work. Certainly, there is a large group of important studies in the field of which I am partially or totally ignorant.

234   Recent trends in medieval and Renaissance science

This list is meant to be a starting point for further research and is to be used accordingly. Its chronological limits run from the Middle Ages to the first few years of the seventeenth century. Geographically, it includes Western Europe and those areas where the Western languages were functional.

Arts libéraux et philosophie médiévale (1969). Actes du 4° congrès international de philosophie médiévale. Paris; Vrin

Beaujouan, G. (1967). *La Science en Espagne aux 14ᵉ et 15ᵉ siècles*. Paris; Palais de la Découverte

Boas Hall, M. (1962). *The Scientific Renaissance, 1450–1630*. London; Collins

Boas Hall, M. (1979). Il rinascimento scientifico, in *Il Rinascimento. Interpretazioni e problemi*. Bari–Rome; Laterza, 323–352

Buck, A. (1973). Der Wissenschaftsbegriff des Renaissance-Humanismus, *Wolfenbüttler Beiträge*, Vol. 2, 45–63

Bylebyl, J.J. (1979). The School of Padua: Humanistic Medicine in the Sixteenth Century, in *Health, Medicine and Mortality in the Sixteenth Century*. Ed. C. Webster. Cambridge; Cambridge University Press, 335–370

Catalogus Translationum et Commentariorum (1960). Ed. P.O. Kristeller and F.E. Cranz. Washington; Catholic University of America Press. Especially relevant to history of science are the following: Vol. I: Alexander Aphrodisiensis, Aristarchus Samius, Autolycus, and Hypsicles; Vol. II: Olympiodorus, Pappus, Pausanias. Stephanus Byzantius, Strabo, Theophrastus, Lucretius, and Martianus Capella; Vol. III: Dionysius Periegetes, Musici scriptores graeci, Priscianus Lydus, Thessalus astrologus, Columella, and Vitruvius; Vol. IV: Dioscorides, Paulus Aegineta, and Plinius Secundus

Clagett, M. (1959). *The Science of Mechanics in the Middle Ages*. Madison; University of Wisconsin Press

Clagett, M., Ed. (1962). *Critical Problems in the History of Science*. Madison; University of Wisconsin Press

Clagett, M. (1964–80). *Archimedes in the Middle Ages*, 4 Vols. Vol. 1, *The Arabo-Latin Tradition* (1964). Madison; University of Wisconsin Publications in Medieval Science. Vol. 2, *The Translations from the Greek by William of Moerbeke* (1976). 2 Vols. Vol. 3, *The Fate of the Medieval Archimedes 1300 to 1565* (1978). 3 Vols. Vol. 4, *A Supplement on the Medieval Latin Traditions of Conic Sections (1150–1566)* (1980). Philadelphia; American Philosophical Society

Clagett, M. (1979). *Studies in Medieval Physics and Mathematics*. London; Variorum

Clavelin, M. (1968). *La Philosophie naturelle de Galilée*. Paris; Armand Colin

Clulee, N. (1971). John Dee's Mathematics and the Grading of Compound Qualities, *Ambix*, Vol. 18, 178–211

Cochrane, E. (1976). Science and Humanism in the Italian Renaissance, *American Historical Review*, Vol. 81, 1039–57

Copenhaver, B.P. (1978). *Symphorien Champier and the Reception of the Occultist Tradition in Renaissance France*. The Hague; Mouton

Copenhaver, B.P. (1980). Jewish Theologies of Space in the Scientific Revolution: Henry More, Joseph Raphson, Isaac Newton and Their Predecessors, *Annals of Science*, Vol. 37, 489–548

Copernicus, N. (1972–). *Complete Works*. Warsaw; Polish Academy of Science

Crapulli, G. (1969). *Mathesis universalis: genesi di una idea nel XVI secolo*. Rome; Ateneo

Recent trends in medieval and Renaissance science 235

Crombie, A.C., Ed. (1963). *Scientific Change. Historical Studies in the Intellectual, Social and Technical Conditions for Scientific Discovery and Technical Innovation, from Antiquity to the Present*. Symposium on the History of Science, University of Oxford, 9–15 July 1961. London; Heinemann.

Crosby, H.L., Ed. (1955). *Thomas Bradwardine*. Madison; University of Wisconsin Press

Debus, A.G., Ed. (1972). *Science, Medicine and Society in the Renaissance. Essays to Honor Walter Pagel*. 2 Vols. New York; Science History Publications

Debus, A.G. (1977). *The Chemical Philosophy. Paracelsian Science and Medicine in the Sixteenth and Seventeenth Centuries*. 2 Vols. New York; Science History Publications

Dijksterhuis, E.J. (1961). *The Mechanization of the World Picture*. Trans. C. Dikshoorn. Oxford; Clarendon Press

Dilg, P. (1975). Die botanische Kommentariteratur in Italien um 1500 und ihr Einfluss auf Deutschland, in *Der Kommentar in der Renaissance*. Ed. A. Buck and O. Herding. Boppard; Harald Boldt, 225–52

Dionisotti, C. (1955). Ermolao Barbaro e la fortuna di Suiseth, in *Medioevo e Rinascimento: studi in onore di Bruno Nardi*. Ed. T. Gregory. Florence; Sansoni, 219–253

Drake, S. (1970). *Galileo Studies*. Ann Arbor; University of Michigan Press

Drake, S. (1978). *Galileo at Work: His Scientific Biography*. Chicago and London; University of Chicago Press

Drake, S. and Drabkin, I.E. (1969). *Mechanics in Sixteenth-Century Italy*. Madison; University of Wisconsin Press

Duhem, P. (1906–13). *Études sur Léonard de Vinci*. 3 Vols. Paris; Hermann

Duhem, P. (1913–59). *Le Système du monde. Histoire des doctrines cosmologiques de Platon à Copernic*. 10 Vols. Paris; Hermann

Eastwood, B.S. (1967). Grosseteste's 'Quantitative' Law of Refraction: a Chapter in the History of Non-Experimental Science, *Journal of the History of Ideas*, Vol. 28, 403–414

Egmond, W. van (1977). The Commercial Revolution and the Beginnings of Western Mathematics in Renaissance Florence, 1300–1800, University of Indiana PhD thesis

Eisenstein, E.L. (1979). *The Printing Press as an Agent of Change*. Cambridge; Cambridge University Press

Federici Vescovini, G. (1979). *Astrologia e scienza. La crisi dell'aristotelismo sul cadere del Trecento e Biagio Pelacani da Parma*. Florence; Vallecchi

Firenze e la Toscana dei Medici nell'Europa del Cinquecento. [Exhibition catalogue] (1980). *La Rinascita della scienza*. Ed. P. Galluzzi. *Astrologia, magia, e alchimia*. Ed. P. Zambelli. Florence; Electra, 123–243, 309–435

Funkenstein, A. (1971). Some Remarks on the Concept of Impetus and the Determination of Simple Motion, *Viator*, Vol. 2, 329–348

Gagnon, C. (1974). Recherche bibliographique sur l'alchimie médiévale occidentale, *Cahiers d'études médiévales*, Vol. 2, 155–199

Galluzzi, P. (1973). Il 'Platonismo' del tardo Cinquecento e la filosofia di Galileo, in *Ricerche sulla cultura dell'Italia moderna*. Ed. P. Zambelli. Rome and Bari; Laterza, 37–79

Galluzzi, P. (1979). *Momento. Studi galileiani*. Rome; Ateneo and Bizarri

Garin, E. (1969). *L'Età nuova: ricerche di storia della cultura dal XII al XVI secolo*. Naples; Morano

Garin, E. (1975). *Rinascite e rivoluzioni. Movimenti culturali dal XIV al XVII secolo*. Rome and Bari; Laterza

Gilbert, N.W. (1960). *Renaissance Concepts of Method*. New York; Columbia University Press

Gilbert, N.W. (1963). Galileo and the School of Padua, *Journal of the History of Philosophy*, Vol. 1, 223–231

Gille, B. (1964). *Les Ingénieurs de la Renaissance*. Paris; Hermann. Trans. (1966) as *The Renaissance Engineers*. London; Lund Humphries

Goldthwaite, R.A. (1972). Schools and Teachers of Commercial Arithmetic in Renaissance Florence, *Journal of European Economic History*, Vol. 1, 418–433

Grant, E., Ed. (1974). *Source Book in Medieval Science*. Cambridge, Mass.; Harvard University Press

Grant, E. (1981a). *Much Ado about Nothing. Theories of Space and Vacuum from the Middle Ages to the Scientific Revolution*. Cambridge; Cambridge University Press

Grant, E. (1981b). *Studies in Medieval Science and Natural Philosophy*. London; Variorum

Hall, B.S. and West, D., Ed. (1976). *On Pre-Modern Technology and Science. A Volume of Studies in Honor of Lynn White Jr.* Malibu, Calif.; Udena

Halleux, R. (1979). *Les Textes alchimiques*. Turnhout, Belgium; Brepols

Hannaway, O. (1975). *The Chemists and the Word. The Didactic Origins of Chemistry*. Baltimore and London; Johns Hopkins University Press

Hedwig, K. (1977). Forschungsübersicht: Arbeiten zur scholastischen Lichtspeculation. Allegorie–Metaphysik–Optik, *Philosophisches Jahrbuch*, Vol. 84, 102–126

Henry, J. (1979). Francesco Patrizi da Cherso's Concept of Space and Its Later Influence, *Annals of Science*, Vol. 36, 549–575

Hewson, M.A. (1975). *Giles of Rome and the Medieval Theory of Conception*. London; Athlone

Hutton, S. (1977). Some Renaissance Critiques of Aristotle's Theory of Time, *Annals of Science*, Vol. 34, 345–363

Jardine, N. (1976). Galileo's Road to Truth and the Demonstrative Regress, *Studies in the History and Philosophy of Science*, Vol. 7, 277–318

Jardine, N. (1979). The Forging of Modern Realism: Clavius and Kepler against the Sceptics, *Studies in the History and Philosophy of Science*, Vol. 10, 141–173

Jayawardene, S.A. (1978). Western Scientific Manuscripts before 1600: a Checklist of Published Catalogues, *Annals of Science*, Vol. 35, 143–172

Keller, A.G. (1975). Mathematicians, Mechanics and Experimental Machines in Northern Italy in the Sixteenth Century, in *The Emergence of Science in Western Europe*. Ed. M.P. Crosland. London; Macmillan, 15–34

Kepler Festschrift (1971). Regensburg; Naturwissenschaftslichen Verein

Kepler und Tübingen. (1971). Tübingen; Universität Tübingen

Kibre, P. (1975–). Hippocrates Latinus. Repertorium of Hippocratic Writings in the Latin Middle Ages, *Traditio*, Vol. 31–

Koyré, A. (1957). *From the Closed World to the Infinite Universe*. Baltimore; Johns Hopkins University Press

Krafft, F. (1970). Die Stellung der Technik zur Naturwissenschaft in Antike und Neuzeit, *Technikgeschichte*, Vol. 37, 189–209

Krafft, F. (1975). Renaissance der Naturwissenschaften – Naturwissenschaften der Renaissance. Ein Überblick über die Nachkriegsliteratur, *Humanismusforschung seit 1945*. Boppard; Harald Boldt, 111–183

Lemay, R. (1962). *Abu Ma 'Shar and Latin Aristotelianism in the Twelfth Century*. Beirut; Catholic Press

Lesky, E. (1957). Harvey und Aristoteles, *Sudhoffs Archiv*, Vol. 41, 289–311, 349–378

Lewis, C. (1980). *The Merton Tradition and Kinematics in Late Sixteenth and Early Seventeenth Century Italy*. Padua; Antenore

Lind, L.R. (1975). *Pre-Vesalian Anatomy*. Philadelphia; American Philosophical Society

Lindberg, D.C. (1970). *Theories of Vision from Al-Kindi to Kepler*. Madison; University of Wisconsin Press

Lindberg, D.C., Ed. (1978). *Science in the Middle Ages*. Chicago and London; University of Chicago Press

Lohr, C.H. (1967–74). Medieval Latin Aristotle Commentaries, *Traditio*, Vols. 23–30 *passim*

Lohr, C.H. (1974–). Renaissance Latin Aristotle Commentaries, *Studies in the Renaissance*, Vol. 21, 228–289; *Renaissance Quarterly*, Vol. 28–

Maccagni, C., Ed. (1967). *Atti del primo convegno internazionale di ricognizione delle fonti per la storia della scienza italiana. I secoli XIV–XVI*. Florence; Barbèra

Maccagni, C., Ed. (1972). *Saggi su Galileo Galilei*, Vol. 2. Florence; Barbèra

McMullin, E., Ed. (1967). *Galileo Man of Science*. New York; Basic Books

McVaugh, M.R. (1969). Quantified Medical Theory and Practice at Fourteenth-Century Montpellier, *Bulletin of the History of Medicine*, Vol. 43, 397–413

Maeyama, Y. and Saltzer, W., Ed. (1977). *Prismata. Naturwissenschaftsgeschichtliche Studien. Festschrift für Willy Hartner*. Wiesbaden; Steiner

Maier, A. (1949–58). *Studien zur Naturphilosophie der Spätscholastik*. 5 Vols. Rome; Edizioni di Storia e Letteratura

Marangon, P. (1977). *Alle origini dell'aristotelismo padovano (sec. XII–XIII)*. Padua; Antenore

Martin, R.N.D. (1976). The Genesis of a Medieval Historian: Pierre Duhem and the Origins of Statics, *Annals of Science*, Vol. 33, 119–129

Masotti, A. (1962). *Studi su Niccolò Tartaglia*. Brescia; Ateneo di Brescia

Mélanges Alexandre Koyré (1964). 2 Vols. Paris; Hermann

Molland, A.G. (1968–9). The Geometrical Background to the Merton School, *British Journal for the History of Science*, Vol. 4, 108–125

Molland, A.G. (1978). An Examination of Bradwardine's Geometry, *Archive for the History of the Exact Sciences*, Vol. 19, 113–175

Moody, E.A. (1975). *Studies in Medieval Philosophy, Science and Logic*. Berkeley, Los Angeles and London; University of California Press

Murdoch, J.E. (1974). Philosophy and the Enterprise of Science in the Later Middle Ages, in *The Interaction between Science and Philosophy*. Ed. Y. Elkana. Atlantic Highlands; Humanities, 51–113

Murdoch, J.E. and Sylla, E.D., Ed. (1975). *The Cultural Context of Medieval Learning*. Dordrecht and Boston; Reidel

Naylor, R.H. (1976). Galileo: the Search for the Parabolic Trajectory, *Annals of Science*, Vol. 33, 153–72

North, J.D., Ed. (1976). *Richard of Wallingford, An Edition of His Writings with Introductions, English Translation and Commentary*. 3 Vols. Oxford; Clarendon Press

Olmi, G. (1976). *Ulisse Aldrovandi. Scienza e natura nel secondo Cinquecento*. Trent; Libera Università

Pagel, W. (1958). *Paracelsus. An Introduction to Philosophical Medicine in the Era of the Renaissance*. Basle; Karger

Pagel, W. (1967). *William Harvey's Biological Ideas: Selected Aspects and Historical Background*. Basle; Karger

Pagel, W. (1969–70). William Harvey Revisited, *History of Science*, Vol. 8, 1–31; Vol. 9, 1–41

Pedersen, O. and Pihl, M. (1974). *Early Physics and Astronomy*. London; Macdonald and James

Pesenti Marangon, T. (1976–7). Michele Savonarola a Padova, *Quaderni per la storia dell'Università di Padova*, Vol. 9–10, 45–102

Plochmann, G.K. (1963). William Harvey and His Methods, *Studies in the Renaissance*, Vol. 10, 192–210

Poppi, A. (1972). *LaDottrinadella scienza di Giacomo Zabarella*. Padua; Antenore

Poulle, E. (1980). *Les Instruments de la théorie des planètes selon Ptolémée: Equatoires et horlogerie planétaire du XIIIe au XVIe siècle.* 2 Vols. Geneva; Droz. Paris; Librairie H. Champion

Purnell, F.J. (1972). Jacopo Mazzoni and Galileo, *Physis*, Vol. 14, 273–294

Randall, J.H. (1961). *The School of Padua and the Emergence of Modern Science.* Padua; Antenore

Reeds, K. (1976). Renaissance Humanism and Botany, *Annals of Science*, Vol. 33, 519–542

Righini Bonelli, M.L. and Settle, T.B. (1979). Egnatio Danti's Great Astronomical Quadrant, *Annali dell'Istituto e Museo di Storia della Scienza*, Vol. 4, 3–13

Righini Bonelli, M.L. and Shea, W.R., Ed. (1975). *Reason, Experiment and Mysticism in the Scientific Revolution.* New York; Science History Publications

Rose, P.L. (1975). *The Italian Renaissance of Mathematics.* Geneva; Droz

Rose, P.L. and Drake, S. (1971). The Pseudo-Aristotelian *Questions in Mechanics* in Renaissance Culture, *Studies in the Renaissance*, Vol. 18, 65–104

Rosen, E. (1961). Renaissance Science as Seen by Burckhardt and His Successors, in *The Renaissance: a Reconsideration of the Theories and Interpretations of the Age.* Ed. T. Helton. Madison; University of Wisconsin Press, 77–103

Rossi, P. (1970). *Philosophy, Technology and the Arts in the Early Modern Era*, Trans. S. Attanasio. New York; Harper and Row

Rossi, P. (1974). *Francesco Bacone: dalla magia alla scienza*, rev. edn. Turin; Einaudi. English transl. of 1st edn (1968). London; Routledge and Kegan Paul. Chicago; University of Chicago Press

Sarton, G. (1957). *Appreciation of Ancient and Medieval Science during the Renaissance (1450–1600).* Philadelphia; University of Pennsylvania Press

Sarton, G. (1957). *Six Wings. Men of Science in the Renaissance.* Bloomington; Indiana University Press. London; The Bodley Head

Schmitt, C.B. (1979). Filosofia e scienza nelle università italiane del XVI secolo, *Il Rinascimento: interpretazioni e problemi.* Rome–Bari; Laterza, 353–398

Schmitt, C.B. (1981). *Studies in Renaissance Philosophy and Science.* London; Variorum

Schmitz, R. and Krafft, F., Ed. (1980). *Humanismus und Naturwissenschaften.* Boppard; Harald Boldt

Schüling, H. (1969). *Die Geschichte der axiomatischen Methode im 16. und beginnenden 17. Jahrhundert.* Hildesheim; Olms

La Science au seizième siècle (1960). Paris; Hermann

Settle, T.B. (1961). An Experiment in the History of Science, *Science*, Vol. 133, 19–23

Settle, T.B. (1966). Galilean Science. Essays in the Mechanics and Dynamics of the Discorsi, Cornell University PhD thesis

Settle, T.B. (1971). Ostilio Ricci. A Bridge between Alberti and Galileo, *XIIe Congrès international d'histoire des sciences* (Paris 1968). *Actes*, Vol. IIIB, 121–126

Shumaker, W. (1972). *The Occult Sciences in the Renaissance.* Berkeley, Los Angeles and London; University of California Press

Singleton, C.S., Ed. (1967). *Art, Science and History in the Renaissance.* Baltimore; Johns Hopkins University Press

Siraisi, N.G. (1973). *Arts and Sciences at Padua. The Studium at Padua before 1350.* Toronto; Pontifical Institute of Medieval Studies

Siraisi, N.G. (1981). *Taddeo Alderotti and His Pupils. Two Generations of Italian Medical Learning.* Princeton; Princeton University Press

Le Soleil à la Renaissance. Science et mythe (1965). Brussels; Presses universitaires de Bruxelles

Stannard, J. (1969). P.A. Mattioli: Sixteenth-Century Commentator on Dioscorides, (University of Kansas) *Bibliographical Contributions*, Vol. 1, 59–81

Steneck, H.H. (1976). *Science and Creation in the Middle Ages. Henry of Langenstein (d. 1397) on Genesis.* Notre Dame and London; University of Notre Dame Press

Stillwell, M.B. (1970). *The Awakening Interest in Science during the First Century of Printing, 1450–1550; an Annotated Checklist of First Editions Viewed from the Angle of their Subject Content.* New York; Bibliographical Society of America

Stock, B. (1972). *Myth and Science in the Twelfth Century; a Study of Bernard Sylvester.* Princeton; Princeton University Press

Studia Copernicana (1970–). Wrocław, Warsaw and Cracow; Polish Academy of Sciences. 21 Vols to date

Swerdlow, N.W. (1976). Pseudodoxia Copernicana, *Archives Internationales d'Histoire des Sciences*, Vol. 26, 108–158

Sylla, E.D. (1971). Medieval Quantification of Qualities: the Merton School, *Archive for the History of the Exact Sciences*, Vol. 8, 9–39

Symposium on Copernicus (1973). *Proceedings of the American Philosophical Society*, Vol. 117, 413–550

Temkin, O. (1973). *Galenism: Rise and Decline of a Medical Philosophy.* Ithaca and London; Cornell University Press

Thorndike, L.T. (1923–58). *A History of Magic and Experimental Science.* 8 Vols. New York; Columbia University Press

Truesdell, C. (1968). *Essays in the History of Mechanics.* Berlin; Springer Verlag

Tugnoli Pattaro, S. (1981). *Metodo e sistema delle scienze nel pensiero di Ulisse Aldrovandi.* Bologna; Editrice CLUEB

Vasoli, C. (1974). *Profezia e ragione.* Naples; Morano

Victor, S.K. (1979). *Practical Geometry in the Middle Ages.* Philadelphia; American Philosophical Society

Walker, D.P. (1958). *Spiritual and Demonic Magic from Ficino to Campanella.* London; Warburg Institute

Walker, D.P. (1978). *Studies in Musical Science in the Late Renaissance.* London; Warburg Institute

Wallace, W.A. (1972–4). *Causality and Scientific Explanation.* 2 Vols. Ann Arbor; University of Michigan Press

Wallace, W.A. (1981). *Prelude to Galileo. Essays on Medieval and Sixteenth-Century Sources of Galileo's Thought.* Dordrecht and Boston; Reidel

Weisheipl, J. (1965). The Principle *Omne quod movetur ab alio movetur* in Medieval Physics, *Isis*, Vol. 56, 26–45

Weisheipl, J.A., Ed. (1980). *Albertus Magnus and the Sciences.* Toronto; Pontifical Institute of Medieval Studies

Westman, R.S. (1975a). The Melanchthon Circle, Rheticus and the Wittenberg Interpretation of Copernican Theory, *Isis*, Vol. 66, 165–193

Westman, R.S., Ed. (1975b). *The Copernican Achievement.* Berkeley, Los Angeles and London; University of California Press

Westman, R.S. (1980). The Astronomer's Role in the Sixteenth Century: a Preliminary Survey, *History of Science*, Vol. 18, 105–147

Westman, R.S. and McGuire, J.E. (1977). *Hermeticism and the Scientific Revolution.* Los Angeles; W.A. Clark Memorial Library

White, L. (1962). *Medieval Technology and Social Change.* London; Oxford University Press

White, L. (1978). *Medieval Religion and Technology.* Berkeley, Los Angeles and London; University of California Press

Wightman, W. (1962). *Science and the Renaissance*. 2 Vols. Edinburgh and London; Oliver and Boyd

Wilson, C. (1956). *William Heytesbury. Medieval Logic and the Rise of Mathematical Physics*. Madison; University of Wisconsin Press

Wisan, W.L. (1974). The New Science of Motion: a Study of Galileo's *De motu locali, Archive for the History of the Exact Sciences*, Vol. 13, 103–306

Wisan, W.L. (1978). Galileo's Scientific Method: a Re-examination, in *New Perspectives on Galileo*. Ed. R.E. Butts and J.C. Pitt. Dordrecht and Boston; Reidel, 1–57

Witt, R.G. (1977). Salutati and Contemporary Physics, *Journal of the History of Ideas*, Vol. 38, 667–672

Yates, F.A. (1964). *Giordano Bruno and the Hermetic Tradition*. London; Routledge and Kegan Paul

Zambelli, P. (1973). Il Problema della magia naturale nel Rinascimento, *Rivista critica di storia della filosofia*, Vol. 28, 271–296

Zambelli, P. (1978). Aut Diabolus aut Achillinus. Fisionomia, astrologia e demonologia nel metodo di un aristotelico, *Rinascimento*, Vol. 18, 59–86

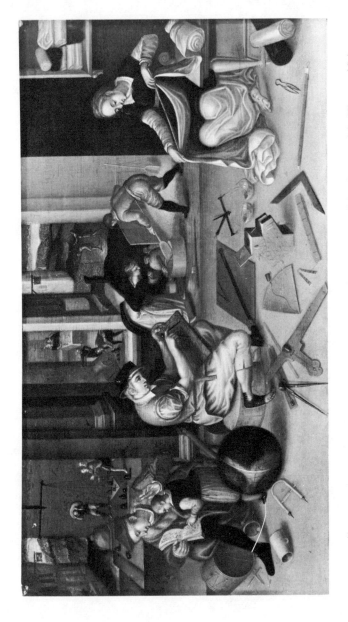

Plate 5. The Measurers. An oil by Hendrik van Balen (1560–1632). By courtesy of the Museum of the History of Science, Oxford University

13

Scientific instruments

G.L'E. Turner

Science is the study that leads to discriminative knowledge (*scientia*) of the material world based on observation, experiment and induction. The *ad hoc* solving of practical problems in man's dealings with nature must be distinguished from the use of reason applied to the complexities of the material world. Some elementary classifying may be carried out without the help of instruments; nevertheless, modern science cannot exist without them. (For a general conspectus of the range of scientific instruments, see Turner 1980a; Michel 1967 selects the most decorative pieces.) Instruments and manipulative skills are the basic necessities for measuring and provoking phenomena, and are in themselves neutral. A brass astrolabe, incorporating a means for measuring the elevation angle of stars or the altitude of the sun, as well as a stereographic representation of the globe and of the heavens, can be used equally well for telling the time, finding the latitude, and collecting data for casting horoscopes (Maddison 1966; Michel 1947; National Maritime Museum 1976).

It is well known that observatories were constructed in the ancient world, and the stone circles, such as Stonehenge, have been identified as such (Thom 1971; Wood 1978). Not generally known is that a Greek, geared, calendar computer of about 80 BC exists (Price 1975). Starting with this Greek instrument, King and Millburn (1979) deal most thoroughly with the evolution of all kinds of planetary models, including the astrolabe and the astronomical clock. They devote a chapter to the Astrarium of Giovanni de' Dondi, the subject of a separate work by Bedini and Maddison (1966). A medieval planetary computer called an equatorium also had its origins in Hellenistic times (North 1969; Poulle 1980). The remarkable fourteenth-century astronomical clock of Richard of Wallingford, together with his albion (a computing device), are the subject of the monumental work by North (1976). Chaucer's astrolabe treatise was published in modern English, with commentary, by Gunther (1929), and a manuscript on an equatorium possibly by Chaucer was published by Price (1955).

The convenient and ubiquitous sundial – only displaced by the electric telegraph as the check on clocks and watches – must be the oldest of scientific instruments. It is to be found in a great variety of types and sizes (Gibbs 1976; Körber 1965; Maddison 1963; Portaluppi 1968; Rohr 1970; Van Cittert-Eymers 1972).

The Italian Renaissance of the fifteenth century laid the foundation of a modern science that was to be free from the magic inherent in alchemy and astrology. Towards the end of this century, the Portuguese for the first time used astronomical navigation with the aid of instruments on their voyages of discovery; this was to be developed markedly in the following century (Maddison 1969). Outstanding products of the early sixteenth century were two books published in 1543, *De Revolutionibus Orbium Coelestium* by Nicholas Copernicus (1473–1543) and *De Humani Corporis Fabrica* by Andreas Vesalius (1514–1564). Copernicus's work incorporated no new observations; its importance lay in a change of viewpoint, the realization that the planetary system was simpler to describe if the sun and not the earth were regarded as central. Vesalius wrote about his own carefully observed discoveries of the human body. Copernicus was followed by Tycho Brahe (1546–1601), an outstanding observational astronomer whose instruments, used with the unassisted eye, were constructed by a remarkable group of German craftsmen (Thoren 1973; Mackensen 1980). Kepler's name might well have been lost along with those of other mathematicians of his time, were it not for Tycho's observations, which were made possible by the superb instruments at his disposal. This is not in any way to belittle the importance of concept and theory, but simply to stress that the design, the craft techniques of the workshop, and the way in which instruments were used must also be taken into account in studying the development of science. Moreover, their capability at any given time can constitute a technical frontier, which makes it possible to understand why a certain discovery was delayed, or a sudden breakthrough occurred. The accuracy of angular measure obtained by Tycho was about one minute of arc, which may be contrasted with the ten minutes of Ulugh Beg, in about AD 1440, and the twenty minutes of Hipparchus, in about 130 BC (Pledge 1939: 291). With improved construction techniques and telescopic sights, John Flamsteed (1646–1719) was able to improve on Tycho by a factor of five, with an accuracy of about fifteen seconds. (For Greenwich, see Chapman 1976; Howse 1975; in general, Donnelly 1973.)

Vesalius was followed by William Harvey (1578–1657), who propounded the theory of the circulation of the blood. The flow of the blood was to be observed directly by means of the microscopes of the second half of the seventeenth century. These new optical instruments, the microscope and the telescope, were the invention of Dutch spectacle makers in about 1600, and added to man's experience the new dimensions of the very small and the very distant (Drake 1976; North 1974; Turner 1969a; Van Helden 1977; Van Zuylen 1981).

Trade and exploration during the sixteenth century encouraged the development and teaching of the mathematics of navigation, and the improvement of such instruments as the mariner's astrolabe, the quadrant and the compass (Anderson 1972; Maddison 1963; McConnell 1980). The problem of finding the longitude was understood in principle, but could not be solved because there was no mechanism capable of being carried on board ship that would keep the time at the port of departure. Christiaan Huygens (1629–1695) attempted a sea-going pendulum clock, but the solution had to wait for John Harrison (1693–1776) in the mid-eighteenth century (Howse 1980; Quill 1966). On land there was marked development of surveying instruments (Eden 1975; Richeson 1966; Roche 1981). The military surveyor or engineer required instruments in the construction of fortifications, and the gunner required levels, range-finders and calipers to assist him in blowing them up (Hall 1952; Galileo 1978; Wunderlich 1977). Navigational and topographical instruments, as well as charts and globes (which, like the instruments, involve accurate engraving on brass or copper), were required in large numbers, and this caused the establishment of several centres in Western Europe where instrument makers congregated (May 1973; Stimson 1976; Taylor 1971; Tyacke and Huddy 1980; Waters 1958).

Francis Bacon (1561–1626) was the man who contributed so much to the change in scientific method that he may be said to herald modern experimental science. Bacon stressed the need to test by works, since an explanation that cannot be tested is useless because it must lack a basis in the real world, the yardstick by which scientific truth is recognized. It is hardly surprising, then, that the Royal Society, founded some forty years after Bacon's *Novum Organum* (1620) was published, has as its motto: *Nullius in verba*.

On the Continent and in England groups of men learned in literature and science came together during the early years of the seventeenth century; this resulted in the foundation of the great academies in Italy, France and England. The Royal Society was notable for setting up the post of curator of experiments, whose duty was to provide 'three or four considerable experiments' each day the Society met. Robert Hooke (1635–1703) was the first curator, having previously been assistant to Robert Boyle (1627–1691). Hooke knew and advised most of the instrument makers of London, and his inventiveness and their skill helped to inspire and provide for the new interest in natural philosophy. Hooke's work with the microscope and Newton's work on optics and astronomy stimulated the optical instrument trade to provide for the awakened imaginations of men at about the turn of the century. Newton's work on mechanics also had the effect of creating a demand for demonstrations of many elementary and complex effects. Meteorological instruments were soon needed in the new observatories in Paris, Greenwich and elsewhere to refine the angular measurements, and so the barometer and thermometer were developed (Bolle, 1982; Goodison 1977; Habenicht and Holland 1977; Middleton 1964, 1966, 1969a,b).

The eighteenth century saw scientific societies proliferate throughout Europe, such was the interest in experimental natural philosophy; philosophical cabinets, composed of instruments and natural history specimens, multiplied with the societies. Private collections continued to be formed in a tradition started as a result of the explorations of the sixteenth century, and examples that are still largely preserved are the King George III collection in the Science Museum, London, Teyler's Museum in Haarlem, and the Harvard College collection in Cambridge, Massachusetts (Bologna 1980; Brown 1959; Carvalho 1978; Chaldecott 1951; Grötzsch 1978; Hughes 1980; Pipping 1977; Turner and Levere 1973; Wheatland 1968). In 1700, John Keill (1671–1721) was giving lecture–demonstrations in Oxford, an example soon followed in London. Demonstrations of the workings of a wide range of apparatus were advertised; a course of instruction might cover twelve weeks and cost two or three guineas. In 1717, Willem 's Gravesande (1688–1742) was elected professor of astronomy and natural philosophy in Leyden. He based his teaching on Newton's principles, using elaborate apparatus to illustrate them. This apparatus was extensively copied and continued in scarcely altered form, especially the mechanics and optics, into twentieth-century school teaching.

During the eighteenth century, scientific instruments were made not only for the lecture–demonstration business, but also for people to use in their homes. The most popular domestic instruments were the microscope (Millburn 1976; Turner 1980b, especially ch. 10), used for looking at fleas, hair and wood, and telescopes for observing sunspots and the moon. The next favoured were the electrostatic generator to make hair stand on end (Hackmann 1973, 1978, 1979), and the air-pump, used to evacuate a chamber containing a mouse or a cat. However futile this activity may seem at first glance, it did two things: it disseminated an interest and knowledge of things scientific, and it provided a very considerable market, especially among the many wealthy English of the later eighteenth century. The well-supported London trade not only supplied the world with its excellent products, but could also sustain the making of large, complex, difficult pieces, such as Ramsden's theodolite – a product of his improved dividing engine – and the Harrison chronometers (Brown 1978, 1979; Calvert 1971; Millburn 1976; Taylor 1954, 1966; Turner 1976). These chronometers, made after years of applied physical research, were to improve the accuracy of navigation quite suddenly by a factor of 100, a most far-reaching and dramatic discontinuity (Davies 1978). Some map engravers also made instruments (Fordham 1976; Tyacke 1978). The origins of the London instrument-making trade, which arose in the sixteenth century, must be sought on the Continent (Daumas 1972), and London's subsequent influence on Scotland (Bryden 1972) and on North America (Bedini 1964, 1975) can readily be seen. During the eighteenth century, London supplied much of the world (for a Russian example see Chenakal 1972), and for best results an agent or go-between would be employed (Turner 1974).

The nineteenth century opened with the advantages to manufacturing of the new machine tools and processes of the industrial revolution (Musson and Robinson 1969), and soon benefited from new instruments. Accuracy of measurement markedly improved, as with precision balances for chemical work (Stock 1969). Following the issue of new standards for weights and measures in England in 1824, the old apothecaries' and coin balances were gradually superseded, and large numbers of more accurate sub-standards for length and volume were manufactured (Crawforth 1979; Kisch 1965; Koning and Houben 1980).

Throughout the eighteenth century, surgery improved greatly, and teaching colleges were set up in Paris, Berlin, Vienna and

Edinburgh. The Royal College of Surgeons of London was not, however, founded until 1800. Naturally, this activity generated a demand for instruments, which was met by cutlers; the trade in surgical instruments has always been quite separate from that in other scientific instruments (Belloni 1971; Bennion 1979). By the beginning of the twentieth century, physics had intruded into medical research, and a useful guide has been provided by Van Spronsen (1973). Drug jars form another group of objects that can reveal important historical information, and they are conventionally placed in the broad category of scientific instruments (Drey 1978; Hill and Drey 1980). Chemical glassware is also to be included (Anderson 1978; Hill 1971); but in chemistry, too, physical methods of analysis have become more and more important (Szabadvary 1966).

Optical instruments were late in achieving their full potential because of the poor quality of optical glass. To obtain better images from the telescope, in the late seventeenth century Gregory and Newton devised forms of reflecting telescope that used a concave metal objective, so avoiding the use of a glass objective lens. The late eighteenth century saw the greatest use of the reflector, made by such renowned craftsmen as James Short and Edward Nairne (Turner 1969b, 1979). Great efforts to improve optical glass were made in the middle of the nineteenth century. A pioneer in the production of this material was the German, Fraunhofer (Roth 1976), and the man responsible for achieving the desired technical perfection in glass for lenses in the 1880s was Schott of Jena (Körber 1975).

Lenses were used in the camera obscura, both in static and portable forms, and this ancient device eventually developed in the 1830s into the first photographic cameras. The Science Museum, London, has a particularly fine collection representing all aspects of photography, and Thomas (1969) has written an excellent introduction to photographic equipment and catalogue of the collection. Fox Talbot, the British pioneer, is the subject of a biography (Arnold 1978), and Wall (1978) has produced a directory of photographic collections for the Royal Photographic Society.

A detailed survey of sources and modern studies for optical instruments has been made by Turner (1969a). This covers modern studies of the eye (an essential component) glass, and spectacles, as well as the telescope, the microscope and photography. The reprint (Turner 1980b: ch. 2) extends the bibliography for microscopy to 1979. An outline of the history of the microscope, particularly suitable for students and fully illustrated, has been written by Turner (1981). A collection of a dozen catalogues for the period 1854 to 1910 of the Parisian microscope-making firm of Nachet has been reprinted by Brieux (1979). This publication (and one on precision instruments, Brieux 1980) underlines the value to students of scientific instruments of all old catalogues, from which new developments and refinements of design can often be dated.

Instruments used in the preparation of specimens for microscopy, such as the microtome, have received remarkably little attention. This has been remedied by Bracegirdle (1978), who has studied the development of the microtome in detail, drawing on museums in Europe and on the nineteenth-century literature in particular. His book includes an evaluation of the literature and many references.

The first electron microscope was made in Berlin in 1931 by Ernst Ruska, and two years later a new model could give high magnifications. The early history of this remarkable invention has been written by Ruska himself (1980).

The laboratory-based electron microscope can be seen as symptomatic of the radical change in the operation of science that took place during the later nineteenth and early twentieth centuries. In a word, it became professionalized. The 'scientific gentleman' of the eighteenth century, who contributed to new knowledge and might even become a Fellow of the Royal Society, disappeared. Scientific societies flourished, some for amateurs bent on recreation, others for the professionals. Technical training became formalized, first with the mechanics institutes and then with the municipal universities. Science left the home, the club and the popular lecture hall, and flourished in laboratories and classrooms.

Instrument-making involves technical, economic and social factors in addition to the science it embodies. The complexity of these interactions can only be hinted at in this short essay, but one significant aspect is increasing accuracy of measurement, which requires either the refinement of a single concept or new concepts that radically alter the manner of making the measurement. The balance may be cited as an example in which the principle of comparing one mass with another is very old, and increasing accuracy is effected by refinements in engineering the instrument. On the other hand, time-telling devices show marked differences – discontinuities in fact – in the manner in which time is measured. From shadow, through clepsydra-orifice, verge and foliot, pendulum, piezo-electric effect, to the frequency of the caesium atom, we have a series of seemingly unrelated devices that could make some people doubt if they all measure the same thing.

In chemistry, the new ideas of Lavoisier, Dalton and Davy made it imperative that the chemical balance be greatly refined in its capacity to make delicate measurements. Skinner produced a chart showing the sensitivity of a balance against date (published in Pledge 1939: 126). His figures were based on actual weighing with reconditioned instruments of the relevant periods. He was able to show that accuracy had increased by 1,000 from 1550 to 1930, and a hundred-fold from 1825 to 1930. In spite of certain problems in ensuring that meaningful results are obtained when using old instruments, this is a particularly important and fruitful line of research that has, unfortunately, been too little pursued. The only recent work on the accuracy of the balance is that of Iwata (1975), whose graph of increasing accuracy of measurement of mass was entirely based on assessment of the printed literature. Such an approach may be satisfactory for a technically advanced period such as the past 100 years, but needs experimental support for earlier periods.

Accuracy of time measurement is vital for the astronomer, and, with the marine chronometer, for the navigator and the hydrographer. For the physicist, accuracy to seconds and part-seconds is frequently required. The illuminating chart drawn by Ward (1961: 8) shows that the first pendulum clock, that of Huygens, increased accuracy some 500-fold, and from 1660 to 1960, accuracy increased over one million-fold, with the arrival of the caesium-atom clock. A chart on similar lines was drawn by Mineur (Pledge 1939: 291), which shows the accuracy of astronomical angular measurement over 2000 years.

A study that was part experimental and partly based on examination of the literature was that of Turner (1967b), who prepared charts showing the increase in the resolving power of the optical microscope during the nineteenth century, the period when it became established as a vital scientific instrument. It was not until the beginning of the century that geometrical and technical optics became sufficiently advanced to correct the aberrations of the microscopic image, with their consequent limitation on the resolution of fine detail. Improvement in objective lens design was rapid from 1830, but a standard was then needed to facilitate the comparison of lenses; this was provided by the resolution test plates of the German, Friedrich Nobert. The figures of performance of many objective lenses produced between 1830 and 1880 were plotted against the date of manufacture, and *Figure 13.1* shows that the most rapid improvement took place about 1850.

With the core of the development established, it becomes possible to assess a discovery in a new way. If a certain resolution produced by manufacturers is closely followed by a discovery requiring that degree of resolution, then the research is keeping pace with the instrument. It is also possible to establish the date before which it was impossible to have made the discovery. On the other hand, if a discovery is made long after the necessary resolution was attainable, then it is likely that a conceptual difficulty hindered the research. Bacteriology developed very closely with the development of the microscope. An example is the study of pleomorphism, or the varieties that occur within a single

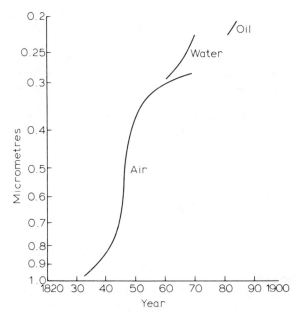

Figure 13.1 The increase in resolution of microscope objectives during the nineteenth century

type of bacterium. Some pleomorphs may be a fifth to a tenth of the size of the more usual form, and the resolution and clarity of image needed to observe them were realized in the apochromatic objective lens systems first marketed by Zeiss in 1886. By around 1900, there were claims by scientists that bacteria underwent sudden changes to entirely different shapes, so a time lag of some fifteen years can be established. The study of metallography, the crystal structure of metals, provides an example of the conceptual block effect. The crystals in metals may often be measured in millimeters, and satisfactory work in the examination of metal structure can be done with a resolution of 10 micrometres, which was attainable throughout the eighteenth century. Yet metals continued to be thought amorphous until they were examined by Henry Sorby in the mid-nineteenth century.

The varied examples described above serve to demonstrate what may be described as the technical frontiers of science. Limitations may be placed on scientists by the quality of the tools available to them, or they may be limited in their discoveries by their own capacity to formulate a theory.

Museums and libraries

For many purposes, the instruments themselves are the primary source. Guides to museums are variable in the information provided, not every country may have one, and they tend to become dated. A comprehensive guide to world museums is Hudson and Nicholls (1975), a large work with subject index, but unfortunately all the museums' names have been translated into English and the originals are not given.

Since the 1950s, a number of national inventories have been in preparation under the general guidance of the Commission pour l'inventaire mondial des appareils scientifiques d'intérêt historique, a group set up by the International Union of the History and Philosophy of Science. The following countries have published inventories in one form or another: Belgium, Italy, France, Poland, Russia, Portugal (for details, see Turner 1969a). Regrettably, these are far too restricted in coverage; probably nor more than a tenth of the instruments actually in the country concerned is mentioned. (For a review of the French inventory, see Turner 1967a.) The British inventory (Science Museum, to be published) was planned on a different basis and is a guide of first importance: it lists all the locations and the complete holdings of the smaller museums, and provides an outline of the contents of the major museums such as the Science Museum, London, and the Museum of the History of Science, Oxford.

Some museums have published catalogues of all or, more usually, of part of their holdings (e.g. Bonelli 1968; Brachner and Seeberger 1976; Chaldecott 1951; Engberts 1970; Horský and Škopová 1968; Middleton 1969b; Turner and Levere 1973; Ward 1981).

There are certain libraries that must be visited by any student. The Library of the Science Museum, London, is particularly strong on early and modern periodical literature, exhibition catalogues, trade catalogues and trade cards, prints, plans, and drawings. With the opening in November 1980 of the Wellcome Medical Museum at the Science Museum, it is now possible to study medical instruments together with associated literature. The Museum of the History of Science, Oxford, contains the largest specialist library of early and modern works on astronomical, mathematical and optical instruments, and there is a similar, though less extensive, library at the Whipple Museum of the History of Science, Cambridge. The Rare Books Library at the Smithsonian Institution, Washington DC, together with other central and departmental libraries, make the Smithsonian the obvious centre for the study of instruments in the United States. In the Netherlands, the library of the Boerhaave Museum, Leyden, has books and periodicals concerned with modern studies on instruments, as well as archival material. The Teyler's Museum, Haarlem, has the most complete stock of eighteenth- and nineteenth-century scientific periodicals from all over the world, and a collection of books to match.

There is no general bibliography on scientific instruments, although there are a few on restricted topics (Maddison 1963; Turner 1969a). For a full discussion on the general bibliographies and sources for the history of science, see chapter 10 in the present volume. There are some guide books that a research worker could, with profit, acquire for his own library. Collison (1962) provides a guide to subject bibliographies, and Collison (1964) leads the reader through the maze of the history of encyclopaedias. The value of encyclopaedias, especially their plates, for the study of instruments must be stressed. Ferguson (1968) gives far more than its title, *Bibliography of the History of Technology*, would suggest. There are chapters on government records, illustrations, manuscripts, directories and much else, apart from the subject fields, which include, if briefly, scientific instruments.

Bibliography

Anderson, R.G.W. (1972). *The Mariner's Astrolabe*. Edinburgh; Royal Scottish Museum

Anderson, R.G.W. (1978). *The Playfair Collection and the Teaching of Chemistry at the University of Edinburgh 1713 – 1858*. Edinburgh; Royal Scottish Museum

Arnold, H.J.P. (1978). *William Henry Fox Talbot, Pioneer of Photography and Man of Science*. London; Hutchinson Benham

Bedini, S.A. (1964). *Early American Scientific Instruments and their Makers*. Washington DC; Smithsonian Institution

Bedini, S.A. (1975). *Thinkers and Tinkers: Early American Men of Science*. New York; Charles Scribner's Sons

254   Scientific instruments

Bedini, S. and Maddison, F.R. (1966). Mechanical Universe: The Astrarium of Giovanni de' Dondi, *Transactions of the American Philosophical Society*, new ser., Vol. 56, part 5

Belloni, L. (1971). *Lo Strumentario chirurgico di Giovanni Alessandro Brambilla*. Florence; Istituto e Museo di Storia della Scienza di Firenze

Bennion, E. (1979). *Antique Medical Instruments*. London; Sotheby Parke Bernet. Berkeley; University of California Press

Bolle, B. (1982). *Barometers*. Watford, Herts; Argus Books

Bologna, Comune di (1980). *Macchine scuola industria: Dal mestiere alla professionalità operaia* (1° centenario dell'Istituto Tecnico Industriale Aldini Valeriani). Bologna; Società editrice il Mulino

Bonelli, M.L.R. (1968). *Il Museo di Storia della Scienza a Firenze*. Milan; Electa Editrice

Bracegirdle, B. (1978). *A History of Microtechnique: The Development of the Microtome and the Development of Tissue Preparation*. London; Heinemann

Brachner, A. and Seeberger, M. (1976). *Joseph von Fraunhofer 1787–1826. Ausstellung zum 150. Todestag*. Munich; Deutsches Museum

Brieux (1979). *Maison Nachet: Catalogues de fonds de 1854 à 1910*. Introduction by G.L'E. Turner. Paris; Editions Alain Brieux

Brieux (1980). *L'Industrie française des instruments de précision: catalogue 1901 – 1902*. Paris; Editions Alain Brieux

Brown, L.A. (1959). *Early Philosophical Apparatus at Transylvania College (and Relics of the Medical Department)*. Lexington, Ky; Transylvania College Press

Brown, J. (1978). *Mathematical Instrument-Makers in the Grocers' Company 1688–1830*. London; Science Museum Monographs, HMSO

Brown, J. (1979). Guild Organisation and the Instrument-Making Trade, 1550–1830, *Annals of Science*, Vol. 36, 1–34

Bryden, D.J. (1972). *Scottish Scientific Instrument-Makers 1600–1900*. Royal Scottish Museum Information Series, Technology 1. Edinburgh; Royal Scottish Museum

Calvert, H.R. (1971). *Scientific Trade Cards in the Science Museum Collection*. London; HMSO

Carvalho, R. de (1978). *História do Gabinete de Física da Universidade de Coimbra*. Coimbra; Universidade de Coimbra

Chaldecott, J.A. (1951). *Handbook of the King George III Collection of Scientific Instruments*. London; HMSO

Chapman, A. (1976). Astronomia practica: the Principal Instruments and their Uses at the Royal Observatory, *Vistas in Astronomy*, Vol. 20, 141–156

Chenakal, V.L. (1972). The Astronomical Instruments of John Rowley in Eighteenth Century Russia, *Journal for the History of Astronomy*, Vol. 3, 119–135

Cittert-Eymers, J.G. van (1972). *Zonnewijzers aan en bij Gebouwen in Nederland*. Zutphen; Thieme

Collison, R. (1962). *Bibliographies: Subject and National. A Guide to their Contents, Arrangement and Use*, 2nd edn. New York; Hafner. Also (1968). London; Crosby, Lockwood and Son

Collison, R. (1964). *Encyclopaedias: Their History Throughout the Ages*. New York; Hafner. 2nd edn (1966)

Crawforth, M.A. (1979). *Weighing Coins: English Folding Gold Balances of the 18th and 19th Centuries*. London; Cape Horn Trading Coy

Daumas, M. (1972). *Scientific Instruments of the 17th and 18th Centuries and their Makers*. Trans. M. Holbrook. London; Batsford

Davies, A.C. (1978). The Life and Death of a Scientific Instrument: the Marine Chronometer, 1770–1920, *Annals of Science*, Vol. 35, 509–525

Donnelly, M.C. (1973). *A Short History of Observatories*. Eugene; University of Oregon Books

Drake, S. (1976). Galileo's First Telescopic Observations, *Journal for the History of Astronomy*, Vol. 7, 153–168

Drey, R.E.A. (1978). *Apothecary Jars: Pharmaceutical Pottery and Porcelain in Europe and the East 1150–1850*. London; Faber and Faber

Eden, P. (1975). *Dictionary of Land Surveyors and Local Cartographers of Great Britain and Ireland 1550–1850*. 3 Parts. Folkestone; W. Dawson and Sons

Engberts, E. (1970). *Descriptive Catalogue of Telescopes in the National Museum of the History of Science, Leyden*. Leyden; Museum Boerhaave

Ferguson, E.S. (1968). *Bibliography of the History of Technology*. Society for the History of Technology, Monograph 5, Cambridge, Mass.; Society for the History of Technology and MIT Press

Fordham, H.G. (1976). *John Cary: Engraver, Map, Chart and Print-seller and Globe-maker 1754 to 1835*. Folkestone; Dawson and Sons. Reprint of (1925) edn.

Galileo Galilei (1978). *Operations of the Geometric and Military Compass*. Trans. S. Drake from 1606 edn. Washington DC; Dibner Library and Smithsonian Institution Press

Gibbs, S.L. (1976). *Greek and Roman Sundials*. New Haven; Yale University Press

Goodison, N. (1977). *English Barometers 1680–1860: A History of Domestic Barometers and their Makers and Retailers*, 2nd edn. Woodbridge; Antique Collectors' Club

Grötzsch, H. (1978). *Dresden Mathematisch-Physikalischer Salon*. Leipzig; VEB E.A. Seemann Verlag

Gunther, R.T. (1929). *Chaucer and Messahalla on the Astrolabe. Now printed in full for the first time with the original illustrations*. Early Science in Oxford, V. Oxford; printed for the subscribers at the University Press

Habenicht, W. and Holland, R. (1977). *Alte Quecksilber Barometer, Ihre Schönheit und Funktion*. Bremen; Anker-Druk

Hackmann, W.D. (1973). *John and Jonathan Cuthbertson: The Invention and Development of the Eighteenth Century Plate Electrical Machine*. Leyden; Museum Boerhaave

Hackmann, W.D. (1978). *Electricity from Glass: the History of the Frictional Electrical Machine 1600–1850*. Alphen aan den Rijn; Sijthoff and Noordhoff

Hackmann, W.D. (1979). The Relationship between Concept and Instrument Design in Eighteenth-century Experimental Science, *Annals of Science*, Vol. 36, 205–224

Hall, A.R. (1952). *Ballistics in the Seventeenth Century*. Cambridge; Cambridge University Press

Helden, A. van (1977). The Invention of the Telescope, *Proceedings of the American Philosophical Society*, Vol. 67, part 4

Hill, C.R. (1971). *Chemical Apparatus: Catalogue 1 Museum of the History of Science*. Oxford; Museum of the History of Science

Hill, C.R. and Drey, R.E.A. (1980). *Drug Jars: Catalogue 3 Museum of the History of Science*. Oxford; Museum of the History of Science

Horský, Z. and Škopová, O. (1968). *Astronomy Gnomonics: A Catalogue of Instruments of the 15th to the 19th Centuries in the Collections of the National Technical Museum, Prague*. Prague; National Technical Museum

Howse, D. (1975). *The Buildings and Instruments*. Vol. 3 of *Greenwich Observatory*. London; Taylor and Francis

Howse, D. (1980). *Greenwich Time and the Discovery of the Longitude*. Oxford; Oxford University Press

Hudson, K. and Nicholls, A. (1975). *The Directory of Museums*. London; Macmillan

Hughes, B. (1980). *Catalog of the Scientific Apparatus at the College of Charlston: 1800–1940*. Charlston, SC; College of Charlston Library Associates

Iwata, S. (1975). Development of Sensitivity of the Precision Balance, in *Travaux du 1er congrès international de la métrologie historique, Zagreb, 28–30 octobre 1975*. Ed. Z. Herkov. Zagreb; Académie Yougoslave des Sciences et des Arts, Institut d'Histoire.

King, H.C. and Millburn, J.R. (1979). *Geared to the Stars: the Evolution of Planetariums, Orreries and Astronomical Clocks*. Toronto; Toronto University Press. Bristol; Adam Hilger

Kisch, B. (1965). *Scales & Weights: A Historical Outline*. Yale Studies in the History of Science and Medicine, Vol. 1. New Haven, Conn.; Yale University Press

Koning, D.A.W. and Houben, C.M.M. (1980). *2000 Jaar gewichten in de Nederlanden. Stelsels, ijkwegen, vormen, makers, merken, gebruik*. Lochem; De Tijdstroom

Körber, H.-G. (1965). *Zur Geschichte der Konstruktion von Sonnenuhren und Kompassen des 16. bis 18. Jahrhunderts*. Veröffentlichungen des Staatlichen Mathematisch-Physikalischen Salons Dresden-Zwinger, Vol. 3. Berlin; VEB Deutscher Verlag der Wissenschaften

Körber, H.-G. (1975). Otto Friedrich Schott, in *Dictionary of Scientific Biography*. Ed. C.C. Gillispie. New York; Charles Scribner's Sons, Vol. 12: 211–212

McConnell, A. (1980). *Geomagnetic Instruments Before 1900*. London; Harriet Wynter

Mackensen, L. von (1980). *Die erste Sternwarte Europas mit Ihren Instrumenten and Uhren: 400 Jahr Jost Bürgi in Kassel*. Munich; Callwey

Maddison, F.R. (1963). Early Astronomical and Mathematical Instruments. Brief Survey of Sources and Modern Studies, *History of Science*, Vol. 2, 17–50

Maddison, F.R. (1966). *Hugo Helt and the Rojas Astrolabe Projection*. Coimbra; Agrupamento de Estudos de Cartografia Antiga, series sep. XII

Maddison, F.R. (1969). *Medieval Scientific Instruments and the Development of Navigational Instruments in the XV and XVI Centuries*. Coimbra; Agrupamento de Estudos de Cartografia Antiga, series sep. XXX

May, W.E. (1973). *A History of Marine Navigation*. Henley-on-Thames; G.T. Foulis and Co.

Michel, H. (1947). *Traité de l'astrolabe*. Paris; Gauthiers-Villars. Reprinted (1976) with preface and notes by F.R. Maddison. Paris; Librairie Alain Brieux

Michel, H. (1967). *Scientific Instruments in Art and History*. Trans. R.E.W. Maddison and F.R. Maddison. London; Barrie and Rockliff

Middleton, W.E.K. (1964). *The History of the Barometer*. Baltimore, Johns Hopkins University Press

Middleton, W.E.K. (1966). *A History of the Thermometer and its Uses in Meteorology*. Baltimore, Johns Hopkins University Press

Middleton, W.E.K. (1969a). *Invention of the Meteorological Instruments*. Baltimore, Johns Hopkins University Press

Middleton, W.E.K. (1969b). *Catalog of Meteorological Instruments in the Museum of History and Technology*. Washington DC; Smithsonian Institution Press

Millburn, J.R. (1976). *Benjamin Martin: Author, Instrument-Maker and 'Country Showman'*. Leyden; Noordhoff International Publishing

Musson, A.E. and Robinson, E. (1969). *Science and Technology in the Industrial Revolution*. Manchester; Manchester University Press

National Maritime Museum (1976). *The Planispheric Astrolabe*. London; HMSO

North, J. (1969). A Post-Copernican Equatorium, *Physis: Rivista Internazionale di Storia della Scienza*, Vol. 11, 418–457

North, J. (1974). Thomas Harriot and the First Telescopic Observations of Sunspots, in *Thomas Harriot Renaissance Scientist*. Ed. J.R. Shirley. Oxford; Clarendon Press

North, J.D., Ed. (1976). *Richard of Wallingford: An Edition of his Writings with Introductions, English Translation and Commentary*. 3 Vols. Oxford; Clarendon Press

Pipping, G. (1977). *The Chamber of Physics. Instruments in the History of Sciences Collections of the Royal Swedish Academy of Sciences, Stockholm.* Stockholm; Almqvist and Wiksell

Pledge, H.T. (1939). *Science since 1500*. London; HMSO .

Portaluppi, P. (1968). *Gnomonica Atellana: le Meridiane dell'Arte, l'Arte delle Meridiane.* Milan; Studio Atellano

Poulle, E. (1980). *Les Instruments de la théorie des planètes selon Ptolémée: Équatoires et horlogerie planétaire du XIIIᵉ au XVIᵉ siècle.* 2 Vols. Geneva; Librairie Droz. Paris; Librairie H. Champion

Price, D.J. (1955). *The Equatorie of the Planetis edited from Peterhouse MS 75.I.* Cambridge; Cambridge University Press

Price, D.J. de Solla (1975). *Gears from the Greeks. The Antikythera Mechanism – a Calendar Computer from ca. 80 B.C.* New York; Science History Publications

Quill, H. (1966). *John Harrison the Man who Found Longitude*. London; John Baker

Richeson, A.W. (1966). *English Land Measuring to 1880: Instruments and Practice*. Cambridge, Mass.; MIT Press

Roche, J.J. (1981). The Radius Astronomicus in England, *Annals of Science*, Vol. 38, 1–32

Rohr, R.R.J. (1970). *Sundials, History, Theory, and Practice*. English translation, Toronto and Buffalo; University of Toronto Press

Roth, G.D. (1976). *Joseph von Fraunhofer: Handwerker, Forscher, Akademiemitglied, 1787–1826.* Stuttgart; Wissenschaftliche Verlagsgesellschaft

Ruska, Ernst (1980). *The Early Development of Electron Lenses and Electron Microscopy*. Trans. T. Mulvey. Stuttgart; Hirzel Verlag

Spronsen, J.W. van (1973). *Historie van de Scheikunde in Europese Musea.* Leyden; Museum Boerhaave

Stimson, A. (1976). The Influence of the Royal Observatory at Greenwich upon the Design of 17th and 18th Century Angle-Measuring Instruments at Sea, *Vistas in Astronomy*, Vol. 20, 123–130

Stock, J.T. (1969). *Development of the Chemical Balance: A Science Museum Survey.* London; HMSO

Szabadváry, F. (1966). *A History of Analytical Chemistry*. Oxford; Pergamon Press

Taylor, E.G.R. (1954). *The Mathematical Practitioners of Tudor and Stuart England.* Cambridge; Cambridge University Press for the Institute of Navigation

Taylor, E.G.R. (1966). *The Mathematical Practitioners of Hanoverian England 1714–1840.* Cambridge; Cambridge University Press for the Institute of Navigation

Taylor, E.G.R. (1971). *The Haven-Finding Art: a History of Navigation from Odysseus to Captain Cook*, revised edn. London; Hollis and Carter for the Institute of Navigation

Thom, A. (1971). *Megalithic Lunar Observatories*. Oxford; Clarendon Press

Thomas, D.B. (1969). *The Science Museum Photography Collection*. London; HMSO

Thoren, V.E. (1973). New Light on Tycho's Instruments, *Journal for the History of Astronomy*, Vol. 4, 25–45

Turner, G.L'E. (1967a). Review of *Inventaire des instruments scientifiques conservés en France*, in *Archives internationales d'histoire des sciences*, Vol. 20, 135–137

Turner, G. L'E. (1967b). The Microscope as a Technical Frontier in Science, *Proceedings of the Royal Microscopical Society*, Vol. 2, 175–199. Reprinted in Turner (1980b) ch. 9

Turner, G. L'E. (1969a). The History of Optical Instruments. A Brief Survey of Sources and Modern Studies, *History of Science*, Vol. 8, 53–93. Reprinted in Turner (1980b) ch. 2

Turner, G. L'E. (1969b). James Short, FRS, and his Contribution to the Construction of Reflecting Telescopes, *Notes and Records of the Royal Society*, Vol. 24, 91–108

Turner, G. L'E. (1974). The Portuguese Agent: J.H. de Magellan, *Antiquarian Horology*, Vol. 9, 74–76

Turner, G. L'E. (1976). The London Trade in Scientific Instrument-Making in the 18th Century, *Vistas in Astronomy*, Vol. 20, 173–182

Turner, G. L'E. (1979). The Number Code on Reflecting Telescopes by Nairne and Blunt, *Journal for the History of Astronomy*, Vol. 10, 177–184

Turner, G. L'E. (1980a). *Antique Scientific Instruments*. Poole; Blandford Press

Turner, G. L'E. (1980b). *Essays on the History of the Microscope*. Oxford; Senecio Publishing Co.

Turner, G. L'E. (1981). *Collecting Microscopes*. London; Studio Vista

Turner, G. L'E. and Levere, T.H. (1973). *Van Marum's Scientific Instruments in Teyler's Museum*. Vol. 4 of *Martinus van Marum: Life and Work*. Ed. R.J. Forbes. 6 Vols (1969–76). Leyden; Noordhoff International Publishing for the Hollandsche Maatschappij der Wetenschappen

Tyacke, S. (1978). *London Map-sellers 1660–1720*. Tring; Map Collector Publications

Tyacke, S. and Huddy, J. (1980). *Christopher Saxton and Tudor Map-making*. British Library Series No. 2. London; British Library

Wall, J. (1978). *Directory of British Photographic Collections*. London; Heinemann, for the Royal Photographic Society

Ward, F.A.B. (1961). *Handbook of the Collection Illustrating Time Measurement. Part 1: Historical Review*, 4th edn amended. London; HMSO

Ward, F.A.B. (1981). *A Catalogue of European Scientific Instruments in the Department of Medieval and Later Antiquities of the British Museum*. London; British Museum Publications

Waters, D.W. (1958). *The Art of Navigation in England in Elizabethan and Early Stuart Times*. London; Hollis and Carter

Wheatland, D.P. (1968). *The Apparatus of Science at Harvard, 1765–1800*. Cambridge, Mass.; Harvard University Press

Wood, J.E. (1978). *Sun, Moon and Standing Stones*. Oxford; Oxford University Press

Wunderlich, H. (1977). *Kursächsische Feldmesskunst, artilleristische Richtverfahren und Ballistik in 16. und 17. Jahrhundert*. Berlin; VEB Deutscher Verlag der Wissenschaften

Zuylen, J. van (1981). The Microscopes of Antoni van Leeuwenhoek, *Journal of Microscopy*, Vol. 121, 309–328

14

Mathematical sciences

S.A. Jayawardene

Introduction

Historians of mathematics have proudly traced the origins of their discipline to Eudemus of Rhodes, a pupil of Aristotle, whose histories of arithmetic, geometry and astronomy have unfortunately not been preserved. Moritz Cantor (1902), in his address to the Second International Congress of Mathematicians held in Paris in 1900, gave a brief sketch of the history of the historiography of mathematics from Eudemus to his own time. Other accounts can be found in the concluding chapters of the histories of Smith (1923–5) and Loria (1950). These and more recent accounts are listed in the latest survey made by Struik (1980).

The subject is dealt with in greater detail by Cantor (1880–1908) and Günther in the last three volumes of Cantor's *Vorlesungen*. In it they included editions of classical texts, editions of collected works of recently deceased mathematicians, and mathematical dictionaries.

A review of the principal works in the history of mathematics has been given by Loria (1946: 15–60), while Kenneth May (1973: 590–7) has compiled a bibliography from 1615 to 1968. Biobibliographical notices of 126 historians of mathematics have been included in a checklist covering some 800 historians of science compiled by Jayawardene and Lawes (1979).

The historiography of mathematics from Bernardino Baldi (1553–1617) to Kenneth May (1915–1977). Periodicals in the history of mathematics

Baldi's *Vite de' matematici*, the lives of 202 mathematicians, written during the years 1587—95 but not published during his lifetime, is considered to be the first great European history of mathematics (see Rose 1975: 253–69; Bilinski 1977). His *Cronica de' matematici* (1707) contained brief notes on 366 mathematicians. Pietro Cossali's *Origine, trasporto in Italia, primi progressi in essa dell'algebra* (1797–9) is still used by historians of Renaissance mathematics. Montucla's *Histoire des mathématiques* (1799–1802) has been reprinted (1960) and also translated into Italian (1879).

During the nineteenth century, Libri's *Histoire* (1865: ii, 202–14, 287–480; iii, 282–343) and the studies of Chasles (1843), Curtze (Günther 1903) and Boncompagni (Galli 1893–4) brought into the limelight a large number of unpublished mathematical texts in European libraries. Special periodicals for the history of mathematics were founded.

In 1859 Moritz Cantor joined the editorial board of the newly established *Zeitschrift für Mathematik und Physik* (64 Vols, 1856–1917). Its section devoted to reviews (Literaturzeitung) carried half-yearly lists of current contents of mathematical journals (Abhandlungsregister), arranged by subject (including the history of mathematics). In 1875, articles on the history of mathematics were included in this section and it was renamed 'Historische-literarische Abteilung'. In 1877 a supplement was added – *Abhandlungen zur Geschichte der Mathematik* – intended for long articles on the history and bibliography of mathematics. When Cantor retired in 1900, the new editorial board stopped publication of the historical section, and the *Abhandlungen* was separated from the *Zeitschrift*. The thirty issues of the *Abhandlungen*, from 1877 to 1913, contain some of the most important historical monographs written at the time. Cantor's monumental work, however, was his *Vorlesungen* (1880–1908), a revision of his Heidelberg lectures on the history of mathematics.

The first independent journal for the history of mathematics, *Bullettino di bibliografia e storia delle scienze matematiche e fisiche*, was started by Baldassarre Boncompagni in 1868. During the twenty years of its life, it carried articles on the history of mathematics, editions of manuscripts, biobibliographies and studies of primary sources. Each volume contained some 800 pages.

(Boncompagni's habit of making changes in the text while in press resulted in variant copies.) The twenty volumes, which deserve a subject index and an index of manuscripts, have been reprinted by Johnson (*Bullettino Reprints*).

The gap left by the *Bullettino* was partly filled by the *Bibliotheca Mathematica* (1884–1915) of Gustav Eneström. Published on a modest scale from 1884 to 1899 (the first three volumes were mere bibliographies issued as supplements to *Acta Mathematica*), it became the foremost journal for the history of mathematics on the cessation of the historical section of the *Zeitschrift für Mathematik und Physik* in 1900. Although it was no equal to Boncompagni's *Bullettino* in size, the *Bibliotheca Mathematica* contained a current bibliography of the literature of the history of mathematics, and news of the profession; its articles complemented the monographs in Cantor's *Abhandlungen*. Unfortunately it ceased publication in 1915.

Loria's *Bollettino di bibliografia e storia delle scienze matematiche* (21 Vols, 1898–1921; Turin and Palermo) was modest in comparison with its predecessors. Each volume consisted of some 120 pages and contained book reviews and a few short articles. In 1913, George Sarton, then a young man of independent means with no commitments other than his dedication to the history of science, began publishing *Isis* (Thackray and Merton 1972). Among the thirty-two members forming the Comité de patronage of the journal were eight distinguished historians of mathematics – Cantor, Favaro, Günther, Heath, Heiberg, Loria, Smith and Zeuthen. Most important for the historian of mathematics was the current *Critical Bibliography* that *Isis* carried at frequent intervals, and that now appears annually as a separate issue of the journal. In 1930 a companion journal *Osiris* was established to contain longer articles.

In 1932, *Scripta Mathematica*, a journal devoted to the philosophy, history and expository treatment of mathematics, was founded by Jekuthiel Ginsburg of Yeshiva College, New York. On the editorial board there were, besides Gino Loria, three American professors, D.E. Smith, R.C. Archibald and L.C. Karpinski, well-known for fostering the study, in the United States, of the history of mathematics. Their influence can be seen in the bibliographical articles published in the journal. Two of its sections – 'Notes and queries', 'Bibliographical and historical notes' – were edited by Archibald. Notes and articles on recreational mathematics appeared frequently in it. Carl Boyer, who joined the editorial board in 1947, assisted with the book review section and became solely responsible for it in 1949 on the death of the review-editor L.G. Simons. With the passing of Archibald, Karpinski and Ginsburg, the journal's interest in the history of mathematics waned, but the book review section under Boyer (until the journal ceased in 1973) continued to give adequate coverage to the subject.

Two other journals devoted mainly to the history of mathematics are *Istoriko-matematicheskie issledovaniia* (1948–) and *Archive for History of Exact Sciences* (1960–) edited by C.A. Truesdell. Until recently, articles in the first were restricted to the history of mathematics in Russia and the Orient. In 1979 a sixty-year survey of Soviet research in the history of mathematics was made by Yushkevich. The second journal is similar to the *Abhandlungen* and contains articles of monographic length.

Historia Mathematica began publication in 1974 under the editorship of Kenneth May. It was the result of five years of preparation during which a permanent Commission was established and a newsletter, *Notae de Historia Mathematica* (1971–3), published. The journal was preceded by the Commission's *World Directory of Historians of Mathematics* (May and Gardner 1972) and May's *Bibliography and Research Manual of the History of Mathematics* (1973). The journal has maintained the traditions of its distinguished predecessors. One of its features is the 'Abstracts' department in which the current literature of the history of mathematics is recorded. May's death in 1977 was a great loss to the profession (Dauben *et al.* 1978). Fortunately, by transferring editorial responsibility for the journal to younger hands, he had ensured that it would not suffer the fate of the journals of Boncompagni and others.

The new journals of interest to us are *Annals of the History of Computing* (1979–) and *Gaṇita Bhāratī*, Bulletin of the Indian Society for History of Mathematics (1979–). In 1980 the annual *History and Philosophy of Logic*, of relevance to the history of foundations of mathematics, began publication under the editorship of Ivor Grattan-Guinness. The Unione Matematica Italiana has recently started publication of the half-yearly *Bollettino di storia delle scienze matematiche*. I hope it will be a worthy successor to Boncompagni's *Bullettino* of a hundred years ago.

General histories of mathematics. Source books.

The hazards of writing a general history of mathematics are reflected in Eneström's additions and corrections to the second edition of Cantor's *Vorlesungen* (Eneström *et al.* 1900–14), and in Bruins' review (1969) of Boyer's *History of Mathematics* (1968). Since Montucla and Cantor, no one has attempted writing a general history on the same scale. The only extensive accounts written since then are by Loria (1950), Yushkevich (1970–2) and Kline (1972). Hofmann's 416-page history (1953–7) in three small paperbacks contained a vast amount of bibliographical information.

Many histories have been written with the needs of teachers and students in mind. Smith's history of elementary mathematics (1923–5) in two volumes – one chronological, the other topical – is illustrated and full of bibliographical detail. Archibald's *Outline* (1932) was based on two summer-school lectures to teachers of engineering. The sixth edition (1949), revised to meet the needs of teachers of the history of mathematics, contains a long literature list and notes. More recent textbooks written for classroom use are the histories of Boyer (1968) and Eves (1976). Among popular works are the concise histories of Ball (1888) and Struik (1948). The last two have gone through several editions, been reprinted many times and translated into more than one language. Other histories worth noting are those of Cajori (1919), Enriques (1938) and Carruccio (1958, 1964). The *Isis Cumulative Bibliography* has provided full bibliographical details of most of these works and indicated some reviews (Whitrow 1972–6: iii, 99–101). May (1973: 590–7) has listed about 150 general histories of mathematics from Heilbronner (1742) and Montucla (1799–1802) to Loria (1950) and Boyer (1968).

No account of general histories of mathematics can fail to mention the multi-volume *Histoire générale des sciences* edited by Taton (1957–64), with several chapters devoted to the history of mathematics. It has been translated into English.

The need for a systematic treatment of the history of mathematics by subject was met by Tropfke (1921–4, 1930–7, 1980). The fourth edition of his history is being completely rewritten under the editorship of Kurt Vogel. Smith's history (1923–5: ii) contained a study of ten special topics of elementary mathematics. Separate studies of mathematical topics are listed by Russo (1969: 142–4).

Many source books have been published, giving students access to major primary sources. The best known among them is the series *Ostwalds Klassiker der exakten Wissenschaften* (1889–. Leipzig; Engelmann) founded by Wilhelm Ostwald. Each volume contains extracts from one of the classics of science in German translation, with copious notes. Of the 250 volumes in the first

series, about 80 contain the work of mathematicians and mathematical physicists from Archimedes to Einstein. It is now continued in separate GDR and Federal German series. Source
books devoted solely to mathematics have been compiled by
Wieleitner (1927–9), Smith (1929), Newman (1956), Struik (1969)
and Birkhoff (1973).

Mathematics from the Renaissance to the end of the eighteenth century

From the catalogues of surviving manuscripts in European libraries, and from the bibliographies of early printed books, we can
form an idea of the mathematical knowledge that the Renaissance
inherited from the Middle Ages (Jayawardene 1978; Stillwell
1970). Broadly speaking, the texts fall into the following groups:
arithmetic (computi, theoretical arithmetics, algorisms and practical arithmetics), geometry (Euclid, Archimedes, Pappus, Apol-
lonius), trigonometry, mechanics.

It took a long time for medieval Western Europe, used to the
Roman number system and the abacus (or counting-board), to
accept the decimal place system. The Hindu–Arabic numerals and
the rules of algebra were introduced to Europe through Latin
translations of the works of Al-Khowarizmi and the *Liber abbaci*
of Leonardo of Pisa (Boncompagni 1857). Italian merchants gave
up the use of the abacus long before the rest of Europe; but the
word *abbaco* (*abaco*) continued to be used in popular parlance to
mean arithmetic.

Leonardo's *Liber abbaci* served as a model for generations of
maestri d'abbaco who taught arithmetic to merchant apprentices in
the commercial cities of Central and Northern Italy. It was in their
schools and in their manuals that the rules of algebra were kept
alive until they joined the mainstream of knowledge in the *Summa
de arithmetica, geometria, proportioni et proportionalita* (1494) of
Luca Pacioli. The success of the Italian mathematicians of the
sixteenth century in finding methods of solving the cubic and
quartic equations prompted Girolamo Cardano to write his treatise on algebraic equations, *Artis magnae sive de regulis algebraicis
liber unus* (1545; transl. 1968). Some years later, Rafael Bombelli
published his *Algebra* (1572), a systematic presentation of the
subject, free from its practical applications. What had begun as a
collection of rules for solving arithmetical problems was now an
independent discipline.

The major contribution of the German mathematicians of the

Renaissance (Rudolf, Stiefel and others) was to algebraic notation. It was Viète, however, who took the significant step of
distinguishing between unknown quantities and parameters, and
providing separate symbols for them. He made it possible to work
with a more general form of equation without specific numerical
coefficients (Viète 1973).

The early years of the seventeenth century saw advances made
in algebraic notation and in the theory of equations by Harriot and
Girard, and a theory of numbers developed by Fermat. The first
logarithmic tables, using the correspondence between an arithmetic and a geometric progression, were published by Napier in 1614.
The geometric interpretation of algebraic operations and the use
of algebra for solving geometrical problems, expounded by Descartes in his *La géométrie* (1637), and the study of loci by Fermat
were the basis of the new analytical geometry (Boyer 1956).

The development of algebraic symbolism helped to establish
trigonometry as an analytical science in the seventeenth century
(Braunmühl 1900–3; Karpinski 1946). It had already become
independent of astronomy with the publication of Regiomontanus'
De triangulis omnimodis (1533).

The knowledge of mechanics that the Renaissance inherited
came down in several traditions, which were assimilated, criticized
and tested by the mathematicians of the sixteenth century. Chief
among them were Tartaglia, Stevin, Galileo and Kepler. The first
half of the seventeenth century, dominated by Galileo, Kepler and
Descartes, saw the study of natural phenomena being reduced to a
mathematical science ('La natura è scritta in lingua matematica').
With the publication of Newton's *Principia* in 1687, this mechanization of the world picture was complete (Dijksterhuis 1961).

The greatest achievement of the seventeenth century was the
'invention' of the calculus by Leibniz and Newton. By the end of
the sixteenth century, a vast store of mathematical knowledge was
available. The works of Archimedes, Euclid, Hero, Pappus and
Diophantus had been published. With its transformation from
l'arte della cosa to *ars analytica*, algebra had become a sophisticated mathematical tool. Mathematicians – from Stevin and
Valerio to Torricelli and Pascal – applied new techniques to the
study of old problems (determining centres of gravity, constructing
tangents, rectification, quadrature and cubature). The result was a
change from the geometrical method of exhaustion to the algor-
ithms of the calculus, culminating in the discovery that integration
and differentiation were inverse procedures (Edwards 1979).

By the turn of the century the mathematical activity of Newton
and Leibniz had waned. True enough, some of their work was

published only in the early years of the century. Meanwhile, the calculus in whose creation they had played a vital part made rapid progress and gave rise to new branches of analysis in the hands of their successors. Taylor, Cotes, Maclaurin, the Bernoullis, d'Alembert, Clairaut and the mathematicians of the French revolution contributed largely to these developments. Towering above them was one man whose work has enriched almost every branch of mathematics, Leonhard Euler (Eneström 1910–13).

Outstanding among the work of the French mathematicians of the second half of the eighteenth century were the *Mécanique analitique* (1788) of Lagrange, the *Géométrie descriptive* (1798) of Monge, the *Mécanique céleste* (1799–1825) and *Théorie analytique des probabilités* (1812) of Laplace. Monge was responsible for the revival of geometry at the newly founded Ecole Polytechnique in Paris. By now the academies of Berlin and St Petersburg had lost their importance and mathematical activity had shifted to the technical colleges and universities. The arrival in Göttingen of the young Gauss in 1795 and the composition of his now famous thesis on the fundamental theorem of algebra mark the dawn of a new era (Klein 1926–7, i: 1–7).

Excellent surveys of the development of mathematics from the Renaissance through the scientific revolution to the end of the eighteenth century are found in the *Histoire générale des sciences* (Taton 1957–64). A more extensive account is given by Kline (1972). Struik (1969) gives extracts from classic texts, translated into English, with annotations. The *Dictionary of Scientific Biography* (Gillispie 1970–80) contains up-to-date articles on the leading mathematicians of the period.

Zoubov's study (1968) of Leonardo da Vinci, which has been translated into English, contains a chapter on the mathematical sciences and an introduction to the extensive bibliography of works about him. A facsimile edition of his *Codex Atlanticus* in the Ambrosian Library in Milan was published from 1973 to 1975.

Surveys of algebraical texts from Pacioli to the end of the eighteenth century have been made by Vivanti (1924) and Karpinski (1944). Russo (1959) has analysed the development of algebra in the sixteenth century. The influence of practical arithmetics on Bombelli's *Algebra* (1572) and the study of this work by Leibniz are analysed in two papers commemorating the fourth centenary of its publication (Jayawardene 1973; Hofmann 1972). The Ateneo di Brescia has published facsimile editions of Tartaglia's *Quesiti et inventioni diverse* (1959) and of the *Cartelli di sfida matematica* (1974) exchanged between Ferrari and Tartaglia, with introductory essays and copious annotations by Arnaldo

Masotti. Let us hope that similar editions of Tartaglia's other works will follow. The *Ars magna* of Cardano has been translated into English (1968), and his *Opera omnia* reprinted (1967); there is a recent study of his posthumous *Sermo de plus et minus* (Tanner 1980b).

Reich and Gericke have translated the algebra of Viète (1973) and provided a historical outline of alphabetical notation in arithmetic and algebra, followed by an annotated bibliography of his works. Harriot's manuscripts are being studied at present and annual seminars have been held since 1966 (Tanner 1980a). On Descartes, there are recent studies by Molland (1976) and Lenoir (1979). A critical guide to the Descartes literature is found in Sebba's (1964) bibliography and in the 'Bulletin cartésien' of the Equipe Descartes (1972–4). Mahoney's *The Mathematical Career of Pierre Fermat 1601–1665* (1973) has been analysed by Itard (1974a,b) and Weil (1973). The emergence of probability in the second half of the seventeenth century has been studied by Hacking (Knobloch 1980).

Selections from the mechanics of Tartaglia, Benedetti, Guido Ubaldo and Galileo have been published in translation, with a long introduction and bibliography by Drake and Drabkin (see Schmitt 1970). Editions of the collected works of Huygens (1888–1950) and Stevin (1955–66) have been completed (Dijksterhuis 1970). Martha List's supplement to Caspar's bibliography of Kepler has been published by Beer and Beer (1975: 955–1010) along with other papers presented at the symposia held in 1971 to commemorate the fourth centenary of Kepler's birth.

Newtonian studies, revived some forty years ago, became a veritable industry in the 1960s. The tercentenary of Newton's *annus mirabilis* was celebrated in 1966 and a critical edition of his *Principia* was brought out by Koyré and Cohen in 1971–2. The editing of his correspondence by Turnbull, Scott, Hall and Tilling (successively) has been completed (Turnbull *et al.* 1959–77; see Whiteside 1979). The monumental task of editing Newton's mathematical papers undertaken by Whiteside – one of the biggest historiographical projects of our time – is almost complete (Westfall 1978). A new bibliography of works by and about Newton has been compiled by Wallis and Wallis (1977). Other works of interest are a reconstructed catalogue of Newton's library (Harrison 1978) and a biography by Westfall (1980).

Hofmann's study of Leibniz's early years in Paris has been revised and translated into English (1974). The third centenary of his departure from Paris was commemorated by a symposium held in Chantilly by the Leibniz-Gesellschaft (1978). Bibliographies of works by and about Leibniz (K. Müller 1967: 7–10) are now brought up to date by a current bibliography in *Studia Leibnitiana* (1969–). The index to Gerhardt's edition of the mathematical papers and correspondence of Leibniz, compiled by Hofmann (1977) for his own use, has been published.

A survey of mathematical developments in the eighteenth century has been made by Scott (1948). Nielsen (1929, 1935) has given biobibliographical notes on 228 French mathematicians of the eighteenth and early nineteenth centuries. A biobibliography of British mathematicians up to 1850 is being compiled by Wallis (1974) – similar to that for Italy by Riccardi (1870–80).

Bibliographies of Euler's works have been compiled by Eneström (1910–13) and Truesdell (1972). The publication of his collected works and correspondence continues (Habicht 1977). Several volumes of the *Opera Omnia* (1911–) contain valuable introductory articles on the history of aspects of eighteenth-century mathematics; in particular, there is an outline of the history of seventeenth- and eighteenth-century acoustics in Truesdell's introduction to volume 11 of series 2 (see Lindsay 1972).

Mathematics of the nineteenth century

The history of nineteenth-century mathematics, were it to be written on the same scale as Cantor's *Vorlesungen* (which ended at 1799), would, according to an estimate by Cajori (1918), require about fifteen volumes. Cantor himself thought that it should be written as a series of monographs, each dealing with a special subject, and completed by a separate volume devoted to the history of mathematical ideas. The increased mathematical activity of the century was mainly due to: the democratization of learning; the educational reforms in France following the Revolution; the foundation of the École Polytechnique and the École Normale in Paris where special emphasis was given to the study of mathematics; the university reforms in Germany; the professionalization of mathematics. The need for communication among mathematicians resulted in an increase in the number of mathematical journals and in the formation of national mathematical societies. Among the bibliographical works to appear were Poggendorff's *Handwörterbuch* (1863–), the Royal Society's *Catalogue* (1867–1925), and the *Jahrbuch über die Fortschritte der Mathematik* (1871–1944). By the end of the century the International Congress of Mathematicians had held its first two meetings. It was to the second Congress, held in Paris in 1900, that Hilbert read his well-known paper on the future problems of mathematics (1902).

The advances in nineteenth-century mathematics include:

* further developments in algebra, leading to the study of linear and vector algebra, and also of algebraic structures;
* advances in the theory of numbers by Gauss, Galois and others;
* arithmetization of analysis, leading to set topology, the theory of functions and functional analysis; the improvement of rigour in analysis; complex variable analysis;
* differential equations, including both general theory and methods of solution (exact and numerical);
* the development of mathematical physics, including both terrestrial and celestial mechanics; the establishment of the new disciplines of heat diffusion, optics, and electricity and magnetism;
* the revival of geometry (synthetic, analytical, differential) begun by Monge and his pupils, the rise of non-Euclidean and algebraic geometry, culminating in the work of Gauss, Riemann, Klein and Hilbert (Klein 1974; Toretti 1978);
* development of set theory and of algebraic and mathematical logic.

The history of mathematics of this period was sketched in a series of lectures on selected topics by Felix Klein (1926–7) who had himself lived through the second half of the century and had personally known many of the protagonists (Wieleitner 1927–8; Sarton 1936a: 50–1). Good surveys are found in Taton (1957–64) and Morris Kline (1972). More recent accounts are a work in French edited by Dieudonné (see Grattan-Guinness 1979) and one in Russian by Kolmogorov and Yushkevich (1978). Grattan-Guinness' bibliographical essay (1977) includes a survey of historical studies of: logic and set theory; number and number theory; algebra; calculus and mathematical analysis; mathematical physics and mechanics; probability and statistics. To these may be added the recent special studies of analysis (Manning 1974–5; Dugac 1976), differential geometry (Reich 1973; Vincensini 1972), and differential equations (Dobrovolskii 1974).

Two workshops on the history of modern mathematics have been held recently (Birkhoff 1975; Mehrtens 1980). On the mathematicians themselves there are: bibliographical notes by Sarton (1936a: 49–53, 67–98); biographical notices and articles (Eneström 1901; Gillispie 1970–80, xvi: 250); a study by Biermann (1973); and biographies (Grattan-Guinness 1977: 68; Dauben

1979). Editions of collected works and correspondence are listed by Müller (1909: 17–20) and Grattan-Guinness (1977: 65–7).

Among subjects whose development since the Renaissance has been studied are: foundational aspects of calculus (Grattan-Guinness 1980); calculus of variations (Goldstine 1980); graph theory (Biggs, Lloyd and Wilson 1976); algebraic geometry (Dieudonné 1974); topology (Pont 1973); linear and vector algebra (Crowe 1967). Recent studies in the history of probability theory have been surveyed by Knobloch (1980).

In the late 1890s a group of mathematicians led by Felix Klein, Heinrich Weber and Franz Meyer began the compilation of the *Encyklopädie der mathematischen Wissenschaften mit Einschluss ihrer Anwendungen* (1898–1935). Their aim was to provide a concise and comprehensive account of every branch of mathematics, while surveying the literature of the subject from the beginning of the nineteenth century. It took three generations of mathematicians (German and foreign) nearly forty years to prepare and publish the 23-volume work (Sarton 1936a: 56–7). A new edition in French (see Russo 1969: 138), started in 1904, was only partly prepared before its abandonment in 1914 on the death of the general editor, Jules Molk. As for the second German edition begun in 1939 (see Ore 1942), only a few parts of the first volume have been published so far.

Mathematical education

Although the teaching of mathematics has been the subject of study by historians (Günther 1887; Yeldham 1936), one aspect of it that deserves separate investigation is the interaction between teachers (lectures, textbooks, seminars) on the one hand, and the developments in mathematics on the other. For example, it is in the medieval *trattati d'abbaco* – manuals written for the use of merchant apprentices – that we see the first attempts (unsuccessful) at solving the cubic equation. It was a disputation between two teachers of mathematics, Tartaglia and Antonio Maria Fiore, that triggered off the events leading up to Cardano writing his *Ars magna* (Bortolotti 1927). The teaching of mathematics at Cambridge and in German universities has been studied by Ball (1889) and Lorey (1916) respectively. Biermann (1973) has made a detailed investigation of the teaching of mathematics at the University of Berlin from its inception in 1810 up to 1920.

During the nineteenth century, the links between mathematical developments and instruction became closer with the rejuvenation of education in France by the founding of the École Polytechnique and the development of other specialist *écoles* and *lycées* (Taton 1954; Klein 1926–7, i: 63–87). Mathematicians like Monge, de Prony, Ampère, and especially Cauchy, developed new mathematical ideas for teaching purposes or at least presented new systematizations of existing theories (Taton 1964). The tradition continued in the hands of men such as Bertrand, Hermite, Poincaré and Borel, and down to the Bourbaki school of our times (Dieudonné 1970, 1979).

In Germany, the Prussian reforms in education, which accompanied the foundation of the University of Berlin in 1810, introduced the idea that a professor had a dual function to perform — that of researcher and teacher — and established the seminar as a form of academic instruction. The seminars of Jacobi and Neumann in Königsberg (Volkmann 1896) and of Kummer, Weiersrass and Kronecker in Berlin (Biermann 1973: 59–120) attracted students from all over Germany, and became the training ground of future teachers and professors (Klein 1926–7, i: 112–14, 282–4). Students from abroad flocked to study under Felix Klein, both at Leipzig and at Göttingen, where he was successively professor since 1880. His eminent role as an educationist is seen in the series of special lectures he gave in Göttingen to prospective teachers of mathematics and in the reports of the International Mathematik-Unterrichts Kommission (Lorey 1926a,b). Developments in education in other countries were influenced by the French and German models.

As for the teaching of the history of mathematics, our information is somewhat scanty. From reports in Bibliotheca Mathematica (1887–1909) it would appear that courses of lectures on the history of mathematics were offered from time to time at universities on the Continent and in the United States. Better known are Moritz Cantor's lectures in Heidelberg and Anton von Braunmühl's seminar at the Technische Hochschule in Munich. In the early years of this century doctoral students were writing dissertations under the direction of David Eugene Smith at Columbia and Louis Karpinski at Michigan. There have been long traditions of teaching the subject at undergraduate level in the United States and the USSR. However, the picture should not be distorted. In some countries (the UK is a good example), there is a long, flourishing tradition of a- or even anti-historical attitudes to history – which, being a tradition, ironically has its own history.

The study of the history of mathematics

Guides

By the turn of the century the history of mathematics had been established as an independent discipline, thanks mainly to the work of Boncompagni, Cantor and Eneström. All that the historian of mathematics now needed was a guide to the literature of his subject. In April 1908, at the Fourth International Congress of Mathematicians held in Rome, Gino Loria (1909) read a paper to the historical section on the need to provide a bibliographic manual for students starting research in the history of mathematics. About the same time, Felix Müller (1909) was working on a guide to the literature of mathematics and of its history. Loria (1908–9) developed his ideas further in a paper in the *Bibliotheca Mathematica*. He was urged by colleagues to put his proposals into action and promote the collective preparation of a work of reference. The outbreak of the 1914–18 war made such an enterprise impracticable. In 1916, Loria wrote a guide all by himself, revising it thirty years later (1946). In the meantime Sarton published *The Study of the History of Mathematics* (1936a), an introduction to the methodology of the subject followed by a brief guide to the literature. A complement to this work was his *Study of the History of Science* (1936b). The bibliography in the last work was amplified in Sarton's *Horus* (1952). Many of the topics treated in the latter work are of interest to the historian of mathematics.

The guides of Loria and Sarton were restricted to bibliographical works and secondary sources. For primary sources one had to turn to Felix Müller's *Führer* (1909), Poggendorff's *Handwörterbuch* (1863–), special bibliographies and library catalogues. A guide that includes primary sources is François Russo's *Eléments de bibliographie de l'histoire des sciences et des techniques* (1969). Among the sources listed by him are the major works of mathematics followed by studies relating to them, including articles in journals.

A brief guide to the literature of the history of mathematics by Grattan-Guinness (1977) was included in *Uses of Mathematical Literature*, a reference work intended primarily for students of mathematics and non-specialists.

The need to provide students and teachers of mathematics with a basic knowledge of the history of their subject has prompted Rogers (1979) to compile a resource file containing a partly annotated list of some 450 titles in English inclusive of primary sources.

Sources

The frequent need for the historian to consult original sources has led some scholars – Curtze, Björnbo, Thorndike, Clagett, and others – to devote much of their time to examining and cataloguing manuscripts (see Günther 1903; Jayawardene 1978). In a study of the migrations of manuscripts, the formation of libraries and the relations between humanists and mathematicians in Italy, Rose (1975) has surveyed the work of generations of Renaissance scholars. A first attempt at bibliographic control of inventories of Western scientific manuscripts before 1600 has been made by Jayawardene (1978). Van Egmond (1976) has catalogued some 200 manuscripts of practical arithmetic in the libraries of Rome, Tuscany and New York. The need for a register of medieval mathematical manuscripts has been stressed at international gatherings by Gino Arrighi (1967). Only in 1981 did he succeed, with the collaboration of Laura Toti Rigatelli and Raffaella Franci of the University of Siena, in setting up a Centre for the Study of Medieval Mathematics. A group of German scholars led by Menso Folkerts in Munich (1977) is making a survey of medieval Western mathematical manuscripts in European libraries.

Suter (1900) and Sezgin (1974), in their biobibliographical surveys, have listed Arabic manuscripts of mathematics and astronomy. A corresponding census of Sanskrit texts has been made by Pingree (1970–6). Articles and reports on collections of manuscripts and archives are published frequently in the 'Sources' department of *Historia Mathematica* (1974–).

Books and manuscripts collected by humanists and bibliophiles have found their way, by gift and purchase, into libraries and have been made accessible to scholars. Among collections of interest to the historian of mathematics are: the Crawford collection at the Royal Observatory, Edinburgh (Forbes 1972–3); the Turner collection at the University of Keele (Shapin and Hill 1972–3); the Graves collection at University College London (Dorling 1976); and the De Morgan collection at the University of London Library. Among collections abroad are the Mittag-Leffler Library in Djursholm-Stockholm (Grattan-Guinness 1971), and the collections at Brown, Columbia, and Wisconsin Universities. Two remarkable collections that have been dispersed are those of Libri (Fumagalli 1963) and Boncompagni.

Bibliographies (retrospective and current)

Systematic bibliography, which began in the sixteenth century with Symphorien Champier, Otto Brunfels and Conrad Gesner, reached a peak in the nineteenth century when a large number of specialized retrospective bibliographies made their appearance. Malclès (1962: 95–103) has listed them in her survey of the history of bibliography. Among them are several bibliographies of mathematics: Rogg (1830), Halliwell (1839), De Morgan (1847), Sohncke (1854), Riccardi (1870–80), and Erlecke (1873). Also of interest to the historian of mathematics is Houzeau and Lancaster's monumental *Bibliographie générale de l'astronomie* (1882–9). Most important among these works are the Royal Society's *Catalogue of Scientific Papers* (1867–1925) and Poggendorff's *Biographisch-literarisches Handwörterbuch* (1863–). Of these two, the first covers the periodical literature of the nineteenth century; it has a subject index for mathematics, mechanics and physics. The second, now in its seventh series, serves as a biographical dictionary and a bibliography; it is especially useful for the nineteenth century.

The rapid growth of scientific literature in the nineteenth century also necessitated the publication of *current* subject bibliographies. Of these, the most important for mathematics was the *Jahrbuch über die Fortschritte der Mathematik* (68 vols, 1871–1944) founded by Ohrtmann (F. Müller 1904). Its coverage included history, philosophy and pedagogy. Eneström's *Bibliotheca Mathematica* (1884–1915) started as a bibliography of mathematical literature in *Acta Mathematica*; after it became an independent journal, it carried a current bibliography in the history of mathematics.

The *Revue semestrielle des publications mathématiques* (1893–1934) was a half-yearly index of articles in journals, with brief annotations, published by the Société de Mathématique d'Amsterdam. The abstracting and indexing of mathematical literature is now done by two serials, *Zentralblatt für Mathematik* (1931–), founded by Otto Neugebauer (edited by him until 1938), and *Mathematical Reviews* (1940–), founded by the American Mathematical Society (Boas 1979). Both have sections, though not extensive, devoted to the history of mathematics; *Mathematical Reviews* has improved its coverage in recent years. The historian of mathematics can supplement these bibliographies with material provided by the *International Catalogue of Scientific Literature* (1902–18), the *Isis Critical Bibliography* (1913–), the history of science section of *Bulletin signalétique* (1953–) and the abstracts department of *Historia Mathematica* (1974–). For the nineteenth century, especially for the period prior to the publication of the *Jahrbuch*, the historian can use the index to the Royal Society's *Catalogue of Scientific Papers*, and the half-yearly lists of current contents of periodicals in the *Zeitschrift für Mathematik und Physik*.

Kenneth May (1973) has cumulated the entries relating to the history of mathematics in the major serial bibliographies published since 1871. In spite of many minor errors inherent in a work produced in a short time at little expense, it is an essential reference tool that could at times save a researcher the labour of examining some 250 issues of serial bibliographies. A useful complement to it is the *Isis Cumulative Bibliography* (Whitrow 1972–6) where the entries are more detailed than in May's work.

Conclusion

My survey of the historiography of mathematics began with the *Vite de' matematici* of Bernardino Baldi, written about 400 years ago. His modern counterparts have contributed biobibliographical articles on some 850 mathematicians to the sixteen-volume *Dictionary of Scientific Biography* (Gillispie 1970–80), recently completed with an excellent index. Another work just added to the varied collection of reference tools that the historian of mathematics is fortunate in having is the *Annotated Bibliography in the History of Mathematics* (1982). Compiled by some fifty specialists under the direction of Joseph W. Dauben, editor of *Historia Mathematica*, it is dedicated to the memory of Kenneth May. It is gratifying to note that this work will, together with Kenneth May's *Bibliography* (1973), provide the complete bibliographic manual that Gino Loria dreamt of seventy-five years ago.

Acknowledgements

I am very grateful to Ivor Grattan-Guinness for criticizing the original draft of this chapter, and helping me with his specialist knowledge of nineteenth-century mathematics and the history of mathematical education.

Bibliography

Abhandlungen zur Geschichte der Mathematik (1877–1913). Leipzig; Teubner
Archibald, R.C. (1932). *Outline of the History of Mathematics*. Lancaster, Pa.; The Lancaster Press. 6th edn (1949)
Arrighi, G. (1967). Le Matematiche, *Atti del primo Convegno Internazionale di*

Ricognizione delle Fonti per la Storia della Scienza Italiana: i Secoli XIV–XVI, Pisa, 14–16 settembre 1966. Ed. C. Maccagni. Florence; Barbèra, 109–132

Baldi, B. (1707). *Cronica de' Matematici, ovvero dell'istoria delle vite loro.* Urbino; A.A. Monticelli

Ball, W.W.R. (1888). *A Short Account of the History of Mathematics.* London; Macmillan and Company

Ball, W.W.R. (1889). *A History of the Study of Mathematics at Cambridge.* Cambridge; Cambridge University Press

Beer, A. and Beer, P., Ed. (1975). Kepler: Four Hundred Years: Proceedings of Conferences held in Honour of Johannes Kepler, *Vistas in Astronomy,* Vol. 18, 1–1034. Oxford, Pergamon Press

Bibliotheca Mathematica (1884–1915). 1st Series, 3 Vols. (1884–86) as Supplement to *Acta Mathematica;* Stockholm. 2nd Series, 13 Vols. (1887–99); Stockholm. 3rd Series, 14 Vols. (1900–14); Leipzig

Biermann, K.R. (1973). *Die Mathematik und ihre Dozenten an der Berliner Universität 1810–1920. Stationen auf dem Wege eines mathematischen Zentrums von Weltgeltung.* Berlin; Akademie Verlag

Biggs, N.L., Lloyd, E.K. and Wilson, R.J. (1976). *Graph Theory: 1736–1936.* Oxford; Clarendon Press

Bilinski, B. (1977). *Prolegomena alle* Vite dei matematici *di Bernardino Baldi (1587–1596): manoscritti Rosminiani–Celli già Albani-Boncompagni.* Accademia Polacca delle Scienze, Biblioteca e Centro di Studi a Roma, Conferenze e Studi 71. Wroclaw; Ossolineum

Birkhoff, G., Ed. (1973). *A Source Book in Classical Analysis.* Cambridge, Mass.; Harvard University Press

Birkhoff, G., Ed. (1975). Proceedings of the American Workshop on the Evolution of Modern Mathematics, *Historia Mathematica,* Vol. 2, 425–615

Boas, R.P. (1979). Award for Distinguished Services to Otto Neugebauer, *American Mathematical Monthly,* Vol. 86, 77–78

Bombelli, R. (1572). *L'Algebra.* Bologna; Giovanni Rossi

Boncompagni, B., Ed. (1857). *Scritti di Leonardo Pisano.* Vol. 1, *Il liber abbaci.* Rome; privately published

Bortolotti, E. (1927). Disputazioni matematiche nel secolo XVI, *Bollettino della Unione Matematica Italiana,* Vol. 6, 23–27

Boyer, C.B. (1956). *History of Analytical Geometry.* The Scripta Mathematica Studies No. 6 and 7. New York; Scripta Mathematica

Boyer, C.B. (1968). *A History of Mathematics.* New York; John Wiley

Braunmühl, A. von (1900–3). *Vorlesungen über Geschichte der Trigonometrie.* Leipzig; Teubner. Reprinted (1971) Wiesbaden; Dr Martin Sändig OHG

Bruins, E.M. (1969). Review of C.B. Boyer (1968), *Janus,* Vol. 56, 63–77

Bullettino Reprints (1964). 20 Vols. New York; Johnson Reprint Company

Cajori, F. (1890). *The Teaching and History of Mathematics in the United States.* US Bureau of Education, Circular of Information No. 3. Washington DC; Government Printing Office

Cajori, F. (1918). Plans for a History of Mathematics in the Nineteenth Century, *Science,* new ser., Vol. 48, 279–284

Cajori, F. (1919). *A History of the Conception of Limits and Fluxions in Great Britain, from Newton to Woodhouse.* Chicago and London; The Open Court

Cantor, M. (1880–1908). *Vorlesungen über Geschichte der Mathematik.* 4 Vols. Leipzig; Teubner. Vol. 1, from the beginning to 1200. 1st edn (1880); 2nd edn (1894); 3rd edn (1907). Vol. 2, 1200–1668. 1st edn (1892); 2nd edn (1899–1900), reprinted (1913). Vol. 3, 1668–1758. 1st edn (1898); 2nd edn with corrections (1901). Vol. 4, 1759–1799 (1908) under Cantor's direction by S. Günther, F.

Cajori, E. Netto, V. Bobynin, A. von Braunmühl, G. Loria, G. Vivanti, C.R. Wallner

Cantor, M. (1902). Sur l'historiographie des mathématiques, *Compte rendu du deuxième congrès international des mathématiciens (Paris, 6–12 août 1900).* Paris; Gauthier–Villars, 27–42

Cardano, G. (1967). *Opera omnia.* 10 Vols. New York; Johnson Reprint Corporation. First published (1663)

Cardano, G. (1968). *The Great Art or the Rules of Algebra.* Trans. and Ed., T. R. Witmer. Cambridge. Mass.; MIT Press

Carruccio, E. (1958). *Matematica e logica nella storia e nel pensiero contemporanei.* Turin; Gheroni

Carruccio, E. (1964). *Mathematics and Logic in History and in Contemporary Thought.* Trans. Isabel Quigly. London; Faber and Faber

Chasles, M. (1843). Histoire de l'arithmétique, *Compte rendu hebdomadaire des séances de l'Académie des Sciences,* Vol. 16, 156–174, 218–246, 281–299, 1393–1420

Cossali, P. (1797–9). *Origine, trasporto in Italia, primi progressi in essa dell'algebra.* 2 Vols. Parma; Tipografa Reale

Crowe, M.J. (1967). *A History of Vector Analysis.* Notre Dame, Ill.; University of Notre Dame Press

Dauben, J.W. (1979). *Georg Cantor: his Mathematics and Philosophy of the Infinite.* Cambridge, Mass.; Harvard University Press

Dauben, J.W. (1982). *Annotated Bibliography in the History of Mathematics.* New York; Garland Press (in press)

Dauben, J.W. *et al.* (1978). Kenneth O. May, 1915–1977, *Historia Mathematica,* Vol. 5, 1–12

Descartes, R. (1637). *La géométrie* (published with *Discours de la méthode pour bien conduire la raison,* etc.). Leyden; I. Maire

De Morgan, A. (1847). *Arithmetical Books from the Invention of Printing to the Present Time.* London; Taylor and Walton

Dieudonné, J. (1970). The Work of Nicholas Bourbaki, *American Mathematical Monthly,* Vol. 77, 134–145

Dieudonné, J. (1974). *Cours de géométrie algébrique. 1. Aperçu historique sur le développement de la géometrie algébrique.* Paris; Presses Universitaires de France

Dieudonné, J. (1979). *Panorama des mathématiques pures: le choix bourbachique,* 2nd edn. Paris; Gauthier-Villars

Dijksterhuis, E.J. (1961). *The Mechanization of the World Picture.* Trans. C. Dikshoorn. Oxford; Clarendon Press

Dijksterhuis, E.J. (1970). *Simon Stevin: Science in the Netherlands around 1600.* The Hague; Martinus Nijhoff

Dobrovolskii, V.A. (1974). *Ocherki Razvitiya Analiticheskoi Teorii Differenzial-nykh Uravnenii* [Essays on the development of the analytical theory of differential equations]. Kiev; Vishcha Shkola

Dorling, A.R. (1976). The Graves Mathematical Collection in University College London, *Annals of Science,* Vol. 33, 307–309

Dugac, P. (1976). Problèmes de l'histoire de l'analyse mathématique au XIXe siècle: cas de Karl Weierstrass et de Richard Dedekind, *Historia Mathematica,* Vol. 3, 5–19

Edwards, C.H. (1979). *The Historical Development of the Calculus.* New York; Springer

Encyklopädie der mathematischen Wissenschaften mit Einschluss ihrer Anwendungen (1898–1935). 23 Vols. Herausgegeben im Auftrage der Akademien der

Wissenschaften zu Berlin, Göttingen, Heidelberg, Leipzig, München und Wien sowie unter Mitwirkung zahlreicher Fachgenossen. Leipzig and Berlin; B.G. Teubner

Eneström, G. (1901). Bio-bibliographie der 1881–1900 verstorbenen Mathematiker, *Bibliotheca Mathematica*, ser. 3, Vol. 2, 326–350

Eneström, G. (1910–13). Verzeichnis der Schriften Leonhard Eulers, *Jahresbericht der deutschen Mathematiker-Vereinigung*, Ergänzungsband 4, 1–388

Eneström, G. *et al.* (1900–14). Kleine Bemerkungen zur zweiten (letzten) Auflage von Cantors *Vorlesungen über Geschichte der Mathematik*, *Bibliotheca Mathematica*, ser. 3, Vols 1–14 [some 800 pages of additions and corrections]

Enriques, F. (1938). *Le Matematiche nella storia e nella cultura*. Bologna; Zanichelli

Equipe Descartes (1972–4). Bulletin cartésien: bibliographie critique des études cartésiennes, *Archives de philosophie*, Vol. 35, 263–319, Vol. 36, 431–495; Vol. 37, 453–497

Erlecke, A. (1873). *Bibliotheca Mathematica. Systematische Verzeichnis der bis 1870 in Deutschland auf den Gebieten der Arithmetik,...erschienenen Werke.* Halle a.S.; Erlecke

Euler, L. (1911–). *Opera omnia.* Edited by the Euler Committee of the Swiss Academy of Sciences. 4 Series, 74 Vols. to date. Basle; Birkhäusser Verlag

Eves, H. (1976). *An Introduction to the History of Mathematics*, 4th edn. New York; Holt, Rinehart and Winston

Ferrari, L. and Tartaglia, N. (Facsimile 1974). *Cartelli di sfida matematica.* Riproduzione in facsimile delle edizioni originali 1547–1548. Brescia; Ateneo di Brescia

Folkerts, M. (1977). Vorarbeiten zur Erfassung der mittelalterlichen mathematischen Handschriften Westeuropas, *Abstracts of Scientific Section Papers, XVth International Congress of the History of Science.* Edinburgh; Edinburgh University Press, 18–19

Forbes, E.G. (1972–3). The Crawford collection of books and manuscripts on the history of astronomy, mathematics, etc., at the Royal Observatory, Edinburgh, *British Journal for the History of Science*, Vol. 6, 459–461

Fumagalli, G. (1963). *Guglielmo Libri.* Ed. B. Maracchi Biagiarelli. Florence; Olschki, 175–176

Galli, I. (1893–4). Elogio del Principe Don Baldassarre Boncompagni, *Atti dell' Accademia Pontificia de' Nuovi Lincei*, Vol. 47, 161–186 [Bibliography 171–186]

Gauss, K.F. (1799). *Demonstratio nova theorematis omnem functionem algebraicam rationalem integram unius variabilis in factores reales primi vel secundi gradus resolvi posse.* Helmstadt; C.G. Fleckeisen

Gillispie, C.C., Ed. (1970–80). *Dictionary of Scientific Biography.* 16 Vols. New York; American Council of Learned Societies, Charles Scribner's Sons

Goldstine, H.H. (1980). *History of the Calculus of Variations from the Seventeenth through the Nineteenth Century.* New York; Springer

Grattan-Guinness, I. (1971). Materials for the History of Mathematics in the Institut Mittag-Leffler, *Isis*, Vol. 62, 363–374

Grattan-Guinness, I. (1977). History of Mathematics, in *Uses of Mathematical Literature.* Ed. A.R. Dorling. London; Butterworths, 60–77

Grattan-Guinness, I. (1979). Review of J. Dieudonné, Ed., *Abrégé d'histoire des mathématiques 1700–1900* (2 Vols, Paris; Hermann, 1978), *Annals of Science*, Vol. 36, 653–655

Grattan-Guinness, I., Ed. (1980). *From the Calculus to Set Theory, 1630–1910: an Introductory History.* London; Duckworths

Günther, S. (1887). *Geschichte des mathematischen Unterrichts im deutschen Mittelalter bis zum Jahre 1525.* Berlin; A. Hofmann

Günther, S. (1903). Maximilian Curtze, *Bibliotheca Mathematica*, ser. 3, Vol. 4, 65–81 [includes a bibliography]

Habicht, W. (1977). Die Serien I–III der Euler-Edition der Schweizerischen Naturforschenden Gesellschaft: eine Übersicht, *Verhandlungen der Naturforschenden Gesellschaft in Basel*, Vol. 86, 77–85

Halliwell, J.O. (1839). *Rara mathematica, or a collection of treatises on the mathematics and subjects connected with them from ancient unedited manuscripts.* London; J.W. Parker

Harrison, John (1978). *The Library of Isaac Newton.* Cambridge; Cambridge University Press

Heilbronner, J.C. (1742). *Historia Matheseos universae a mundo condito ad seculum* PCN XVI. Leipzig; Gleditsch

Hilbert, D. (1902). Sur les problèmes futurs des mathématiques, *Compte rendu du deuxième congrès international des mathématiciens (Paris, 6–12 août 1900). Procès-verbaux et communications.* Paris; Gauthier-Villars, 58–114. German original in *Göttinger Nachrichten* (1900) 44–63, 213–297. English transl. (1902) in *Bulletin of the American Mathematical Society*, 2nd ser. Vol. 8, 437–479

Hofmann, J.E. (1953–7). *Geschichte der Mathematik.* 3 Parts. Sammlung Göschen 226, 875, 882. Berlin; Walter de Gruyter

Hofmann, J.E. (1972). Bombelli's Algebra – eine genialische Einzelleistung und ihre Einwirkung auf Leibniz, *Studia Leibnitiana*, Vol. 4, 196–252

Hofmann, J.E. (1974). *Leibniz in Paris, 1672–1676: his Growth to Mathematical Maturity.* Cambridge; Cambridge University Press

Hofmann, J.E. (1977). *Register zu Gottfried Wilhelm Leibniz. Mathematische Schriften und der Briefwechsel mit Mathematikern (herausgegeben von C.I. Gerhardt).* Hildesheim; Georg Olms Verlag

Houzeau, J.C. and Lancaster, A. (1882–9). *Bibliographie générale de l'astronomie.* Brussels; F. Hayez and X. Havermans

Huygens, C. (1888–1950). *Oeuvres complètes.* 22 Vols. The Hague; Nijhoff

International Catalogue of Scientific Literature 1901–1914 (1902–18). Section A, *Mathematics*; Section B, *Mechanics.* 28 Vols. London; The Royal Society for the International Council

Isis Critical Bibliography. Bibliographie analytique des publications relatives à l'histoire de la science (afterwards: Critical Bibliography of the History of Science and its Cultural Influences), *Isis*, 1–, 1912–

Itard, J. (1974a). A propos d'un livre sur Pierre Fermat, *Revue d'histoire des sciences*, Vol. 27, 335–346

Itard, J. (1974b). Review of M.S. Mahoney (1973), *Historia Mathematica*, Vol. 1, 470–476

Jackson, L.L. (1906). *The Educational Significance of Sixteenth Century Arithmetic.* New York; Teachers College, Columbia University

Jayawardene, S.A. (1973). The Influence of Practical Arithmetics on the *Algebra* of Rafael Bombelli, *Isis*, Vol. 64, 510–523

Jayawardene, S.A. (1978). Western Scientific Manuscripts before 1600: a Checklist of Published Catalogues, *Annals of Science*, Vol. 35, 143–172

Jayawardene, S.A. and Lawes, J. (1979). Biographical Notices of Historians of Science: a Checklist. For Kurt Vogel on his 90th Birthday (30 September 1978), *Annals of Science*, Vol. 36, 315–394

Karpinski, L.C. (1944). Algebraical Works to 1700, *Scripta Mathematica*, Vol. 10, 149–169

Karpinski, L.C. (1946). Bibliographical Check List of All Works on Trigonometry Published up to 1700 A.D., *Scripta Mathematica*, Vol. 12, 267–283

Klein, F. (1926–7). *Vorlesungen über die Entwicklung der Mathematik im 19. Jahrhundert.* Ed. R. Courant, O. Neugebauer and S. Cohn-Vossen. Die

Grundlehren der mathematischen Wissenschaften in Einzeldarstellungen, 24–25. 2 Vols. Berlin; Julius Springer

Klein, F. (1974). *Le Programme d'Erlangen: considérations comparatives sur les recherches géométriques modernes* [includes: F. Russo, Groupes et géométrie: la genèse du programme d'Erlangen de Félix Klein, *Conférence du Palais de la Découverte*, D. 129 (1929)]. Paris; Gauthier-Villars

Klemm, F. (1966). Die Rolle der Mathematik in der Technik des 19 Jahrhunderts, *Technikgeschichte*, Vol. 33, 72–90

Kline, M. (1972). *Mathematical Thought from Ancient to Modern Times.* New York; Oxford University Press

Knobloch, E. (1980). Review of Ian Hacking, *The Emergence of Probability* (Cambridge; Cambridge University Press, 1975), *Historia Mathematica*, Vol. 7, 212–216

Kolmogorov, A.N. and Yushkevich, A.P., Ed. (1978). *Matematika XIX Veka* [Mathematics in the nineteenth century]. Moscow; Nauka

Koyré, A. and Cohen, I.B. (1971–2). *Isaac Newton's Principia.* 3 Vols. Cambridge; Cambridge University Press

Lacroix, S.F. (1805). *Essai sur l'enseignement en général, et sur celui des mathématiques en particulier.* Paris; Courcier

Lagrange, J.L. (1788). *Mécanique analitique.* Paris; La Veuve Desaint

Laplace, P.S. (1799–1825). *Traité de mécanique céleste.* Paris; Duprat

Leibniz-Gesellschaft (1978). Leibniz à Paris (1672–1676): Symposium de la G.W. Leibniz-Gesellschaft (Hannover) et du Centre National de la Recherche Scientifique (Paris) à Chantilly (France) du 14 au 18 Novembre 1976, *Studia Leibnitiana Supplementa*, Vols 17 and 18

Lenoir, T. (1979). Descartes and the Geometrization of Thought; the Methodological Background of Descartes' Géométrie, *Historia Mathematica*, Vol. 6, 355–379

Leonardo da Vinci (facsimile 1973–5). *Il codice atlantico.* 12 Vols. Florence; Barbèra

Libri, G. (1865). *Histoire des sciences mathématiques en Italie, depuis la renaissance des lettres jusqu'à la fin du dix-septième siècle*, 2nd edn. 4 Vols. Halle; H.W. Schmidt

Lindsay, R.B., Ed. (1972). *Acoustics: Historical and Philosophical Development.* Bechmark Papers in Acoustics. Stroudsburg, P.; Dowden, Hutchinson and Ross

Lorey, W. (1916). *Das Studium der Mathematik an den deutschen Universitäten seit Anfang des 19. Jahrhunderts.* Abhandlungen über den mathematischen Unterricht in Deutschland 3, No. 9. Leipzig; Teubner

Lorey, W. (1926a). Felix Klein, *Leopoldina*, Vol. 1, 136–151

Lorey, W. (1926b). Felix Kleins Persönlichkeit und seine Bedeutung für die mathematischen Unterricht, *Sitzungsberichte der Berliner Mathematischen Gesellschaft*, Vol. 25, 54–68

Loria, G. (1908–9). Développements relatifs au projet d'un 'Manuel pour les recherches sur l'histoire des mathématiques', *Bibliotheca Mathematica*, ser. 3, Vol. 9, 227–236

Loria, G. (1909). Sur les moyens pour faciliter et diriger les études sur l'histoire des mathématiques, in *Atti del IV Congresso Internazionale dei Matematici (Roma, 6–11 aprile 1908).* Ed. G. Castelnuovo. Vol. 3, 541–548. Rome; Tipografia della R. Accademia dei Lincei

Loria, G. (1946). *Guida allo studio della storia delle matematiche*, 2nd edn. Milan; Hoepli. 1st edn (1916)

Loria, G. (1950). *Storia delle matematiche*, 2nd edn. Milan; Hoepli. 1st edn (1929–33). Turin; Società Tipografica Editrice-Nazionale

Mahoney, M.S. (1973). *The Mathematical Career of Pierre de Fermat 1601–1665.* Princeton, NJ; Princeton University Press

Malclès, L.-N. (1962). *La bibliographie,* 2nd edn. 'Que sais-je?', No. 708. Paris; Presses Universitaires de France

Manning, K.R. (1974–5). The Emergence of the Weierstrassian Approach to Complex Analysis, *Archive for History of Exact Sciences,* Vol. 14, 298–383

May, K.O. (1973). *Bibliography and Research Manual of the History of Mathematics.* Toronto; University of Toronto Press

May, K.O. and Gardner, C.M. (1972). *World Directory of Historians of Mathematics.* Toronto; Historia Mathematica

Mehrtens, H. (1980). Workshop on the Social History of [19th Century] Mathematics, *Historia Mathematica,* Vol. 7, 75–79

Molland, A.G. (1976). Shifting the Foundations: Descartes's Transformation of Ancient Geometry, *Historia Mathematica,* Vol. 3, 21–49

Monge, G. (1798). *Géométrie descriptive, leçons données aux Écoles normales, l'an 3 de la République.* Paris; Baudouin

Montucla, J.E. (1799–1802). *Histoire des mathématiques.* 4 Vols. Paris; H. Agasse. Reissued (1960). Paris; A. Blanchard

Müller, F. (1904). Das Jahrbuch über die Fortschritte der Mathematik, 1869–1904, *Bibliotheca Mathematica,* ser. 3, Vol. 5, 292–297

Müller, F. (1909). *Führer durch die mathematische Literatur, mit besonderer Berücksichtigung der historisch wichtigen Schriften.* Abhandlungen zur Geschichte der mathematischen Wissenschaften, 27. Leipzig; Teubner

Müller, K. (1967). *Leibniz-Bibliographie: die Literatur über Leibniz.* Veröffentlichungen des Leibniz-Archivs, 1. Frankfurt am Main; Klostermann

Newman, J.R., Ed. (1956). *The World of Mathematics: a Small Library of the Literature of Mathematics from A'h-mosé the Scribe to Albert Einstein.* 4 Vols. New York; Simon and Schuster

Newton, I. (1687). *Philosophiae naturalis principia mathematica.* London; Royal Society

Nielsen, Niels (1929). *Géomètres français sous la Révolution.* Copenhagen; Levin and Munksgaard

Nielsen, Niels (1935). *Géomètres français du dix-huitième siècle.* Copenhagen; Levin and Munksgaard

Ore, Oystein (1942). Review of *Enzyklopädie der mathematischen Wissenschaften* ... (2nd edn. Leipzig; Teubner, 1939), *Bulletin of the American Mathematical Society,* Vol. 48, 653–658

Pacioli, L. (1494). *Summa de arithmetica, geometria, proportioni et proportionalita.* Venice; Paganino de Paganini

Pingree, D. (1970–6). Census of the Exact Sciences in Sanskrit, *Memoirs of the American Philosophical Society,* Vol. 81, 1–60; Vol. 86, 1–147; Vol. 111, 1–208

Poggendorff, J.C. (1863–). *Biographisch-literarisches Handwörterbuch (zur Geschichte) der exakten Naturwissenschaften.* Vols 1–4, Leipzig; Verlag von Johann Ambrosius Barth. Vol. 5, Leipzig and Berlin; Verlag Chemie. Vol. 6, Berlin; Verlag Chemie. Vols VIIA and VIIB, Berlin; Akademie Verlag (In progress)

Pont, J.C. (1973). *La topologie algébrique des origines à Poincaré.* Paris; Presses Universitaires de France

Regiomontanus (1533). *De triangulis omnimodis libri quinque.* Nuremberg; Johann Petreius

Reich, K. (1973). Die Geschichte der Differentialgeometrie von Gauss bis Riemann (1828–1868), *Archive for History of Exact Sciences,* Vol. 11, 273–382

Riccardi, P. (1870–80). *Biblioteca matematica italiana dalla origine della stampa ai primi anni del sec XIX.* 3 Vols. Modena; Soliani. Revised edn (1952). Milan; Görlich

Rogers, L.F. (1979). *Finding Out in the History of Mathematics: a Resource File of Bibliographic, Audio-visual and Other Materials ... for Students and Teachers.* Leicester; Leapfrogs

Rogg, I. (1830). *Bibliotheca Mathematica. Handbuch der Mathematischen Literatur vom Anfange der Buchdruckerkunst bis zum Schlusse des Jahres 1830.* Berlin; Rogg, Tübingen, Fuess

Rose, P.L. (1975). *The Italian Renaissance of Mathematics.* Geneva; Droz

Royal Society of London (1867–1925). *Catalogue of Scientific Papers, 1800–1900.* 19 Vols. *Subject Index (Pure Mathematics, Mechanics, Physics).* 3 Vols. London; HMSO. Cambridge; Cambridge University Press (from Vol. 9)

Russo, F. (1959). La constitution de l'algèbre au XVIe siècle: étude de la structure d'une évolution, *Revue d'histoire des sciences,* Vol. 12, 193–208

Russo, F. (1969). *Eléments de bibliographie de l'histoire des sciences et des techniques.* 2nd revised edn. Paris; Hermann. 1st edn (1954). *Histoire des sciences et des techniques: bibliographie.*

Sarton, G. (1936a). *The Study of the History of Mathematics.* Cambridge, Mass.; Harvard University Press. Reprinted (1957). New York; Dover Publications

Sarton, G. (1936b). *The Study of the History of Science.* Cambridge, Mass.; Harvard University Press. Reprinted (1957). New York; Dover Publications

Sarton, G. (1952). *A Guide to the History of Science (Horus): a First Guide for the Study of the History of Science, with Introductory Essays on Science and Tradition.* Waltham, Mass.; Chronica Botanica

Schmitt, C.B. (1970). A Fresh Look at Mechanics in 16th-Century Italy. Essay review of Stillman Drake and I.E. Drabkin, *Mechanics in Sixteenth-Century Italy* (Madison; University of Wisconsin Press, 1969), *Studies in History and Philosophy of Science,* Vol. 1, 161–173

Scott, J.F. (1948). Mathematics through the Eighteenth Century, *Philosophical Magazine,* commemoration No., 67–91

Sebba, G. (1964). *Bibliotheca Cartesiana: a Critical Guide to the Descartes Literature,* 1800–1960. The Hague; Martinus Nijhoff

Sezgin, F. (1974). *Geschichte des arabischen Schrifttums.* Vol. 5, *Mathematik bis ca. 430H.* Leyden; Brill

Shapin, S. and Hill, S. (1972–3). The Turner Collection of the History of Mathematics at the University of Keele, *British Journal for the History of Science,* Vol. 6, 336–337

Smith, D.E. (1923–5). *History of Mathematics.* Vol. 1, *General Survey of the History of Elementary Mathematics;* Vol. 2, *Special Topics of Elementary Mathematics.* Boston; Ginn and Co. Reprinted (1958). New York; Dover Publications

Smith, D.E. (1929). *A Source Book in Mathematics.* New York; McGraw-Hill. Reprinted in 2 Vols (1959). New York; Dover Publications

Sohncke, L.A. (1854). *Bibliotheca Mathematica. Verzeichnis der Bücher über die gesammten Zweige der Mathematik,... welche in Deutschland und dem Auslande vom Jahre 1830 bis Mitte des Jahres 1854 erschienen sind.* 388 pp. Leipzig; Englemann

Stevin, S. (1955–66). *The Principle Works.* 5 Vols. Amsterdam; Swets and Zeitlinger

Stillwell, M.B. (1970). *The Awakening Interest in Science During the First Century of Printing, 1450–1550; an Annotated Checklist of First Editions Viewed from the Angle of their Subject Content.* New York; Bibliographical Society of America

Struik, D.J. (1948). *A Concise History of Mathematics.* New York; Dover Publications

Struik, D.J. (1969). *A Source Book in Mathematics, 1200–1800.* Source Books in the History of Science. Cambridge, Mass.; Harvard University Press

Struik, D.J. (1980). The Historiography of Mathematics from Proklos to Cantor, *NTM Schriftenreihe für Geschichte der Naturwissenschaften, Technik und Medizin*, Vol. 17, 1–22

Suter, H. (1900). *Die Mathematiker und Astronomen der Araber und ihre Werke*. Abhandlungen zur Geschichte der mathematischen Wissenschaften, 10. Leipzig; Teubner. Supplement (1902) in *Abhandlungen*, Vol. 14, 157–185. Reprinted (1963). Ann Arbor, Mich.; University Microfilms

Tanner, R.C.H. (1980a). The Ordered Regiment of the Minus Sign: Off-beat Mathematics in Harriot's Manuscripts, *Annals of Science*, Vol. 37, 127–158

Tanner, R.C.H. (1980b). The Alien Realm of the Minus: Deviatory Mathematics in Cardano's Writings, *Annals of Science*, Vol. 37, 159–178

Tartaglia, N. (facsimile 1959). *Quesiti e inventioni diverse*. Riproduzione infacsimile dell'edizione del 1554. Brescia; Ateneo di Brescia

Taton, R. (1954). Sylvestre-François Lacroix (1765–1843), mathématicien, professeur et historien des sciences, *Actes du VIIe congrès international d'histoire des sciences (Jerusalem, 1953)*. Paris; Hermann, 588–593

Taton, R., Ed. (1957–64). *Histoire générale des sciences*. 4 Vols. Paris: Presses Universitaires de France. Trans. A.J. Pomerans (1963) as *A General History of the Sciences*. London; Thames and Hudson. New York; Basic Books

Taton, R. (1964). L'Ecole Polytechnique et le renouveau de la géométrie analytique, in *Mélanges Alexandre Koyré*. 2 Vols. Paris; Hermann, Vol. 1: 552–564

Thackray, A. and Merton, R.K. (1972). On Discipline Building: the Paradoxes of George Sarton, *Isis*, Vol. 63, 473–495

Torretti, R. (1978). *Philosophy of Geometry from Riemann to Poincaré*. Episteme 7. Dordrecht; D. Reidel

Tropfke, J. (1921–4) *Geschichte der Elementarmathematik in systematischer Darstellung mit besonderer Berücksichtigung der Fachwörter*, 2nd edn. 7 Vols. 3rd edn. (1930–7). 4 Vols only. Berlin; De Gruyter

Tropfke, J. (1980). *Geschichte der Elementarmathematik*, 4th edn. Vol. 1, *Arithmetik und Algebra*, revised edn by K. Vogel, K. Reich, H. Gericke. Berlin; De Gruyter

Truesdell, C.A. (1972). Leonard Euler, Supreme Geometer (1707–1783), in *Irrationalism in the 18th Century*. Ed. H.E. Pagliaro. Cleveland; Press of Case Western Reserve University, 51–95

Turnbull, H., Scott, J., Hall, A.R. and Tilling, L., Ed. (1959–77). *Correspondence of Isaac Newton*. 7 Vols. Cambridge; Cambridge University Press

Van Egmond, W. (1976). The Commercial Revolution and the Beginnings of Western Mathematics in Renaissance Florence, 1300–1500, University of Indiana PhD Thesis

Viète, F. (1973). *Einführung in die neue Algebra*. Trans. and Ed. K. Reich and H. Gericke. Munich; Werner Fritsch

Vincensini, P. (1972). La géométrie differentielle aux XIXe siècle (avec quelques réflexions générales sur les mathématiques), *Scientia*, Vol. 107, 617–696

Vivanti, G. (1924). I Principali trattati di algebra dalle origini della stampa al 1800, *Periodico di matematica*, ser. 4, Vol. 4, 277–306

Volkmann, P. (1896). *Franz Neumann. *11.September 1798, †23.Mai 1895. Ein Beitrag zur Geschichte deutscher Wissenschaft. Dem Andenken an den Altmeister der mathematischen Physik gewidmete Blätter*. Leipzig; B.G. Teubner

Wallis, P.J. (1974). A Biobibliography of British Mathematics and its Applications up to 1850, *Historia Mathematica*, Vol. 1, 449–454

Wallis, P.J. and Wallis, R. (1977). *Newton and Newtoniana, 1672–1975: a Bibliography*. Folkestone; Dawson and Project for Historical Biobibliography

Weil, A. (1973). Review of M.S. Mahoney (1973), *Bulletin of the American Mathematical Society*, Vol. 79, 1138–1149

Westfall, R.S. (1978). Award of the 1977 Sarton Medal to D.T. Whiteside, *Isis*, Vol. 69, 86–87

Westfall, R.S. (1980). *Never at Rest: a Biography of Isaac Newton* (with a bibliographical essay). Cambridge; Cambridge University Press

Whiteside, D.T. (1979). Essay Review of A. Rupert Hall and Laura Tilling (eds), *The Correspondence of Isaac Newton. VII: 1718–1727* (Cambridge; Cambridge University Press, 1977 [1978]), *Annals of Science*, Vol. 36, 539–542

Whitrow, M., Ed. (1972–6). *Isis Cumulative Bibliography: A Bibliography of the History of Science formed from Isis Critical Bibliographies 1–90, 1913–65*. 3 Vols. London; Mansell

Wieleitner, H. (1927–8). Review of Felix Klein (1926–7), *Isis*, Vol. 9, 447–449; Vol. 10, 505–506

Wieleitner, H. (1927–9). *Mathematische Quellenbücher*. 4 Vols. Berlin; Otto Salle

Woodward, R.S. (1900). The Century's Progress in Applied Mathematics, *Bulletin of the American Mathematical Society*, Vol. 6, 133–163

Yeldham, F.A. (1936). *The Teaching of Arithmetic through 400 Years, 1535–1935*. London; Harrap

Yushkevich, A.P., Ed. (1970–2). *Istoriya matematiki s drevneichikh vremen do nachala XIX stoletiya* [History of mathematics from ancient times to the beginning of the XIXth century]. 3 Vols. Moscow; Nauka

Zoubov, V.P. (1968). *Leonardo da Vinci*. Trans. from the Russian by D.H. Kraus, Cambridge, Mass.; Harvard University Press

15

History of physical science

Simon Schaffer

It is symptomatic that the scope of the physical sciences is difficult to define. The processes by which particular areas of nature have been divided and subjected to investigation by specific groups of practitioners have not been thoroughly investigated by historians of science. Historians have tended to assume the existence of well-defined areas – electricity, optics, astronomy, mechanics – and then documented the successive development of theories about these phenomena. In fact, the effect of the scientific revolution was different for different areas of practice: astronomy existed as a well-defined research area; chemistry and mechanics were radically transformed; electricity and magnetism were summoned into existence (Pecheux and Fichant 1974; Westman 1975; Heilbron 1979). Thus there is an important relation between the division of labour and the new map of physical nature in the seventeenth century (Stone 1965; Barnes 1974; Zilsel 1942; Dickson 1979). This was reflected in the attempts of men like John Dee, Francis Bacon and Thomas Hobbes actually to draw such maps (Jardine 1974). This is noted by Adam Smith, in 1763 the Professor of Moral Philosophy in the University of Glasgow, who wrote that 'in opulent or commercial societies...to think or to reason comes to be, like every other employment, a particular business which is carried on by a very few people, who furnish the public with all the thought and reason possessed by the vast multitudes that labour'. Smith explained that only a small part of each individual's knowledge would really be generated from

285

personal experience and he wrote that 'all the rest has been purchased, in the same manner as his shoes and stockings, from those whose business it is to make up and prepare for market that particular species of goods' (Scott 1937: 344–5). The history of physical sciences has only recently begun to accept Smith's argument, and to treat knowledge of physical nature as a species of goods that is marketed and consumed within widely different cultural contexts. The outline of a history of physical science was given in 1767 by Joseph Priestley, who argued that this kind of history 'enjoys, in some measure, the advantages of both civil and natural history,....the idea of continual rise and improvement is conspicuous in the whole study' (Priestley 1767: ii–iv). In using the history of electricity to display the theatre of nature and the progress of the mind (McEvoy 1979), Priestley also declared his intention to 'take no notice of the mistakes, misapprehensions and altercations of electricians, except so far as I apprehended a knowledge of them might be useful to their successors' (Priestley 1767: ix). The establishment of nineteenth-century history of science involved a further development of the heroic mode of writing. Many of these texts are still of enormous use to the student: successive generations tended to celebrate the monuments of their perceived past (Fischer 1801–8; de Candolle 1873; Heller 1882–4; Rosenberger 1882–90) and documented their chronological succession, often with considerable bibliographical detail (Delambre 1821; Grant 1852; Todhunter 1873; Mottelay 1922). Many texts within this tradition are surveyed accessibly in Brush (1972). Yet here the social processes of the generation of knowledge were viewed as obstacles or aids to the march of mind: 'universal history', wrote Carlyle, 'the history of what man has accomplished in this world, is at bottom the history of Great Men who have worked here. They were the leaders of men, these great ones; the modellers, patterns, and in a wide sense creators of whatsoever the mass of men contrived to do or to attain' (Carlyle 1841: 1). Evidently this model of the history of the physical sciences did its own work: for Pierre Duhem it showed the continuity between the allegedly secular achievements of modern science and the glories of medieval Catholic culture (Duhem 1969).

To examine the way in which the knowledge of physical nature has been produced, marketed and consumed, it is (as has been argued in chapter 1) necessary to break with this dominant mode in the history of physics, and to investigate the relation between the practice and the social place of physical scientists (Ben-David 1971; Barnes 1974; Merton 1970). It is necessary to reject the claim that the motive for scientific work is merely the spirit of free enquiry (Clark 1937; Hall 1963). It is necessary, finally, to use lessons from philosophers and cultural historians that successive patterns of technique may be highly differentiated and may carry with them rules that define the world in which they operate and that enforce this definition and identification politically as 'well as epistemologically (Bachelard 1934; Kuhn 1969; Williams 1981). In this survey, some indications will be given as to possible approaches that might use this understanding.

New philosophy and new sciences

The scientific revolution is usually understood as the founding act of the new physical sciences of the seventeenth century. Historians have characterized this revolution as a series of massive displacements within the realm of ideas (Rossi 1975; Dijksterhuis 1961; Cohen 1981); the mathematization of nature; the emphasis on experience; the break-up of the medieval cosmos (Koyré 1957). However, these displacements reflect a crisis in the status and place of knowledge in the early seventeenth century. The growth of scepticism (Popkin 1964), the impact of the Tridentine reforms on the Italian universities (Schmitt 1975), and the humanist demolition of the authority of medieval scholastic texts (Mandrou 1973), were all further aspects of this crisis (Rabb 1975). Schmitt in chapter 12 discusses the preconditions for the scientific revolution, and, in particular, interpretations of Galileo's contribution. The acceptable places where knowledge could be produced and marketed changed. Specifically, the mathematization of nature was fraught with the problems of 'high' and 'low' knowledge (Ginzburg 1980). As Heilbron has argued, because mathematics was associated with the 'mixed mathematics' of the artisan teachers and engineers, any such move was bound to be 'uncomfortable' (Heilbron 1979: 11). Several sources for mathematical practice could be used – all of them posed problems of status. The artisans of Northern Italy and their contemporaries in the Low Countries, such as Tartaglia, Benedetti, Stevin, Drebbel and de Caus, combined work on problems in engineering, hydrostatics, architecture and practical geometry with ideologies drawn from appreciation of authorities like Archimedes and Vitruvius (Keller 1975; Drake and Drabkin 1969). It has often been pointed out that there may be close connections between the artisans and the new philosophy (Bernal 1969b); but this idea was challenged using citations of mechanical philosophers who sought to distance themselves from the artisans (Hall 1952; compare Duhem 1905–6). Similarly, the 'Yates thesis', which claims important sources for a mathematical natural philosophy in the Hermetic tradition (Yates 1964; Debus 1968), has been contested in the work of Westman (1977) on the relation between Hermeticism and Copernicanism. It is more plausible to interpret the debates between mechanical philosophers, theologians, astronomers and chemical philosophers in terms of conflicting roles and practices in the production of natural knowledge for an audience, rather than in terms of abstracted incoherent 'traditions' (Debus 1975). In England, for example, the artisans drew encouragement from John Dee's preface to Henry Billingsley's translation of Euclid in 1570 (Taylor 1954) and from the Vitruvian notion of a combination between astronomy, architecture and practical mathematics (Bennett 1975). They *also* needed institutional support through places such as Gresham College in London, and attracted suspicion precisely because of the mixture of epistemological and social reform (Webster 1975). It was in such a context that Bacon's text might be seen as a radical new map for natural knowledge (Farrington 1951; Hill 1965: ch. 2) and that William Gilbert's seminal text on magnetism, *De magnete*, could be interpreted as the work of, variously, a Renaissance amateur, a chemical philosopher and a progressive empiricist (Roller 1959; Abromitis 1977).

The new sciences organized nature under old headings in new ways: hydrostatics, mechanics, optics, pneumatics. Galileo recommended his Archimedean choice of 'two new sciences' in these terms (Galileo 1638: xix–xxi; compare Drake and Drabkin 1960). Galileo's career, involving a shift from university to Ducal court, perfectly represents this new orientation (Drake 1978). Drake has shown that these new sciences, in the case of Galileo, were not a trivial consequence of his endorsement of heliocentrism, but a true break in natural philosophy (Drake 1970; Drake 1976; compare Geymonat 1957; Clavelin 1968; Shea 1972). Koyré argued that Galileo's selection of the method of mathematical abstraction was a consequence of his Platonist rejection of common experience (Koyré 1943). In this Koyré was following Bachelard's argument that modern science was formed by breaking with the obstacle of common experience (Bachelard 1934: ch. 3). Settle (1961, 1967) showed convincingly, however, that Galileo's published experiments could be successfully performed, and we must understand now that Galileo's innovation lay in the selection of targets for research and the deployment of these results in a new context.

More illuminatingly, Bachelard (1951: ch.5) argued that the instrumental production of new phenomena was a central site of struggle within the new sciences. Considerable attention has been paid to scientific instruments and the new philosophy (Heilbron 1979; Bradbury 1967; King 1965; Middleton 1964; Middleton 1966). In some of the new sciences there was a clear connection between technologies of glass and theoretical development. In optics and astronomy this connection was fraught with difficulty: technicians contested the rights of theoreticians to dictate standards of practice (van Helden 1970). The theoretical development of optics by Kepler, Snel, Descartes and the practitioners in Italy and England such as Grimaldi and Hooke involved both the analysis of new phenomena (such as the work of Huygens on double refraction), and an increase in the wonder of the phenomena themselves, including such celebrated anomalies as the behaviour of Iceland crystal, the effects of diffraction and the marvels of the microscope (Ronchi 1970; Sabra 1967; Lohne and Sticker 1969). Turner discusses microscopy and instruments in chapter 13.

In all this there was a need for a common vocabulary in which practitioners could describe the phenomena they were producing for patrons and audiences. This has attracted the attention of historians to a philosophical analysis of the idealist component of the mechanical philosophy (Burtt 1932; Strong 1936). More rewardingly, historians have drawn attention to institutional and practical contexts in which a peculiar combination of mechanist vocabulary and mathematical analysis emerged. In optics, the 'kinematic' programme dominated the practice developed at the scientific societies of the later seventeenth century (Badcock 1962; Shapiro 1973); the other important area of mechanical interpretation remained pneumatics, with an equal dependence on the technology of display. The use of the air-pump and the barometric tube was an important resource: it was through the Italian and French experiments of 1644–47 that Pascal was able to argue persuasively that this new ontology was a viable mode of explanation, and that it was firmly rooted in common experience: 'let all the disciples of Aristotle collect the profoundest writings of their master and his commentators in order to account for this if they can', he wrote. 'If they cannot, let them learn that experiment is the true master one must follow in physics' (Pascal 1937: 75; Koyanagi 1978). Yet *in fact* the claim for experience was an ideological move in a contest against the philosophy of the schools (Brockliss 1981). Empiricism was not obviously or inevitably the way forward: it was a cultural claim of a particular group of practitioners. As the place of Cartesian philosophy at the centre of this claim demonstrated, this was no assertion of naive empiricism against obscurantism (Mouy

1934; Rogers 1972; Pacchi 1973; Gaukroger 1980). The difficulty in assigning even such a natural philosopher as Christiaan Huygens to a 'Cartesian' or 'empiricist' tradition shows the impossibility of a purely intellectualist analysis of these allegiances (Dugas 1954b; Westman 1980b). In mechanics itself the work of Galileo's disciples was important precisely because of their ability to cope with apparently exclusive modes of analysis of natural phenomena. In France, Descartes, Peiresc, Pascal, Fermat and Gassendi all followed this lead in theories of impact and local motion: what mattered was the activity of Marin Mersenne in the coordination and spreading of a successful programme of research into a problem that had been expropriated from the universities (Lenoble 1943; Mahoney 1973). Furthermore, the transformation of the analysis of local motion into a high-status practice outside such a framework gave considerable assistance to the development of a coherent mechanical vocabulary for other kinds of phenomena (Hall 1952; Westfall 1971, 1977).

The mechanical philosophy therefore found its place in new kinds of social context and involved new kinds of natural phenomena in specific shared vocabularies. These practices could only with difficulty dissociate themselves from the subversive implications of an atheist and atomist mechanism: this was the task that writers like Gassendi and Charleton set themselves (Kargon 1966; Webster 1967b; Gelbart 1971). In turn, the new places of social production, the scientific societies, would have to respond to the criticisms that their practitioners would attract. While these societies have been studied by historians (Webster 1967b; Middleton 1971; Hahn 1971; Hoppen 1970), less attention has been paid to the relation between the political and religious attack on the societies and on their natural philosophical practice (Jacob and Jacob 1971; Webster 1967a). It is clear that the combination of 'the real, the mechanical, the experimental Philosophy' (Hooke 1665) with these conflicts dominated the place of the understanding of physical nature.

Astronomy and the Newtonian apotheosis

Conventionally, historians have focused their reading of the scientific revolution on changes in astronomy. In the late sixteenth century, astronomy already had a recognizable social place and institutional form (Westman 1980a). Changes in this place and form were accompanied by a change in the astronomical gaze produced by Galileo's deployment of the telescope (Drake 1976;

van Helden 1974b), and by the profound reorientation in astronomical practice registered in the texts Kepler produced as Imperial Mathematician at Prague. The scale of this change has drawn historians to the study of the philosophical and methodological aspects of his work (Holton 1973; Beer and Beer 1975; Urban and Sutter 1975). Considerable attention has also been paid to the detailed practice of his work on the physical structure of the heavens and its mathematical analysis (Wilson 1970; Gingerich 1972; Koyré 1973; Krafft 1973). Less attention has been paid to the consequences of the application of a physics to the heavens for the structures of astronomical organization. The combination of the mechanical philosophy, with its utilitarian claims and its ambitions to offer a causal analysis of planetary motion (Armitage 1950), with the new state observatories in France and in England was very powerful in its effects on the direction of astronomy (Forbes 1975). Similarly, there has been little attention given to the Jesuit astronomers who dominated astronomical theories at the mid-century. There was an important division of labour between positional astronomy, which continued to adopt pre-Keplerian modes of 'saving the phenomena', and philosophical astronomy, which sought to give true physical causes for planetary motion; this, too, had important consequences for the organization of the observatories (Russell 1964; Whiteside 1964; Thoren 1974). The Cartesian philosophers adopted the vortex theory of planetary motions, which, while integrating planetary astronomy within natural philosophy, nevertheless reinforced this division because of the comparative inability of a vortex theory to generate an adequate positional model (Aiton 1972). Furthermore, as van Helden (1974a) has shown, the application of Cartesian physics by Huygens to the problem of the ring of Saturn was an excellent example of such a division.

In this context, Newton's intervention appears as a synthesis of mathematical and inductive approaches to nature (Butts and Davis 1970; Cohen 1981). This simplistic characterization has been demolished by the recent publication and examination of much manuscript material (Hall and Hall 1962; Turnbull *et al.* 1959–77; Whiteside 1967– ; Dobbs 1975), and by a more thorough biographical study (Manuel 1968; Westfall 1980). While Newton's mathematical reputation has emerged untarnished, it is now rather clearer that Newton's relationship with the mechanical philosophy needs profound revision, and that a socio-political interpretation of his 'success' is a viable project. The mechanical philosophy had established itself in England through the work of Robert Boyle and his contemporaries with a relatively desiccated vocabulary of matter in motion, and this vocabulary was applied to terrestrial phenomena such as pneumatics and local motion (Hall 1966). The fundamental claim of this practice was that it could produce and then analyse phenomena in terms familiar to every observer, who would thus be impressed with the wise order of nature (J.R. Jacob 1977). Newton's work, in total contrast, mobilized concepts of activity and power in matter, and of action in the heavens, in order to reinforce and strengthen this claim. Natural philosophy now demonstrated God's power directly because it dealt with the powers in matter and produced them before an audience (Whiteside 1970; Dobbs 1975; Heimann and McGuire 1971; Kubrin 1967). At the same time, the mathematical power of the analysis made by Newton of both celestial and terrestrial phenomena (Whiteside 1964) ultimately legitimated the full development of a mathematical physics. However, this physics had to find a social place, and Newton's programmes were constructed around a wide range of social contexts (M.C. Jacob 1976). Natural philosophy, as interpreted by the readers of the Queries to Newton's *Opticks* (1730) and of other texts, would work through instruments upon inert matter in order to produce those active powers that could best exemplify the place of the divine in nature: 'by this we learn, that Nature being but a little adjuvated or seconded with Art can work wonders', as a representative text of seventeenth-century technical education put it (Bate 1654: 132), and 'if natural Philosophy in all its Parts,' wrote Newton in 1706, 'by pursuing this Method, shall at length be perfected, the Bounds of Moral Philosophy will be also enlarged' (Newton 1730: 405). Such a practice, therefore, had obvious social uses, and it could be practised within specific contexts as public lectures in natural philosophy developed through the eighteenth century (Gibbs 1961; Rowbottom 1968). Alternatively, the high status of the display of rational and mathematical order in nature that could be inferred from the *Principia* was connected with new practices in mathematics and astronomy that would pose important problems for the analytical and celestial mechanics of the eighteenth-century scientific academies (Truesdell 1968; Wilson 1980).

Natural philosophy

The image of 'two Newtons', that of the *Principia* and that of the *Opticks*, has dominated the historiography of eighteenth-century science (Buchdahl 1961; Guerlac 1965; Casini 1969). In this it has distracted attention from other intellectual traditions, particularly that of the Wolffian disciples of Leibniz (Barber 1955; Elkana 1971; Heilbron 1979: 46). More importantly, it has ignored the differing contexts in which physical nature was investigated and the differing practices adopted (Schaffer 1980b). I have indicated that natural philosophy was constructed as a practice that would impress an audience with the power of active principles, such as those of heat, light and electricity (Schofield 1970; Beer 1978; Millburn 1976; Allan and Schofield 1980). The social contexts of these practices – the philosophical societies and the public lectures of the eighteenth century – must be understood on their own terms in order to understand the rationale of this form of natural philosophy. Some historians have condemned this work as chaotic (Kuhn 1970); in fact there was a rational practice at the heart of experimental natural philosophy that guided its research programmes, particularly in the field of electricity. Electrical and magnetic phenomena were understood as manifestations of active principles that could then be accounted for using a range of possible physical causal agents (Cohen 1956; Home 1977; Heilbron 1979). Furthermore, electrical practice specifically mobilized the instrumental display that had been inherent in earlier forms of natural philosophy: electricians of the eighteenth century depended upon the drama produced in the spectacle of the Leyden Jar and similar machines for the compulsion of electrical theory (Finn 1971; Hackmann 1978). Thus, although the theoretical developments – the distinction between conductors and insulators, the development of the condenser, the Franklinian theory of charge – have the appearance of random productions from a chaotic theoretical base, in fact there was a structure in this form of practice that distances it from electrical *science* as it was later constituted.

One important development in electrical and natural philosophical practice was the construction of a 'philosophical history', which was important for the Scots and for Priestley and his colleagues amongst the Dissenting academies and philosophical societies in England. The importance of the single experiment was devalued, and, using claims about the psychological constitution of the mind of the audience, the author would arrange series of experiments designed to recapitulate in the mind of the observer the actual progress of science (McEvoy and McGuire 1975; McEvoy 1979). This interpretation stresses the social context of their work in small groups such as the Lunar Society at Birmingham (Schofield 1963), and draws attention away from the philosophical and theological interpretation generally offered to give some kind of coherence to this practice (Schofield 1970; Heimann and McGuire 1971). Instead, we can begin to see the way in which active powers in matter and in the mind were mobilized by these electricians for specific purposes in the moral order (Shapin 1980).

Academic physics

In Europe, the dominant mode of social organization of natural philosophy was the scientific academy, following the model of the Paris Academy of Sciences. In this context the mathematical analysis of the Leibnizian and Newtonian patterns could be more fittingly adopted. The 'resistance' of French writers to Newtonianism must be interpreted in this light, rather than in that adopted by Brunet (1931) for whom the 'progressive' Newtonian programme replaced the 'conservative' Cartesian one. Barber (1955) also drew attention to the more complex intellectual traditions at work in academic France. The role of the Dutch natural philosophers in their universities was crucial in this respect (Ruestow 1973; Maclean 1972; Hackmann 1975; Brunet 1926). In Holland, the university professors combined aspects of the public lecturing traditions of Britain and were in close contact with the academies in France and Germany. Furthermore, specific academic organizations fostered highly identified social groups within academic physics, centred around the prize competitions of the eighteenth century (Calinger 1969). Such competitions dominated the practice of the academic physicists in the work they developed on problems in mechanics and astronomy. One dominant area of concern – the *vis viva* controversy – was with the ontology of the new mechanics; academic physicists found themselves questioning more explicitly the ontology they had inherited from the seventeenth century (Hankins 1965; Laudan 1968; Iltis 1971, 1973).

In celestial mechanics and the problems of resisted motion, as Whiteside (1975) has argued, the Newtonian legacy was neither necessarily successful nor dominant, particularly in the research programme to construct an adequate theory of the moon's motion. It was at scientific academies that rival constraints operated on the method and concerns of analytic celestial mechanics. On the one hand, it was suggested by Hessen (1931) that the concerns that Newton had registered in his *Principia* were a reflection of the technical *needs* of the late seventeenth century; in the case of lunar theory, this 'need' was represented by the desire for an adequate means to find the longitude (Forbes 1975). At the same time, the work of the astronomers in the continental academies increasingly combined complex models of analysis to develop such a theory and a campaign directed at state patrons to support astronomical expeditions allegedly designed to measure the fundamental astronomical parameters: these included the expeditions to Lapland and Peru in the 1730s, to the Cape in 1750, and the Venus expeditions of the 1760s (Woolf 1959).

Within the academies, debates over analysis of planetary motion inevitably raised fundamental issues about the epistemology and method of classical mechanics, such as the struggles between Buffon, Clairaut' and D'Alembert about the prediction of the return of Halley's Comet in 1759 and the attempt to correct the Newtonian lunar theory by a change in the inverse square law of gravitation (Waff 1975; Wilson 1980; Hankins 1970; Briggs 1964).

Finally, as Truesdell has most notably argued, the development of rational mechanics in the eighteenth century owed surprisingly little to some general 'Newtonian' conception of such practice. The rational mechanics developed by men like the Bernoullis, Maupertuis, D'Alembert and Euler was, if anything, a fundamental break with such a tradition, and the problems it set itself on rigid bodies, resisted and unresisted motion and fall, on hydrostatics and local motion, took these practices into a highly sophisticated academic area where the applied utility of mathematical physics was far from obvious, and where the community of active members was small (Truesdell 1954, 1960). The successful institutionalization of rational mechanics in the state academies of the eighteenth century depended upon a relatively small group. In Russia, for example, the Academy was divorced from society, and the influence of, say, Newtonian ideas remained at this élite level (Boss 1972). Home has analysed this trajectory for the career of Aepinus, a member of the St Petersburg group, whose work on the mathematical theory of electricity represented a fundamental rupture with the natural philosophical exploitation of the dramatic power of electrical phenomena (Home 1973, 1979). Similarly in England, the isolation of Henry Cavendish from the public sites of production and his own unwillingness to publish his research drew him closer to the analytic mode of investigating electricity (McCormmach 1969; Cavendish 1879; Dorling 1974). Cavendish's discovery of the inverse square law for electricity is in marked contrast to the forms of work practised by many of his contemporaries in natural philosophy, including one of the earliest mathematical analyses of experimental error.

Thus both for astronomers – such as John Michell, with whom Cavendish collaborated (McCormmach 1968) – and for natural philosophers, the social context of the production and dissemination of knowledge seemed to affect profoundly the character of their work. Emerson has attempted a geographical classification of the forms that such an 'enlightenment' took (Emerson 1973); it is clear that in several cases, such as that of the polymath Johann Heinrich Lambert, who worked on optics, mechanics, cosmology and cometography, there were tensions inherent in the switch between public natural philosophy and organized academic physics; in his search for recognition by the Berlin Academy, Lambert had to choose carefully the right form of practice for acceptance (Berger 1959).

In this context the development of career structures was to become a vital factor in the formation of physical science. In France, the proliferation of sets of competing organizations gave these problems of support and prestige an important role (Hahn 1975; Crosland 1975). The professionalization and institutionalization of *savants* in the Ancien Regime did not and could not by itself produce the classical professional physicist of the nineteenth century. In the case of a practitioner such as Coulomb (Gillmor 1971), there is a clear relation between his work on electrostatics and the relative status of engineering and physics in such a context. Within the physical sciences, it was a dominantly French achievement that formalized mathematical analysis of electricity, mechanics and planetary motion. The publication of Lagrange's *Méchanique analytique* and Laplace's *Mécanique céleste* may stand as the marks of this achievement. At the same time, particularly under the impact of the Revolutionary crisis of the 1790s, it was accepted that this did not offer a complete account of physical nature. The Mesmerist associations of some of the Revolutionary leadership, or the functions of cometography as a philosophical and moral theatre for astronomy, indicated that other functions were demanded (Darnton 1968). Practices involving animal magnetism, heat and electricity, particularly in the work of practitioners such as Volta and Galvani (Gliozzi 1966), certainly represented a sustained attempt to continue some of the practices of eighteenth-century natural philosophy. Laplace's collaboration with Lavoisier on problems of heat and motion was representative of an attempt to reorient the character of such philosophy (Guerlac 1976). Finally, in the hands of such able practitioners and entrepreneurs as Laplace and Biot, the academic and analytic model of mathematical physics that Laplace drew from the high status of his successes in astronomy was explicitly developed as a programme to be copied generally. Disciples such as Fourier or Poisson explored a wide variety of phenomena with mathematical theories of heat and optics as well as the traditional areas of astronomy and mechanics (Herivel 1975). In astronomy, furthermore, the German school of practitioners, such as Gauss, Olbers and Bessel, had effectively come to dominate the field through a successful application of analysis to planetary motion and to that of the comets: the publication *Theoria motus corporum coelestium* (1809) by Gauss (see Davies 1963) and extended work by Legendre and others marked this achievement, just as the programmes in Laplacian physics dominated the practices in France (Fox 1974; Frankel 1977).

German physics and classical physics

The dominance exercised by the German physicists over the structure of classical physics has drawn historians' attention towards its roots in philosophical and institutional reform in the German states from 1790. In 1813 Humphry Davy reported Laplace's contempt for matter theory: 'he treated my idea in a tone bordering on contempt, as if angry that any results in chemistry could, even in their future possibilities be compared with his own labours' (Davy 1839–40: i, 168). The Laplacian attempt to fix the status of scientific hierarchies was subverted by the changes in Germany, which included the development of *Naturphilosophie* through the work of philosophers like Schelling and Fichte and practitioners such as Ritter and Oersted. Although the real ideological importance of *Naturphilosophie* has been challenged (Gower 1973), it is clear that these changes had important effects both on a reorientation of the relative status of mathematical and physical analysis and on the organization of research (Snelders 1970; Knight 1975). At the same time, the destruction of the eighteenth-century German state system and its replacement by active reformist bureaucracy had equally crucial effects (Turner 1971; Farrar 1975). The new German university systems, and their associated research and teaching laboratories on the model established by Liebig for chemistry at Giessen, were the true institutional model for classical physics (Morrell 1972). Two notions of physical science coexisted uneasily in this context; both the work of Oken and his collaborators in the establishment of Associations for the Advancement of Science, and that of Liebig, Siemens and Helmholtz in the research and teaching institutions, particularly around the Physical Society of Berlin, came to dominate nineteenth-century physics and its public face.

This reorientation in turn changed the areas of concern in nature to which physicists would direct their attention. Physicists emerged as 'sages' (Knight 1967) and, in the context of a British scientific community dominated by the methodological schemata derived from the philosophical history of the Scots, this represented a radical transformation (Olson 1975). The 'Romantic' physics of the turn of the nineteenth century drew its violent critics; Ault (1974) recently explained how we can read the polemic of William Blake against the 'water-wheels of Newton' within this context of the growing power of physical science and the Romantic response. In the reconstructed field of optics, for example, the eighteenth century in Britain has too often been condemned as unproductive precisely because of its remarkable distance from the early nineteenth-century work of the Laplacians and the convergent physics of the Germans (Cantor 1978). The reception of a mathematical and empirical wave theory of light in Britain has now been thoroughly analysed using the understanding historians have gained of these problems of politics and method: the struggles surrounding the work of Thomas Young involve much more, therefore, than the assertion of truth through demonstrative experiment (Wood and Oldham 1954; Cantor 1975; Frankel 1976; Worrall 1976). The problems involved in the adoption of French physical theory and practice in England, disseminated by advocates of analytical mechanics and of the Laplacian programme, were made more complex by the necessary restructuring of a British scientific community that was held by many to be in decline (Crosland and Smith 1978). Similarly in France, the teaching and research system in mathematical physics was by no means conspicuously successful (Shinn 1979; Fox and Weisz 1980). Thus classical physics emerged following a German model of concern with problems of heat, pneumatics and optics in radically different contexts from either natural philosophy or academic science.

Classical physics has often been characterized in terms of its concerns with the synthesis and identification of a wide variety of physical phenomena within a single scheme of understanding (Sharlin 1966). The programme of the 'unification of science' was not specific enough to guide practical research, but insofar as it was institutionalized in the physics laboratories and disseminated in the public associations it did offer a guiding ideology (Cannon 1978). Obvious examples of the success of this guide must include research into forms of radiation like light, including the work of Herschel, Ritter and their successors on infrared, ultraviolet and the spectroscope (Lovell 1968; McGucken 1969). The impetus for work on the conservation of energy stemmed from the necessary reinterpretation of a wide variety of sources provided from within both natural philosophy and academic physics. Three such sources might be identified: the practice of pneumatics, which had been developed in natural philosophy and then transformed in kinematic terms by Dalton, Charles, Gay-Lussac and Regnault (Fox

1971); the work by the natural philosophers on animal heat and the connections between heat and vitality established by the school of Lavoisier, which changed the status and place of chemistry (Knight 1967; Levere 1971); and the changes in the practice of electricity and magnetism (Brush 1976). For Bachelard, the work of men like Fourier in the Laplacian tradition on problems of thermal conduction represented the best example of the break between pre-scientific natural philosophical understanding of vitality and the formalization of mathematical analysis (Bachelard 1927). The 'discovery' of the conservation of energy in the 1840s has drawn obsessive attention from historians precisely because of the problems inherent in the production of new phenomena, the philosophical problems of interpretation, and the relation between the technical structures in the early nineteenth century and the actual theoretical development of thermodynamics (Hiebert 1962; Carnot 1979).

Kuhn (1959) stressed the simultaneity of the work of men like Joule, Mayer and Helmholtz and thus stressed the common resources available to physicists at this time. But Elkana (1974) and Heimann (1974a,b) have emphasized that physicists discovered different entities, and that 'it is only under the influence of the hindsight gained from their pooled results that their discoveries seem identical' (Elkana 1974: 189). Certain obvious social factors were at work in this programme: Bernal (1969a: ch. 2) drew attention to the importance of energy accounting in steam technology and to the way in which mathematical analysis was provided by the new institutional forms available, for example to Carnot at the École Polytechnique or to Joule through his collaboration with William Thomson.

Similarly, in the violent priority disputes surrounding this work, the relative questions of philosophical and social status were crucial. Mayer published his work in Liebig's *Annalen der Chimie* in 1842; Mayer and Helmholtz had both been trained as physicians rather than physicists; while it was possible for Clausius to establish the mathematical basis of a dynamical theory of heat, both Joule (at Manchester) and Grove (at the London Institution) developed their ideas before a public audience. The success of the professional academics, such as Thomson (at Glasgow) and Helmholtz, was also affirmed (Helmholtz 1971). Joule's only public exposition of his work, for example, was in front of an audience at St Anne's Church reading room in Manchester in April 1847 (Watson 1947: 383). Evidently the social context of classical physics still divided into places of public dissemination of knowledge and the professional sites of production of that knowledge. This division of labour was crucial in the case of Manchester

(Kargon 1977) and at the Royal Institution in London (Berman 1978), and it dominated the development of a mechanical and dynamic 'map' for physics in Britain in the first half of the nineteenth century (Smith 1976, 1978). Historians are therefore beginning to investigate this division as it affected the growth of mechanics' institutes and institutions that placed science in culture (Shapin and Barnes 1977).

In electricity and magnetism, this division had its effects. The mathematical theories of electricity stemming from the academic work of Aepinus and Coulomb reached their culmination in the classic papers of Ampère in 1822 (Brown 1969). For the French there was an axiomatic distinction between the agencies of electricity and magnetism, and the prime criterion for success was the effective mathematical description of the phenomena (Hamamdjian 1971). Caneva (1978) has convincingly traced the social factors at work in the transformation of these views into classical electrodynamics in the German context: it is clear both for Oersted and for Faraday that complex social and philosophical stimuli dominated any commitment to a 'convergent' approach to such phenomena. For Faraday, there has been considerable debate (Williams 1965: ch.2; Agassi 1971; Heimann 1971) about the roots of his notions of matter and force and their connection with his work in electrochemistry and electromagnetism (Guralnik 1979). His position at the Royal Institution (Jeffreys, 1960) was fundamental in the development of an understanding of electromagnetism that seemed to owe little to the practices of the French and the Germans. Maxwell wrote to him in 1857 in terms that demarcate this project from that of his contemporaries (Williams 1965: 512): 'Now as far as I know you are the first person to whom the idea of bodies acting at a distance by throwing the surrounding medium into a state of constraint has arisen, as a principle to be actually believed in.' In these contrasts historians have tried to trace a coherent route for the origins of field theory (Whittaker 1951; Hesse 1961; Williams 1966) while at the same time analysing the philosophical claims competing physicists made to justify the models they constructed of the field itself.

The fundamental problem areas of early nineteenth-century astronomy can similarly be divided between positional and natural philosophical concerns. The former included the culmination of the analytical programme of the French and German astronomers, including the discovery of the planet Neptune – represented as a triumph of Newtonian theory – and the establishment of stellar parallax (Struve 1959). At the same time, philosophical astronomy, under the influence of Laplace's speculation on the nebular origin of the solar system and William Herschel's natural history of the heavens, raised the ideologically sensitive issue of the history and development of the universe as a whole (Merleau-Ponty 1976; Numbers 1977; Brooke 1979; Schaffer 1980a). The importance of these practices for other areas, particularly natural history and thermodynamics, has recently been stressed (Burchfield 1975). Above all, the spectacular developments of instrumentation, including the giant reflectors of the Herschels and the Earls of Rosse, the spectrometer and the application of the camera to stellar astronomy by men like Kirchhoff and Huggins (King 1955), cannot be understood as a purely autonomous development. In physics and astronomy, instruments were deployed for specific theoretical tasks, and the difficulty historians have experienced in accounting for anomalous instrumental reports in the nineteenth century is a consequence of this fact.

The end of classical physics

The processes by which classical physics broke with the forms of production typical of the scientific academies and the natural philosophers must be traced through the career structures of physics and astronomy (Mendelsohn 1964). Three areas within this problem have drawn attention from historians: the massive development of public patronage for science, connected with the programmes of 'Humboldtian' science in geomagnetism or astronomy (Cawood 1979; Cannon 1978); the philosophical basis of the successes of classical field theory, particularly in the methodology of electrodynamics and thermodynamics (Berkson 1974; Heimann 1970, 1972; Kargon 1969; Doran 1975); and the social context of reorganized physics towards the end of the century (Sviedrys 1970; Wynne 1979). There was, above all, an increasing understanding of the place of physical science in the natural and cultural struggle, well documented in Basalla *et al.* (1970). Norman Lockyer told the readers of *Nature* in 1901 that

> the enormous and unprecedented progress in science during the last century has brought about a perfectly new state of things, in which the 'struggle for existence' which Darwin studied in relation to organic forms is now seen, for the first time, to apply to organised communities... It is a struggle in which the fittest to survive is no longer indicated by his valour and muscle and powers of endurance, but by those qualities in which the most successful differs from the rest (Basalla *et al.* 1970: 492).

With physical science as such a resource, the 'industrialisation of the mind' became inevitable (Sohn-Rethel 1978: ch. 24).

Such an argument has not been fully applied to the development of physics after the revolutions associated with the foundations of relativity and quantum theory (Weiner 1977; Hermann 1977). The development of quantum theory can be traced through collections of printed and manuscript material now assembled by T.S. Kuhn and his colleagues (Kuhn *et al.* 1967). The history itself has concentrated on the series of specific effects whose production was held to destroy the classical synthesis (Kangro 1970; Kuhn 1978; Stuewer 1975) and in terms of detailed studies of the principal actors in the foundation of quantum theory (Meyer-Abich 1965; Hermann 1977; Mendelssohn 1973; Kangro 1970; Heilbron 1974). Einstein, by contrast, has suffered from the treatment meted out to the folk-heroes of modern science (Aichelburg and Sexl 1979; French 1979; Woolf 1980), though some attempt has been made elsewhere to relate the development of relativity theory to social factors (Feuer 1971), and the ether-drift experiments performed after 1880 have been fully documented by Swenson (1972). Most attention has been attracted by Forman's effort (1971, 1969) to relate the development of an acausal quantum theory to the hostile environment in which Weimar physics found itself. This attempt has been criticized by Hendry (1980), although the information available in recent surveys of the physics community in 1900 (Pyenson and Skopp 1977; Forman *et al.* 1975; Malley 1979) provides historians with plentiful data on which to base new assessments of the social basis of the new physics (Bunge and Shea 1979; Kevles 1978). In astronomy, too, the development of 'big science' of the twentieth century has had profound effects on the practice of the 'professionals': the celebrated case of the 'discovery' of internal motions in spiral nebulae (Hetherington 1975) or the development of radio astronomy (Edge and Mulkay 1976) have enabled some historians to examine afresh the social construction of astronomy and astrophysics.

Now that these forms of scientific activity can be seen as forms of production (Sklair 1973: ch. 3), we can, as historians of physical science, recognize as the natural philosopher George Gordon recognized that physical science and its practitioners 'are a party, produced and subsisting upon the same motives as other parties, and altogether of the same nature with them;....and he knows but little of the affairs of the learned world who knows not how considerable that party is in it' (Gordon 1719: preface); and in this perspective there seem to be grounds for a fruitful collaboration between historians and sociologists of the physical sciences (Collins 1975; Pinch 1977).

Bibliography

Abromitis, L. (1977). William Gilbert as Scientist, Brown University PhD thesis

Agassi, J. (1971). *Faraday as a Natural Philosopher*. Chicago and London; University of Chicago Press

Aichelburg, P.C. and Sexl, R.U., Ed. (1979). *Albert Einstein: his Influence on Physics, Philosophy and Politics*. Wiesbaden; Vieweg

Aiton, E.J. (1972). *The Vortex Theory of Planetary Motions*. London; Macdonald

Allan, D.G.C. and Schofield, R.E. (1980). *Stephen Hales: Scientist and Philanthropist*. London; Scolar Press

Armitage, A. (1950). 'Borell's Hypothesis' and the Rise of Celestial Mechanics, *Annals of Science*, Vol. 6, 268–282

Ault, D.D. (1974). *Visionary Physics: Blake's Response to Newton*. Chicago; University of Chicago Press

Bachelard, G. (1927). *Étude sur l'évolution d'un problème de physique: la propagation thermique dans les solides*. Paris; Vrin

Bachelard, G. (1934). *Le Nouvel esprit scientifique*. Paris; Presses Universitaires de France

Bachelard, G. (1951). *L'Activité rationaliste de la physique contemporaine*. Paris; Presses Universitaires de France

Badcock, A.W. (1962). Physical Optics at the Royal Society, *The British Journal for the History of Science*, Vol. 1, 99–116

Barber, W.H. (1955). *Leibniz in France from Arnauld to Voltaire. A Study in French Reactions to Leibnizianism, 1670–1760*. Oxford; Clarendon Press

Barnes, B. (1974). *Scientific Knowledge and Sociological Theory*. London and Boston; Routledge and Kegan Paul

Basalla, G., Coleman, W. and Kargon, R.H., Ed. (1970). *Victorian Science*. Garden City, NY; Doubleday Anchor

Bate, John (1654). *The Mysteries of Nature and Art*, 3rd edn. London; printed by R. Bishop for A. Crook. 1st edn (1634)

Beer, A. and Beer, P., Ed. (1975). Kepler: Four Hundred Years: Proceedings of Conferences held in Honour of Johannes Kepler, *Vistas in Astronomy*, Vol. 18. Oxford; Pergamon Press

Beer, P., Ed. (1978). *Newton and the Enlightenment*. Oxford; Pergamon Press

Ben-David, J. (1971). *The Scientist's Role in Society; A Comparative Study*. Englewood Cliffs, NJ; Prentice Hall

Bennett, J.H.A. (1975). Christopher Wren: Astronomy, Architecture, and the Mathematical Sciences, *Journal for the History of Astronomy*, Vol. 6, 149–184

Berger, P. (1959). J.H. Lamberts Bedeutung in der Naturwissenschaft des 18 Jahrhunderts, *Centaurus*, Vol. 6, 157–254

Berkson, W. (1974). *Fields of Force. The Development of a World View from Faraday to Einstein*. London; Routledge and Kegan Paul

Berman, M. (1978). *Social Change and Scientific Organisation: the Royal Institution 1799–1844*. Ithaca, NY; Cornell University Press. London; Heinemann Educational Books

Bernal, J.D. (1969a). *Science and Industry in the Nineteenth Century*. Bloomington; Indiana University Press. 1st edn (1953)

Bernal, J.D. (1969b). *Science in History*, 3rd revised edn. 4 Vols. London; G.A. Watts and Co. 1st edn (1954)

Beyerchen, A.D. (1977). *Scientists under Hitler: Politics and the Physics Community in the Third Reich*. New Haven, Conn.; Yale University Press

Boss, V. (1972). *Newton and Russia: The Early Influence 1698–1796*. Cambridge, Mass.; Harvard University Press

Bradbury, S. (1967). *Evolution of the Microscope*. Oxford; Pergamon Press

Briggs, J.M. (1964). D'Alembert: Philosophy and Mechanics in the Eighteenth Century, *Colorado University Studies in History*, Vol. 3, 38–56

Brockliss, L.W.B. (1981). Aristotle, Descartes, and the New Science: Natural Philosophy at the University of Paris 1600–1740, *Annals of Science*, Vol. 38, 33–69

Brooke, J.H. (1979). Nebular Contraction and the Expansion of Naturalism, *The British Journal for the History of Science*, Vol. 12, 200–211

Brown, T.M. (1969). The Electric Current in Early Nineteenth Century French Physics, *Historical Studies in the Physical Sciences*, Vol. 1, 61–103

Brunet, P. (1926). *Les Physiciens hollandais et la méthode expérimentale en France au 18e siècle.* Paris; Blanchard

Brunet, P. (1931). *L'Introduction des théories de Newton en France au 18e siècle.* Paris; Blanchard

Brush, S.G., Ed. (1972). *Resources for the History of Physics. Guide to Books and Audiovisual Materials.* Hanover, NH; University Press of New England

Brush, S.G. (1976). *The Kind of Motion We Call Heat: A History of the Kinetic Theory of Gases in the Nineteenth Century.* 2 Vols. Amsterdam and New York; North Holland Publishing Company

Buchdahl, G. (1961). *The Image of Newton and Locke in the Age of Reason.* London and New York; Sheed and Ward

Bunge, M.A. and Shea, W.R., Ed. (1979). *Rutherford and Physics at the Turn of the Century.* London; Dawson. New York; Science History Publications

Burchfield, J.D. (1975). *Lord Kelvin and the Age of the Earth.* New York; Science History Publications

Burtt, E.A. (1932). *The Metaphysical Foundations of Modern Physical Science*, 2nd revised edn. London; Routledge and Kegan Paul. Ist edn (1924)

Butts, R.E. and Davis, J.W., Ed. (1970). *The Methodological Heritage of Isaac Newton.* Oxford; Basic Blackwell

Calinger, R.S. (1969). The Newtonian–Wolffian Controversy, 1740–1759, *Journal of the History of Ideas*, Vol. 30, 319–330

Candolle, A. de (1873). *Histoire des sciences et des savants depuis deux siècles.* Geneva; H. Georg

Caneva, K.L. (1978). From Galvanism to Electrodynamics: The Transformation of German Physics and Its Social Context, *Historical Studies in the Physical Sciences*, Vol. 9, 63–159

Cannon, S.F. (1978). *Science in Culture: the Early Victorian Period.* New York; Dawson and Science History Publications

Cantor, G.N. (1975). The Reception of the Wave Theory of Light in Britain: A Case Study Illustrating the Role of Methodology in Scientific Debate, *Historical Studies in the Physical Sciences*, Vol. 6, 109–132

Cantor, G.N. (1978). The Historiography of 'Georgian' Optics, *History of Science*, Vol. 16, 1–21

Carlyle, T. (1841). *On Heroes, Hero-Worship, and the Heroic in History.* London; J. Chapman. Ist edn (1840)

Carnot, S. (1979). *Réflexions sur la puissance motrice du feu.* Ed. R. Fox. Paris; Vrin

Casini, P. (1969). Le Newtonianisme au siècle des lumières, *Dix-huitième Siècle*, Vol. 1, 139–159

Cavendish, H. (1879). *The Electrical Researches of Henry Cavendish.* Ed. J.C. Maxwell. Cambridge; Cambridge University Press

Cawood, J. (1979). The Magnetic Crusade: Science and Politics in Early Victorian Britain, *Isis*, Vol. 70, 493–518

Clark, G.N. (1937). *Science and Social Welfare in the Age of Newton.* Oxford; Clarendon Press

Clavelin, M. (1968). *La Philosophie naturelle de Galilée.* Paris; Armand Colin

Cohen, I.B. (1956). *Franklin and Newton.* Philadelphia; American Philosophical Society. 2nd edn (1966). Cambridge, Mass.; Harvard University Press

Cohen, I.B. (1981). *The Newtonian Revolution.* Cambridge; Cambridge University Press

Collins, H.M. (1975). The Seven Sexes: A Study in the Sociology of a Phenomenon, or the Replication of an Experiment in Physics, *Sociology*, Vol. 9, 205–224

Crosland, M.P. (1975). The Development of a Professional Career in Science in France, in *The Emergence of Science in Western Europe.* Ed. M.P. Crosland. London; Macmillan, 139–160

Crosland, M.P. and Smith, C. (1978). The Transmission of Physics from France to Britain, 1800–1840, *Historical Studies in the Physical Sciences*, Vol. 9, 1–61

Darnton, R. (1968). *Mesmerism and the End of the Enlightenment in France.* Cambridge, Mass.; Harvard University Press

Davies, C.H. (1963). *Theory of the Motion of the Heavenly Bodies.* New York: Dover. A translation of Gauss, *Theoria motum corporum coeaestium in sectionibus conicis solem ambientum.* Hamburg; Perthes and Besser

Davy, H. (1839–40). *Collected Works.* Ed. J. Davy. 9 Vols. London; Smith and Elder and Co.

Debus, A.G. (1968). Mathematics and Nature in the Chemical Texts of the Renaissance, *Ambix*, Vol. 15, 1–28

Debus, A.G. (1975). The Chemical Debates of the 17th Century: the Reaction to Robert Fludd and J.B. van Helmont, in *Reason, Experiment and Mysticism in the Scientific Revolution.* Ed. M. Righini Bonelli and W.R. Shea. New York; Science History Publications, 19–48

Delambre, J.B.J. (1821). *Histoire de l'astronomie moderne.* 2 Vols. Paris; Courcier

Dickson, D. (1979). Science and Political Hegemony in the 17th Century, *Radical Science Journal*, No. 8, 7–38

Dijksterhuis, E.J. (1961). *The Mechanization of the World Picture.* Trans. C. Dikshoorn. Oxford; Clarendon Press

Dobbs, B.J.T. (1975). *The Foundations of Newton's Alchemy: or 'the Hunting of the Greene Lyon'.* Cambridge; Cambridge University Press

Doran, B.G. (1975). Origins and Consolidation of Field Theory in Nineteenth Century Britain; from the Mechanical to the Electromagnetic View of Nature, *Historical Studies in the Physical Sciences*, Vol. 6, 133–260

Dorling, J. (1974). Henry Cavendish's Deduction of the Electrostatic Inverse Square Law from the Result of a Single Experiment, *Studies in the History and Philosophy of Science*, Vol. 4, 327–348

Drake, S. (1970). *Galileo Studies: Personality, Tradition, and Revolution.* Ann Arbor; University of Michigan Press

Drake, S. (1976). Galileo's First Telescopic Observations, *Journal for the History of Astronomy*, Vol. 7, 153–168

Drake, S. (1978). *Galileo at Work: His Scientific Biography.* Chicago: University of Chicago Press

Drake, S. and Drabkin, I.E., Ed. (1960). *Galileo on Motion, and on Mechanics.* Madison; University of Wisconsin Press

Drake, S. and Drabkin, I.E., Ed. (1969). *Mechanics in Sixteenth-Century Italy.* Madison; University of Wisconsin Press

Dugas, R. (1954a). *La Mécanique au 17e siècle.* Neuchâtel; Griffon

Dugas, R. (1954b). Sur le Cartesianisme de Huygens, *Revue d'Histoire des Sciences*, Vol. 7, 22–33

Duhem, P. (1905–6). *Les Origines de la statique.* 2 Vols. Paris; Hermann

Duhem, P. (1969). *To Save the Phenomena; an Essay on the Idea of Physical*

Theory from Plato to Galileo. Trans. E. Doland and C. Maschler. Chicago and London; University of Chicago Press. Ist French edn (1908)

Edge, D.O. and Mulkay, M.J. (1976). *Astronomy Transformed. The Emergence of Radio Astronomy in Britain*. New York and London; John Wiley

Elkana, Y. (1971). Newtonianism in the Eighteenth Century, *British Journal for the Philosophy of Science*, Vol. 22, 297–306

Elkana, Y. (1974). *The Discovery of the Conservation of Energy*. London; Hutchinson. Cambridge, Mass.; Harvard University Press

Emerson, R. (1973). The Enlightenment and Social Structures, in *City and Society in the Eighteenth Century*. Ed. P.S. Fritz and D. Williams. Toronto; Hakkert, 99–124

Farrar, W.V. (1975). Science and the German University System 1790–1850, in *The Emergence of Science in Western Europe*. Ed. M.P. Crosland. London; Macmillan, 179–192

Farrington, B. (1951). *Francis Bacon, Philosopher of Industrial Science*. London; Lawrence and Wishart. Ist edn (1949)

Feuer, L.S. (1971). The Social Roots of Einstein's Theory of Relativity, *Annals of Science*, Vol. 27, 277–298 and 313–344

Finn, B.S. (1971). Influence of Experimental Apparatus on 18th Century Electrical Theory, *Proceedings of the International Congress of the History of Science: Paris, 1968*. Vol. 10A, 51–55

Fischer, J.K. (1801–8). *Geschichte der Physick*. 8 Vols. Göttingen; J.F. Röwer

Forbes, E.G. (1975). *Greenwich Observatory: Origins and Early History (1675–1835)*. London; Taylor and Francis

Forman, P. (1969). Reception of an acausal quantum mechanics in Germany and Britain, Ed. S.H. Manskopf in *The Reception of Unconventional Science*. Colorado; Westview Press, 11–50

Forman, P. (1971). Weimar Culture, Causality and Quantum Theory, 1918–1927: Adaptation by German Physicists and Mathematicians to a Hostile Intellectual Environment, *Historical Studies in the Physical Sciences*, Vol. 3, 1–115

Forman, P., Heilbron, J.L. and Weart, S.R. (1975). Physics circa 1900, *Historical Studies in the Physical Sciences*, Vol. 5, 1–185

Fox, R. (1971). *The Caloric Theory of Gases: from Lavoisier to Regnault*. Oxford; Clarendon Press

Fox, R. (1974). The Rise and Fall of Laplacian Physics, *Historical Studies in the Physical Sciences*, Vol. 4, 89–136

Fox, R. and Weisz, G. (1980). *The Organization of Science and Technology in France, 1808–1914*. Cambridge; Cambridge University Press

Frankel, E. (1976). Corpuscular Optics and the Wave Theory of Light: the Science and Politics of a Revolution in Physics, *Social Studies of Science*, Vol. 6, 141–184

Frankel, E. (1977). J.B. Biot and the Mathematization of Experimental Physics in Napoleonic France, *Historical Studies in the Physical Sciences*, Vol. 8, 33–72

French, A.P., Ed. (1979). *Einstein: a Centenary Volume*. Cambridge, Mass.; Harvard University Press. London; Heinemann

Galileo Galilei (1638). *Dialogues Concerning Two New Sciences*. Trans. H. Crew and A. de Salvio (1954). New York; Dover Publications

Gaukroger, S., Ed. (1980). *Descartes: Philosophy, Mathematics and Physics*. Brighton; Harvester Press

Gelbart, N.R. (1971). The Intellectual Development of Walter Charleton, *Ambix*, Vol. 18, 149–168

Geymonat, L. (1957). *Galileo Galilei*. Milan; Einaudi

Gibbs, F.W. (1961). Itinerant Lecturers in Natural Philosophy, *Ambix*, Vol.8, 111–117

Gillmor, C.S. (1971). *Coulomb and the Evolution of Physics and Engineering in Eighteenth Century France*. Princeton; Princeton University Press

Gingerich, O. (1972). Johannes Kepler and the New Astronomy, *Quarterly Journal of the Royal Astronomical Society*, Vol. 13, 346–373

Ginzburg, C. (1980). *The Cheese and the Worms: the Cosmos of a Sixteenth Century Miller*. Trans. J. and A. Tedeschi. London; Routledge and Kegan Paul. Baltimore; Johns Hopkins University Press. Originally published (1976) as *Il Formaggio e i vermi*. Turin; Giulio Einaudi

Gliozzi, M. (1966). Il Volta della seconda maniera, *Cultura e Scuola*, Vol. 5, 235–239

Gordon, G. (1719). *Remarcks upon the Newtonian Philosophy*, 2nd edn. London; J. Peele

Gower, B. (1973). Speculation in Physics; the History and Practice of *Naturphilosophie*, *Studies in History and Philosophy of Science*, Vol. 3, 301–356

Grant, R. (1852). *History of Physical Astronomy*. London; Bohn

Guerlac, H. (1965). Where the Statue Stood: Divergent Loyalties to Newton in the 18th Century, *Aspects of the Eighteenth Century*. Ed. E.R. Wasserman. Baltimore; Johns Hopkins Press, 317–334

Guerlac, H. (1976). Chemistry as a Branch of Physics: Laplace's Collaboration with Lavoisier, *Historical Studies in the Physical Sciences*, Vol. 7, 193–276

Guralnik, S.M. (1979). The Contexts of Faraday's Electrochemical Laws, *Isis*, Vol. 70, 59–75

Hackmann, W.D. (1975). The Growth of Science in the Netherlands in the Seventeenth and Early Eighteenth Centuries, in *The Emergence of Science in Western Europe*. Ed. M. Crosland. London; Macmillan, 89–110

Hackmann, W.D. (1978). *Electricity from Glass: the History of the Frictional Electrical Machine 1600–1850*. Alphen-aan-den-Rijn; Sijthoff and Noordhoff

Hahn, R. (1971). *The Anatomy of a Scientific Institution: the Paris Academy of Sciences 1666–1803*. Berkeley; University of California Press

Hahn, R. (1975). Scientific Careers in Eighteenth Century France, in *The Emergence of Science in Western Europe*. Ed. M.P. Crosland. London; Macmillan, 127–138

Hall, A.R. (1952). *Ballistics in the Seventeenth Century*. Cambridge; Cambridge University Press

Hall, A.R. (1963). Merton Revisited: or, Science and Society in the Seventeenth Century, *History of Science*, Vol. 2, 1–16

Hall, A.R. (1966). Mechanics and the Royal Society 1668–70, *The British Journal for the History of Science*, Vol. 3, 24–38

Hall, A.R. and Hall, M.B. (1962). *Unpublished Scientific Papers of Isaac Newton*. Cambridge; Cambridge University Press

Hamamdjian, P.G. (1971). Genèse des idées d'Ampère en Electromagnétisme, *Proceedings of the 12th International Congress of the History of Science*, Vol. 5, 29–34

Hankins, T.L. (1965). Eighteenth-Century Attempts to Resolve the Vis Viva Controversy, *Isis*, Vol. 56, 281–297

Hankins, T.L. (1970). *Jean d'Alembert: Science and the Enlightenment*. Oxford; Clarendon Press

Heilbron, J.L. (1974). *H.G.J. Moseley: the Life and Letters of an English Physicist 1887–1915*. Berkeley; University of California Press

Heilbron, J.L. (1979). *Electricity in the Seventeenth and Eighteenth Centuries*. Berkeley; University of California Press

Heimann, P.M. (1970). Maxwell and the Modes of Consistent Representation, *Archive for History of Exact Sciences*, Vol. 6, 171–213

Heimann, P.M. (1971). Faraday's Theories of Matter and Electricity, *The British Journal for the History of Science*, Vol. 5, 235–257

Heimann, P.M. (1972). The Unseen Universe: Physics and the Philosophy of Nature in Victorian Britain, *The British Journal for the History of Science*, Vol. 6, 73–79

Heimann, P.M. (1974a). Helmholtz and Kant: the Metaphysical Foundations of *Über die Erhaltung der Kraft*, *Studies in History and Philosophy of Science*, Vol. 5, 205–238

Heimann, P.M. (1974b). Conversion of Forces and the Conservation of Energy, *Centaurus*, Vol. 18, 147–161

Heimann, P.M. and McGuire, J.E. (1971). Newtonian Forces and Lockean Powers: Concepts of Matter in Eighteenth Century Thought, *Historical Studies in the Physical Sciences*, Vol. 3, 233–306

Helden, A. van (1970). Eustachio Divini versus Christiaan Huygens: a Reappraisal, *Physis*, Vol. 12, 36–50

Helden, A. van (1974a). 'Annulo Cingitur': the Solution of the Problem of Saturn, *Journal for the History of Astronomy*, Vol. 5, 155–174

Helden, A. van (1974b) The Telescope in the 17th Century, *Isis*, Vol. 65, 38–58

Heller, A. (1882–4). *Geschichte der Physik*. 2 Vols. Stuttgart; F. Enke

Helmholtz, H. von (1971). *Selected Writings*. Ed. R. Kahl. Middletown, Conn.; Wesleyan University Press

Hendry, J. (1980). Weimar Culture and Quantum Causality, *History of Science*, Vol. 18, 155–180

Herivel, J. (1975). *Joseph Fourier: The Man and The Physicist*. Oxford: Clarendon Press

Hermann, A. (1977). *Die Jahrhundertwissenschaft: Werner Heisenberg und die Physik seiner Zeit*. Stuttgart; Deutsche Verlags-Anstalt

Hesse, M.B. (1961). *Forces and Fields: the Concept of Action at a Distance in the History of Physics*. London; Nelson

Hessen, B. (1931). The Social and Economic Roots of Newton's *Principia*, *Science at the Cross Roads*. 2nd edn (1971). Ed. P.G. Werskey. London; Frank Cass, 149–212

Hetherington, N.S. (1975). The Simultaneous 'Discovery' of Internal Motions in Spiral Nebulae, *Journal for the History of Astronomy*, Vol. 6, 115–125

Hiebert, E.N. (1962). *Historical Roots of the Principle of the Conservation of Energy*. Madison; University of Wisconsin Press

Hill, J.E.C. (1965). *Intellectual Origins of the English Revolution*. Oxford; Clarendon Press

Holton, G. (1973). Kepler's Universe: its Physics and Metaphysics, in *Thematic Origins of Scientific Thought*. Cambridge, Mass.; Harvard University Press, 69–91

Home, R.W. (1973). Science as a Career in Eighteenth Century Russia: the Case of Aepinus, *Slavonic and Eastern European Review*, Vol. 51, 75–94

Home, R.W. (1977). 'Newtonianism' and the Theory of the Magnet, *History of Science*, Vol. 15, 252–266

Home, R.W., Ed. (1979). *F.U.T. Aepinus, 'Essay on the Theory of Electricity and Magnetism'*. Princeton, NJ; Princeton University Press

Hooke, R. (1665). *Micrographia*. London; Jo. Martyn and Ja. Allestry, Printers to the Royal Society. Reprinted (1961). New York; Dover Publications

Hoppen, K.T. (1970). *The Common Scientist in the Seventeenth Century: a Study of the Dublin Philosophical Society 1683–1708*. London; Routledge and Kegan Paul

Iltis, C. (1971). Leibniz and the Vis Viva Controversy, *Isis*, Vol. 62, 21–35

Iltis, C. (1973). The Leibnizian–Newtonian Debates: Natural Philosophy and Social Psychology, *The British Journal for the History of Science*, Vol. 6, 343–377

Jacob, J.R. (1977). *Robert Boyle and the English Revolution.* New York; Burt Franklin

Jacob, J.R. and Jacob, M.C. (1971). Scientists and Society: the Saints Preserved, *Journal of European Studies*, Vol. 1, 87–90

Jacob, M.C. (1976). *The Newtonians and the English Revolution 1689–1720.* Hassocks; Harvester Press. Ithaca, NY; Cornell University Press

Jardine, L. (1974). *Francis Bacon; Discovery and the Art of Discourse.* Cambridge; Cambridge University Press

Jeffreys, A.E. (1960). *Michael Faraday. A List of His Lectures and Published Writings.* London; Royal Institution

Kangro, H. (1970). *Vorgeschichte des Planckschen Strahlungsgesetzes.* Wiesbaden; F. Steiner

Kargon, R.H. (1966). *Atomism in England, from Hariot to Newton.* Oxford; Oxford University Press

Kargon, R.H. (1969). Model and Analogy in Victorian Science: Maxwell's Critique of the French Physicists, *Journal of the History of Ideas*, Vol. 30, 423–436

Kargon, R.H. (1977). *Science in Victorian Manchester: Enterprise and Expertise.* Manchester; Manchester University Press

Keller, A.G. (1975). Mathematicians, Mechanics, and Experimental Machines in Northern Italy in the Sixteenth Century, in *The Emergence of Science in Western Europe.* Ed. M.P. Crosland. London; Macmillan, 15–34

Kevles, D.J. (1978). *The Physicists: The History of a Scientific Community in Modern America.* New York; Knopf

King, H.C. (1965). *History of the Telescope.* London; Griffin

Knight, D.M. (1967). *Atoms and Elements. A Study of Theories of Matter in the 19th Century.* London; Hutchinson

Knight, D.M. (1975). German Science in the Romantic Period, in *The Emergence of Science in Western Europe.* Ed. M.P. Crosland. London; Macmillan, 161–178

Koyanagi, K. (1978). Pascal et l'expérience du vide dans le vide, *Japanese Studies in the History of Science*, Vol. 17, 105–127

Koyré, A. (1939). *Études Galiléennes.* 3 Vols. Paris; Hermann

Koyré, A. (1943). Galileo and Plato, *Journal of the History of Ideas*, Vol. 4, 400–428

Koyré, A. (1957). *From the Closed World to the Infinite Universe.* Baltimore; Johns Hopkins University Press

Koyré, A. (1973). *The Astronomical Revolution.* London; Methuen. 1st French edn (1961)

Krafft, F. (1973). Johannes Keplers Beitrag zur Himmelsphysik, in *Internationales Kepler-Symposium, Weil-der-Stadt.* Ed. F. Krafft, K. Meyer, B. Sticker. Hildesheim; Gerstenberg, 55–139

Kubrin, D. (1967). Newton and the Cyclical Cosmos: Providence and the Mechanical Philosophy, *Journal of the History of Ideas*, Vol. 28, 325–346

Kuhn, T.S. (1959). Energy Conservation as an Example of Simultaneous Discovery, in *Critical Problems in the History of Science.* Ed. M. Clagett. Madison; University of Wisconsin Press, 321–356

Kuhn, T.S. (1970). *The Structure of Scientific Revolutions*, 2nd edn. Chicago and London; University of Chicago Press. 1st edn (1962)

Kuhn, T.S. (1978). *Black Body Theory and the Quantum Discontinuity, 1894–1912.* Oxford; Oxford University Press

Kuhn, T.S., Heilbron, J.L. and Forman, P., Ed. (1967). *Sources for the History of Quantum Physics.* Philadelphia; American Philosophical Society

Laudan, L.L. (1968). The Vis Viva Controversy, a Post-Mortem, *Isis*, Vol. 59, 131–143

Lenoble, R. (1943). *Mersenne ou la naissance du mécanisme.* Paris; Vrin

Levere, T.H. (1971). *Affinity and Matter: Elements of Chemical Philosophy 1800–1865.* Oxford; Oxford University Press

Lohne, J.A. and Sticker, B. (1969). *Newtons Theorie des Prismenfarben*. Munich; Werner Fritsch

Lovell, D.J. (1968). Herschel's Dilemma in the Interpretation of Thermal Radiation, *Isis*, Vol. 59, 46–60

McCormmach, R. (1968). John Michell and Henry Cavendish: Weighing the Stars, *The British Journal for the History of Science*, Vol. 4, 126–155

McCormmach, R. (1969). Henry Cavendish: A Study of Rational Empiricism in 18th Century Natural Philosophy, *Isis*, Vol. 60, 293–306

McEvoy, J.G. (1979). Electricity, Knowledge, and the Nature of Progress in Priestley's Thought, *British Journal for the History of Science*, Vol. 12, 1–30

McEvoy, J.G. and McGuire, J.E. (1975). God and Nature: Priestley's Way of Rational Dissent, *Historical Studies in the Physical Sciences*, Vol. 6, 325–404

McGucken, W. (1969). *Nineteenth Century Spectroscopy*. Baltimore and London; Johns Hopkins University Press

Maclean, J. (1972). Science and Theology at Groningen University, 1698–1702, *Annals of Science*, Vol. 29, 187–201

Mahoney, M.S. (1973). *The Mathematical Career of Pierre de Fermat*. Princeton, NJ; Princeton University Press

Malley, M. (1979). The Discovery of Atomic Transmutation: Scientific Styles and Philosophies in France and Britain, *Isis*, Vol. 70, 213–223

Mandrou, R. (1973). *Des humanistes aux hommes de science (XVIe et XVIIe siècles)*. Paris; Editions du Seuil

Manuel, F. (1968). *A Portrait of Isaac Newton*. Cambridge, Mass.; Harvard University Press. Reprinted (1980). London; Frederick Mulder

Mayer, J.R. (1842). Bemerkung über die Kräfte der unbelebten Natur. *Annalen der Chemie*, Vol. 42, 233–244

Mendelsohn, E. (1964). The Emergence of Science as a Profession in Nineteenth Century Europe, in *The Management of Scientists*. Ed. K. Hill. Boston; Beacon Press, 3–48

Mendelssohn, K. (1973). *The World of Walther Nernst: the Rise and Fall of German Science 1864–1941*. London; Macmillan. Pittsburg; University of Pittsburg Press

Meyer-Abich, K.M. (1965). *Korrespondenz, Individualität, und Komplementarität*. Wiesbaden; F. Steiner

Merleau-Ponty, J. (1976). Situation et rôle de l'hypothèse cosmogonique dans la pensée cosmologique de Laplace, *Revue d'Histoire des Sciences*, Vol. 29, 21–49

Merton, R.K. (1970). *Science, Technology and Society in Seventeenth Century England*, 2nd edn. New York; Harper and Row

Middleton, W.E.K. (1964). *The History of the Barometer*. Baltimore; Johns Hopkins University Press

Middleton, W.E.K. (1966). *History of the Thermometer and its Uses in Meteorology*. Baltimore; Johns Hopkins University Press

Middleton, W.E.K. (1971). *The Experimenters: a Study of the Accademia del Cimento*. Baltimore; Johns Hopkins University Press

Millburn, J.R. (1976). *Benjamin Martin: Author, Instrument-Maker and 'Country Showman'*. Leyden; Noordhoff International Publishing

Morrell, J.B. (1972). The Chemist Breeders: the Research Schools of Liebig and Thomas Thomson, *Ambix*, Vol. 19, 1–46

Mottelay, P.F., Ed. (1922). *Bibliographical History of Electricity and Magnetism. Chronologically Arranged*. London; C. Griffin

Mouy, P. (1934). *Le Développement de la physique Cartesienne 1646–1712*. Paris; Vrin

Newton, Isaac (1730). *Opticks*, 4th edn. London; William Innys. Reprinted (1952). New York; Dover Books

Numbers, R.L. (1977). *Creation by Natural Law: Laplace's Nebular Hypothesis in American Thought.* Seattle; University of Washington

Olson, R. (1975). *Scottish Philosophy and British Physics 1750–1880.* Princeton, NJ; Princeton University

Pacchi, A. (1973). *Cartesio in Inghilterra. Da More a Boyle.* Bari; Laterza

Pascal, Blaise (1937). *The Physical Treatises of Pascal.* Trans. I.H. Bard and G.H. Spiers. New York; Columbia University Press

Pecheux, M. and Fichant, M. (1974). *Sur l'histoire des sciences. Cours de philosophie pour scientifiques.* Paris; Maspéro. 1st edn (1970)

Pinch, T.J. (1977). What Does a Proof Do if it Does not Prove?, in *The Social Production of Scientific Knowledge.* Ed. E. Mendelsohn, P. Weingart, R. Whitley. Dordrecht; D. Reidel

Popkin, R.H. (1964). *The History of Scepticism from Erasmus to Descartes.* New York; Humanities Press. 1st edn (1960)

Priestley, J. (1767). *The History and Present State of Electricity.* London; J. Dodsley

Pyenson, L. and Skopp, D. (1977). Educating Physicists in Germany circa 1900, *Social Studies of Science,* Vol. 7, 329–366

Rabb, T.K. (1975). *The Struggle for Stability in Early Modern Europe.* New York; Oxford University Press

Reif, P. (1969). The Textbook Tradition in Natural Philosophy, 1600–1650, *Journal of the History of Ideas,* Vol. 30, 17–32

Rogers, G.A.J. (1972). Descartes and the Method of English Science, *Annals of Science,* Vol. 29, 237–255

Roller, D.H.D.B. (1959). *The De Magnete of William Gilbert.* Amsterdam; Hertzberger

Ronchi, V. (1970). *The Nature of Light: an Historical Survey.* Cambridge, Mass.; Harvard University Press

Rosenberger, F. (1882–90). *Die Geschichte der Physik.* 3 Vols. Brunswick; F. Vieweg

Rossi, P. (1975). Hermeticism, Rationality and the Scientific Revolution, in *Reason, Experiment and Mysticism in the Scientific Revolution.* Ed. M. Righini Bonelli and W. Shea. New York; Science History Publications, 247–273

Rowbottom, M.E. (1968). The Teaching of Experimental Philosophy in England, 1700–1730, *Proceedings of the International Congress of the History of Science 1965,* Vol. 4, 46–53

Ruestow, E.G. (1973). *Physics at Seventeenth and Eighteenth Century Leiden.* The Hague; Martinus Nijhoff

Russell, J.L. (1964). Kepler's Laws of Planetary Motion, 1609–66, *The British Journal for the History of Science,* Vol. 2, 1–24

Sabra, A.I. (1967). *Theories of Light: from Descartes to Newton.* London; Oldbourne

Schaffer, S. (1980a). The Great Laboratories of the Universe: William Herschel on Matter Theory and Planetary Life, *Journal for the History of Astronomy,* Vol. 11, 81–110

Schaffer, S. (1980b). Natural Philosophy, in *The Ferment of Knowledge: Studies in the Historiography of Eighteenth Century Science.* Ed. G.S. Rousseau and R.S. Porter. Cambridge; Cambridge University Press, 55–91

Schmitt, C.B. (1975). Science in Italian Universities in the 16th and the Early 17th Centuries, in *The Emergence of Science in Western Europe.* Ed. M.P. Crosland. London; Macmillan, 35–56

Schofield, R.E. (1963). *The Lunar Society of Birmingham. A Social History of Provincial Science and Industry in Eighteenth Century England.* Oxford; Clarendon Press

Schofield, R.E. (1967). Joseph Priestley, Natural Philosopher, *Ambix*, Vol. 14, 1–15

Schofield, R.E. (1970). *Mechanism and Materialism: British Natural Philosophy in an Age of Reason*. Princeton; Princeton University Press

Scott, W.R. (1937). *Adam Smith as Student and Professor*. Glasgow; Jackson, Son and Company

Settle, T.B. (1961). An Experiment in the History of Science, *Science*, Vol. 133, 19–23

Settle, T.B. (1967). Galileo's Use of Experiment as a Tool of Investigation, in *Galileo Man of Science*. Ed. E. McMullin. New York; Basic Books, 315–337

Shapin, S. (1980). Social Uses of Science, in *The Ferment of Knowledge: Studies in the Historiography of Eighteenth-Century Science*. Ed. G.S. Rousseau and R.S. Porter. Cambridge; Cambridge University Press, 93–139

Shapin, S. and Barnes, B. (1977). Science, Nature and Control: Interpreting Mechanics' Institutes, *Social Studies of Science*, Vol. 7, 31–74

Shapiro, A.E. (1973). Kinematic Optics: A Study of the Wave Theory of Light in the Seventeenth Century, *Archive for History of Exact Sciences*, Vol. 11, 134–266

Sharlin, H.L. (1966). *The Convergent Century: the Unification of Science in Nineteenth Century*. London and New York; Abelard-Schuman

Shea, W.R. (1972). *Galileo's Intellectual Revolution: Middle Period 1610–1632*. London; Macmillan. New York; Science History Publications

Shinn, T. (1979). The French Science Faculty System 1808–1914: Institutional Change and Research Potential in Mathematics and Physical Science, *Historical Studies in the Physical Sciences*, Vol. 10, 271–332

Sklair, L. (1973). *Organised Knowledge: a Sociological View of Science and Technology*. St Albans; Paladin

Smith, C. (1976). 'Mechanical Philosophy' and the Emergence of Physics in Britain: 1800–1850, *Annals of Science*, Vol. 33, 3–29

Smith, C. (1978). A New Chart for British Natural Philosophy: the Development of Energy Physics in the Nineteenth Century, *History of Science*, Vol. 16, 231–279

Snelders, H.A.M. (1970). Romanticism, *Naturphilosophie*, and the Inorganic Natural Sciences 1797–1840, *Studies in Romanticism*, Vol. 9, 193–215

Sohn-Rethel, A. (1978). *Intellectual and Manual Labour: a Critique of Epistemology*. London; Macmillan. Ist edn (1970)

Steffens, H.J. (1979). *James Prescott Joule and the Concept of Energy*. Folkstone; Dawson. New York; Science History Publications

Stone, L. (1965). *The Crisis of the Aristocracy. 1558–1641*. Oxford; Clarendon Press

Strong, E.W. (1936). *Procedures and Metaphysics: a Study in the Philosophy of the Mathematical–Physical Sciences in the Sixteenth and Seventeenth Centuries*. Berkeley; University of California Press

Struve, O. (1959). The First Stellar Parallax Determination, in *Men and Moments in the History of Science*. Ed. H.M. Evans. Seattle; Washington University Press, 177–206

Stuewer, R.H. (1975). *The Compton Effect: Turning Point in Physics*. New York; Science History Publications

Sviedrys, R. (1970). The Rise of Physical Science at Victorian Cambridge, *Historical Studies in the Physical Sciences*, Vol. 2, 127–151

Swenson, L.S. (1972). *The Ethereal Aether: a History of the Michelson–Morley–Miller Aether-Drift Experiments 1880–1930*. Austin; University of Texas Press

Taylor, E.G.R. (1954). *Mathematical Practitioners of Tudor and Stuart England*. Cambridge; Cambridge University Press for the Institute of Navigation

Thoren, V.E. (1974). Kepler's Second Law in England, *The British Journal for the History of Science*, Vol. 7, 243–256

Todhunter, I. (1873). *History of the Mathematical Theories of Attraction and the Figure of the Earth.* 2 Vols. London; Macmillan

Truesdell, C.A. (1954). Rational Fluid Mechanics 1687–1765. *L. Euleri Opera Omnia* (2) Vol. 12. Zürich; Füssli, ix–cxxv

Truesdell, C.A. (1960). Rational Mechanics of Flexible or Elastic Bodies, 1638–1788, *L. Euleri Opera Omnia* (2) Vol. 11, Part 2. Zürich; Füssli

Truesdell, C.A. (1968). *Essays in the History of Mechanics.* Berlin; Springer Verlag

Turnbull, H., Scott, J., Hall, A.R. and Tilling, L., Ed. (1959–77). *Correspondence of Isaac Newton.* 7 Vols. Cambridge; Cambridge University Press

Turner, R.S. (1971). The Growth of Professorial Research in Prussia 1818–1848: Causes and Contexts, *Historical Studies in the Physical Sciences*, Vol. 3, 137–182

Urban, P. and Sutter, B. (1975). *Johannes Kepler 1571–1971: Gedenkschrift der Universität Graz.* Graz; Leykam Verlag

Waerden, B.L. van der (1967). *Sources of Quantum Mechanics.* Amsterdam; North-Holland Publishing Company

Waff, C.B. (1975). Universal Gravitation and the Motion of the Moon's Apogee: the Establishment and Reception of Newton's Inverse Square Law 1687–1749, Johns Hopkins PhD Dissertation

Wallis, P.J. and Wallis, R. (1977). *Newton and Newtoniana 1672–1975. A Bibliography.* Folkestone; Dawson and Project for Historical Biobibliography

Watson, E.C. (1947). Joule's Only General Exposition of the Principle of Conservation of Energy, *American Journal of Physics*, Vol. 15, 383

Webster, C. (1967a). Henry Power's Experimental Philosophy, *Ambix*, Vol. 14, 150–178

Webster, C. (1967b). Origins of the Royal Society, *History of Science*, Vol. 6, 106–128

Webster, C. (1975). *The Great Instauration: Science, Medicine and Reform, 1626–1660.* London; Duckworth

Weiner, C., Ed. (1977). *History of Twentieth Century Physics.* New York; Academic Press

Westfall, R.S. (1971). *Force in Newton's Physics: the Science of Dynamics in the Seventeenth Century.* London; Macdonald. New York; American Elsevier

Westfall, R.S. (1977). *The Construction of Modern Science. Mechanisms and Mechanics.* London and New York; Cambridge University Press

Westfall, R.S. (1980). *Never at Rest: a Biography of Isaac Newton.* Cambridge; Cambridge University Press

Westman, R.S. (1975). The Wittenberg Interpretation of the Copernican Theory, in *The Nature of Scientific Discovery.* Ed. O. Gingerich. Washington; Smithsonian Institution Press, 393–423

Westman, R.S. (1977). Magical Reform and Astronomical Reform: the Yates Thesis Reconsidered, in *Hermeticism and the Scientific Revolution.* Los Angeles; University of California at Los Angeles

Westman, R.S. (1980a). The Astronomer's Role in the Sixteenth Century: a Preliminary Study, *History of Science*, Vol. 18, 105–147

Westman, R.S. (1980b). Huygens and the Problem of Cartesianism, in *Studies on Christiaan Huygens.* Ed. H. Bos, M. Rudwick, H. Snelders and R. Visser. Liss; Swets and Zeitlinger, 83–103

Whiteside, D.T. (1964). Newton's Early Thoughts on Planetary Motion: a Fresh Look, *The British Journal for the History of Science*, Vol. 2, 117–137

Whiteside, D.T. (1967–). *The Mathematical Papers of Isaac Newton.* 8 Vols published so far. Cambridge; Cambridge University Press

Whiteside, D.T. (1970). Before the *Principia*: the Maturing of Newton's Thoughts on Dynamical Astronomy 1664–1684, *Journal for the History of Astronomy*, Vol. 1, 5–19

Whiteside, D.T. (1975). Newton's Lunar Theory: from High Hope to Disenchantment, *Vistas in Astronomy*, Vol. 19, 317–328

Whittaker, E.T. (1951). *History of the Theories of Aether and Electricity*. 2 Vols. London and New York; T. Nelson

Williams, L.P. (1965). *Michael Faraday: a Biography*. New York; Simon and Schuster. London; Chapman and Hall

Williams, L.P. (1966). *The Origins of Field Theory*. New York; Random House

Williams, R. (1981). *Culture*. Glasgow; Fontana

Wilson, C.A. (1970). From Kepler's Laws, So-Called, to Universal Gravitation: Empirical Factors, *Archive for History of Exact Sciences*, Vol. 6, 89–170

Wilson, C.A. (1980). Perturbations and Solar Tables from Lacaille to Delambre: the Rapprochement of Observation and Theory, *Archive for History of Exact Sciences*, Vol. 22, 53–304

Wilson, D.B. (1974). Kelvin's Scientific Realism: the Theological Context, *Philosophical Journal*, Vol. 11, 41–55

Wood, A. and Oldham, F. (1954). *Thomas Young, Natural Philosopher 1773–1829*. Cambridge; Cambridge University Press

Woolf, H. (1959). *The Transits of Venus. A Study of Eighteenth Century Science*. Princeton, NJ; Princeton University Press

Woolf, H., Ed. (1980). *Some Strangeness in the Proportion: Studies in Honor of Albert Einstein*. Reading, Mass.; Addison Wesley

Worrall, J. (1976). Thomas Young and the 'Refutation' of Newtonian Optics: a Case-Study in the Interaction of Philosophy of Science and History of Science, in *Method and Appraisal in the Physical Sciences. The Critical Background to Modern Science, 1800–1905*. Ed. C. Howson. Cambridge; Cambridge University Press, 107–179

Wynne, B. (1979). Physics and Psychics: Science, Symbolic Action and Social Control in Late Victorian England, in *Natural Order*. Ed. B. Barnes and S. Shapin. London; Sage, 167–186

Yates, F. (1964). *Giordano Bruno and the Hermetic Tradition*. London; Routledge and Kegan Paul

Zilsel, E. (1942). The Sociological Roots of Science, *American Journal of Sociology*, Vol. 47, 544–562

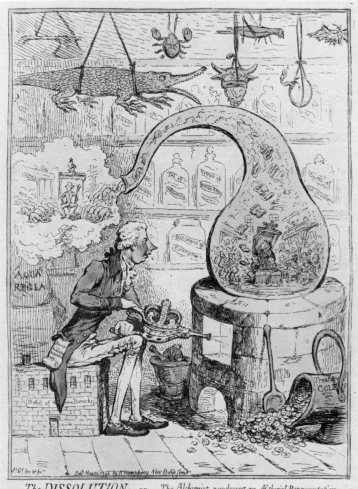

The DISSOLUTION,—or—The Alchymist producing an Æthurial Representation.

Plate 6. Government expenditure depicted as alchemy; an etching by James Gillray, 1796. By courtesy of the Wellcome Trustees

16

History of chemistry

W.H. Brock

Chemistry has had 'a persistent historical tradition' (Debus 1971: 169) ever since the sixteenth century (Debus 1962). Well into the twentieth century it was considered obligatory for chemistry courses to be prefaced by a historical review, the historiographical tones of which have been critically analysed by Weyer (1974). As with the history of medicine, a 'science history' literature is to be found together with a literature published by professional historians. The former finds respectable expression in the Historical Division of the American Chemical Society, the Historical Group of the Royal Chemical Society, in articles written by and for chemists published in *Chemistry*, *Chemistry in Britain*, *Journal of Chemical Education* (Ihde and Kieffer 1975) and other secondary chemistry journals. A symposium on the teaching of the history of chemistry edited by G.B. Kauffman (1971) provides ample justification for the continuation of the tradition. Research by professional historians of chemistry, on the other hand, is to be found in the defunct annual *Chymia* (1948–67), the journal *Ambix* (1937–), which is published by the Society for the History of Alchemy and Chemistry (f. 1936) (1937–75 known as Society for the Study of Alchemy and Early Chemistry), and in general journals of the history of science.

In recent years, in common with other areas of the history of science, historians of chemistry have become much more interested in the social history of chemistry – the development of chemical education, laboratories, institutions, societies and journals, the process of discipline formation and professionalization.

However, apart from entries in a conceptually arranged dictionary (Bynum *et al.* 1981), tantalizing miniatures by Caldin (1959–60, 1961) and Theobald (1976), some positivistic and Lakatosian musings on the phlogiston theory by Musgrave (1976), on Avogadro's hypothesis by Frické (1976), on nineteenth-century organic chemistry by Potter (1953) and Gay (1976), and the superlative pre-war insights of the French historian and philosopher, Hélène Metzger (1918, 1923, 1930a,b, 1935, 1938), the philosophical side of chemistry has been comparatively neglected by historians and philosophers of science. Much influenced by the arguments of Emile Meyerson (1908) that the fundamental concepts of science are those of identity and causality, Metzger's *La Chimie* (1930b) still remains one of the clearest introductions to pre-eighteenth-century chemistry, though she should now be read in conjunction with the remarkable comparative insights opened up by Needham's studies of Chinese science and civilization (Needham 1974, 1976, 1980).

For their comprehensiveness, insights and bibliographical completeness, the synthetic encyclopaedic works of Kopp (1843–7, 1873, 1886), Berthelot (1885, 1887–8, 1889, 1890, 1893, 1906), Partington (1961, 1962, 1964, 1970) and Ihde (1964) are the recommended starting points for any serious investigation. The third and fourth volumes of Kopp's *Geschichte* (1843–7), for example, are still worth consulting for treatments of the history of individual chemical substances – an interesting method of writing history that, apart from the history of elements by Weeks (1968), of alum by Singer (1948), of common salt by Multhauf (1978) and of *aqua ardens* (or alcohol) by Gwei-Djen *et al.* (1972) and Needham (1980), has remained under-cultivated. Ihde (1964) provides a particularly strong bibliography for nineteenth- and twentieth-century topics and should be consulted in conjunction with this chapter, which will, for convenience, adopt a division of the subject by period.

Early chemistry

As the science that deals with the properties and reactions of matter, chemistry may be said to have originated in the integration of the interests of various groups and practitioners, namely artisans and technologists, natural philosophers, alchemists and iatrochemists. The integration of these groups is the subject of two exemplary studies by Multhauf (1966, 1978). The origins and development of applied chemistry were surveyed comprehensively by Partington (1935, 1960) from literary sources. Archaeological insights opened up by Berthelot (1906) have been continued by Forbes (1955), Tylecote (1965, 1976) and Halleux (1974). Note also the economic perspective on early technology suggested by Singer (1948) and Multhauf (1978). Because of its importance, much attention has been paid to the surviving archaeological and manuscript evidence for distillation (Forbes 1948; Taylor 1930, 1937, 1945, 1951; Gwei-Djen *et al.* 1972). Butler and Needham (1980), Needham (1980), as well as Mahdihassan (1979), have produced convincing evidence that distillation was a familiar skill amongst early Chinese and Indian technologists. An excellent key to the complicated obsolete terminology of early chemical laboratory procedures has been provided by Eklund (1975). (For further consideration of India, see chapter 22 and for China see chapter 23.)

Although the Greeks knew of no subject called chemistry, the matter theories of both the atomists and the Aristotelians were to play major roles in providing a theoretical structure for later chemistry. Multhauf (1966) again provides a good overview, while more specialized studies are available by Sambursky (1956), Dijksterhuis (1961) and Bolzan (1976). Partington's treatment (1970), which was published posthumously, is unfortunately exceedingly literary and unhelpful, but its place is handsomely filled by the fifth 'volume' of Needham's ambitious investigation of science and civilization in China. This volume is appearing in six parts. Part 1, of which only portions have appeared as a Newcomen Society monograph (Needham 1958), concerns iron and steel manufacture, pyrotechnics, textiles, mining, salt-production and ceramics; Part 2 (Needham 1974) deals with alchemy and includes an eighty-three-page bibliography of books and articles in Western languages; Part 3 (Needham 1976) is a general survey of Chinese chemistry from antiquity to the twentieth century; and Part 4 (Needham 1980) deals particularly with chemical apparatus. A final Part 5 on physiological alchemy will complete the 'volume'. Because of its readability, bibliographical strength and extensive digressions into, and discussions of, Western chemistry, Needham and his collaborators have provided by far the most interesting, comprehensive and exciting account of pre-seventeenth-century chemistry available.

The literature on alchemy is very large indeed, and is best approached through Needham (1974) or Coudert (1980), and two excellent analytical bibliographies by Halleux (1979) and Pritchard (1980). Halleux provides 'an inventory of problems' connected with alchemy and 'a balance sheet of scholarship'; Pritchard gives more than 3400 references to English-language writings on alchemy, including theses, published between 1597 and 1978. Sheppard (1970) has examined the various suggestions concerning the origins of alchemy, and stressed that it was a cultural trait of most societies. Following Eliarde (1956), he defines alchemy as

> a cosmic art by means of which parts of that cosmos – mineral and animal – can be liberated from their temporal existence and attain states of perfection, gold in the case of metals, and for humans longevity, immortality and, finally, redemption. Such accomplishments can be brought about on the one hand by use of a material substance (elixir) or, on the other, by revelatory knowledge (gnosis) or psychological enlightenment (Sheppard 1979).

Such a definition allows for the difference between an exoteric alchemy concerned with gold-making and an esoteric alchemy concerned with spiritual and religious perfection. The latter 'traditional' school, which has been interpreted psychologically by Jung (1944), reviewed by Martin (1975) and sumptuously illustrated by Fabricius (1976), continues to thrive amongst modern Hermeticists who interpret alchemy as a revealed occult knowledge handed down through initiation.

Graeco-Roman–Egyptian alchemy is examined in the writings of Sherwood Taylor (1930, 1937, 1951) and in a much criticized but stimulating book by Hopkins (1934); Islamic alchemy is best approached through the writings of Holmyard (1927, 1957), Ruska (1924, 1931) and Plessner (1954, 1969); and Chinese practice in the work of Needham previously cited. Information on alchemical symbolism, which is to be found in an *Ambix* report (Report 1937), the popular writings of Read (1936) and in an essay on egg symbolism by Sheppard (1958), has been summarized by Crosland (1962a), though the exact relationship between alchemical symbolism and chemical conceptualization still remains unexplored. Hill (1975) has issued a valuable warning against the misinterpretation of artists' representations of alchemical laboratories and workshops.

Needham (1974: 10) has introduced a terminology that is bound to be influential. He identifies 'aurifiction', 'aurifaction' and 'macrobiotics' as 'key operational conceptions' that are 'applicable to all the aspects of early chemistry in every civilisation'. Aurifiction, or gold-faking, which is the imitation of gold or other precious materials – whether as a deliberate deception or not depending upon the circumstances (compare modern synthetic products) – is associated with technicians and artisans. Aurifaction, or gold-making, is 'the belief that it is possible to make gold (or "a gold", or an artificial "gold") indistinguishable from or as good as (if not better than), natural gold, from other quite different substances'. This, suggests Needham, tended to be the conviction of natural philosophers who, coming from a different social class than the aurifictors, either knew nothing of assaying tests for gold, or rejected their validity. Finally, macrobiotics is 'the belief that it is possible to prepare, with the aid of botanical, zoological, mineralogical, and above all chemical, knowledge, drugs or elixirs which will prolong human life beyond old age, rejuvenating the body' (Needham 1974: 11). Concern with macrobiotics, or iatrochemistry, appears to have entered 'Europe only with the transmission of Arabic chemical knowledge from the +12th century onward'. On the other hand, claims have been made on etymological grounds by Mahdihassan (1976, 1977) that the term *elixir* was used by the Greeks. Despite some reservations by Multhauf (1975) concerning the universal applicability of Needham's terms and of his sociological approach, Needham's global perspective must be the starting point for any future research into alchemy and early chemistry.

Iatrochemistry and Paracelsianism

The use in the Latin West of mineral or chemical medicinal remedies instead of the traditional Galenic plant substances, was due to Arabic influences. Besides Needham (1976), there is a good introduction to the subject by Multhauf (1966) who also provides a sympathetic overture to any study of the subject's principal protagonist, Paracelsus. The latter is the subject of an important book by Walter Pagel (1958), who is himself honoured in a useful *Festschrift* of essays on science, medicine and society during the Renaissance (Debus 1972). The myriad faces of Paracelsianism, and in particular the 'English compromise' whereby chemical remedies came to be adopted in the English pharmacopoeia without commitment to Paracelsus's cosmology, are the subjects of a large number of papers by A.G. Debus, which he has synthesized in two books (Debus 1965, 1977). Interesting remnants of Paracelsian cosmology have been detected by Rees (1975a,b, 1977a,b) in Francis Bacon's plans for a Great Instauration of Learning. Essays by Rattansi (1964), Howe (1965), Webster (1965–6), Debus (1967) and Pagel (1973) focus on the sources drawn on by, and the influence of, J.B. van Helmont. Paracelsus's and van Helmont's significance in the controversies between 'ancients' and 'moderns' is vividly seen in the debate between Webster and Ward edited by Debus (1970), and in its widest context in Webster's monumental portrait of seventeenth-century science (Webster 1975). A fine monograph by Hannaway (1975) explores how the anti-Paracelsianism of Libavius encouraged the emergence of a chemical textbook tradition.

Chemistry and the scientific revolution

Although Marie Boas in her biography of Robert Boyle (Boas 1958), which is more readable than that by Maddison (1969), argued that seventeenth-century chemistry did undergo a change in methods and aims comparable to the 'scientific revolution' in mechanics and cosmology, most historians of chemistry have felt it more meaningful to speak of an eighteenth-century chemical revolution (George 1952). Some of the reasons for the postponement of this revolution were first analysed by Metzger (1930b) – namely the complexity of chemistry's subject matter, the absence of clear criteria for the purity of substances, the failure to imagine a gaseous state of matter, and the large number of competing theories of the elements used to explain chemical reactivity. A history of the concept of purity is a major lacuna in the history of chemistry, though some suggestions may be found in Caldin (1961) and in Szabadváry's very useful survey of analytical chemistry (Szabadváry 1960). The significance of the development of the concept of a gaseous state of matter for the limiting conceptualizations that were possible to seventeenth-century chemists compared with their successors a century later is now fully realized. Here the works of Pagel (1962), Crosland (1962b), Gough (1968–9, 1969), Fichman (1971) and Siegfried (1972) are particularly important. However, since these historians have concentrated on Lavoisier's gas theory, whereby when caloric was added to a substance it caused either expansion or a change of physical state, further investigation of how seventeenth- and early eighteenth-century chemists thought of air seems desirable (Rappaport 1961).

The various theories of elements, ranging from Helmont's unique Water, through Sylvius's acid and alkali, the Paracelsian Tria Prima, the Aristotelian Four Elements, and the more pragmatic theories of five or six elements, have been explored individually or collectively by many writers, including Debus (1967, 1977), Boas (1956, 1958), Howe (1965), Webster (1965–6) and de Milt (1941). Robert Boyle's devastating critique of such theories is best read in the clearer preliminary version of his *Sceptical Chymist* published by Boas (1954). Boyle's reason for rejecting his contemporaries' support for a doctrine of elements lay in his adoption of corpuscular mechanical explanations. The revival of such explanations of chemical change as reshufflings of invariant parts rather than transmutations has been explored critically by Boas (1952) and Kargon (1966). Good integrations of the large journal literature on seventeenth-century chemistry are to be found in Multhauf (1966) and Westfall (1971: ch. 4), while the adoption of atomistic explanations on the Continent is best traced through a brilliant study of Jungius by Kangro (1968). Westfall (1972: 183–98) is tempted to see Newton's interest in alchemy and chemistry as a fusion between mechanism and Hermeticism. Support for such a view comes from the elaborate studies of Newton's alchemical manuscripts by Dobbs (1975) and Figala (1977), both of whom provide citations to a large earlier literature on Newton's chemical interests. Newton's dream of a quantified chemistry, and his influence upon eighteenth-century matter theory, have been investigated most fully by Thackray (1970a); while Duncan (1962; 1970) has closely documented practical chemists' attempts to tabulate chemical reactivities in terms of affinity.

The chemical revolution

In retrospect it seems clear that the necessary and sufficient conditions for a chemical revolution were: (1) the demonstration by Stephen Hales in 1727 that air participated in chemical reactions; (2) the demonstration by Joseph Black and others that atmospheric air was not elementary – leading in the hands of Lavoisier to the concept of a gaseous state; (3) the application of the balance by Lavoisier with the gaseous state in mind; (4) the demonstration in 1771 by Guyton de Morveau that metals increased in weight during calcination; and (5) the replacement of the older views of chemical composition especially associated with Stahl – which are described by Metzger (1930a), Oldroyd (1973), and Cassebaum and Kauffman (1976) – by Lavoisier's views of elements, oxides and binary salts. The best and most exciting introduction to these matters is the work of Henry Guerlac, all of whose essays, with one exception (1976), have been conveniently collected in book form (1977). These should be studied in conjunction with Guerlac's analysis of the reasons why Lavoisier moved into the field of research on combustion (1961a) and his biography of Lavoisier (1973). The 1975 reprint of the latter contains a critical bibliography of Lavoisier studies, which may be supplemented by Smeaton (1963). Guerlac (1977) provides penetrating insight into Lavoisier's career and particularly the influence on him of such British chemists as Hales, Black, Cavendish and Priestley. As Perrin (1979) points out, however, much remains to be done on the middle and late portions of Lavoisier's life and on placing Lavoisier in the broader perspective of the development of European chemistry in the eighteenth century. Several useful attempts at placing Lavoisier within the Enlightenment tradition have been made by Crosland (1963, 1980) who, like Christie (1983), feels that the importance of combustion and the overthrow of phlogiston has been greatly overemphasized by historians – as, for example, in the scholarly investigations of Partington and McKie (1937, 1938, 1939–40), Rappaport (1961) or Perrin (1969). In recent years, historians have tried alternatively to interpret eighteenth-century chemistry as part of natural history, and therefore as concerned with problems of classification and language (Smeaton 1954; Crosland 1962a, 1963, 1980; Toulmin and Goodfield 1962); or concerned with elements and composition (Siegfried and Dobbs 1968; Oldroyd 1973; Perrin 1973), or acidity (Le Grand 1972; Crosland 1973). Christie (1983), for example, whose perspective is Scottish rather than French and whose focus is Black rather than Lavoisier, suggests that 'the Chemical Revolution... was to do with a general theory of the aeriform state and a particular theory of acidity'. By also emphasizing that the precise meaning of Lavoisier's revolution is a function of contemporaries' perceptions, Christie is able to show that much work remains to be done concerning the reception of the new chemistry in England, Scotland, Germany, Sweden and the United States.

A good deal of interesting work is already available on chemistry in Scotland (Christie 1974; Morrell 1969), where a Newtonian concern with the forces and powers of matter was quite strong (Donovan 1975, 1976a,b). There are important studies of Cullen's and Black's chemistry lectures by Crosland (1959, 1962a), Wightman (1955, 1956) and McKie (1959, 1960, 1962, 1965, 1966, 1967). Priestley's chemistry has also been placed in a philosophical and theological context in a sustained epistemological analysis by McEvoy (1978, 1979).

Although, unlike Newton, Lavoisier left no 'ism', the significance of his quantitative and pragmatic programme for chemistry has been suggested by Crosland (1967a), who has also published definitive studies of Lavoisier's pupil, Berthollet (Crosland 1967b), and of Berthollet's pupil, Gay-Lussac (Crosland 1978). The suasive function of Lavoisier's emphasis on experiments and lecture demonstrations, which often involved complicated apparatus, has been examined by Levere (1973); its role in Fourcroy's chemistry course at the École Polytechnique, and its possible connection with that school's decline as a chemistry teaching and research establishment, are discussed by Langins (1981).

Apart from isolated studies of the German chemical community, and of Boerhaave, Scheele and Bergman by Hufbauer (1971), Gibbs (1957–8), Boklund (1968), Cassebaum and Kauffman (1976), Love (1972) and Smeaton (1954), eighteenth-century German, Dutch and Scandinavian chemistry has not been assimilated into a European context. Similarly, apart from some work by Frick (1973) and Debus (1981), the persistence of Hermetic currents alongside mechanical–experimental explanations also awaits integration.

The nineteenth century

Research on nineteenth-century chemistry has concentrated so far on the impact of electrochemistry and its influence on the development of the atomic-molecular theory; on the many attendant difficulties of the latter as well as the conception of the chemical element; on the development of organic chemistry and its transformation from a system of classification into a structural theory; and on the organization of, and teaching of, chemistry during the period. Very little work of substance, and readability, has been published on the history of physical chemistry.

Volta's discovery of the electric pile and electrolysis in 1800 sounded 'an alarm bell' for European chemists, and led to the discovery of several new elements as well as the development of electrical (electrochemical) explanations of chemical reactions and reactivity. A series of papers by Russell (1959, 1963a,b) examines in considerable detail the emergence of the electrochemical systems of Humphry Davy in England and of Berzelius in Sweden. The good, but conventional biography of Davy by Hartley (1966b) should be supplemented by the more romantic approach adopted by Treneer (1963) and by an appreciation of Davy's transcendentalism and anti-materialism explored by Siegfried (1959, 1967) and Knight (1978). Particular facets of Davy's many-sided talents, which are listed by Fullmer (1967, 1969), are also celebrated in a volume of essays delivered at the Davy bicentenary conference (Forgan 1980). Faraday's elegant discovery of electrochemical laws, and his adoption of an electrolytic terminology of ions and cathodes are best studied in the much-praised biography of Faraday by Williams (1965: chs 2, 3, 6). Very little satisfactory work has been published on the history of the ionic theory, though Berry

(1946: ch. 7) and two studies by Wolfenden (1972) and Dolby (1976) are stimulating starting points for future investigations.

The centenary of the birth of Dalton (Greenaway 1966; Smyth 1966; Patterson 1970) in 1966 stimulated the publication of a large literature concerned with the origin of the atomic theory. This literature is best approached through the work of Thackray (1966a,b, 1970a, 1972), who has argued (1966a, 1972) that Dalton's unique contribution was to develop 'a calculating system for deriving... weights from chemical data'. In so doing, Thackray suggests, Dalton owed little or nothing to the ideas of his predecessors such as Richter – as Guerlac (1961b), Siegfried (1963b) and Mauskopf (1969c) had suggested. In particular, although Dalton's data drew on the analytical materials that had been thrown up in the controversy between Proust and Berthollet (Kapoor 1965), he avoided Berthollet's 'Newtonian Dream' to quantify the short-range forces of chemical affinity (Thackray 1968: 92–108). Particular aspects of Thackray's treatment of Dalton's theory of mixed gas have been criticized by Fleming (1974) and Cole (1978); while Mauskopf (1969a) has 'exhumed' some doubts concerning the origins of Dalton's theory, namely the theory's relationship with the crystallographic concept of '*molécule intégrante*' developed earlier by René Haüy.

Mauskopf (1969b, 1970, 1976) has also assessed the continuing significance of the crystallographic tradition (Burke 1966; Goodman 1969) in the development of chemistry up to mid-century. Avogadro's use of the French terminology of 'integrant molecules' is considered by Coley (1964), while his place within the Newtonian dynamic, and therefore anti-Daltonian, tradition is made plain by Fox (1971). Morselli (1980) has published the preliminary version of Avogadro's famous essay of 1811, and this deserves further study. The pseudo-problem of why Avogadro's hypothesis was ignored for so long (Coley 1964; Frické 1976) has probably been settled once and for all by Brooke (1981) and Fisher (1982). The Karlsruhe conference of 1860 on atomic weights, at which Cannizzaro 'revived' Avogadro's hypothesis, has been described by Milt (1948) and Hartley (1966a).

The grand dualistic electrochemical theory erected by Berzelius on the basis of Dalton's atomism (Russell 1968) is best grasped through Berzelius's *Essai* of 1818, which has been edited by Russell (1972). There is only one short biography of Berzelius in English by Jorpes (1966); hence apart from Swedish studies of Berzelius's atomism by Eriksson (1965–6) and Lundgren (1979), the massive Swedish biography by Söderbaum (1929–31) must be consulted, together with Partington (1964: 142–77) and the splendid edition of Berzelius's foreign correspondence also edited by Söderbaum (1912–35). A biography begun by the late Sir Harold Hartley (1971: 134–52) is to be completed by C.A. Russell.

Dalton's 'bulldog' was Thomas Thomson, whose receptiveness towards Dalton's theory is analysed by Mauskopf (1969c). Thomson's similar enthusiastic support for Prout's hypothesis that atomic weights were integers is investigated by Brock (1968), while his failure to develop a research school at the University of Glasgow has been elegantly explained by Morrell (1972). The emergence of Prout's hypothesis (Brock 1969a) that the number of elements could be reduced to one or two basic substances and that there is a basic unity of matter is best seen in the context of the unsettling effects of Lavoisier's operational definition of the chemical element (Siegfried 1963a, 1964; Usselman 1978), and seems to form a leitmotiv in nineteenth-century matter theory (Farrar 1965; Brock and Knight 1965; Brock 1967a; Knight 1967, 1978). Two valuable collections of sources on matter theory and the classification of the elements have been assembled by Knight (1968, 1970), who has also published an important study of the persistence of speculative (or transcendental) chemistry during the century (Knight 1978). The diverse speculative and observational streams leading to Mendeleev's announcement of the periodic law have been reviewed by van Spronsen (1969) and Rawson (1974), though there has been no satisfactory study of the reception and use of the periodic table by chemists in the decades following 1869 (J.R. Smith 1976). The scepticism that many chemists showed towards the existence of atoms has attracted much attention (Brock and Knight 1965; Brock 1967a; Knight 1967, 1978; Post 1968; Buchdahl 1959–60; Nye 1972, 1976). On the other hand, the ways in which chemical atomism was actually used have begun to be explored by Rocke (1975, 1978), who differentiates this more practical form of atomism from 'the highly controversial physical atomic theory which made statements about the intimate mechanical nature of substances'. The fusion of these two chemical and physical views in the 1860s by Cannizzaro (Hartley 1966a), Williamson (Harris and Brock 1974), Clausius and Maxwell still awaits further study, though it clearly depended upon the development of organic chemistry (Levere 1971; Rocke 1975). The reception of atomism in France and Germany has been briefly discussed by Crosland (1968) and Rocke (1979) respectively, but much remains untold.

The main hindrance to the emergence of organic chemistry seems to have been analytical (Szabadváry 1960; Brock 1967b) and not due to the assumption of vitalistic explanations demarcating between inorganic and organic chemistry – as traditional historical accounts of Wöhler's synthesis of urea in 1828 tended to imply (Lipman 1964; Brooke 1968; Russell 1976). In a thesis and a series of papers Brooke (1969, 1973, 1975) has demonstrated the importance that the inorganic model of chemical composition assumed in explaining, by analogy, the composition of, and ways of classifying, organic compounds. That classification rather than composition and structure formed the goal of most organic chemists before the 1870s was noticed by Kapoor (1969a, 1969b) and powerfully argued by Fisher (1973, 1974). The theory of chemical combination (Benfey 1963), or valency, has been comprehensively surveyed by Palmer (1965) and Russell (1971, 1976). Russell's biography of Frankland (1978), who first articulated the idea of 'combining power' in 1852, is eagerly awaited. Russell (1971) and Larder (1967) examine the introduction of graphical formulae by Crum Brown and Frankland, the ramifications of which deserve further exploration (Ramsay 1974a,b). The triumphant explanation of stereoisomerism by van't Hoff and Le Bel has been analysed philosophically by Gay (1978) and celebrated in a centenary monograph (Ramsay 1974b). The importance of synthesis, whether to eradicate the possibility of vital forces in organic chemistry (as with Berthelot) or to throw light on the real structure of organic compounds, has been stressed by Brooke (1971) and Russell (1976). Whether valency was constant or variable formed an interesting debating ground between inorganic and organic chemists (Russell 1971; Kauffman 1972) and was only resolved when models of the internal structure of the atom, such as those of Lewis and Kossel, became available in the twentieth century (Kohler 1972, 1975a,b). The central significance of Werner's model of coordination compounds for directing much of the course of early twentieth-century chemistry has been emphasized by Kauffman (1966, 1968, 1976, 1978). For the transformation of animal and vegetable chemistry (Coley 1967, 1973; Fruton 1972) into biochemistry, see chapters 18.

Physical chemistry has received little serious attention from professional historians of chemistry and much of the basic information has to be gleaned from general histories such as Partington (1964), Ihde (1964), Findlay and Williams (1965) or Berry (1946, 1954). An exemplary essay by Holmes (1962) on the law of mass action connects Kapoor's epistemological analysis of Berthollet (Kapoor 1965) with mid-century discussions of equilibria. The latter form the context for the development of an understanding of indicators (Baker 1964) and the debates over the theory of solutions (Dolby 1976). Some interesting reflections on the rise of physical chemistry, its institutionalization and transmission from Germany to America have been made by Dolby (1977a,b). Apart from studies by Brock (1969b), Sutton (1974, 1976) and DeKosky (1973, 1980), the focus of research on the development of spectroscopy has been physical and astronomical (McGucken 1969). Fresh light has been thrown on Joule and the development of thermodynamics by Forrester (1976), who argues that Joule was a chemist in education, research interests and inclination.

The emergence of the discipline of chemistry in Great Britain and of the (Royal) Chemical Society of London is the subject of a thesis by Bud (1980) and of a valuable study by Russell *et al.* (1977). The seminal influence of Liebig (Brock 1981) on the institutionalization of chemistry is suggested by the investigation of the necessary and sufficient conditions for the creation of a research school published by Morrell (1972). The failure of the University of Cambridge to develop such a school during the nineteenth century has been explained by Roberts (1980). The training of pharmacists appears to have been significant for the establishment of laboratories in Germany (Pohl 1972; Gustin 1975), and further research is needed on the relationship between pharmacy and chemistry in other countries. The Royal College of Chemistry, which, under its director, A.W. Hofmann (Bentley 1970, 1972), was modelled on the chemistry laboratory at Giessen, has been analysed prosopographically by Roberts (1973, 1976), who reveals how widespread support for chemistry was during the 1840s (Brock 1978). International comparisons concerning the chemical professions and their interactions are made possible for France (Crosland 1978), Germany (Ruske 1967; Hufbauer 1971; Gustin 1975) and America (Hannaway 1976; Skolnik and Reese 1976; Servos 1980; Thackray *et al.* 1981).

Much work still remains to be done on the history of chemical publications (including textbooks) and chemical instrument and materials suppliers such as Griffins (Griffin 1970). In particular, apart from the existing studies of *Nicholson's Journal* (Lilley 1948), Rozier's *Observations* (Neave 1948, 1951, 1952; McKie 1958) and the *Annales de Chimie* (Court 1972), and the fairly factual accounts of national chemical society publications by Watchurst (1974), Hückel (1967) and Bud (1980), a detailed history of Crookes's *Chemical News* is a desideratum. Similarly, as a seminal article by Fullmer (1980) demonstrates, the role of chemists as witnesses in legal cases ranging from insurance and patent claims (Wood 1975) to murder trials cries out for examination. Storrs (1966, 1968) and Crosland (1978) have shown that historians can learn much from technical literature; but, apart from studies by German historians (Zimmermann 1965; Schmauderer 1971), chemical patent literature remains unexamined.

The twentieth century

Needless to say, research on the development of twentieth-century chemistry has been left largely to chemists. For example, a special issue of *Chemical and Engineering News* (1976) contains reviews by chemists of 'progress' in inorganic, physical, organic and analytical chemistry, each of which could, with the bibliographies suggested by Ihde (1964), form a starting point for deeper research by professional historians. Trenn (1974) has compared Ramsay's speculative 'alchemical' interpretation of radioactivity with the more cautious experimental approach of Rutherford. The emergence of the electronic theory of valency has been imaginatively reconstructed by R.E. Kohler (1971, 1972, 1975a, 1975b), but the autobiography of one of its main protagonists in applying it to organic chemistry is deeply disappointing (Robinson 1976). Charting the contributions of Ingold (Shoppee 1972) to the study of the mechanisms of chemical change, and the bitter controversies he and Robinson created, is rendered difficult by the destruction of his papers (Bykov 1965). Three inevitably rather technical papers by Ballhausen (1979), which describe the gradual penetration of quantum mechanics into chemistry, suggest that a study of Sidgwick's career would be useful (L.E. Sutton 1975). Reminiscences by Pauling (1970) are also relevant. The retrospectively puzzling failure to prepare rare gas compounds until the 1960s is explained by Hein (1966) and Gay (1977). Marxist difficulties (comparable to Lysenkoism in biology) concerning the acceptability of 'resonance' have been investigated by Graham (1964) and Kaufman (1977). Oral history has been put to good use by Ettre and Zlatkins (1979) and Ewald (1962) in celebrations of the history of chromotography and crystallography.

Twentieth-century chemical education in England, and the associated growth of laboratories, have been studied by Brock (1973), Brock and Meadows (1977) and Chilton and Coley (1980). The American experience of chemistry has been treated exhaustively using a large number of 'indicators' of change and performance (Thackray *et al.* 1981). The connection between some of America's larger research schools and the world of industry is being explored by Servos (1976, 1980).

Chemical industry

Ihde (1964: 800–4, 816–20) provides particularly good bibliographies of the development of chemical industry since 1800. For the eighteenth century the work of the Clows (1952), Schofield (1963) and Musson and Robinson (1969) will be found particularly interesting. The alkali industry, which formed the basis of the heavy chemical industry in most countries, has been particularly well served by historians. The Leblanc process has been analysed by Multhauf (1971), Gillispie (1957) and Mathews (1976); it has been placed in a French context by J.G. Smith (1979), and in an English interdisciplinary one by Warren (1980), who demonstrates the great significance of the switch from the Leblanc to the Solvay process. Borscheid (1976) and the massive studies by Haynes (1945, 1948, 1949, 1954) throw light on the emergence and development of the German and American systems. The development of dyestuffs chemistry, and its significant connection with the state of university and technical education, form the subject of monographs by Beer (1959) and Haber (1958, 1971, 1973). Food analysis and its relation to the rise of food processing industries is of importance. There are excellent business histories of Unilever and Imperial Chemical Industries by Wilson (1954) and Reader (1970–5), and a study of polyvinyl chloride by Kaufman (1969). The development of the chemical industry on Tyneside is the subject of an introductory essay by Campbell (1968) and of a large unpublished prosopographical investigation by Russell *et al.*

Bibliography

Ambix (1937–). *The Journal of the Society for the History of Alchemy and Chemistry*. Index to Vols 1–17 (1937–70) in Vol. 17 (1970) and to Vols 18–27 (1971–80) in Vol. 27 (1980)

Anderson, R.G.W. (1978). *The Playfair Collection and the Teaching of Chemistry at the University of Edinburgh 1713–1858*. Edinburgh; Royal Scottish Museum

Baker, A.A. (1964). A History of Indicators, *Chymia*, Vol. 9, 147–168

Ballhausen, C.J. (1979). Quantum Mechanics and Chemical Bonding in Inorganic Complexes, *Journal of Chemical Education*, Vol. 56, 215–218, 294–297, 357–361

Beardsley, E.H. (1964). *The Rise of the American Chemistry Profession 1850–1900*. Gainesville; University of Florida Press

Beer, J.J. (1959). *The Emergence of the German Dye Industry*. Urbana; University of Illinois

Benfey, O.T., Ed. (1963). *Classics in the Theory of Chemical Combination*. New York; Dover

Bentley, J. (1970). The Chemical Department of the Royal School of Mines. Its Origins and Development under A.W. Hofmann, *Ambix*, Vol. 17, 153–181

Bentley, J. (1972). Hofmann's return to Germany from the Royal College of Chemistry, *Ambix*, Vol. 19, 197–203

Berry, A.J. (1946). *Modern Chemistry*. Cambridge; Cambridge University Press
Berry, A.J. (1954). *From Classical to Modern Chemistry*. Cambridge; Cambridge University Press. Reprinted (1968). New York; Dover
Berthelot, M. (1885). *Les Origines de l'alchimie*. Paris; G. Steinheil
Berthelot, M. (1887–8). *Collection des anciens alchimistes Grecs*. 3 Vols. Paris; G. Steinheil
Berthelot, M. (1889). *Introduction à l'étude de la chimie des anciens et du moyen âge*. Paris; G. Steinheil
Berthelot, M. (1890). *La Révolution chimique. Lavoisier*. Paris; F. Alcan. 2nd edn (1902)
Berthelot, M. (1893). *Histoire des sciences. La chimie au moyen âge*. 3 Vols. Paris; Imprimerie Nationale
Berthelot, M. (1906). *Archéologie et histoire des sciences*. Paris; Gauthier-Villars
Boas, M. (1952). The Establishment of the Mechanical Philosophy, *Osiris*, Vol. 10, 412–541
Boas, M. (1954). An Early Version of Boyle's *Sceptical Chymist*, *Isis*, Vol. 45, 153–168
Boas, M. (1956). Acid and Alkali in 17th Century Chemistry, *Archives Internationales d'Histoire des Sciences*, Vol. 9, 13–28
Boas, M. (1958). *Robert Boyle and 17th Century Chemistry*. Cambridge; Cambridge University Press
Boklund, U. (1968). *Carl Wilhelm Scheele. His Work and Life*. 2 Vols. Stockholm; Roos Boktryckeri
Bolzan, J.E. (1976). Chemical Combination according to Aristotle, *Ambix*, Vol. 23, 134–144
Borscheid, P. (1976). *Naturwissenschaft, Staat und Industrie in Baden 1848–1914*. Stuttgart; Ernst Klett
Brock, W.H. (1967a). *The Atomic Debates*. Leicester; Leicester University Press
Brock, W.H. (1967b). An Attempt to Establish the First Principles of the History of Chemistry, *History of Science*, Vol. 6, 156–169
Brock, W.H. (1968). Dalton versus Prout. The Problem of Prout's Hypotheses, in *John Dalton and the Progress of Science*. Ed. D.S.L. Cardwell. Manchester; Manchester University Press, 240–258
Brock, W.H. (1969a). Studies in the History of Prout's Hypotheses, *Annals of Science*, Vol. 25, 49–80, 127–137
Brock, W.H. (1969b). Lockyer and the Chemists. The First Dissociation Hypothesis, *Ambix*, Vol. 16, 81–99
Brock, W.H., Ed. (1973). *H.E. Armstrong and the Teaching of Science 1880–1930*. Cambridge; Cambridge University Press
Brock, W.H. (1978). The Society for the Perpetuation of Gmelin. The Cavendish Society, 1846–1872, *Annals of Science*, Vol. 35, 599–617
Brock, W.H. (1981). Liebigiana. Old and New Perspectives, *History of Science*, Vol. 19, 201–218
Brock, W.H. and Knight, D.M. (1965). The Atomic Debates, *Isis*, Vol. 56, 5–25. Reprinted with corrections in Brock (1967a), 1–30
Brock, W.H. and Meadows, A.J. (1977). Physics, Chemistry and Higher Education in the UK, *Studies in Higher Education*, Vol. 2, 109–124
Brooke, J.H. (1968). Wohler's Urea, and its Vital Force? – A Verdict from the Chemists, *Ambix*, Vol. 15, 84–114
Brooke, J.H. (1969). The Role of Analogical Argument in the Development of Organic Chemistry, University of Cambridge PhD Thesis
Brooke, J.H. (1971). Organic Synthesis and the Unification of Chemistry – A Reappraisal, *British Journal for the History of Science*, Vol. 5, 363–392

Brooke, J.H. (1973). Chlorine Substitution and the Future of Organic Chemistry, *Studies in the History and Philosophy of Science*, Vol. 4, 47–94

Brooke, J.H. (1975). Laurent, Gerhardt and the Philosophy of Chemistry, *Historical Studies in the Physical Sciences*, Vol. 6, 405–430

Brooke, J.H. (1981). Avogadro's Hypothesis and its Fate. A Case Study in the Failure of Case Studies, *History of Science*, Vol. 19, 235–273

Buchdahl, G. (1959–60). Sources of Scepticism in Atomic Theory, *British Journal for the Philosophy of Science*, Vol. 10, 120–134

Bud, R. (1980). The Discipline of Chemistry. The Origins and Early Years of the Chemical Society of London, University of Pennsylvania PhD Thesis

Burke, J.G. (1966). *Origins of the Science of Crystals*. Berkeley and Los Angeles; University of California Press

Butler, A.R. and Needham, J. (1980). An Experimental Comparison of the East Asian, Hellenistic and Indian (Gandhāran) Stills in Relation to the Distillation of Ethanol and Acetic Acid, *Ambix*, Vol. 27, 69–76

Bykov, G.V. (1965). Historical Sketch of the Electron Theories of Organic Chemistry, *Chymia*, Vol. 10, 199–254

Bynum, W.F., Browne, E.J. and Porter, R.S., Ed. (1981). *Dictionary of the History of Science*. London; Macmillan

Caldin, E.F. (1959–60). Theories and the Development of Chemistry, *British Journal for the Philosophy of Science*, Vol. 10, 209–222

Caldin, E.F. (1961). *The Structure of Chemistry*. London and New York; Sheed and Ward

Campbell, W.A. (1968). *A Century of Chemistry on Tyneside 1868–1968*. Newcastle; Dept of Inorganic Chemistry, University of Newcastle

Cassebaum, H. and Kauffman, G.B. (1976). The Analytical Concept of a Chemical Element in the Work of Bergman and Scheele, *Annals of Science*, Vol. 33, 447–456

Chemical and Engineering News (1976). Centennial American Chemical Society 1876–1976, Vol. 54, No. 15, 6 April

Chilton, D. and Coley, N.G. (1980). The Laboratories of the Royal Institution in the Nineteenth Century, *Ambix*, Vol. 27, 173–203

Chirnside, R.C. and Hamence, J.H. (1974). *The 'Practising Chemists'. A History of the Society for Analytical Chemistry 1874–1974*. London; Society for Analytical Chemistry

Christie, J.R. (1974). The Origins and Development of the Scottish Scientific Community 1680–1760, *History of Science*, Vol. 12, 122–141

Christie, J.R. (1983). The Chemical Revolution in Scotland, *Ambix*, Vol. 30, in press

Chymia (1948–67). Annual Studies in the History of Chemistry. Philadelphia; University of Pennsylvania Press. London; Oxford University Press

Clow, A. and Clow, N.L. (1952). *The Chemical Revolution*. London; Batchworth

Cole, T., Jr. (1978). Dalton, Mixed Gases, and the Origin of the Chemical Atomic Theory, *Ambix*, Vol. 25, 117–130

Coley, N.G. (1964). The Physico-Chemical Studies of Amedeo Avogadro, *Annals of Science*, Vol. 20, 195–210

Coley, N.G. (1967). The Animal Chemistry Club. Assistant Society to the Royal Society, *Notes and Records of the Royal Society of London*, Vol. 22, 173–185

Coley, N.G. (1973). *From Animal Chemistry to Biochemistry*. Amersham, Bucks; Hulton Educational

Coudert, A. (1980). *Alchemy. The Philosopher's Stone*. London; Wildwood House. Sydney; Bookwise

Court, S. (1972). The *Annales de Chimie*, 1789–1815, *Ambix*, Vol. 19, 113–128

Crosland, M.P. (1959). The Use of Diagrams as Chemical Equations in the Lecture Notes of William Cullen and Joseph Black, *Annals of Science*, Vol. 15, 75–90

Crosland, M.P. (1962a). *Historical Studies in the Language of Chemistry*. London, Melbourne and Toronto; Heinemann. Reprinted (1978). New York; Dover

Crosland, M.P. (1962b). The Development of the Concept of the Gaseous State as a Third State of Matter, *Proceedings of the 10th International Congress of the History of Science, Ithaca, New York, 1962*, Vol. 2, 851–854

Crosland, M.P. (1963). The Development of Chemistry in the 18th Century, *Studies on Voltaire and the 18th Century*, Vol. 24, 369–441

Crosland, M.P. (1967a). *Les Héritiers de Lavoisier*. Paris; Palais de Découverte

Crosland, M.P. (1967b). *The Society of Arcueil. A View of French Science at the Time of Napoleon*. London; Heinemann

Crosland, M.P. (1968). The First Reception of Dalton's Atomic Theory in France, in *John Dalton and the Progress of Science*. Ed. D.S.L. Cardwell. Manchester; Manchester University Press, 274–289

Crosland, M.P. (1973). Lavoisier's Theory of Acidity, *Isis*, Vol. 64, 306–325

Crosland, M.P. (1978). *Gay-Lussac Scientist and Bourgeois*. Cambridge; Cambridge University Press

Crosland, M.P. (1980). Chemistry and the Chemical Revolution, in *The Ferment of Knowledge*. Ed. G.S. Rousseau and R.S. Porter. Cambridge; Cambridge University Press, 389–416

Dean, P.A.W. and Usselman, M.C. (1979). The Synthetic Palladium of Richard Chenevix, *Ambix*, Vol. 27, 100–115

Debus, A.G. (1962). An Elizabethan History of Medical Science, *Annals of Science*, Vol. 18, 1–29

Debus, A.G. (1965). *The English Paracelsians*. London; Oldbourne

Debus, A.G. (1967). Fire Analysis and the Elements in the 16th and 17th Centuries, *Annals of Science*, Vol. 23, 127–147

Debus, A.G., Ed. (1970). *Science and Education in the 17th Century. The Webster–Ward Debate*. London; Macdonald. New York; American Elsevier

Debus, A.G. (1971). The History of Chemistry and the History of Science, *Ambix*, Vol. 18, 169–177

Debus, A.G., Ed. (1972). *Science, Medicine and Society in the Renaissance. Essays to Honor Walter Pagel*. 2 Vols. New York; Science History Publications

Debus, A.G. (1977). *The Chemical Philosophy. Paracelsian Science and Medicine in the Sixteenth and Seventeenth Centuries*. 2 Vols. New York; Science History Publications

Debus, A.G. (1981). The Paracelsians in 18th Century France, *Ambix*, Vol. 28, 36–54

DeKosky, R.K. (1973). Spectroscopy and the Elements in the late 19th Century. The Work of Sir William Crookes, *British Journal for the History of Science*, Vol. 6, 400–423

DeKosky, R.K. (1980). George Gabriel Stokes, Arthur Smithells and the Origin of Spectra and Flames, *Ambix*, Vol. 27, 103–123

Dijksterhuis, E.J. (1961). *The Mechanization of the World Picture*. Trans. C. Dikshoorn. Oxford; Clarendon Press

Dobbs, B.J.T. (1975). *The Foundations of Newton's Alchemy: or 'The Hunting of the Greene Lyon'*. Cambridge; Cambridge University Press

Dolby, R.G.A. (1976). Debates over the Theory of Solution. A Study of Dissent in Physical Chemistry in the English-Speaking World in the late 19th and early 20th Centuries, *Historical Studies in the Physical Sciences*, Vol. 7, 297–404

Dolby, R.G.A. (1977a). The Transmission of Science, *History of Science*, Vol. 15, 1–43

Dolby, R.G.A. (1977b). The Transmission of Two New Scientific Disciplines from Europe to North America in the late 19th Century, *Annals of Science*, Vol. 34, 287–310

Donovan, A.L. (1975). *Philosophical Chemistry in the Scottish Enlightenment*. Edinburgh; Edinburgh University Press

Donovan, A.L. (1976a). Pneumatic Chemistry and Newtonian Natural Philosophy, *Isis*, Vol. 67, 217–228

Donovan, A.L. (1976b). Chemistry and Philosophy in the Scottish Enlightenment, *Studies on Voltaire and the 18th Century*, Vol. 152, 587–605

Duncan, A.M. (1962). Some Theoretical Aspects of 18th Century Tables of Affinity, *Annals of Science*, Vol. 18, 177–194, 217–232

Duncan, A.M. (1970). The Function of Affinity Tables and Lavoisier's List of Elements, *Ambix*, Vol. 17, 28–42

Eklund, J. (1975). *The Incompleat Chymist. An Essay on the 18th Century Chemist in his Laboratory, with a Dictionary of Obsolete Chemical Terms*. Washington; Smithsonian Institution

Eklund, J. (1976). Of a Spirit in the Water. Some Early Ideas on the Aerial Dimension, *Isis*, Vol. 67, 527–550

Eliarde, M. (1956). *Forgerons et alchimistes*. Paris; Flammarion. English trans. (1962) as *The Forge and the Crucible*. New York; Harper

Eriksson, G. (1965–6). Berzelius och Atomtheorin, *Lychnos*, 3–37

Ettre, L.S. and Zlatkins, S., Ed. (1979). *75 Years of Chromotography – A Historical Dialogue*. Amsterdam; Elsevier

Ewald, P.P., Ed. (1962). *50 Years of X-Ray Diffraction*. Utrecht; International Union of Crystallography

Fabricius, J. (1976). *Alchemy. The Medieval Alchemists and their Royal Art*. Copenhagen; Rosenkilde and Bagger

Farrar, W.V. (1965). 19th Century Speculations on the Complexity of the Chemical Elements, *British Journal for the History of Science*, Vol. 2, 297–323

Fichman, M. (1971). French Stahlism and Chemical Studies of Air (1750–1770), *Ambix*, Vol. 18, 94–122

Figala, K. (1977). Newton as Alchemist, *History of Science*, Vol. 15, 102–137

Findlay, A. and Williams, T. (1965). *A Hundred Years of Chemistry*, 3rd edn. London; Methuen

Fisher, N.W. (1973). Organic Classification before Kekulé, Part I and Part II, *Ambix*, Vol. 20, 106–31, 209–33

Fisher, N.W. (1974). Kekulé and Organic Classification, *Ambix*, Vol. 21, 29–52

Fisher, N.W. (1975). Wislicenus and Lactic Acid. The Chemical Background to van't Hoff's Hypotheses, in Ramsay (1974b) 33–54

Fisher, N.W. (1982). Avogadro, the Chemists and the Historians, *History of Science*, Vol. 20, 77–102

Fleming, R.S. (1974). Newton, Gases and Daltonian Chemistry. The Foundations of Combinations in Definite Proportions, *Annals of Science*, Vol. 31, 561–574

Forbes, R.J. (1948). *A Short History of the Art of Distillation*. Leyden; Brill. Reprinted (1970)

Forbes, R.J. (1955). *Studies in Ancient Technology*. Vol. 1, *Bitumen and Petroleum in Antiquity; The Origin of Alchemy; Water Supply*. Leyden; Brill

Forgan, S., Ed. (1980). *Science and the Sons of Genius. Studies on Humphry Davy*. London; Science Reviews Ltd

Forrester, J. (1976). Chemistry and the Conservation of Energy. The Work of James Prescott Joule, *Studies in the History and Philosophy of Science*, Vol. 6, 273–313

Fox, R. (1971). *The Caloric Theory of Gases: From Lavoisier to Regnault*. Oxford; Clarendon Press

Frick, K.R.H. (1973). *Die Erleuchteten: gnostisch-theosophische und alchemistis-chrosencreuzererische Geheim-gesellschaften bis zum Ende des 18. Jahrhunderts.* Graz; Akademisch Druck u. Verlaganstalt

Frické, M. (1976). The Rejection of Avogadro's Hypotheses, in *Method and, Appraisal in the Physical Sciences. The Critical Background to Modern Science, 1800–1905.* Ed. C. Howson. Cambridge; Cambridge University Press, 277–307

Fruton, J.S. (1972). *Molecules and Life. Historical Essays on the Interplay of Chemistry and Biology.* New York and London; Wiley Interscience

Fullmer, J.Z. (1967). Davy's Biographers, *Science*, Vol. 155, 285–291

Fullmer, J.Z. (1969). *Sir Humphry Davy's Published Works.* Cambridge, Mass.; Harvard University Press

Fullmer, J.Z. (1980). Technology, Chemistry, and the Law in Early 19th Century England, *Technology and Culture*, Vol. 21, 1–28

Gay, H. (1976). Radicals and Types. A Critical Comparison of the Methodologies of Popper and Lakatos and their Use in the Reconstruction of some 19th Century Chemistry, *Studies in the History and Philosophy of Science*, Vol. 7, 1–51

Gay, H. (1977). Nobel's Gas Compounds. A Case Study in Scientific Conservatism and Opportunism, *Studies in the History and Philosophy of Science*, Vol. 8, 61–70

Gay, H. (1978). The Asymmetric Carbon Atom, *Studies in the History and Philosophy of Science*, Vol. 9, 207–238

George, P. (1952). The Scientific Movement and the Development of Chemistry in England, as seen in the Papers published in the *Philosophical Transactions* from 1664/5 until 1750, *Annals of Science*, Vol. 8, 302–322

Gibbs, F.W. (1957–8). Boerhaave's Chemical Writings, *Ambix*, Vol. 6, 117–135

Gillispie, C.C. (1957). The Discovery of the Leblanc Process, *Isis*, Vol. 48, 152–170

Goodman, D.C. (1969). Problems in Crystallography in the Early 19th Century, *Ambix*, Vol. 16, 152–166

Gough, J.B. (1968–9). Lavoisier's Early Career in Science. An Examination of Some New Evidence, *British Journal for the History of Science*, Vol. 4, 52–57

Gough, J.B. (1969). Nouvelle contribution à l'étude de l'evolution des idées de Lavoisier sur la nature de l'air et sur le calcination des métaux, *Archives Internationales d'Histoire des Sciences*, Vol. 22, 267–275

Graham, L.R. (1964). A Soviet Marxist View of Structural Chemistry. The Theory of Resonance Controversy, *Isis*, Vol. 55, 20–31

Greenaway, F. (1966). *John Dalton and the Atom.* London; Heinemann

Griffin, Charles, and Co. Ltd (1970). *Catalogue of Books. 150th Anniversary Issue 1820–1970, With a Short Historical Retrospect.* London; Charles Griffin

Guerlac, H. (1961a). *Lavoisier – The Crucial Year. The Background and Origin of his first Experiments on Combustion in 1772.* New York; Cornell

Guerlac, H. (1961b). Some Daltonian Doubts, *Isis*, Vol. 52, 544–554

Guerlac, H. (1973). Lavoisier, in *Dictionary of Scientific Biography*. Ed. C.C. Gillispie. Vol. 8, 66–91. Reprinted as *Antoine-Laurent Lavoisier* (1975). New York; Scribner's

Guerlac, H. (1976). Chemistry as a Branch of Physics. Laplace's Collaboration with Lavoisier, *Historical Studies in the Physical Sciences*, Vol. 7, 193–276

Guerlac, H. (1977). *Essays and Papers in the History of Modern Science.* Baltimore and London; Johns Hopkins University Press

Gustin, B.H. (1975). The Emergence of the German Chemical Profession, 1790–1867, University of Chicago PhD Thesis

Gwei-Djen, L., Needham, J. and Needham, D.M. (1972). The Coming of Ardent Water, *Ambix*, Vol. 19, 69–112

Haber, L.F. (1958). *The Chemical Industry during the Nineteenth Century. A Study of the Economic Aspect of Applied Chemistry in Europe and North America.* Oxford; Clarendon Press

Haber, L.F. (1971). *The Chemical Industry 1900–1930. International Growth and Technological Change.* Oxford; Clarendon Press

Haber, L.F. (1973). Government Intervention at the Frontiers of Science. British Dyestuffs and Synthetic Organic Chemicals, 1914–1939, *Minerva*, Vol. 11, 79–93

Halleux, R. (1974). *Le Problème des métaux dans la science antique.* Paris; Société d'Edition les Belles Lettres

Halleux, R. (1979). *Les Textes alchimiques.* Turnhout, Belgium; Brepols

Hannaway, O. (1975). *The Chemists and the Word. The Didactic Origins of Chemistry.* Baltimore and London; The Johns Hopkins University Press

Hannaway, O. (1976). The German Model of Chemical Education in America. Ira Remsen at Johns Hopkins (1876–1913), *Ambix*, Vol. 23, 145–164

Harris, J. and Brock, W.H. (1974). From Giessen to Gower Street. Towards a Biography of Alexander W. Williamson, *Annals of Science*, Vol. 33, 95–130

Hartley, Sir H. (1966a). Stanislao Cannizzaro, F.R.S. (1826–1910) and the First International Chemical Conference at Karlsruhe in 1860, *Notes and Records of the Royal Society of London*, Vol. 21, 56–63. Reprinted in Hartley (1971), 185–194

Hartley, Sir H. (1966b). *Humphry Davy.* London; Nelson. Reprinted (1971). London; S.R. Publishers

Hartley, Sir H. (1971). *Studies in the History of Chemistry.* Oxford; Clarendon Press

Haynes, W. (1945). *The World War I Period, 1912–1922.* Vols 2–3 of *American Chemical Industry.* New York; van Nostrand

Haynes, W. (1948). *The Merger Era, 1923–1929.* Vol. 4 of *American Chemical Industry.* New York; van Nostrand

Haynes, W. (1949). *The Chemical Companies.* Vol. 6 of *American Chemical Industry.* New York; van Nostrand

Haynes, W. (1954). *Background and Beginnings; Decade of New Products, 1930–1939.* Vols 1 and 5 of *American Chemical Industry.* New York; van Nostrand

Hein, H. (1966). The Chemistry of Noble Gases – A Modern Case History in Experimental Science, *Journal of the History of Ideas*, Vol. 27, 417–428

Hill, C.R. (1971). *Chemical Apparatus. Catalogue I. Museum of the History of Science.* Oxford; Museum of the History of Science

Hill, C.R. (1975). The Iconography of the Laboratory, *Ambix*, Vol. 22, 102–110

Holmes, F.L. (1962). From Elective Affinities to Chemical Equilibria. Berthollet's Law of Mass Action, *Chymia*, Vol. 8, 105–146

Holmyard, E.J. (1927). An Essay on Jabir ibn Hayyan, in *Studien zur Geschichte der Chimie.* Ed. J. Ruska. Berlin; Springer, 28–37

Holmyard, E.J. (1957). *Alchemy.* Harmondsworth; Penguin Books. Reprinted (1968)

Hopkins, A.J. (1934). *Alchemy, Child of Greek Philosophy.* New York; Columbia University Press. Reprinted (1967). New York; AMS Press

Howe, H.M. (1965). A Root of van Helmont's Tree, *Isis*, Vol. 56, 408–419

Hückel, W. (1967). 100 Years of the *Berichte*, *Berichte*, Vol. 100, 1–39

Hufbauer, K. (1971). Social Support for Chemistry in Germany during the 18th Century. How and Why did it Change?, *Historical Studies in the Physical Sciences*, Vol. 3, 205–232

Ihde, A. (1964). *The Development of Modern Chemistry.* New York, Evanston and London; Harper and Row

Ihde, A.J. and Kieffer, W.F. (1975). *Selected Readings in the History of Chemistry.* Reprints from *Journal of Chemical Education*, 1933–63. Easton, Pa.; Journal of Chemical Education

Jorpes, J.E. (1966). *Jac. Berzelius. His Life and Work.* Stockholm; Almqvist and Wiksell

Jung, C. (1944). *Psychologie und Alchemie.* Zürich; Raschev. Rev. edn (1952). English trans. (1953) as *Psychology and Alchemy.* London; Routledge and Kegan Paul

Kangro, H. (1968). *Joachim Jungius' Experimente und Gedanken zur Begründung der Chemie als Wissenschaft.* Wiesbaden; Franz Steiner

Kapoor, S. (1965). Berthollet, Proust and Proportions, *Chymia*, Vol. 9, 53–110

Kapoor, S. (1969a). Dumas and Organic Classification, *Ambix*, Vol. 16, 1–65

Kapoor, S. (1969b). The Origins of Laurent's Organic Classification, *Isis*, Vol. 60, 477–527

Kargon, R.H. (1966). *Atomism in England from Hariot to Newton.* Oxford; Clarendon Press

Kauffman, G.B. (1966). *Alfred Werner, Founder of Co-ordination Chemistry.* Berlin; Springer-Verlag

Kauffman, G.B. (1968). *Classics in Co-ordination Chemistry, Part I, The Selected Papers of Alfred Werner.* New York; Dover

Kauffman, G.B., Ed. (1971). *Teaching the History of Chemistry.* Budapest; Akadémiai Kiadó

Kauffman, G.B. (1972). Werner, Kekulé, and the Demise of the Doctrine of Constant Valency, *Journal of Chemical Education*, Vol. 49, 813–817

Kauffman, G.B. (1976). *Classics in Co-ordination Chemistry. Part II, Selected Papers (1789–1899).* New York; Dover

Kauffman, G.B. (1978). *Classics in Co-ordination Chemistry. Part 3, 20th Century Papers.* New York; Dover

Kaufman, J. (1977). Criticism of the Theory of Resonance in Organic Chemistry 1944–1956, *Synthesis* (Cambridge), Vol. 4, 44–59

Kaufman, M. (1969). *The History of Polyvinyl Chloride.* London; MacLaren

Knight, D.M. (1967). *Atoms and Elements. A Study of Theories of Matter in the 19th Century.* London; Hutchinson

Knight, D.M., Ed. (1968). *Classical Scientific Papers. Chemistry.* London; Mills and Boon

Knight, D.M., Ed. (1970). *Classical Scientific Papers – Chemistry Second Series – on the Nature and Arrangement of the Chemical Elements.* London; Mills and Boon

Knight, D.M. (1978). *The Transcendental Part of Chemistry.* Folkestone; Dawson

Kohler, R.E., Jr. (1971). The Origin of G.N. Lewis's Theory of the Shared Pair Bond, *Historical Studies in the Physical Sciences*, Vol. 3, 343–376

Kohler, R.E., Jr. (1972). Irving Langmuir and the 'Octet' Theory of Valence, *Historical Studies in the Physical Sciences*, Vol. 4, 39–87

Kohler, R.E., Jr. (1975a). The Lewis–Langmuir Theory of Valence and the Chemical Community, 1920–1928, *Historical Studies in the Physical Sciences*, Vol. 6, 431–468

Kohler, R.E., Jr. (1975b). G.N. Lewis's Views on Bond Theory 1900–1916, *British Journal for the History of Science*, Vol. 8, 233–239

Kohler, R.E. (1975c). Lavoisier's Rediscovery of the Air from Mercury Calx. A Reinterpretation, *Ambix*, Vol. 22, 52–57

Kopp, H.F.M. (1843–7). *Geschichte der Chemie.* 4 Vols. Brunswick; F. Vieweg und Sohn

Kopp, H.F.M. (1873). *Die Entwicklung der Chemie in der neueren Zeit.* Munich; R. Oldenbourg

Kopp, H.F.M. (1886). *Die Alchemie in älterer und neuerer Zeit.* Heidelberg; C. Winter

Langins, J. (1981). The Decline of Chemistry at the Ecole Polytechnique, *Ambix*, Vol. 28, 1–19

Larder, D.F. (1967). Alexander Crum Brown and his Doctoral Thesis of 1861, *Ambix*, Vol. 14, 112–132

Le Grand, H.E. (1972). Lavoisier's Oxygen Theory of Acidity, *Annals of Science*, Vol. 29, 1–18

Levere, T.H. (1971). *Affinity and Matter. Elements of Chemical Philosophy 1800–1865.* Oxford; Oxford University Press

Levere, T.H. (1973). The Interaction of Ideas and Instruments in van Marum's Work on Chemistry and Electricity, in *Martinus van Marum. Life and Work.* Vol. 4, *Van Marum's Scientific Instruments in Teyler's Museum.* Ed. G. L'E. Turner and T.H. Levere. Leyden; Noordhoff, 103–122

Lilley, S. (1948). Nicholson's Journal 1797–1813, *Annals of Science*, Vol. 6, 78–101

Lindeboom, G.A. (1968). *Hermann Boerhaave. The Man and his Work.* London; Methuen

Lipman, T.O. (1964). Wöhler's Preparation of Urea and the Fate of Vitalism, *Journal of Chemical Education*, Vol. 41, 452–458

Love, R. (1972). Some Sources of Boerhaave's Concept of Fire, *Ambix*, Vol. 19, 157–174

Lundgren, A. (1979). *Berzelius och den kemiska atomteorin* (with English summary). Uppsala; Uppsala University. Stockholm; Almqvist and Wiksell

McEvoy, J.G. (1978). Joseph Priestley, 'Aerial Philosopher', Metaphysics and Methodology in Priestley's Chemical Thought from 1772 to 1781, Parts 1–4, *Ambix*, Vol. 25, 1–55, 93–116, 153–175

McEvoy, J.G. (1979). Joseph Priestley, Part 5, *Ambix*, Vol. 26, 16–38

McGucken, W. (1969). *Nineteenth-Century Spectroscopy.* Baltimore and London; Johns Hopkins University Press

McKie, D. (1958). 'Observations' of the Abbé François Rozier (1734–93), *Annals of Science*, Vol. 13, 73–89

McKie, D. (1959). On Some Ms Copies of Black's Chemical Lectures, II, *Annals of Science*, Vol. 15, 65–74

McKie, D. (1960). Some Ms Copies of Black's Chemical Lectures, III, *Annals of Science*, Vol. 16, 1–10

McKie, D. (1962). Some Ms Copies of Black's Chemical Lectures, IV, *Annals of Science*, Vol. 18, 87–98

McKie, D. (1965). Some Ms Copies of Black's Chemical Lectures, V, *Annals of Science*, Vol. 21, 209–256

McKie, D. (1966). [Thomas Cochrane's] *Notes from Doctor Black's Lectures on Chemistry, 1767–8.* Wilmslow, Cheshire; ICI Ltd

McKie, D. (1967). Some Ms Copies of Black's Chemical Lectures, VI, *Annals of Science*, Vol. 23, 1–34

Maddison, R. (1969). *The Life of the Honorable Robert Boyle, F.R.S.* London; Taylor and Francis

Mahdihassan, S. (1976). Early Terms for Elixir hitherto unrecognised in Greek Alchemy, *Ambix*, Vol. 23, 129–133

Mahdihassan, S. (1977). Elixirs of Mineral Origin in Greek Alchemy, *Ambix*, Vol. 24, 133–142

Mahdihassan, S. (1979). Distillation Assembly of Pottery in Ancient India, *Vishveshvaranand Indological Journal*, Vol. 17, 264–266

Martin, L.H. (1975). A History of the Psychological Interpretation of Alchemy, *Ambix*, Vol. 22, 10–20

Mathews, M.H. (1976). Development of the Synthetic Alkali Industry in Great Britain by 1823, *Annals of Science*, Vol. 33, 371–382

Mauskopf, S.H. (1969a). Haüy's Model of Chemical Equivalence. Daltonian Doubts Exhumed, *Ambix*, Vol. 17, 182–191

Mauskopf, S.H. (1969b). The Atomic Structural Theories of Ampère and Gaudin. Molecular Speculation and Avogadro's Hypothesis, *Isis*, Vol. 60, 61–74

Mauskopf, S.H. (1969c). Thomson Before Dalton, *Annals of Science*, Vol. 25, 229–242

Mauskopf, S.H. (1970). Minerals, Molecules and Species, *Archives Internationales d'Histoire des Sciences*, Vol. 23, 185–206

Mauskopf, S.H. (1976). Crystals and Compounds. Molecular Structure and Composition in 19th Century French Science, *Transactions of the American Philosophical Society*, Vol. 66, Part 3, July

Melhardo, E.M. (1981). *Jacob Berzelius. The Emergence of his Chemical System.* Stockholm; Almqvist & Wiksell

Metzger, H. (1918). *La Genèse de la science des cristaux.* Paris; Alcan. Reprinted (1969). Paris; Albert Blanchard

Metzger, H. (1923). *Les Doctrines chimiques en France du debut du XVIIe à la fin du XVIIIe siècle.* Paris; Presses Universitaires de France. Reprinted (1969). Paris; Librairie Scientifique

Metzger, H. (1930a). *Newton, Stahl, Boerhaave et la doctrine chimique.* Paris; Alcan

Metzger, H. (1930b). *La Chimie.* Part 4 of *La Civilisation européenne.* Ed. E. Cavaignac. Paris; E. de Brocard

Metzger, H. (1935). *La Philosophie de la matière chez Lavoisier.* Paris; Hermann et Cie

Metzger, H. (1938). *Attraction universelle et religion naturelle chez quelques commentateurs anglais de Newton.* Paris; Hermann et Cie

Meyerson, E. (1908). *Identité et réalité.* Paris; F. Alcan. 3rd edn (1926). Trans. K. Loewenberg (1930) as *Identity and Reality.* London and New York; George Allen and Unwin. Reprinted (1964)

Milt, C. de (1941). The Five Element Theory, *Journal of Chemical Education*, Vol. 18, 503–505

Milt, C. de (1948). Carl Weltzein and the Congress at Karlsruhe, *Chymia*, Vol. 1, 153–169

Morrell, J.B. (1969). Practical Chemistry in the University of Edinburgh, 1799–1843, *Ambix*, Vol. 16, 66–80

Morrell, J.B. (1972). The Chemist Breeders. The Research Schools of Liebig and Thomas Thomson, *Ambix*, Vol. 19, 1–46

Morris, R.J. (1969). Lavoisier on Fire and Air. The Memoir of July 1772, *Isis*, Vol. 60, 374–380

Morselli, M.A. (1980). The Manuscript of Avogadro's *Essai* (1811), *Ambix*, Vol. 27, 147–172

Multhauf, R.P. (1966). *The Origins of Chemistry.* London; Oldbourne

Multhauf, R.P. (1971). The French Crash Program for Saltpeter Production 1776–94, *Technology and Culture*, Vol. 12, 163–181

Multhauf, R.P. (1975). Aurification, Aurifaction and Macrobiotics, Essay Review of Needham (1974), *Ambix*, Vol. 22, 218–220

Multhauf, R.P. (1978). *Neptune's Gift. A History of Common Salt.* Baltimore and London; The Johns Hopkins Press

Musgrave, A. (1976). Why did Oxygen surplant Phlogiston? Research Programmes and the Chemical Revolution, in *Method and Appraisal in the Physical Sciences. The Critical Background to Modern Science, 1800–1905.* Ed. C. Howson. Cambridge; Cambridge University Press, 181–209

Musson, A.E. and Robinson, E. (1969). *Science and Technology in the Industrial Revolution.* Manchester; Manchester University Press

Neave, E.W.J. (1948). Chemistry in Rozier's Journal, Part I, The Editors, *Annals of Science*, Vol. 6, 416–421

Neave, E.W.J. (1951). Chemistry in Rozier's Journal, Parts II–VII, *Annals of Science*, Vol. 7, 101–106, 144–148, 284–299, 393–400

Neave, E.W.J. (1952). Chemistry in Rozier's Journal – [Parts] VIII and IX, *Annals of Science*, Vol. 8, 28–45

Needham, J. (1958). *The Development of Iron and Steel Technology in China.* London; Newcomen Society. Reprinted (1964). Cambridge; Heffer

Needham, J. (1974). *Spagyrical Discovery and Invention. Magisteries of Gold and Immortality.* Vol. 5, Part 2 of *Science and Civilisation in China.* Cambridge; Cambridge University Press

Needham, J. (1976). *Spagyrical Discovery and Invention. Historical Survey from Cinnabar to Elixirs to Synthetic Insulin.* Vol. 5, Part 3 of *Science and Civilisation in China.* Cambridge; Cambridge University Press

Needham, J. (1980). *Spagyrical Discovery and Invention. Apparatus, Theories and Gifts.* Vol. 5, Part 4 of *Science and Civilisation in China.* Cambridge; Cambridge University Press

Nye, M.J. (1972). *Molecular Reality. A Perspective on the Scientific Work of Jean Perrin.* New York; Science History Publications

Nye, M.J. (1976). The 19th Century Atomic Debates and the Dilemma of 'Indifferent Hypotheses', *Studies in the History and Philosophy of Science*, Vol. 7, 245–268

Oldroyd, D.R. (1973). An Examination of Stahl's *Philosophical Principles of Universal Chemistry*, *Ambix*, Vol. 20, 36–52

Pagel, W. (1958). *Paracelsus. An Introduction to Philosophical Medicine in the Era of the Renaissance.* Basle; S. Karger

Pagel, W. (1962). The 'Wild Spirit' (gas) of van Helmont and Paracelsus, *Ambix*, Vol. 10, 1–13

Pagel, W. (1973). The Spectre of van Helmont and the Idea of Continuity in the History of Chemistry, in *Changing Perspectives in the History of Science. Essays in Honour of Joseph Needham.* Ed. M. Teich and R. Young. London; Heinemann, 100–109

Palmer, W.G. (1965). *A History of the Concept of Valency to 1930.* Cambridge; Cambridge University Press

Partington, J.R. (1935). *Origins and Development of Applied Chemistry.* London; Longmans

Partington, J.R. (1960). *A History of Greek Fire and Gunpowder.* Cambridge; Heffer

Partington, J.R. (1961). *A History of Chemistry.* Vol. 2 [1600–1800]. London; Macmillan. Reprinted (1969)

Partington, J.R. (1962). *A History of Chemistry.* Vol. 3 [1600–1800]. London; Macmillan. Reprinted (1970)

Partington, J.R. (1964). *A History of Chemistry.* Vol. 4 [19th and 20th centuries]. London; Macmillan. Reprinted (1972)

Partington, J.R. (1970). *A History of Chemistry.* Vol. 1, Part 1, Theoretical Background. London; Macmillan [Part 2 was not published]

Partington, J.R. and McKie, D. (1937). Historical Studies on the Phlogiston Theory. I. The Levity of Phlogiston, *Annals of Science*, Vol. 2, 361–404

Partington, J.R. and McKie, D. (1938). Ibid., II. The Negative Weight of Phlogiston; III. Light and Heat in Combustion, *Annals of Science*, Vol. 3, 1–58, 337–371

Partington, J.R. and McKie, D. (1939–40). Ibid., IV. Last Phases of the Theory, *Annals of Science*, Vol. 4, 113–149

Patterson, E.C. (1970). *John Dalton and the Atomic Theory*. Garden City, NY; Doubleday

Pauling, L. (1970). 50 Years of Progress in Structural Chemistry and Molecular Biology, *Daedulus*, Vol. 99, 988–1014

Perrin, C.E. (1969). Prelude to Lavoisier's Theory of Calcination. Some Observations on *Mercurius Calcinatus per se*, *Ambix*, Vol. 16, 140–151

Perrin, C. (1973). Lavoisier's Table of the Elements. A Reappraisal', *Ambix*, Vol. 20, 95–105

Perrin, C.E. (1979). Review of Guerlac (1977), *Ambix*, Vol. 26, 137–138

Plessner, M. (1954). The Place of the *Turba Philosophorum* in the Development of Alchemy, *Isis*, Vol. 45, 331–338

Plessner, M. (1969). Geber and Jabir ibn Hayyan. An Authentic 16th Century Quotation from Jabir, *Ambix*, Vol. 16, 113–118

Pohl, D. (1972). Zur Geschichte der pharmazeutischen Privatinstitute in Deutschland von 1779 bis 1873, University of Marburg PhD Thesis

Post, H.R. (1968). Atomism 1900, *Physics Education*, Vol. 3, 1–13

Potter, O. (1953). Auguste Laurent's Contributions to Chemistry, *Annals of Science*, Vol. 9, 271–280

Pritchard, A. (1980). *Alchemy. A Bibliography of English-Language Writings*. London and Boston; Routledge and Kegan Paul with the Library Association

Ramsay, O.B. (1974a). Molecules in Three Dimensions, *Chemistry*, Vol. 47, January, 6–9; February, 6–11. Reprinted as 'Molecular Models in the Early Development of Stereochemistry' in Ramsay (1974b)

Ramsay, O.B., Ed. (1974b). *Van't Hoff–Le Bel Centennial*. Washington; American Chemical Society

Rappaport, R. (1961). Rouelle and Stahl – The Phlogistic Revolution in France, *Chymia*, Vol. 7, 73–102

Rattansi, P.M. (1964). The Helmontian–Galenist Controversy in Restoration England, *Ambix*, Vol. 12, 1–23

Rawson, D.C. (1974). The Process of Discovery. Mendeleev and the Periodic Law, *Annals of Science*, Vol. 31, 181–204

Read, J. (1936). *Prelude to Chemistry*. London; Bell

Read, J. (1947). *Humour and Humanism in Chemistry*. London; Bell

Reader, W.J. (1970–5). *Imperial Chemical Industries. A History*, Vol. 1, *The Forerunners 1870–1926*. Vol. 2, *The First Quarter of the Century 1926–1952*. London; Oxford University Press

Rees, G. (1975a). Francis Bacon's Semi-Paracelsian Cosmology, *Ambix*, Vol. 22, 81–101

Rees, G. (1975b). Francis Bacon's Semi-Paracelsian Cosmology and the Great Instauration, *Ambix*, Vol. 22, 161–173

Rees, G. (1977a). The Fate of Bacon's Cosmology in the 17th Century, *Ambix*, Vol. 24, 27–38

Rees, G. (1977b). Matter Theory. A Unifying Factor in Bacon's Natural Philosophy?, *Ambix*, Vol. 24, 110–125

Report (1937). Report of a Discussion upon Chemical and Alchemical Symbolism, *Ambix*, Vol. 1, 61–77

Roberts, G.K. (1973). The Royal College of Chemistry (1845–1853). A Social History of Chemistry in Early-Victorian England, Johns Hopkins University PhD Thesis

Roberts, G.K. (1976). The Establishment of the Royal College of Chemistry. An Investigation of the Social Context of Early-Victorian Chemistry, *Historical Studies in the Physical Sciences*, Vol. 7, 437–486

Roberts, G.K. (1980). The Liberally-Educated Chemist. Chemistry in the Cambridge Natural Science Tripos, 1851–1914, *Historical Studies in the Physical Sciences*, Vol. 11, 157–183

Robinson, Sir R. (1976). *Memoirs of a Minor Prophet. 70 Years of Organic Chemistry*. Vol. 1. Amsterdam, Oxford and New York; Elsevier

Rocke, A.J. (1975). Origins of the Structural Theory in Organic Chemistry, University of Wisconsin PhD Thesis

Rocke, A.J. (1978). Atoms and Equivalents. The Early Development of the Chemical Atomic Theory, *Historical Studies in the Physical Sciences*, Vol. 9, 225–263

Rocke, A.J. (1979). The Reception of Chemical Atomism in Germany, *Isis*, Vol. 70, 519–536

Ruska, J. (1924). *Arabische Alchemisten*. 2 Vols. Heidelberg; Winter. Reprinted (1967). Wiesbaden; Sändig

Ruska, J. (1931). Turba Philosophorum. Ein Beitrag z. Geschichte d. Alchemie, *Quellen und Studien zur Geschichte der Naturwissenschaften*, Vol. 1, 1–368

Ruske, W. (1967). *100 Jahre Deutsche Chemische Gesellschaft*. Weinheim; Verlag Chemie

Russell, C.A. (1959). The Electrochemical Theory of Sir Humphry Davy, *Annals of Science*, Vol. 15, 1–13, 15–25

Russell, C.A. (1963a). The Electrochemical Theory of Berzelius, *Annals of Science*, Vol. 19, 117–126, 127–145

Russell, C.A. (1963b). The Electrochemical Theory of Sir Humphry Davy. Part III, *Annals of Science*, Vol. 19, 255–271

Russell, C.A. (1968). Berzelius and the Development of the Atomic Theory, in *John Dalton and the Progress of Science*. Ed. D.S.L. Cardwell. Manchester; Manchester University Press, 259–273

Russell, C.A. (1971). *The History of Valency*. Leicester; Leicester University Press

Russell, C.A. (1972). Introduction to the Reprint Edition, J.J. Berzelius, *Essai sur la théorie des proportions chimiques*. New York; Johnson Reprint Corporation

Russell, C.A. (1973a). *Coal the Basis of 19th Century Technology*, AST 281, Unit 4, *Science and the Rise of Technology since 1800*. Milton Keynes; Open University Press. Corrected reprint (1976)

Russell, C.A. (1973b). Petroleum, Unit 12 of *The New Chemical Industry*, AST 281, *Science and the Rise of Technology since 1800*. Milton Keynes; Open University Press: Corrected reprint (1976)

Russell, C.A. (1976). *The Structure of Chemistry*. Units 1–3, *The Nature of Chemistry*, S304 (S351). Milton Keynes; The Open University Press

Russell, C.A. (1978). Edward Frankland and the Cheapside Chemists of Lancaster. An Early Victorian Pharmaceutical Apprenticeship, *Annals of Science*, Vol. 35, 253–273

Russell, C.A., Coley, N.G. and Roberts, G.K. (1977). *Chemists by Profession. The Origins of the Royal Institute of Chemistry*. Milton Keynes; Open University Press

Sambursky, S. (1956). *The Physical World of the Greeks*. London; Routledge and Kegan Paul

Schmauderer, E. (1971). Der Einfluss der Chemie auf die Entwicklung des Patentwesens in der zweiten Hälfte des 19. Jahrhunderts, *Veröffentlichungen des Forschungsinstituts des Deutschen Museums für die Geschichte der Naturwissenschaften und die Technik*, Reihe A. Kleine Mitteilungen No. 89, 144–176

Schofield, R.E. (1963). *The Lunar Society of Birmingham. A Social History of Provincial Science and Industry in Eighteenth Century England*. Oxford; Clarendon

Servos, J.W. (1976). The Knowledge Corporation. A.A. Noyes and Chemistry at the California Institute of Technology 1915–1930, *Ambix*, Vol. 23, 175–186

Servos, J.W. (1980). The Industrial Relations of Science. Chemistry at MIT, *Isis*, Vol. 71, 531–549

Sheppard, H.J. (1958). Egg Symbolism in Alchemy, *Ambix*, Vol. 6, 140–148

Sheppard, H.J. (1970). Alchemy. Origin or Origins, *Ambix*, Vol. 17, 69–84

Sheppard, H.J. (1979). The Cultural Values involved in the Study of Alchemy, unpubl. talk given at British Society for the History of Science meeting, Leicester, 6–8 April

Shoppee, C.W. (1972). Christopher Kelk Ingold, *Biographical Memoirs of Fellows of the Royal Society*, Vol. 18, 349–412

Siegfried, R. (1959). The Chemical Philosophy of Humphry Davy, *Chymia*, Vol. 5, 193–201

Siegfried, R. (1963a). The Discovery of Potassium and Sodium and the Problem of the Chemical Elements, *Isis*, Vol. 54, 247–258

Siegfried, R. (1963b). Further Daltonian Doubts, *Isis*, Vol. 54, 480–481

Siegfried, R. (1964). The Phlogistic Conjectures of Humphry Davy, *Chymia*, Vol. 9, 117–124

Siegfried, R. (1967). Boscovich and Davy. Some Cautionary Remarks, *Isis*, Vol. 58, 236–238

Siegfried, R. (1972). Lavoisier's View of the Gaseous State and its Early Application to Pneumatic Chemistry, *Isis*, Vol. 63, 59–78

Siegfried, R. and Dobbs, B.J. (1968). Composition, a Neglected Aspect of the Chemical Revolution, *Annals of Science*, Vol. 24, 275–294

Singer, C. (1948). *The Earliest Chemical Industry. An Essay in the Historical Relations of Economics and Technology Illustrated from the Alum Trade.* London; Folio Society

Skolnik, H. and Reese, K.M. (1976). *A Century of Chemistry. The Role of Chemists and the American Chemical Society.* Washington DC; American Chemical Society

Smeaton, W.A. (1954). The Contributions of P.J. Macquer, T.O. Bergman and L.B. Guyton de Morveau to the Reform of Chemical Nomenclature, *Annals of Science*, Vol. 10, 87–106

Smeaton, W.A. (1963). New Light on Lavoisier. The Research of the Last Ten Years, *History of Science*, Vol. 2, 51–69

Smith, J.G. (1979). *The Origins and Early Development of the Heavy Chemical Industry in France.* Oxford; Clarendon Press

Smith, J.R. (1976). Philosophy of Chemistry. Problems Arising from the Work of D. Mendeleev, University of London PhD Thesis

Smyth, A.L. (1966). *John Dalton 1766–1844. A Bibliography of Works By and About Him.* Manchester; Manchester University Press

Söderbaum, H.G., Ed. (1912–35). *Jac. Berzelius Bref.* 6 Vols. Stockholm and Uppsala; Almqvist and Wiksell

Söderbaum, H.G. (1929–31). *Jac. Berzelius Levnadsteckning.* 3 Vols. Uppsala; K. Svenska Vetenskapsakademien

Spronsen, J.W. van (1969). *The Periodic Systems of Chemical Elements. A History of the First Hundred Years.* Amsterdam; Elsevier

Stock, J.T. (1969). *Development of the Chemical Balance: A Science Museum Survey.* London; HMSO

Storrs, F.C. (1966). Lavoisier's Technical Reports 1768–1794, Part I, *Annals of Science*, Vol. 22, 251–275

Storrs, F.C. (1968). Lavoisier's Technical Reports, Part II, *Annals of Science*, Vol. 24, 179–198

Sutton, L.E. (1975). Sidgwick, in *Dictionary of Scientific Biography*. Ed. C.C. Gillispie. New York; American Council of Learned Societies, Charles Scribner's Sons, Vol. 12, 418–420

Sutton, M.A. (1974). Sir John Herschel and the Development of Spectroscopy in Britain, *British Journal for the History of Science*, Vol. 7, 42–60

Sutton, M.A. (1976). Spectroscopy and the Chemists. A Neglected Opportunity?, *Ambix*, Vol. 23, 16–26

Szabadváry, F. (1960). *Az analitikai kémia módszereinek Kialakulása*. Budapest; Akadémai Kiadó. English edn (1966). *History of Analytical Chemistry*. Oxford; Pergamon Press

Taylor, F.S. (1930). A Survey of Greek Alchemy, *Journal of Hellenistic Studies*, Vol. 50, 109–139

Taylor, F.S. (1937). The Origins of Greek Alchemy, *Ambix*, Vol. 1, 30–47

Taylor, F.S. (1945). The Evolution of the Still, *Annals of Science*, Vol. 5, 185–202

Taylor, F.S. (1951). *The Alchemists*. London; Heinemann. Reprinted (1976). St Albans; Paladin

Thackray, A. (1966a). The Origins of Dalton's Chemical Atomic Theory. Daltonian Doubts Resolved, *Isis*, Vol. 57, 35–55

Thackray, A. (1966b). The Emergence of Dalton's Chemical Atomic Theory 1801–08, *British Journal for the History of Science*, Vol. 3, 1–23

Thackray, A. (1968). Quantified Chemistry – the Newtonian Dream, in *John Dalton and the Progress of Science*. Ed. D.S.L. Cardwell. Manchester; Manchester University Press, 92–108

Thackray, A. (1970a). *Atoms and Powers. An Essay on Newtonian Matter Theory and the Development of Chemistry*. Cambridge, Mass.; Harvard University Press. London; Cambridge University Press

Thackray, A. (1970b). Introduction to reprint of H.E. Roscoe and A. Harden, *A New View of the Origin of Dalton's Atomic Theory*. New York; Johnson Reprint Corporation

Thackray, A. (1972). *John Dalton. Critical Assessments of his Life and Science*. Cambridge, Mass.; Harvard University Press

Thackray, A., Sturchio, J., Carroll, P.T. and Bud, R.F. (1981). *Science in America 1876–1976. An Historical Application of Science Indicators*. Boston, Mass.; Reidel

Theobald, D.W. (1976). The Philosophy of Chemistry, *Chemical Society Reviews*, Vol. 5, 202–213

Toulmin, S. and Goodfield, J. (1962). *The Architecture of Matter*. London; Hutchinson

Treneer, A. (1963). *The Mercurial Chemist. A Life of Sir Humphry Davy*. London; Methuen

Trenn, T.J. (1974). The Justification of Transmutation. Speculations of Ramsay and the Experiments of Rutherford, *Ambix*, Vol. 21, 53–77

Tylecote, R.F. (1965). The Development of Iron Smelting Techniques in Great Britain, *Organon*, Vol. 2, 155–178

Tylecote, R.F. (1976). *A History of Metallurgy*. London; The Metals Society

Usselman, M.C. (1978). The Wollaston/Chenevix Controversy over the Elemental Nature of Palladium, *Annals of Science*, Vol. 35, 551–579

Warren, K. (1980). *Chemical Foundations. The Alkali Industry in Britain to 1926*. Oxford; Clarendon Press

Watchurst, E.C. (1974). *The Journal of the Chemical Society*, 1862–1900. Enquiries into Some Aspects of 19th Century Chemical Publishing, University of Bristol MSc Dissertation

Webster, C. (1965–6). Water as the Ultimate Principle of Nature. The Background to Boyle's *Sceptical Chymist*, *Ambix*, Vol. 13, 96–107

Webster, C. (1975). *The Great Instauration. Science, Medicine and Reform, 1626–1660*. London; Duckworth

Weeks (1968). *Discovery of the Elements*, 7th edn, rev. by H.M. Leicester. Easton, Pa.; Journal of Chemical Education

Westfall, R.S. (1971). *The Construction of Modern Science. Mechanism and Mechanics*. New York; Wiley. Cambridge; Cambridge University Press

Westfall, R.S. (1972). Newton and the Hermetic Tradition, in *Science, Medicine and Society in the Renaissance. Essays to Honor Walter Pagel*. Ed. A.G. Debus. 2 Vols. New York; Science History Publications, 183–198

Westfall, R.S. (1975). The Role of Alchemy in Newton's Career, in *Reason, Experiment and Mysticism in the Scientific Revolution*. Ed. M.L.R. Bonelli and W.R. Shea. New York; Science History Publications, 189–232

Weyer, J. (1974). *Chemiegeschichtsschreibung von Wiegleb (1790) bis Partington (1970). Eine Untersuchung über ihre Methode, Prinzipien und Ziele*. Hildesheim; Verlag Dr H.A. Gerstenberg

Wightman, W.P.D. (1955). William Cullen and the Teaching of Chemistry, I, *Annals of Science*, Vol. 11, 154–165

Wightman, W.P.D. (1956). William Cullen and the Teaching of Chemistry, II, *Annals of Science*, Vol. 12, 192–205

Williams, L.P. (1965). *Michael Faraday*. London; Chapman and Hall

Wilson, C. (1954). *The History of Unilever*. 2 Vols. London; Cassell

Wolfenden, J.H. (1972). The Anomaly of Strong Electrolytes, *Ambix*, Vol. 19, 175–196

Wood, R.D. (1975). The Involvement of Sir John Herschel in the Photographic Patent Case, *Talbot v. Henderson*, 1854, *Annals of Science*, Vol. 32, 239–264

Zimmermann, P.A. (1965). *Patentwesen in der Chemie*. Ludwigshafen; BASF

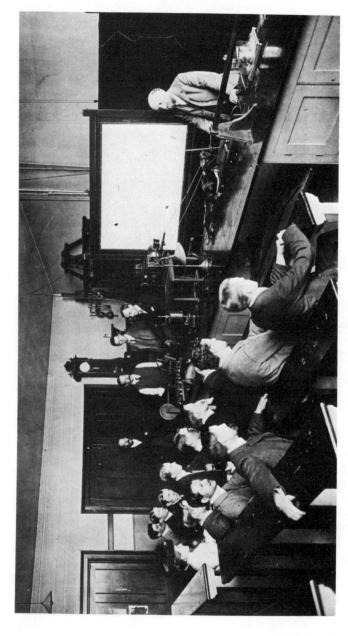

Plate 7. A provocation to anti-vivisectionists. The 'brown dog experiment' at University College London, 2 February 1903. From right to left behind the bench are W.M. Bayliss, E.H. Starling and H.H. Dale. By courtesy of the Wellcome Trustees

17

Life sciences: natural history

David Elliston Allen

There is probably no area of the history of science that has developed more untypically than the study of those aspects of botany and zoology that are focused on the field rather than on the laboratory – and that correspond more or less to what has traditionally been known (on one of its narrower definitions) as 'natural history'. The reason for this is simple. The preponderant concerns of this scientific sector are, and always have been, the classification and the distribution of organisms, and these are studies that by their very character have been productive of theory only sparsely. So long as historians of science have been for the most part 'internalist' in their orientation, there has consequently been distinctly little in this sector to tempt their intellectual appetites and, with the one great exception of evolutionary theory, 'natural history' has been largely avoided by them.

To some extent this avoidance may also have arisen from the fact that most recruits to the history of science have been scientists by training and have naturally gravitated to those disciplines that loom largest at the present day in numbers and in academic standing. By contrast taxonomy, in particular, has declined to a small-scale, low-status, even eccentric-seeming activity. For reasons that are not altogether clear, there has furthermore long been a disproportionately small recruitment of historians of science (as opposed to historians of medicine, that specialist enclave that has stood well apart) from the ranks of the life sciences, with a marked under-representation as a result of biological topics of any kind. Even though most historians of biology, in view of their background, are likely to prefer to concern themselves with laboratory-centred developments, had they only been around in greater numbers more attention would surely have spilled over on to the non-experimental aspects – as is certainly suggested by the material that found its way into the *Journal of the History of Biology* once this, very belatedly, was founded.

A further distorting factor, highly peculiar to this area, is the substantially 'historical' character of systematics itself. Quite exceptionally for a present-day scientific discipline, this cannot be pursued without repeated and continual referring back to the past – and often the very distant past. Although generally described as 'history', the kind of work that this involves would be more correctly classed as antiquarianism. Identifying it as a quite distinct scholarly discipline of its own, Allen (1977: 92) has proposed for it the term 'taxonomic archaeology':

> all that remarkably varied delving into the past that has developed as an outgrowth of taxonomy and museum work: the identification of collectors, the reconstruction of the routes of pioneer explorers, the pinpointing of type localities, the more precise annotation of specimens, the inside story of how particular institutions have come by what they have. At one extreme this grades off into work that is full-bloodedly biographical; at the other extreme, particularly in the matter of establishing priority of publication for nomenclatural purposes, it becomes inseparable from bibliography.

The investment of so much professional time and effort in the solving of questions of this type has long since produced a climate of sympathy with historical work of a wider kind. Working taxonomists, for example, played a leading part in the founding in 1936 of the Society for the Bibliography of Natural History, in whose journal, recently renamed *Archives of Natural History*, a good deal of material well outside the bounds of 'taxonomic archaeology' has increasingly been appearing. More important, the needs of professionals in this direction have stimulated the production of a range of 'historical' works of reference that must surely be without parallel in any other history of science area.

The existence of this extra impulse, over and above the ordinary antiquarian current that tends to irrigate every field of learning, is most perfectly exemplified in the publishing of Britten and Boulger's (1893–1908) biographical dictionary of British botanists. Britten was a taxonomist on the staff of the British Museum

(Natural History) and engaged in studying its early botanical collections; Boulger, with a foothold in the literary world through his novelist wife, had been enlisted as chief contributor of the numerous entries on botanists for the *Dictionary of National Biography*. On his own, Boulger would never have felt the inducement sufficient to undertake the enormously useful (but then quite uncommercial) publication that in due course appeared – at first serially, in the pages of the *Journal of Botany*. The best that could otherwise have been expected was the usual type of biographical dictionary limited just to a smallish, select number of comparatively well-known figures. It was the need of the world of botanical practitioners for a guide to the very many who were much more obscure that effected the necessary mutation.

In botany, biographical dictionaries have since become an outstanding speciality. After passing into a second and enlarged edition, Britten and Boulger's work has recently been massively extended by Desmond (1977) to take in horticulturists as well. The similar publication by Barnhart (1965), in three volumes and with a predominantly American coverage, was formed from a working file built up in the course of a professional lifetime. The Hunt Botanical Library (1972) has produced a more specialized example, essentially as a guide to its extensive portrait collection, and one of Miss Henrey's (1975) primarily bibliographical volumes is largely given over to accounts of botanical authors too. An index to entomologists' obituaries by Gilbert (1977) is so far the only near-counterpart of these in zoology.

In botany, too, the long-established tradition in Britain of writing county Floras has led in turn to a deeply rooted custom of including in these a section on the more important contributors of records, past as well as present. This descends from the path-breaking *Flora of Middlesex* of Trimen and Dyer (1869), whose lengthy historical appendix, contributed anonymously by the self-effacing W.W. Newbould, has never been surpassed. Work on local Floras also gave impetus to the production by Kent (1958) of an index of all known collections in the British Isles of British vascular plants, which is usefully cross-referenced to the biographical entries in Britten and Boulger. An earlier work by Sherborn (1940) is its very incomplete zoological equivalent.

The importance of tracing, for nomenclatural or other reasons, the often tangled wanderings of specimens from one collection to another has led to the compiling by Chalmers-Hunt (1976) of a register of natural history auctions in Britain; it has also promoted studies of the fate of individual major collections, of which that by Whitehead (1969), on the zoological specimens from Captain

Cook's three Pacific voyages, stands in a class of its own. Various institutions with particularly rich collections, especially in early material, have increasingly been galvanized by such work into bringing out indexes of collectors, which in some cases (e.g. Dandy 1958; Clokie 1964) have extended fairly extensively into the biographical field.

Much of the vast amount of work that has gone into all this biographical indexing activity (of which Boivin, 1977, has supplied a most useful country-by-country summary) has necessarily been derivative. But even where original probing has been attempted, this has seldom been pressed home to the basic level of registration and testamentary records. Only the very few authors who have happened already to have expertise in genealogy, notably Bristowe (1967), Jeffers (1967) and Christy (1919), have consequently achieved a degree of penetration that can be regarded as definitive.

The writing of full-scale biography has long reflected this general lack of sophistication. Only when experienced scholars have come in from other fields to undertake this has the standard been other than modest. The majestic study of John Ray by Raven (1942), surely one of the finest biographies in the English language of a major man of learning, came as a jolt in this respect. R.T. Gunther's (1922) resuscitation of another early figure, John Goodyer, out of mere jottings on odd scraps of paper was an earlier triumph of biographical detective work; and the recent double biography by his son (A.E. Gunther 1975) of two of the past Keepers of the British Museum maintains the family élan in this sphere.

Autobiographies of naturalists are far from numerous and on the whole not of the special value to the historian that they ought to be. Of considerably greater usefulness are published collections of their correspondence: of Linnaeus, for example, by Smith (1821); of Richard Richardson with most of the leading late seventeenth-century figures, by Turner (1835) and, in part, by Nichols (1817–58) too; of Ray, by Lankester (1848) and Gunther (1928); and of Banks, by Dawson (1958). To that fortunate Victorian taste for massive literary entombment we also owe a fair number of examples – though nothing like enough – of that peculiarly rich quarry, the posthumous 'life and letters'. Among the volumes in this genre are those by Smith (1832), Darwin (1887), Babington (1897), Huxley (1900) and (on the botanist Joseph Hooker) Huxley (1918). A reminder that these can nevertheless be deceptive in their richness is salutarily provided in those one or two cases where catalogues have been published of the correspondence in its true entirety. That of Smith's by Dawson (1934) is perhaps the most conspicuous example. In addition, as Browne (1978a) has emphasized in a paper specifically addressed to this point, volumes in the 'life and letters' mode are all too liable to contain errors of transcription and dating and their biographical sections to have been variously distorted in the course of composition. All badly stand in need of the type of searching scrutiny that is commonplace in literary criticism.

Invaluable though published listings like that of Dawson (1934) are, they amount to but the merest scratching on the surface of the vast nether world of non-printed material that survives in this field, much of it still virgin territory for historians. Because questions of nomenclature revolve around establishing priority in print, 'taxonomic archaeologists' have tended on the whole to ignore manuscript material. Natural history librarians, in response, have concerned themselves with printed matter either very largely or altogether exclusively. Now that enquirers after manuscripts show signs at last of becoming more numerous, the recently published results of a survey of the holdings in this respect of British libraries, archives and museums (Bridson, Phillips and Harvey 1980) come at a good moment and should set in train more, and better-directed, searching.

As if to quieten its conscience over the neglect it has long shown on this front, the natural history world has concentrated ever more intensely on its inheritance of books. The outstanding visual appeal of so much of the literature of the subject has long made it a favourite field of the bibliomane, and a special side-branch of connoisseurial scholarship has been called into being as a result. One of the earlier products of this was a bibliography of British ornithology by Mullens and Swann (1917) – appropriately, a leading book-collector and a leading dealer respectively, personifying an interdependence that has proved lastingly fruitful for learning. More recently has come the monumental, three-volume bibliography by Henrey (1975) of British botany and horticulture before 1800. The less ambitious handlist of British natural history up to 1900 published by Freeman (1980) conveniently complements this, while there are also bibliographies of vertebrate zoology (Wood 1931), British Lepidoptera (Lisney 1960) and British local botany (Simpson 1960) for those needing to wander into more specialized sectors. At the other extreme there is the introductory guide by Smit (1974), which ranges across the life sciences as a whole. Natural history illustration, a parallel vein of connoisseurship and not unimportant to historians of science in view of its intimate relationship with taxonomy, has also yielded authoritative surveys or bibliographies by Blunt (1950) and Nissen (1966) in the botanical field and by Anker (1938), Nissen (1953, 1969–78) and Knight (1977) in the zoological. The very many works illustrated by the Sowerby family have also been made the subject of a special bibliography by Cleevely (1974).

Though a great part of this work that lies outside the mainstream of the history of science consists of major, long-term undertakings predestined to appear as monographs, it gives rise to a considerable number of journal articles too. The main outlets for these are *Archives of Natural History* (formerly the *Journal of the Society for the Bibliography of Natural History*), the *Biological Journal of the Linnean Society* (formerly *Proceedings of the Linnean Society*) and the Historical Series of the *Bulletin of the British Museum (Natural History)*; for a period, *Annals of Science* served this function as well. Three other journals (apart from many more local ones) happy to play host to historical material reasonably often are the *Naturalist*, the *Irish Naturalists' Journal* and the *Entomologist's Record*. Articles that appear in such places may be liable to be missed by other historians, but they do have the compensating advantage that the journals may be among those that fall within the coverage of *Biological Abstracts*. Articles relating to British vascular plants are similarly liable to notice in *BSBI Abstracts* (published by the Botanical Society of the British Isles), which for many years has had a 'Historical' section. Brief though they usually are, entries in these are inherently more informative than the mere indexing of titles performed by the *Zoological Record*, the Wellcome Institute's *Current Work in the History of Medicine* and (for the most part) the *Isis Critical Bibliography*, all of which pick up at least a certain proportion of historical items in the natural history field on a regular basis. Far more comprehensive than any of these last were two checklists of current literature produced by Bridson and Harvey (1971, 1973), but these unfortunately have not continued.

The cast of mind of the taxonomist, the librarian and the book-collector is especially conducive to the compiling of indexes and lists but not, alas, to the writing of narrative history. Few general histories have consequently appeared. Indeed of botany there are none at all that are not mainly on its coming into being as an experimental science – unless an exception is made for the very early history by Pulteney (1790). Zoology is notably better covered, with good and recent histories of the pre-Linnean period (Petit and Théodoridès 1962), of ornithology (Stresemann 1951), of entomology (Smith, Mittler and Smith 1973), of ethology (Thorpe 1979), of early marine zoology (Rehbock 1979), and of conchology (Dance 1966). But for natural history as a whole – apart from studies of particular facets, like that of Sheail (1976) of the movement for nature conservation – there have so far been but two attempts at general accounts focused on Britain. That by Raven (1947), hardly the inferior in acumen and thoroughness of his great biography of Ray, regrettably covers the pre-1700 period only; the companion volume on more recent times that he is known to have projected never in the end materialized. His redoubtable strength in the history of ideas would have made this a very different work from the post-1700 general history that has subsequently appeared (Allen 1976). Strongly 'externalist' in its leanings, this concentrates on tracing the rise of an organizational structure and on delineating the social influences, more especially fashions, that have successively propelled the subject to and fro. It constitutes a first try at constructing a framework, of a necessarily very provisional kind, around which the mounting yield from research in this unfamiliarly amorphous (because largely atheoretical) field may be better able to cohere.

A social history approach has similarly been found useful by Lowe (1978) in studying the overall pattern of development of the nineteenth-century local societies. Lowe (1976) and Duff (1980) have gone even further and examined the early history of British ecology from a perspective that is explicitly sociological. Another recent instance of the impingement of social science methods is a monograph by Brockway (1979) in which the overseas role of Kew is considered as an exercise of 'botanical imperialism'.

A related trend, but with a more orthodox, purely historical pedigree, is the use of prosopography as a means of rendering membership lists less bleakly uninformative. In this field, as in most others, histories of societies have till only very recently typically been lacking in incisiveness, ranging from the excessively discreet to the flabbily episodic. That of the Linnean Society by Gage (1938) is perhaps the best of a generally disappointing shelf-ful. Other types of institution have fared hardly better, though at the Royal Botanic Garden, Edinburgh, a long and exceptional tradition of scholarly enquiry into its unusually complicated roots has been brought by Fletcher and Brown (1970) to a befitting culmination. The April 1980 number of the *Journal of the Society for the Bibliography of Natural History* (Vol. 9, Part 4), in which appear the fruits of an international conference on the history of museums, zoos and related institutions, suggests a widening reinvigoration is in prospect.

The advent of prosopography is symptomatic of a new wave of deeper analysis to which a variety of these institutions is being submitted. First employed by Allen (1967) to reconstruct a small, obscure society in the early eighteenth century, the technique is currently being brought to bear on the only slightly less obscure Botanical Society of London, some first results from which are just appearing (Allen 1981). An unusual feature is that these results have been derived in part from information obtained from old herbarium labels – an example of how the inherently antique procedures of taxonomy itself offer useful extra possibilities in this direction. Another way in which the subject's special assets might profitably be exploited by historians would be to put some of its many excellent bibliographical and biographical reference works to auxiliary use as quarries of numerical trend data. A primitive start towards this has been made by Allen (1969: 48,59) as a means of plotting the year-by-year oscillations of the mid-Victorian fern craze. Other steps towards quantification, using more conventional sources, have been made by Lowe (1978) and, more particularly, Beirne (1955). Much more such work is badly needed.

This gradual baring of the institutional and social skeleton, with the aid of instruments appropriate to the very different nature of the subject matter, carries the promise of a comprehensive and well-articulated structure that can substitute for the one built out of theory to which historians are accustomed in other areas of science. For, despite the central position occupied by evolutionary theory in modern systematics, it must be evident that this cannot serve as a sufficient organizing principle inasmuch as its reach scarcely extends, if at all, to many of the subject's most populous corners. Natural history, inconveniently, is an area of cultural behaviour rather than a network of ideas. So dominant has been the 'great ideas' tradition in Anglo-American history of science in the last three decades, however, that academic work in this area has nevertheless been confined more or less exclusively to investigating the genesis and impact of major theory. The shortage of obvious topics has resulted in a great ponding-up of interest in Darwin studies – which, if Greene (1975: 272) is right, is due to go on mounting for a long, long time to come. In the rain-shadow of Darwin studies other figures on the evolutionary landscape – from Wallace and Huxley, Lamarck and Cuvier, down to the entirely overlooked Edward Blyth – have one by one been coming in for a sprinkling of attention; and very recently a trickle of interest has begun to spread still further into such hitherto historical deserts as biogeography (Kinch 1974; Fichman 1977; Nelson 1978; Browne 1978b; Egerton 1980), ecology (Egerton and McIntosh 1977; Worster 1977; Lowe and Worboys 1980) and the theoretical aspects of taxonomy itself (Winsor 1969, 1976; Sloan 1972, 1979;

Farber 1972; Dean 1979, 1980). As evidence of the strength of the current now flowing in this quarter, a new and further crop of specialist research aids (Barrett 1977; Egerton 1977) shows signs of springing up to serve the needs of those who pursue this alternative approach. But it still remains to be seen whether we are moving towards a confluence that will endure, with a great strengthening and enriching as a result of the pre-existing stream of social history intermixed with 'taxonomic archaeology', or whether this outburst of attention is no more than a temporary flash-flood, to be followed by a withdrawal of academic energy to some other, more amenable terrain.

Bibliography

Allen, D.E. (1967). John Martyn's Botanical Society: A Biographical Analysis of the Membership, *Proceedings of the Botanical Society of the British Isles*, Vol. 6, 305–324

Allen, D.E. (1969). *The Victorian Fern Craze: a History of Pteridomania*. London; Hutchinson

Allen, D.E. (1976). *The Naturalist in Britain: a Social History*. London; Allen Lane

Allen, D.E. (1977). Naturalists in Britain: Some Tasks for the Historian, *Journal of the Society for the Bibliography of Natural History*, Vol. 8, 91–107

Allen, D.E. (1981). The Women Members of the Botanical Society of London, 1836–56, *British Journal for the History of Science*, Vol. 13, 240–254

Anker, J. (1938). *Bird Books and Bird Art: an Outline of the Literary History and Iconography of Descriptive Ornithology*. Copenhagen; Levin and Munksgaard

B[abington], A.M., Ed. (1897). *Memorials, Journal and Botanical Correspondence of Charles Cardale Babington...* Cambridge; Macmillan and Bowes

Barnhart, J.H. (1965). *Biographical Notes upon Botanists*. Boston, Mass.; Hall

Barrett, P.H., Ed. (1977). *The Collected Papers of Charles Darwin*. Chicago; Chicago University Press

Beirne, B.P. (1955). Fluctuations in Quantity of Work in British Insects, *Entomologist's Gazette*, Vol. 6, 7–9

Blunt, W. (1950). *The Art of Botanical Illustration*. London; Collins

Boivin, B. (1977). A Basic Bibliography of Botanical Biography and a Proposal for a More Elaborate Bibliography, *Taxon*, Vol. 26, 75–105

Bridson, G. and Harvey, A.P. (1971). A Checklist of Natural History Bibliographies and Bibliographical Scholarship, 1966–1970, *Journal of the Society for the Bibliography of Natural History*, Vol. 5, 428–467

Bridson, G. and Harvey, A.P. (1973). A Checklist of Natural History Bibliographies and Bibliographical Scholarship, 1970–71, *Journal of the Society for the Bibliography of Natural History*, Vol. 6, 263–292

Bridson, G.D.R., Phillips, V.C. and Harvey, A.P. (1980). *Natural History Manuscript Resources in the British Isles*. London; Mansell

Bristowe, W.S. (1967). The Life and Work of a Great English Naturalist, Joseph Dandridge (1664–1746), *Entomologist's Gazette*, Vol. 18, 73–89

Britten, J. and Boulger, G.S. (1893–1908). *A Biographical Index of British and Irish Botanists*. London; Taylor and Francis

Brockway, L.H. (1979). *Science and Colonial Expansion: the Role of the British Royal Botanic Gardens*. New York and London; Academic Press

Browne, J. (1978a). The Charles Darwin–Joseph Hooker Correspondence: an Analysis of Manuscript Resources and their Use in Biography, *Journal of the Society for the Bibliography of Natural History*, Vol. 8, 351–366

Browne, J. (1978b). C.R. Darwin and J.D. Hooker: Episodes in the History of Plant Geography, Imperial College, London University PhD Dissertation

Chalmers-Hunt, J.M. (1976). *Natural History Auctions, 1700–1972: a Register of Sales in the British Isles.* London; Sotheby Parke Bernet

Christy, M. (1919). Samuel Dale (1659?–1739), of Braintree, Botanist, and the Dale Family: Some Genealogy and Some Portraits, *Essex Naturalist*, Vol. 19, 49–69

Cleevely, R.J. (1974). A Provisional Bibliography of Natural History Works by the Sowerby Family, *Journal of the Society for the Bibliography of Natural History*, Vol. 6, 482–559

Clokie, H.N. (1964). *An Account of the Herbaria of the Department of Botany in the University of Oxford.* Oxford; Oxford University Press

Dance, S.P. (1966). *Shell Collecting. An Illustrated History.* London; Faber

Dandy, J.E., Ed. (1958). *The Sloane Herbarium.* London; British Museum (Natural History)

Darwin, F., Ed. (1887). *The Life and Letters of Charles Darwin, Including an Autobiographical Chapter.* 3 Vols. London; Murray

Dawson, W.R. (1934). *Catalogue of the Manuscripts in the Library of the Linnean Society of London. Part I. – The Smith Papers.* London; Linnean Society

Dawson, W.R., Ed. (1958). *The Banks Letters.* London; British Museum (Natural History)

Dean, J. (1979). Controversy over Classification: a Case Study from the History of Botany, in *Natural Order: Historical Studies of Scientific Culture.* Ed. B. Barnes and S. Shapin. Beverly Hills; Sage Publications, 211–230

Dean, J. (1980). A Naturalistic Model of Classification and its Relevance to Some Controversies in Botanical Systematics, 1900–1950, University of Edinburgh PhD Dissertation

Desmond, R. (1977). *Dictionary of British and Irish Botanists and Horticulturists, Including Plant Collectors and Botanical Artists.* London; Taylor and Francis.

Duff, A. (1980). National Styles of Scientific Research: the Early History of Ecology in Britain and the U.S.A., University of Manchester PhD Dissertation

Egerton, F.N. (1977). A Bibliographic Guide to the History of General Ecology and Population Ecology, *History of Science*, Vol. 15, 189–215

Egerton, F.N. (1980). Hewett C. Watson, Great Britain's First Phytogeographer, *Huntia*, Vol. 3, 87–102

Egerton, F.N. and McIntosh, R.P., Ed. (1977). *History of American Ecology.* New York; Arno Press

Farber, P.L. (1972). Buffon and the Concept of Species, *Journal of the History of Biology*, Vol. 5, 259–284

Fichman, M. (1977). Wallace: Zoogeography and the Problem of Land Bridges, *Journal of the History of Biology*, Vol. 10, 45–63

Fletcher, H.R. and Brown, W.H. (1970). *The Royal Botanic Garden, Edinburgh, 1670–1970.* London; HMSO

Freeman, R.B. (1980). *British Natural History Books, 1495–1900. A Handlist.* London; Dawson

Gage, A.T. (1938). *A History of the Linnean Society of London.* London; Linnean Society

Gilbert, P. (1977). *A Compendium of the Biographical Literature on Deceased Entomologists.* London; British Museum (Natural History)

Greene, J.C. (1975). Reflections on the Progress of Darwin Studies, *Journal of the History of Biology*, Vol. 8, 243–274

Gunther, A.E. (1975). *A Century of Zoology at the British Museum through the Lives of Two Keepers, 1815–1914.* London; Dawson

Gunther, R.T. (1922). *Early British Botanists and their Gardens.* Oxford; Oxford University Press

Gunther, R.T., Ed. (1928). *Further Correspondence of John Ray.* London; Ray Society

Henrey, B. (1975). *British Botanical and Horticultural Literature Before 1800.* 3 Vols. London; Oxford University Press

Hunt Botanical Library (1972). *Biographical Dictionary of Botanists Represented in the Hunt Institute Portrait Collection.* Boston, Mass.; Hall

Huxley, L., Ed. (1900). *Life and Letters of Thomas Henry Huxley.* 2 Vols. London; Macmillan

Huxley, L., Ed. (1918). *Life and Letters of Sir Joseph Dalton Hooker.* London; Murray

Jeffers, R.H. (1967). *The Friends of John Gerard (1545–1612): Surgeon and Botanist.* Falls Village, Conn.; Grower Press

Kent, D.H. (1958). *British Herbaria: an Index to the Location of Herbaria of British Vascular Plants.* London; Botanical Society of the British Isles

Kinch, M. (1974). An Assessment of Rival British Theories of Biogeography, 1800–1859, Oregon State University MA Dissertation

Knight, D.M. (1977). *Zoological Illustration: an Essay towards a History of Printed Zoological Pictures.* Folkestone; Dawson

Lankester, E., Ed. (1848). *The Correspondence of John Ray.* London; Ray Society

Lisney, A.A. (1960). *A Bibliography of British Lepidoptera 1608–1799.* London; Chiswick Press

Lowe, P.D. (1976). Amateurs and Professionals: the Institutional Emergence of British Plant Ecology, *Journal of the Society for the Bibliography of Natural History*, Vol. 7, 517–535

Lowe, P.D. (1978). Locals and Cosmopolitans: a Model for the Social Organisation of Provincial Science in the Nineteenth Century, University of Sussex MPhil Dissertation

Lowe, P.D. and Worboys, M. (1980). Ecology as Ideology, in *Rural Sociology of the Advanced Societies.* Ed. S. Buttel and H. Newby. New Jersey; Allanheld Osmun

Mullens, W.H. and Swann, H.K. (1917). *A Bibliography of British Ornithology from the Earliest Times to the End of 1912.* London; Macmillan

Nelson, G. (1978). From Candolle to Croizat: Comments on the History of Biogeography, *Journal of the History of Biology*, Vol. 11, 269–305

Nichols, J. (1817–58). *Illustrations of the Literary History of the Eighteenth Century.* London; the author

Nissen, C. (1953). *Die illustrierten Vogelbücher: ihre Geschichte und Bibliographie.* Stuttgart; Hiersemann

Nissen, C. (1966). *Die botanische Buchillustration: ihre Geschichte und Bibliographie.* Stuttgart; Hiersemann

Nissen, C. (1969–78). *Die zoologische Buchillustration:ihre Geschichte und Bibliographie.* Stuttgart; Hiersemann

Petit, G. and Théodoridès, J. (1962). *Histoire de la zoologie des origines à Linné.* Paris; Hermann

Pulteney, R. (1790). *Historical and Biographical Sketches of the Progress of Botany in England from its Origin to the Introduction of the Linnaean System.* London; Cadell

Raven, C.E. (1942). *John Ray, Naturalist; His Life and Works.* Cambridge; Cambridge University Press

Raven, C.E. (1947). *English Naturalists from Neckam to Ray*. Cambridge; Cambridge University Press

Rehbock, P.F. (1979). The Early Dredgers: 'Naturalizing' in British Seas, 1830–1850, *Journal of the History of Biology*, Vol. 12, 293–368

Sheail, J. (1976). *Nature in Trust: the History of Nature Conservation in Britain*. Glasgow and London; Blackie

Sherborn, C.D. (1940). *Where is the ----- Collection?* Cambridge; Cambridge University Press

Simpson, N.D. (1960). *A Bibliographical Index of the British Flora*. Bournemouth; the author

Sloan, P.R. (1972). John Locke, John Ray, and the Problem of the Natural System, *Journal of the History of Biology*, Vol. 5, 1–53

Sloan, P.R. (1979). Buffon, German Biology, and the Historical Interpretation of Biological Species, *British Journal for the History of Science*, Vol. 12, 109–153

Smit, P. (1974). *History of the Life Sciences: an Annotated Bibliography*. Amsterdam; Asher

Smith, J.E. (1821). *A Selection of the Correspondence of Linnaeus and Other Naturalists*. London; Longman

Smith, P., Ed. (1832). *Memoir and Correspondence of the late Sir James Edward Smith, M.D.* London; Longman

Smith, R.F., Mittler, T.E. and Smith, C.N., Ed. (1973). *History of Entomology*. Palo Alto; Annual Reviews

Stresemann, E. (1951). *Die Entwicklung der Ornithologie von Aristoteles bis zur Gegenwart*. Berlin; F.W. Peters

Thorpe, W.H. (1979). *The Origins and Rise of Ethology. The Science of the Natural Behaviour of Animals*. London; Heinemann Educational. New York; Praeger

Trimen, H. and Dyer, W.T.T. (1869). *Flora of Middlesex*. London; Hardwicke

Turner, D., Ed. (1835). *Extracts from the Literary and Scientific Correspondence of Richard Richardson...* Yarmouth; the author

Whitehead, P.J.P. (1969). Zoological Specimens from Captain Cook's Voyages, *Journal of the Society for the Bibliography of Natural History*, Vol. 5, 161–201

Winsor, M.P. (1969). Barnacle Larvae in the Nineteenth Century: a Case Study in Taxonomic Theory, *Journal of the History of Medicine*, Vol. 24, 294–309

Winsor, M.P. (1976). *Starfish, Jellyfish, and the Order of Life: Issues in Nineteenth-Century Science*. New Haven and London; Yale University Press

Wood, C.A. (1931). *An Introduction to the Literature of Vertebrate Zoology*. London; Oxford University Press

Worster, D. (1977). *Nature's Economy: the Roots of Ecology*. San Francisco; Sierra Club

18

Experimentalism and the life sciences since 1800

Margaret Pelling

The term 'biology', distinguishing and cohering the study of matter endowed with life, came into use in the early nineteenth century. The term's origins are now obscured. Early uses by Roose and Burdach were followed by Treviranus and by Lamarck, as well as by Comte. The connotation that has persisted reflects not the wholeness of life but rather the conviction that the functions of plants, animals and man, and even the attributes thought peculiar to man or to the soul, could be analysed (by man) using the same modes of explanation as the physical sciences. This programme, although interpreted in various degrees, continues to the present day. The development of biology is commonly divided into three phases: the exploratory or taxonomic, the organic (anatomy and physiology), and the molecular or analytic (see e.g. Beck 1958). Hall (1969) gives a similar sequence in terms of the history of ideas. Biologists concerned for the status of their discipline (and historians of biology, see e.g. Mendelsohn 1964b) were reassured by the reflection that, however belatedly, biology had also had its revolutions, equivalent to those of Newton and Einstein: first the Darwinian, and then molecular biology, the triumph of reductionism, which is beginning to find historians (Stent 1969; Olby 1974; Judson 1979; Bearman and Edsall 1980).

Within this tradition most stress is placed on aspects of the scientific method, especially experimentalism, quantification and the definition of standard units (Harré 1969). The analysis of function is given precedence over that of structure; hence experimentation in physiology is perhaps the largest single subject category in modern historical writing on the biological sciences (e.g. Fulton 1931; Rothschuh 1953; Wightman 1956; Brooks and Cranefield 1959; Goodfield 1960; Mendelsohn 1964a, 1965; Schröer 1967; Rapp 1970; Schiller and Schiller 1975; see also chapter 19 below). Medical historians also contribute largely to this literature (see chapter 19 below), because of the status physiology is thought to give to medicine (Bernard 1865; Olmsted 1944; Olmsted and Olmsted 1952). Faber (1923) was a significant attempt to extend experimental status even to the clinical side of medicine, a project that was not uncontroversial. Younger life sciences seek to follow the same path as physiology and biochemistry (Paoloni 1968; Florkin 1972–7; Fruton 1972; Holmes 1974; Kohler 1975; Teich 1980); thus, in a historically based discussion of current research problems in psychology (Postman 1962), the different authors date the history of their research interest from the first experimental approaches to it, consider the difficulties of experimental control and the need to replace or bring into the laboratory old, philosophical categories such as 'reason' and 'imagination', and regret the absence of agreed basic units. Psychology has received a great deal of attention not only through anthropocentrism but also because of the various forms of resistance to the realization of these aims (e.g. Murphy 1928; Murchison 1930–52; Hamlyn 1961; Herrnstein and Boring 1965). Neurology has increasingly emerged as a historical interest, as it promised an experimental if not material basis for activity and coordination, response and behaviour (Frolov 1937; Canguilhem 1955; Gordon-Taylor and Walls 1958; Liddell 1960; Granit 1966; Young 1970; Cranefield 1974).

No single science of biology is any longer recognizable. Fragmentation into sub-disciplines began early and attempts are now made to supply coherence by groupings such as 'life sciences' or the 'behavioural sciences' (Young 1966). A survey textbook emphasizing accessibility, such as Allen (1975), finds little difficulty however in observing a hierarchy in which modern embryology, genetics, evolution, general physiology, biochemistry and molecular biology are given prominence at the expense of such areas as immunology (see Parish 1965), protozoology, bacteriology (see below), ecology (see chapter 19 below), palaeontology (d'Archiac 1847–60; Bowler 1976; Rudwick 1972), ethology (Tinbergen 1951; Klopfer and Hailman 1967), psychology, and anthropology (Penniman 1935; Hodgen 1964; see also below), and the movements arising from these (for example genetical engineering, eugenics, environmentalism, behaviourism). To the observer, the life sciences appear not as a unity but as a pyramid with molecular biology at the apex, sharing the same rarefied atmosphere as modern physics. However, in spite of chronic concern about lack of communication and overspecialization, other parts of the pyramid claim their own justification as specialisms emerging with the increase of knowledge, the acquisition of institutional or professional status, and the application of scientific methods (Hughes 1959, cytology; Penniman 1935, anthropology; Dunn 1965, genetics; Thorpe 1979, ethology; etc.). Histories of specialisms therefore appear in the life sciences as in medicine (see below, chapter 19). Similarly, blameless histories are written of the fruits of the experimental method in areas of practical importance (e.g. McCollum 1957 on nutrition; cf. the broader approach of Blake 1970 on drug safety).

This justificatory line of interpretation has inevitably produced obvious areas of neglect or distortion. As David Allen (chapter 17, p.349) points out, except in relation to Darwinism (Ghiselin 1969; Bowler 1976; Dagognet 1970), the 'descriptive' phases of biology have been reduced to a preliminary, and robbed of intellectual content. Fieldwork and laboratory science have been reclassified as essentially different activities, one 'soft', the other 'hard', in spite of such obvious institutional phenomena as the marine research stations (Lillie 1944; *Colloque international* 1965; Groeben and Müller 1975). Museums are under-recognized as research institutions. Similarly, more attention is given to work carried out on vertebrates or on man than on invertebrates and unicellular organisms (Metchnikoff 1892; Zeiss 1932). Botany, zoology, mineralogy, meteorology and palaeontology have been submerged, often to surface as suitable subjects for study only by historians of Victorian popular taste. The descriptive sciences of man (see above; also Prichard 1813; Weber 1974) have not suffered in this way. Only bacteriology revived the claims of descriptive knowledge, although experimental aspects are now emphasized (Dagognet 1967). The biases of most twentieth-century historians contrast sharply with the historical surveys of areas such as zoology and botany produced by practitioners like Cuvier, de Blainville, Milne Edwards and Geoffroy St Hilaire, and later by Meyer and Carus, as well as with Whewell's unified view of the inductive sciences (1837). There are recent exceptions to this (e.g. Foucault 1966; Farber 1976; Balan 1979; Jordanova and Porter 1979). *A fortiori*, the definition of 'fundamental issues' as the first priority not only lowers the claims of certain subject areas and introduces the danger of anachronism, but justifies the postponement, often to an indefinite period, of any consideration of science's interactions with society.

Biologists themselves have contributed largely and sometimes uncritically to the historical version of this tradition. However biology, being concerned with birth, life and death, and such concepts as growth and development, has within it a historical tendency, at times strongly developed (Temkin 1950) or a matter of debate (Burckhardt 1907b). Biologists have produced much historical writing imbued with a strong sense of purpose, and prominent biologists have become respected historians (for example,) Needham 1931 and Cole 1930, 1944). Practitioners have written to clarify the aims of their subjects (Delage 1895; Thompson 1917); to assert the claims of a particular approach or line of development (von Sachs 1875, botany; Driesch 1914, vitalism; Russell 1930, development; Baker 1948–55, cell theory; Needham 1931 and Oppenheimer 1967, embryology); to improve the image of the biological sciences with the public (Beck 1958); to fulfil a perceived duty of communication (Woodworth 1931, psychology; Conant and Nash 1957); to adjust public expectations to a realistic level (Galdston 1943, chemotherapy); or to make connections with the results of research and public concern (for recent examples see Goodfield 1975, on cancer; Goodfield 1977, on genetic engineering). Others claim historical sophistication as a necessary attribute for experimental research (Boring 1929, 1942, psychology). Many biologists produced, often in later life, works of a more 'speculative' nature, testifying to underlying concerns and to the reality of their interest in issues usually omitted from professional publications (see, for example, Eccles and Gibson 1979, for Sherrington's *Man on his Nature*). The successes of reductionism regularly caused reactions in biologists themselves. Beck (1958) found that his colleagues, repelled by the progressive depersonalizing of nature, were falling prey to degraded forms of supernaturalism, and wrote of the broader issues in the sciences of life to restore to true science its sense of adventure.

Of great value are those reflective works, sometimes of considerable philosophical acuity, that were written to urge a reconsideration of fundamental problems at a time of crisis (Rádl 1909–13; Russell 1916; Woodger 1929; Mainx 1955). Such works show an awareness of the historical as well as the philosophical dimensions of many problems in biology, together with a recognition not only of historical continuity but of the cyclic rather than linear mode of discourse within the subject area so defined. Such studies are often avowedly partisan. Many of their authors were interested in reviving the claims of trends of thought condemned as vitalistic. Of these the most widely respected is Russell (1916). This has proved difficult to supersede; Coleman (1971) is an attempt at popularization. Russell's study of morphology may be compared with that of Crow (1929), who considered that Russell had underestimated the influence of Goethe (Lewes 1855; von Aesch 1941) and the Darwinist Haeckel (Bölsche 1900).

Twentieth-century biologists have readily turned to philosophers of science to support or rationalize their various positions. Recent commentators have urged the claims of the philosophy of biology within the philosophy of science (Grene and Mendelsohn 1976). Beck and others explained the tendencies of the present century in biology as an effect of the scientization of philosophy itself, which had rejected absolutes in favour of logical empiricism and the study of language (see also the autobiographical Dewey 1930). Not necessarily desirable for either biology or the history of biology was the twentieth century's unconscious identification of epistemology with the scientific method, since this led to a failure to recognize that the modern causal mode of explanation was only one of a number of options. Less than justice has been done to those philosophical aspects of biology that are difficult to divorce from social and political events. Within the experimental tradition, historians have chiefly praised the weapons developed by Magendie and elevated by his pupil Bernard (Olmsted 1939, 1944; Olmsted and Olmsted 1952; Schiller 1967; Grmek 1967, 1973; Holmes 1974; Roll-Hansen 1976), although periodically there is significant disagreement over what Bernard meant by 'general physiology' (e.g. Fulton 1931). The emphasis is on methods, schools and discoveries, notwithstanding that Temkin and Olmsted have pointed decisively to the broader political and philosophical relations of French as well as German physiology.

Anglo-Saxon historians have found French developments easier to assimilate than the German, and the influence of the Romantic school and *Naturphilosophie* has been understated, interpreted entirely in the negative sense, or seen as having only the most fortuitous connection with the evolution of the biological sciences. More recently, historians of biology have turned from the disparagement of vitalism to the cautious exploration of shades of opinion and areas of compromise (Hirschfeld 1930; Temkin 1946a; Rothschuh 1953; Mendelsohn 1965; Maulitz 1971; Benton 1974; Culotta 1975; Lenoir 1978, 1980). Major studies of Romanticism (von Aesch 1941) and materialism (Gregory 1977) have been produced, significantly in series devoted to Germanic studies and the history of modern science respectively. As in the case of debates concerning the Puritan Revolution of the seventeenth century, or conflicts between religion and science in the nineteenth (see chapter 1 above), there is the danger that a simplistic account in terms of polarities will be modified only in the cause either of 'latitudinarianism' or of interpretations convinced of the common appreciation of sober scientific fact by rational men of good will.

Schleiden, Henle (Robinson 1921; Rosen 1937) and Virchow are all major, well-known figures, whose range of interests and activities was nonetheless obscured by the influence of political factors. Ackerknecht's study of Virchow (1953) was seen by its author as the first full-length study in any language. Writing during the Cold War, Ackerknecht viewed his subject as the perfect type of the liberal intellectual scientist, universalist and individualist, whose influence was depreciated by both past Nazi and present Soviet regimes. This account may be contrasted with Ackerknecht's pre-war Marxist analysis of the 1848 medical reform movement in which Virchow was prominent (1932). The scientist Virchow has now become a dominant figure (Virchow 1858, 1959), casting into the shade the achievements of contemporaries such as Remak (Kisch 1954). Werskey's collective biography (1978) of J.B.S. Haldane, Hogben, Levy, Bernal and Needham is a reminder of the political commitments of modern scientists.

The historiography of genetics provides a major case study of the interaction of politics and biological science. Historians of science continue to be puzzled by Mendel (Iltis 1924; *Folia Mendeliana* 1966–), his comparative isolation and rediscovery. Later discoveries, however, present few problems of interpretation (Allen 1978). For the geneticist Dunn, modern genetics was perhaps the clearest example among the biological sciences of how scientific knowledge evolves, and thus an example that deserved to establish the credit of biology with physicists (1965). But geneticists were currently working without historical perspective, and a lay public, excited by the inordinately rapid progress of molecular genetics, was unaware that the subject had a history before 1944. Dunn wished to restore an intellectual perspective to the history of genetics that included the central problems in biology, but criticized Barthelmess (1952) for equating genetics with heredity and thus for tracing his subject back before the beginnings of modern science. These firm outlines, and the subject's 'factual foundations', are stressed in Dunn's earlier treatment (1951), written in the context of the Russian outlawing of Mendelian genetics (Hudson and Richens 1946; Medvedev 1969; Joravsky 1970). Another geneticist, Zirkle, produced first a study of plant hybridization (1935; Roberts 1929 is superior), then statements on the relations of politics, science and society (e.g. 1959), and lastly collaborated on a history of biology (Sirks and Zirkle 1964). Western geneticists have been able to denounce the interaction of science and politics as a dangerous aberration; that such interaction in modern science is the exception rather than the rule is the implication of the interest taken by historians in the eugenics movement (see e.g. Farrall 1970; Ludmerer 1972; Searle 1976). The geneticists' histories have helped to create a climate of opinion in which issues raised by the possibility of 'genetic engineering' will be discussed. A recent study of the influence of politics in the funding of medical research (Brown 1979) has aroused considerable hostility. It is nonetheless plain that the modern socio-biological debates reflect an intimacy of relation between biology and society equal to that of their nineteenth-century counterparts (Webster 1981).

With respect to British literature and British subjects, the overriding emphasis has been on Darwin and Darwinism (Fleming 1959; Loewenberg 1965; Ruse 1974; see also chapter 17 above). Rádl observed in 1930 that, at a time when Einstein had replaced Darwin in the mind of the laity and the revolutionary implications of Darwinism for society, politics, philosophy and religion had long faded, the natural sciences continued to dominate Anglo-Saxon intellectual life. Rádl added the rider that the British were in general more interested in what he regarded as technical applications than in the pure sciences. Rádl's views are typical of the scientist–historians, although his Continental stereotype of the British as unphilosophical might be contradicted. J.D. Watson condemned British botanists and zoologists of the 1950s as wasting their time in useless polemics about the origins of life (Watson 1968). Emphases such as Rádl's are now being challenged by rather different perspectives. The role of Darwinism in the loss of religious faith becomes less if it is established that faith itself was less universal, more diverse than was assumed; or if a case can be made out for the influence of other factors in the popularization of materialism, for example phrenology or freethinking. So far, however, the prevailing historiography has introduced diversity only by connecting Darwinism itself with social, political and economic factors (Burrow 1966), or, more commonly, by placing beside Darwin a range of similar deities, such as Charles Lyell, or by asserting the claims of precursors (Glass *et al.* 1959). There is little appreciation even of such complex and accomplished figures as Darwin's opponent Richard Owen (Owen 1894). More balanced perspectives have been suggested by Temkin (1963) or Young (1969); see also chapter 1 above.

The institutional development of laboratory science in England was long delayed (Temkin 1963; see Erman and Horn 1904–5; Sharpey-Schafer 1927; d'Irsay 1933–5; Needham and Baldwin 1949; Bynum n.d., Gougher 1969; Geison 1978). Proper attention has nonetheless been paid to one of its social dimensions, the anti-vivisection movement (Stevenson 1956; French 1975). The British failure to produce institutes has robbed of notice even formally organized series of investigations; of the researchers connected with the Medical Department of the Privy Council from the mid-1850s, only the later careers of John Burdon Sanderson (Sanderson 1911) and J.L.W. Thudichum (Drabkin 1958) have received any attention, except in Lambert (1963). Research conducted on an individual basis is appreciated only in terms of results, as in the case of Charles Bell. The historians of experimentalism have yet to assess the activity of a large number of minor British experimentalists of the first half of the nineteenth century, such as R.D. Grainger. Those not directly concerned in the experimental tradition, but greatly respected by contemporaries – such as the mycologist the Revd Miles Berkeley (Ainsworth 1976), the botanist Frederick Orpen Bower or the early ecologist Arthur George Tansley – will have longer to wait, as will areas of development of great economic importance but considered outside the intellectual arena (or beyond the social pale), such as agriculture (Hall 1905; Russell 1966; Fussell 1971; see especially Orwin and Whetham 1964; Rossiter 1975) and veterinary science.

Bibliography

Ackerknecht, E.H. (1932). Beiträge zur Geschichte der Medizinalreform von 1848, *Sudhoffs Archiv*, Vol. 25, 61–109, 113–183

Ackerknecht, E.H. (1953). *Rudolf Virchow: Doctor, Statesman, Anthropologist.* Madison; University of Wisconsin

Aesch, A.G.F. Gode-von (1941). *Natural Science in German Romanticism.* New York; Columbia University Press

Ainsworth, G.C. (1976). *Introduction to the History of Mycology.* Cambridge; Cambridge University Press

Allen, G.E. (1975). *Life Science in the Twentieth Century.* New York; J. Wiley

Allen, G.E. (1978). *Thomas Hunt Morgan. The Man and His Science.* Princeton, NJ; Princeton University Press

d'Archiac, A. (1847–60). *Histoire des progrès de la géologie de 1834 à 1859.* 8 Vols. Paris; Société géologique de France

Baker, J.R. (1948–55). The Cell Theory: a Restatement, History and Critique, *Quarterly Journal of Microscopical Science*, Vol. 89, 103–125; Vol. 90, 87–108, 331; Vol. 93, 157–190; Vol. 94, 407–440; Vol. 96, 449–481

Balan, B. (1979). *L'Ordre et le temps. L'anatomie comparée et l'histoire des vivants au XIXe siècle.* Paris; J. Vrin

Barthelmess, A. (1952). *Vererbungswissenschaft.* Orbis Academicus Problemgeschichten. Freiburg and Munich; Karl Alber

Bearman, D. and Edsall, J.T., Ed. (1980). *Archival Sources for the History of Biochemistry and Molecular Biology. A Reference Guide and Report.* 1 Vol and microfiche supplement. Boston, Mass.; American Academy of Arts and Sciences. Philadelphia; The American Philosophical Society

Beck, W.S. (1958). *Modern Science and the Nature of Life.* London; Macmillan

Benton, E. (1974). Vitalism in Nineteenth Century Scientific Thought: A Typology and Reassessment, *Studies in the History and Philosophy of Science*, Vol. 5, 17–48

Bernard, C. (1865). *Introduction à l'étude de la médecine expérimentale.* Paris; Baillière. Trans. H.C. Green, introd. L.J. Henderson (1927). New York; Macmillan. New edn (1957). New York; Dover

Blacker, C.P. (1952). *Eugenics, Galton and After.* London; Duckworth

Blake, J.B., Ed. (1970). *Safeguarding the Public: Historical Aspects of Medicinal Drug Control.* Baltimore and London; Johns Hopkins University Press

Boardman, P. (1978). *The Worlds of Patrick Geddes. Biologist, Town Planner, Re-educator, Peace-warrior.* London; Routledge and Kegan Paul

Bölsche, C.E.W. (1900). *Ernst Haeckel. Ein Lebensbild.* Dresden and Leipzig; H. Seeman. Trans. J. McCabe (1906). London; T. Fisher Unwin. New edn (1909) issued for the Rationalist Press Association. London; Watts and Co.

Boring, E.G. (1929). *A History of Experimental Psychology.* New York and London; The Century Co. Repr. [1931]. 2nd edn (1950). New York; Appleton-Century-Crofts

Boring, E.G. (1942). *Sensation and Perception in the History of Experimental Psychology.* New York; D. Appleton-Century

Boring, E.G. (1961). *Psychologist at Large: An Autobiography and Selected Essays.* New York; Basic Books

Bowler, P.J. (1976). *Fossils and Progress. Paleontology and the Idea of Progressive Evolution in the Nineteenth Century.* New York; Science History Publications

Brooks, C.McC. and Cranefield, P.F., Ed. (1959). *The Historical Development of Physiological Thought: A Symposium.* New York; Hafner

Brown, E.R. (1979). *Rockefeller Medicine Men: Medicine and Capitalism in America.* Berkeley; University of California Press

Burckhardt, K.R. (1907a). *Geschichte der Zoologie.* Leipzig; G.J. Göschen. 2nd edn (1921). Ed. H. Erhard. Berlin; de Gruyter

Burckhardt, K.R. (1907b). *Biologie und Humanismus. Drei Reden.* Jena; E. Diederichs

Burkhardt, R.W., Jr. (1977). *The Spirit of System. Lamarck and Evolutionary Biology.* Cambridge, Mass. and London; Harvard University Press

Burrow, J.W. (1966). *Evolution and Society: A Study in Victorian Social Theory.* London; Cambridge University Press. Reprinted (1974)

Bynum, W.F. (n.d.). *A Short History of the Physiological Society 1926–1976.* [London]; the Society

Canguilhem, G. (1952). *La Connaissance de la vie.* Paris; Librairie Hachette. 2nd edn (1965). Paris; J. Vrin. Reprinted (1969)

Canguilhem, G. (1955). *La Formation du concept de réflexe aux XVIIe et XVIIIe siècles.* Paris; Presses Universitaires de France

Canguilhem, G. (1970). *Études d'histoire et de philosophie des sciences.* Paris; J. Vrin

Cannon, W.B. (1945). *The Way of an Investigator. A Scientist's Experiences in Medical Research.* New York; W.W. Norton

Carlson, E.A. (1966). *The Gene: A Critical History.* Philadelphia and London; W.B. Saunders

Carpenter, W.B. (1888). *Nature and Man. Essays Scientific and Philosophical.* London; Kegan Paul, Trench and Co. Republished (1970). Farnborough, Hants; Gregg International

Cole, F.J. (1930). *Early Theories of Sexual Generation.* Oxford; Clarendon Press

Cole, F.J. (1944). *A History of Comparative Anatomy from Aristotle to the Eighteenth Century.* London; Macmillan. 2nd edn (1949)

Coleman, W. (1964). *Georges Cuvier, Zoologist. A Study in the History of Evolution Theory.* Cambridge, Mass.; Harvard University Press

Coleman, W. (1971). *Biology in the Nineteenth Century: Problems of Form, Function and Transformation.* New York; John Wiley. Paperback edn (1977). Cambridge; Cambridge University Press

Colloque international sur l'histoire de la biologie marine. Les grandes expéditions scientifiques et la création des laboratoires maritimes (1965). Supplement 19 of *Vie et Milieu.* Paris; Masson. Banyuls-sur-Mer; Laboratoire Arago

Conant, J.B. and Nash, L.K., Ed. (1957). *Harvard Case Histories in Experimental Science.* 2 Vols. Cambridge, Mass.; Harvard University Press

Cranefield, P.F. (1974). *The Way In and the Way Out. François Magendie, Charles Bell and the Roots of the Spinal Nerves. With a facsimile of Charles Bell's Annotated Copy of his Idea of a New Anatomy of the Brain.* Mount Kisco, NY; Futura

Crow, W.B. (1929). *Contributions to the Principles of Morphology.* London; Kegan Paul, Trench, Trübner and Co.

Culotta, C.A. (1975). German Biophysics, Objective Knowledge, and Romanticism, *Historical Studies in the Physical Sciences*, Vol. 4, 3–38

Dagognet, F. (1967). *Méthodes et doctrine dans l'oeuvre de Pasteur.* Paris; Presses Universitaires de France

Dagognet, F. (1970). *Le Catalogue de la vie. Étude méthodologique sur la taxinomie.* Paris; Presses Universitaires de France

Dawson, W.R. (1946). *The Huxley Papers; A Descriptive Catalogue of the Correspondence, Manuscripts and Miscellaneous Papers of…Thomas Henry Huxley… Preserved in the Imperial College of Science and Technology.* London; Macmillan

Delage, Y. (1895). *La Structure du protoplasma et les théories sur l'hérédité et les grands problèmes de la biologie générale.* Paris; C. Reinwald. 2nd edn (1903) as *L'Hérédité.* Paris; C. Reinwald

Dewey, J. (1930). From Absolutism to Experimentalism, in *Contemporary American Philosophy.* Ed. G.P. Adams and W.P. Montague. 2 Vols. London; George Allen and Unwin. New York; Macmillan, Vol. 2, 13–27

Drabkin, D.L. (1958). *Thudichum. Chemist of the Brain.* Philadelphia; University of Pennsylvania Press

Driesch, H.A.E. (1914). *The History and Theory of Vitalism.* Trans. C.K. Ogden. London; Macmillan

Dunn, L.C., Ed. (1951). *Genetics in the 20th Century: Essays on the Progress of Genetics during its First 50 Years.* New York; Macmillan

Dunn, L.C. (1965). *A Short History of Genetics. The Development of Some of the Main Lines of Thought: 1864–1939.* New York; McGraw Hill

Eccles, J.C. and Gibson, W.C. (1979). *Sherrington. His Life and Thought.* Berlin and New York; Springer

Edwards, H. Milne (1867). *Rapport sur les progrès récents des sciences zoologiques en France.* Paris; L'Imprimerie impériale

Erman, W. and Horn, E., Ed. (1904–5). *Bibliographie der Deutschen Universitäten.* Pt. I, 3 Vols. Leipzig and Berlin; B.G. Teubner

Faber, K.H. (1923). *Nosography in Modern Internal Medicine.* Trans. by the author. London; Oxford University Press. English version expanded from *Annals of Medical History* (1922), Vol. 4, 1–63. 2nd edn (1930). New York; P.B. Hoeber

Farber, P.L. (1976). The Type-Concept in Zoology During the First Half of the Nineteenth Century, *Journal of the History of Biology*, Vol. 9, 93–119

Farley, J. (1977). *The Spontaneous Generation Controversy from Descartes to Oparin*. Baltimore and London; Johns Hopkins University Press

Farrall, L.A. (1970). *The Origins and Growth of the English Eugenics Movement, 1865–1925*. Ann Arbor; University Microfilms

Figlio, K. (1976). The Metaphor of Organisation: A Historiographical Perspective on the Biomedical Sciences of the Early Nineteenth Century, *History of Science*, Vol. 14, 17–53

Fleming, D. (1959). The Centenary of the 'Origin of Species', *Journal of the History of Ideas*, Vol. 20, 437–446

Florkin, M. (1960). *Naissance et déviation de la théorie cellulaire dans l'oeuvre de Théodore Schwann*. Paris; Hermann

Florkin, M. (1972–7). *A History of Biochemistry. Pt I: Proto-biochemistry. Pt II: From Proto-biochemistry to Biochemistry. Pt III: History of the Identification of the Sources of Free Energy in Organisms. Pt IV: Early Studies on Biosynthesis*. Amsterdam; Elsevier. Planned in 5 parts as Vols 30–33 of *Comprehensive Biochemistry*, Ed. M. Florkin and E.H. Stotz

Flugel, J.C. (1933). *A Hundred Years of Psychology 1833–1933*. London; Duckworth. Revised edns (1957, 1964). Paperback edn (1964). London; Methuen University Paperbacks

Folia Mendeliana. Papers Relating to Mendel and to the Early Development of Genetics (1966–). Vol. 1–. Brno; Moravian Museum

Forrester, J. (1980). *Language and the Origin of Psychoanalysis*. New York; Columbia University Press

Foster, W.D. with Dyke, S.C. (1961). *A Short History of Clinical Pathology*. Edinburgh and London; Livingstone

Foucault, M. (1966). *Les Mots et les choses: une archéologie des sciences humaines*. Paris; Gallimard. Trans. (1970) as *The Order of Things*. London; Tavistock

French, R.D. (1975). *Antivivisection and Medical Science in Victorian Society*. Princeton and London; Princeton University Press

Frolov, Y.P. (1937). *Pavlov and his School. The Theory of Conditional Reflexes*. Trans. C.P. Dutt. London; Kegan Paul, Trench, Trübner and Co.

Fruton, J.S. (1972). *Molecules and Life: Historical Essays on the Interplay of Chemistry and Biology*. New York and London; Wiley Interscience

Fulton, J.F. (1931). *Physiology. Clio Medica* Series, Vol. 5. New York; Hoeber

Fussell, G.E. (1971). *Crop Nutrition: Science and Practice before Liebig*. Lawrence, Kansas; Coronado Press. English edn (1978). Lavenham; Tortoise Shell Press

Galdston, I. (1943). *Behind the Sulfa Drugs: A Short History of Chemotherapy*. New York; D. Appleton-Century Co.

Galton, F. (1874). *English Men of Science: Their Nature and Nurture*. London; Macmillan

Geison, G.L. (1978). *Michael Foster and the Cambridge School of Physiology. The Scientific Enterprise in Late Victorian Society*. Princeton; Princeton University Press

Ghiselin, M.T. (1969). *The Triumph of the Darwinian Method*. Berkeley and Los Angeles; University of California Press

Glass, B., Temkin, O. and Straus, W.L., Ed. (1959). *Forerunners of Darwin: 1745–1859*. Baltimore; Johns Hopkins Press

Goodfield, G.J. (1960). *The Growth of Scientific Physiology. Physiological Method and the Mechanist–Vitalist Controversy. Illustrated by the Problems of Respiration and Animal Heat.* London; Hutchinson

Goodfield, G.J. (1975). *Cancer Under Siege.* London; Hutchinson

Goodfield, G.J. (1977). *Playing God. Genetic Engineering and the Manipulation of Life.* London; Hutchinson

Gordon-Taylor, G. and Walls, E.W. (1958). *Sir Charles Bell. His Life and Times.* Edinburgh and London; Livingstone

Gougher, R.L. (1969). Comparison of English and American Views of the German University, 1840–1865: A Bibliography, *History of Education Quarterly*, Vol. 9, 477–491

Gower, B. (1973). Speculation in Physics: The History and Practice of *Naturphilosophie*, *Studies in History and Philosophy of Science*, Vol. 3, 301–356

Granit, R. (1966). *Charles Scott Sherrington: An Appraisal.* London; Nelson

Green, F.H.K. and Covell, G., Ed. (1953). *Medical Research. History of the Second World War. United Kingdom Medical Series.* London; HMSO

Green, J.R. (1909). *A History of Botany 1860–1900 Being a Continuation of Sachs 'History of Botany, 1530–1860'.* Oxford; Clarendon Press

Gregory, F. (1977). *Scientific Materialism in Nineteenth Century Germany.* Dordrecht; D. Reidel

Grene, M. and Mendelsohn, E., Ed. (1976). *Topics in the Philosophy of Biology.* Boston Studies in the Philosophy of Science, Vol. 27. Dordrecht and Boston; D. Reidel

Grmek, M.D. (1967). *Catalogue des manuscrits de Claude Bernard; avec la bibliographie de ses travaux imprimés et des études sur son oeuvre.* Paris; Masson

Grmek, M.D. (1973). *Raisonnement expérimental et recherches toxicologiques chez Claude Bernard.* Hautes études médiévales et modernes, 18. Paris and Geneva; Droz

Groeben, C. and Müller, I. (1975). *The Naples Zoological Station at the Time of Anton Dohrn.* Naples; Stazione Zoologica di Napoli

Hall, A.D. (1905). *The Book of the Rothamsted Experiments.* London; John Murray. 2nd edn, revised E.J. Russell (1917)

Hall, T.S. (1969). *Ideas of Life and Matter. Studies in the History of General Physiology 600 BC–1900 AD.* 2 Vols. Chicago and London; University of Chicago Press

Hamlyn, D.W. (1961). *Sensation and Perception. A History of the Philosophy of Perception.* London; Routledge and Kegan Paul

Haraway, D.J. (1976). *Crystals, Fabrics and Fields. Metaphors of Organicism in Twentieth-Century Developmental Biology.* New Haven and London; Yale University Press

Harré, R., Ed. (1969). *Scientific Thought 1900–1960. A Selective Survey.* Oxford; Clarendon Press

Hearnshaw, L.S. (1964). *A Short History of British Psychology 1840–1940.* London; Methuen

Heinroth, K. (1971). *Oskar Heinroth. Vater der Verhaltensforschung 1871–1945.* Stuttgart; Wissenschaftliche Verlagsgesellschaft

Herrnstein, R.J. and Boring, E.G. (1965). *A Source Book in the History of Psychology.* Cambridge, Mass.; Harvard University Press

Hertwig, O. (1908). *Die Entwicklung der Biologie im Neunzehnten Jahrhundert,* 2nd enlarged edn. Jena; Gustav Fischer. 1st publ. (1900)

Hirschfeld, E. (1930). Romantische Medizin, zu einer künftigen Geschichte der Naturphilosophischen Ära, *Kyklos. Jahrbuch für Geschichte und Philosophie der Medizin,* Vol. 3, 1–89

Hodgen, M.T. (1936). *The Doctrine of Survivals: A Chapter in the History of Scientific Method in the Study of Man*. London; Allenson

Hodgen, M.T. (1964). *Early Anthropology in the Sixteenth and Seventeenth Centuries*. Philadelphia; University of Pennsylvania Press

Holmes, F.L. (1974). *Claude Bernard and Animal Chemistry. The Emergence of a Scientist*. Cambridge, Mass.; Harvard University Press

Hudson, P.S. and Richens, R.H. (1946). *The New Genetics in the Soviet Union*. Imperial Bureau of Plant Breeding and Genetics. Cambridge; School of Agriculture

Hughes, A. (1959). *A History of Cytology*. London and New York; Abelard-Schuman

Iltis, H. (1924). *Gregor Johann Mendel, Leben, Werk und Wirkung*. Berlin; Julius Springer. Trans. E. and C. Paul (1932). London; George Allen and Unwin

d'Irsay, S. (1933–5). *Histoire des universités françaises et étrangères des origines à nos jours*. 2 Vols. Paris; Auguste Picard

Jones, E. (1953–7). *The Life and Work of Sigmund Freud*. 3 Vols. New York; Basic Books. London; Hogarth Press

Joravsky, D. (1970). *The Lysenko Affair*. Cambridge, Mass.; Harvard University Press

Jordanova, L.J. and Porter, R.S., Ed. (1979). *Images of the Earth. Essays in the History of the Environmental Sciences*. The British Society for the History of Science Monographs, Vol. 1. Chalfont St Giles; British Society for the History of Science

Judson, H.F. (1979). *The Eighth Day of Creation. Makers of the Revolution in Biology*. London; Jonathan Cape

Kay, A.W. (1977). *Research in Medicine: Problems and Prospects*. The Rock Carling Fellowship. London; Nuffield Provincial Hospitals Trust.

Kisch, B. (1954). Forgotten Leaders in Modern Medicine. Valentin, Gruby, Remak, Auerbach, *Transactions of the American Philosophical Society*, new ser., Vol. 44, 141–317

Klopfer, P.H. and Hailman, J.P. (1967). *An Introduction to Animal Behaviour: Ethology's First Century*. London; Prentice-Hall. 2nd edn by P.H. Klopfer (1974). New Jersey; Prentice-Hall

Kohler, R.E. (1975). The History of Biochemistry: A Survey, *Journal of the History of Biology*, Vol. 8, 275–318

Latour, B. and Woolgar, S. (1979). *Laboratory Life: The Social Construction of Scientific Facts*. Beverly Hills and London; Sage

Lambert, J. (1963). *Sir John Simon 1816–1904 and English Social Administration*. London; MacGibbon and Kee

Lechevalier, H.A. and Solotorovsky, M. (1965). *Three Centuries of Microbiology*. New York; McGraw-Hill. Revised paperback edn (1974). New York; Dover

Lenoir, T. (1978). Generational Factors in the Origin of 'Romantische Naturphilosophie', *Journal of the History of Biology*, Vol. 2, 57–100

Lenoir, T. (1980). Kant, Blumenbach and Vital Materialism in German Biology, *Isis*, Vol. 71, 77–108

Lewes, G.H. (1855). *The Life and Works of Goethe: with Sketches of his Age and Contemporaries, from Published and Unpublished Sources*. 2 Vols. London; David Nutt. 2nd edn in 1 Vol (1864). London; Smith, Elder and Co. Everyman edn (1908). London; Dent. New York; E.P. Dutton

Liddell, E.G.T. (1960). *The Discovery of Reflexes*. Oxford; Clarendon Press

Lillie, F.R. (1944). *The Woods Hole Marine Biological Laboratory*. Chicago; University of Chicago Press

Loewenberg, B.J. (1965). Darwin and Darwin Studies, 1959–63, *History of Science*, Vol. 4, 15–54

Ludmerer, K. (1972). *Genetics and American Society: A Historical Appraisal*. Baltimore; Johns Hopkins University Press

McCollum, E.V. (1957). *A History of Nutrition: The Sequence of Ideas in Nutrition Investigations*. Boston; Houghton Mifflin

McDougall, W. (1908). *Introduction to Social Psychology*. London; Methuen

Macfarlane, G. (1979). *Howard Florey. The Making of a Great Scientist*. Oxford; Oxford University Press

Mainx, F. (1955). *Foundations of Biology*. Trans. J.H. Woodger. International Encyclopedia of Unified Science. Chicago; University of Chicago Press

Marsh, E.L. and Irvine, L.G. (1895). *Index to the Reports of the Medical Officers to the Privy Council and Local Government Board of England 1858–1893. I. Subjects. II. Authors*. Glasgow; William Hodge for the Police Commissioners of Glasgow

Maulitz, R.C. (1971). Schwann's Way: Cells and Crystals, *Journal of the History of Medicine*, Vol. 26, 422–437

Medvedev, Z.A. (1969). *The Rise and Fall of T.D. Lysenko*. Trans. I.M. Lerner. New York and London; Columbia University Press

Mendelsohn, E. (1964a). *Heat and Life*. Cambridge, Mass.; Harvard University Press

Mendelsohn, E. (1964b). The Biological Sciences in the Nineteenth Century: Some Problems and Sources, *History of Science*, Vol. 3, 39–59

Mendelsohn, E. (1965). Physical Models and Physiological Concepts: Explanation in Nineteenth Century Biology, in *Boston Studies in the Philosophy of Science*, Vol. 2. Ed. R.S. Cohen and M.W. Wartofsky. New York; Humanities Press, 127–150

Metchnikoff, E. (1892). *Lektsii o sravnitelnoi patologii vospaleniy*. St Petersburg; K.L. Rikker. Trans. F.A. and E.H. Starling (1893) as *Lectures on the Comparative Pathology of Inflammation Delivered at the Pasteur Institute in 1891*. London; Kegan Paul, Trench, Trübner and Co. New edn with introduction and bibliography (1968). New York; Dover

Morrell, J.B. (1972). The Chemist Breeders: the Research Schools of Liebig and Thomas Thomson, *Ambix*, Vol. 19, 1–46

Murchison, C., Ed. (1930–52). *A History of Psychology in Autobiography*. 4 Vols. Worcester, Mass.; Clark University Press

Murphy, G. (1928). *An Historical Introduction to Modern Psychology*. London; Routledge and Kegan Paul. Revised 5th edn (1949). Reprinted (1967)

Needham, J. (1929). *The Sceptical Biologist (Ten Essays)*. London; Chatto and Windus

Needham, J. (1931). *Chemical Embryology*. 3 Vols. Cambridge; Cambridge University Press. Part II of Vol. 1 publ. separately (1934) as *A History of Embryology*. Cambridge; Cambridge University Press. 2nd edn (1959), revised with assistance of A. Hughes

Needham, J. and Baldwin, E., Ed. (1949). *Hopkins and Biochemistry 1861–1947. Papers Concerning Sir Frederick Gowland Hopkins ... with a Selection of his Addresses and a Bibliography of his Publications*. Cambridge; Heffer

Nordenskiöld, E. (1920–4). *Biologins Historia*. 3 Vols. Stockholm; Björck and Börjesson. Trans. L.B. Eyre (1928) as *The History of Biology: A Survey*. New York; Tudor

Olby, R.C. (1974). *The Path to the Double Helix*. London; Macmillan

Olmsted, J.M.D. (1939). *Claude Bernard Physiologist*. New York and London; Harper and Brothers

Olmsted, J.M.D. (1944). *François Magendie. Pioneer in Experimental Physiology and Scientific Medicine in XIX Century France*. New York; Schuman

Olmsted, J.M.D. and Olmsted, E.H. (1952). *Claude Bernard and the Experimental Method in Medicine*. Life of Science Library, No. 23. New York; Schuman

Oppenheimer, J.M. (1967). *Essays in the History of Embryology and Biology*. Cambridge, Mass.; The MIT Press

Orwin, C.S. and Whetham, E.H. (1964). *A History of British Agriculture, 1846–1914*. London; Longmans, Green and Co. 2nd edn (1971). Newton Abbot; David and Charles

Owen, R. (1894). *The Life of Richard Owen*. 2 Vols. London; John Murray

Paoloni, C., Ed. (1968). *Justus von Liebig, Eine Bibliographie sämtlicher Veröffentlichungen*. Heidelberg; Carl Winter

Parish, H.J. (1965). *A History of Immunization*. London; Livingstone

Pearson, K. (1914–30). *The Life, Letters and Labours of Francis Galton*. 3 Vols. Vol. 3 in 2 pts. Cambridge; Cambridge University Press

Pearson, K. (1978). *The History of Statistics in the 17th and 18th Centuries Against the Changing Background of Intellectual, Scientific and Religious Thought. Lectures ... given at University College London ... 1921–1933*. Ed. E.S. Pearson. London and High Wycombe; Charles Griffin

Penniman, T.K. (1935). *A Hundred Years of Anthropology*. London; Duckworth. 3rd revised edn (1965), with contributions by B. Blackwood and J.S. Weiner

Postman, L.J., Ed. (1962). *Psychology in the Making. Histories of Selected Research Problems*. New York; Knopf

Prichard, J.C. (1813). *Researches into the Physical History of Man*. London; J. and A. Arch. Facsimile edn (1973) with Introductory Essay, 'From Chronology to Ethnology. James Cowles Prichard and British Anthropology 1800–1850', ix–cx, by G.W. Stocking, Jr. Chicago and London; University of Chicago Press

Prichard, J.C. (1847). *On the Relations of Ethnology to Other Branches of Knowledge*. Edinburgh; Neill

Provine, W.B. (1971). *The Origins of Theoretical Population Genetics*. Chicago; Chicago University Press

Rádl, E. (1909–13). *Geschichte der biologischen Theorien in der Neuzeit*. Pts I and II. Leipzig and Berlin; W. Engelmann. Revised and trans. E.J. Hatfield (1930). London; Oxford University Press

Rapp, D. (1970). *Die Entwicklung der physiologischen Methodik von 1784 bis 1911: Eine quantitative Untersuchung*. Münstersche Beiträge zur Geschichte und Theorie der Medizin, Ed. K.E. Rothschuh *et al.*, No. 2. Münster; Institut für Geschichte der Medizin der Universität Münster

Rather, L.J. (1972). *Addison and the White Corpuscles: An Aspect of Nineteenth-Century Biology*. London; Wellcome Institute of the History of Medicine

Roberts, H.F. (1929). *Plant Hybridization Before Mendel*. Princeton; Princeton University Press

Robinson, V. (1921). *The Life of Jacob Henle*. New York; Medical Life Co.

Roger, J. (1963). *Les Sciences de la vie dans la pensée française du XVIIIᵉ siècle*. Paris; Armand Colin. 2nd edn (1971)

Roll-Hansen, N. (1976). Critical Teleology: Immanuel Kant and Claude Bernard on the Limitations of Experimental Biology, *Journal of the History of Biology*, Vol. 9, 59–91

Romanes, E., Ed. (1896). *The Life and Letters of George John Romanes*. London; Longmans

Rosen, G. (1937). Social Aspects of Jacob Henle's Medical Thought, *Bulletin of the Institute of the History of Medicine*, Vol. 5, 509–537

Rossiter, M.W. (1975). *The Emergence of Agricultural Science. Justus Liebig and the Americans, 1840–1880.* New Haven and London; Yale University Press

Rothschuh, K.E. (1953). *Geschichte der Physiologie.* Berlin; Springer. Revised edn (1972). Trans. and ed. G.B. Risse. New York; Robert E. Krieger. 1st British edn (1973)

Royal Microscopical Society (1929). *Catalogue of the Printed Books and Pamphlets in the Library of the Royal Microscopical Society.* London; the Society

Ruch, T.C. and Fulton, J.F., Ed. (1960). *Medical Physiology and Biophysics.* Philadelphia; Saunders. 18th edn of Howell's *Textbook of Physiology*

Rudwick, M.J.S. (1972). *The Meaning of Fossils. Episodes in the History of Palaeontology.* London; Macdonald. New York; American Elsevier. 2nd edn (1976). New York; Science History Publications

Ruse, M. (1974). The Darwin Industry – A Critical Evaluation, *History of Science,* Vol. 12, 43–58

Russell, E.J. (1966). *A History of Agricultural Science in Great Britain, 1620–1954.* London; George Allen and Unwin

Russell, E.S. (1916). *Form and Function. A Contribution to the History of Animal Morphology.* London; John Murray

Russell, E.S. (1930). *The Interpretation of Development and Heredity; A Study in Biological Method.* Oxford; Clarendon Press. Reprinted (1972). Freeport, NY; Books for Libraries Press

Sachs, J. von (1875). *Geschichte der Botanik von 16. Jahrhundert bis 1860.* Munich; R. Oldenbourg. Trans. H.E.F. Garnsey, revised I.B. Balfour (1890) as *History of Botany, 1530–1860.* Oxford; Clarendon Press. See also Green (1909)

Sanderson, G.B. (1911). *Sir John Burdon Sanderson: A Memoir.* Ed. J.S. Haldane and E.S. Haldane. Oxford; Clarendon Press

Schiller, J. (1967). *Claude Bernard et les problèmes scientifiques de son temps.* Paris; Cedre

Schiller, J. and Schiller, T. (1975). *Henri Dutrochet (Henri du Trochet, 1776–1847). Le Matérialisme mécaniste et la physiologie générale.* Paris; Albert Blanchard

Schiller, J. (1978). *La Notion d'organisation dans l'histoire de la biologie.* Paris; Maloine s.a. éditeur

Schröer, H. (1967). *Carl Ludwig. Begründer der messenden Experimentalphysiologie.* Stuttgart; Wissenschaftliche Verlagsgesellschaft

Schwalbe, J., Ed. (1901). *Virchowbibliographie. 1843–1901.* Berlin; Georg Reimer

Searle, G.R. (1976). *Eugenics and Politics in Britain 1900–1914.* Leyden; Noordhoff International

Sharpey-Schafer, E.A. (1927). *History of the Physiological Society during its First Fifty Years 1876–1926.* London; Supplement to *Journal of Physiology*

Sherrington, C.S. (1946). *The Endeavour of Jean Fernel with a List of the Editions of his Writings.* Cambridge; Cambridge University Press

Shryock, R.H. (1947). *American Medical Research Past and Present.* New York; The Commonwealth Fund

Sirks, M.J. and Zirkle, C. (1964). *The Evolution of Biology.* New York; Ronald Press

Spencer, H. (1904). *An Autobiography.* 2 Vols. London; Williams and Norgate

Stent, G.S. (1969). *The Coming of the Golden Age: A View of the End of Progress.* Garden City, NY; Natural History Press

Stevenson, L.G. (1956). Religious Elements in the Background of the British Anti-Vivisection Movement, *Yale Journal of Biology and Medicine,* Vol. 29, 125–157

Stocking, G.W., Jr. (1965). From Physics to Ethnology: Franz Boas' Arctic Expedition as a Problem in the Historiography of the Behavioral Sciences, *Journal of the History of the Behavioral Sciences,* Vol. 1, 53–66

Strohl, J.E.F. (1936). *Lorenz Oken und Georg Büchner: zwei Gestalten aus der Übergangszeit von Naturphilosophie zu Naturwissenschaft.* Zürich; Verlag der Corona

Sturtevant, A.H. (1965). *A History of Genetics.* New York; Harper and Row

Sulloway, F.J. (1979). *Freud, Biologist of the Mind. Beyond the Psychoanalytic Legend.* London; Burnett Books

Sutherland, G. (1982). *Ability, Merit and Measurement: Mental Testing and English Education.* Cambridge; Cambridge University Press

Teich, M. (1980). A History of Biochemistry [essay review of M. Florkin (1972–7)], *History of Science,* Vol. 18, 46–67

Temkin, O. (1946a). Materialism in French and German Physiology of the Early Nineteenth Century, *Bulletin of the History of Medicine,* Vol. 20, 322–327

Temkin, O. (1946b). The Philosophical Background of Magendie's Physiology, *Bulletin of the History of Medicine,* Vol. 20, 10–35

Temkin, O. (1950). German Concepts of Ontogeny and History around 1800, *Bulletin of the History of Medicine,* Vol. 24, 227–246

Temkin, O. (1963). Basic Science, Medicine and the Romantic Era, *Bulletin of the History of Medicine,* Vol. 37, 97–129

Thompson, D'A. W. (1917). *On Growth and Form.* Cambridge; Cambridge University Press

Thomson, A.L. (1973–5). *Half a Century of Medical Research.* Vol. 1, *Origins and Policy of the Medical Research Council (U.K.).* Vol. II, *The Programme of the Medical Research Council (U.K.).* London; HMSO

Thomson, J.A. (1899). *The Science of Life. An Outline of the History of Biology and its Recent Advances.* London; Blackie and Son

Thorpe, W.H. (1979). *The Origins and Rise of Ethology. The Science of the Natural Behaviour of Animals.* London; Heinemann Educational. New York; Praeger

Tinbergen, N. (1951). *The Study of Instinct.* Oxford; Oxford University Press. 3rd reprinting (1976). New York; Oxford University Press

Tinbergen, N. (1972–3). *The Animal in its World. Explorations of an Ethologist 1932–1972.* 2 Vols. London; George Allen and Unwin

Virchow, R.L.K. (1858). *Die Cellularpathologie in ihrer Begründung auf physiologische und pathologische Gewebelehre.* Berlin; A. Hirschwald. 2nd German edn trans. F. Chance (1863). Philadelphia; J.B. Lippincott. Republ. (1971), with introduction by L.J. Rather. New York; Dover

Virchow, R.L.K. (1959). *Disease, Life and Man: Selected Essays.* Ed. and trans. L.J. Rather. Stanford; Stanford University Press

Vorzimmer, P.J. (1970). *Charles Darwin: The Years of Controversy. The Origin of Species and its Critics, 1859–1882.* Philadelphia; Temple University Press. British edn (1972). London; University of London Press

Wallace, A.R. (1898). *The Wonderful Century. Its Successes and Failures.* London; Swan Sonnenschein

Watermann, R. (1960). *Theodor Schwann: Leben und Werk.* Düsseldorf; L. Schwann Verlag

Watson, J.D. (1968). *The Double Helix. A Personal Account of the Discovery of the Structure of DNA.* New York; Athenaeum. New critical edn by G.S. Stent (1981). London; Weidenfeld and Nicolson

Watson, R.I. (1974–6). *Eminent Contributors to Psychology.* 2 Vols. New York; Springer

Weber, G. (1974). Science and Society in Nineteenth Century Anthropology, *History of Science,* Vol. 12, 260–283

Webster, C., Ed. (1981). *Biology, Medicine and Society 1840–1940.* Cambridge; Cambridge University Press

Werskey, G. (1978). *The Visible College.* London; Allen Lane

Whewell, W. (1837). *History of the Inductive Sciences, From the Earliest to the Present Times*. 3 Vols. London; John W. Parker. 3rd edn (1857). Reprinted (1967). London; Frank Cass

Wightman, W.P.D. (1956). *The Emergence of General Physiology*. Belfast; Queen's University of Belfast

Wilson, E.B. (1925). *The Cell in Development and Heredity*, 3rd revised and enlarged edn. New York; Macmillan. 1st publ. (1896)

Woodger, J.H. (1929). *Biological Principles: A Critical Study*. London; Kegan Paul, Trench, Trübner and Co.

Woodworth, R.S. (1931). *Contemporary Schools of Psychology*. New York; Ronald Press. London; Methuen. 2nd revised edn (1948). New York; Ronald Press. 8th British edn (1951). London; Methuen. 3rd revised edn (1964, 1965), with M.R. Sheehan. New York; Ronald Press. London; Methuen

Young, M.N. (1961). *Bibliography of Memory*. Philadelphia; Chilton Co.

Young, R.M. (1966). Scholarship and the History of the Behavioural Sciences, *History of Science*, Vol. 5, 1–51

Young, R.M. (1969). Malthus and the Evolutionists: The Common Context of Biological and Social Theory, *Past and Present*, No. 43, 109–145

Young, R.M. (1970). *Mind, Brain and Adaptation in the Nineteenth Century. Cerebral Localization and its Biological Context from Gall to Ferrier*. Oxford; Clarendon Press

Zeiss, H. (1932). *Elias Metschnikow. Leben und Werk*. Jena; Gustav Fischer

Zirkle, C. (1935). *The Beginnings of Plant Hybridization*. Philadelphia; University of Pennsylvania Press. London; Oxford University Press

Zirkle, C. (1959). *Evolution, Marxian Biology and the Social Scene*. Philadelphia; University of Pennsylvania Press

19

Medicine since 1500

Margaret Pelling

The history of medicine differs from the history of science in that it cannot be reduced to the history of ideas. First, the relation between doctor and patient remains vital to medicine even though its importance has been denied by the 'scientization' of medical knowledge, and historically was depreciated by those wishing to detach medicine from its origins in the craft tradition. Nonetheless medicine retains a wider dimension of human and social significance that has always been reflected in the writings of practitioners themselves and that, in less favourable climates, has re-emerged in subject areas such as anthropology and sociology. Secondly, the history of medicine is older than the history of science, since the latter has emerged principally as a result of the philosophies of science that became dominant in the nineteenth century. Thirdly, the desire of medical men to be included among the learned professions persists and has always led to an emphasis on literary production. Medical humanism has a long tradition that in more recent times has had such manifestations as the enormous respect accorded by medical men to figures like Oliver Wendell Holmes and Sir William Osler. In addition it has inspired the views of those who in the twentieth century have regarded a strong historical component as an essential part of medical education.

Until very recently most medical history was written by medical men, who saw the historical mode as appropriate for a variety of purposes, the most obvious being that of commemoration, whether of persons or institutions. Enormous numbers of medical biographies exist and few medical institutions are without a chronicle of some kind. Many of these accounts are modest and witness to the local importance of their subjects; they have been despised but may come to be valued as preserving evidence of conditions of medical practice. Medical biography has similarly had dimensions (particularly the moral) that have been underrated. The more prominent sources are informed by two main ideas: the ideal of progress and the advance of knowledge, and the hierarchical nature of the medical profession. The second has very often been regarded as a reflection of the first. The biography of the individual portrays the absolute value of merit, the role of example and the struggle against ignorance; the emergence and endurance of institutions represents the defence of standards, the accumulation of knowledge and the spread of enlightenment.

These emphases have resulted in an overwhelming concentration on the nineteenth and (increasingly) the twentieth centuries. In the nineteenth century real progress was at last made: medicine became scientific, and its personnel became established as a profession. At the same time, enough remained of ignorance and fear for the century to be seen as a theatre in which the last heroic phases of a medicine without antisepsis or anaesthesia confronted the new age. Such works as De Kruif (1926) or Thorwald (1957) have not only had enormous popular appeal; they have inspired generations of medical students. The ideal of the heroic pioneer has been displaced to some extent by that of the hospital doctor. This success, in which the medical profession has finally achieved a supremacy over the rival callings of divinity and law, has brought a certain degree of reaction, with an interest in 'alternative' medicine, folklore, dehospitalized medicine and paramedical groups. This reaction is as yet hardly more than a reflection of the strength of the beneficiaries of the main approach – physicians, and those subject areas of medicine that could be defined scientifically. It can be seen that the history of medicine itself, if not its subject matter, has come to share many of the priorities of the history of science. Practitioners of the latter are inclined to regard the former as a subsidiary subject, once it has been reduced to its essentials, and reference works are commonly organized along these lines (Blake and Roos 1967).

In the early modern period humanist scholars with a university training in medicine played a modest part in catalogues of learned authors, universal bibliographies, or histories intended to establish the antiquity of the universities (e.g. Bale 1548; Brunfels 1530; Gesner 1545–55: see Thornton 1966). This tradition continued into the eighteenth century (Wood 1721; Baillet 1685–6, 1722–30;

Manget 1731) although many of the later compendia were derivative. New ground was broken by Pierre Bayle, whose *Dictionnaire*
of 1697 was translated (1710) and imitated (*Biographia Britannica*,
1747–66, 2nd edn enlarged but incomplete), and for medicine by
Éloy (1755). These authors, while acknowledging the classical
origins of medicine, were equally concerned with its evolution and
with its status as a body of knowledge. In the late eighteenth and
nineteenth centuries this concern was combined with great erudition and an ideal of cultural and human history, by French and
German scholars in particular, in a body of systematic histories,
bibliographies and biographical dictionaries, most of which have
not been superseded. Histories of medicine, which reflected
philosophical developments in other fields, are reviewed in detail
in chapter 2 and readers should refer there for works by such
authors as Sprengel and Daremberg. Here should be mentioned
the major (though incomplete) contribution of the Swiss systemat-
ist, botanist, politician, physician and comparative anatomist
Albrecht von Haller (1771–9). The subject index of Ploucquet
(1808–14; complemented for this period by Callisen 1830–45)
demonstrates the growth of periodical literature as well as contemporary priorities in medicine.

There is no biographical survey in English to match that of
Hirsch (1859–64), which was continued for the nineteenth century
by Julius Pagel (1901). Among English authors Hutchinson
(1799), a friend of Erasmus Darwin, produced a set of biographies
combining the national enthusiasm for 'the numerous natural, and
acquired excellencies of distinguished characters' with a 'history of
the origin and progress of Medical Science', pharmacy, chemistry,
botany and midwifery being included among the 'departments of
philosophical science connected with medicine'. Others (Pettigrew
1840) were more desultory and anecdotal. This is true even of the
indispensable *Roll of the Royal College of Physicians* of Munk
(1878), who cast his subjects where possible in the role of literary
gentlemen. Munk reflected upon character but quoted with
approval Samuel Johnson's dictum, delivered in the latter's life of
the ideal physician Sir Thomas Browne, that 'the physician's part
lies hid in domestic privacy, and silent duties and silent excellencies are soon forgotten'.

The antiquarianism of many nineteenth-century British medical
men, while genuine, nonetheless served professional interests, for
example in distancing the educated medical man from superstitious practices (Pettigrew 1844), or in countering the contemporary trend to division in medicine (Allbutt 1905). Institutional
loyalty and antiquarianism combined could produce such valuable

sources as Young (1890). The best monument to British scholarship remains the *Dictionary of National Biography* (1882–1900),
an enterprise of nearly twenty years that was originally intended to
'exceed in literary value' Continental achievements such as the
Biographie Universelle and the national biographies by then
produced in Sweden, Holland, Austria and Germany. The *Dictionary of National Biography* drew heavily on personal information and unpublished sources. Regarded as a measure of national
distinction, it identified the sixteenth and the nineteenth centuries
as the periods of greatest 'mental and physical activity', ascribing
this in the latter case in part to the 'multiplication of intellectual
callings' and 'specialisation in science and art'. Medical practitioners were naturally included in this middle-class expansion and an
impressive range of biographies was supplied by the physicians
J.F. Payne and Norman Moore and the surgeon D'Arcy Power, all
of whom made other contributions to medical history.

The history of medicine finally became institutionalized in
Germany after 1900 as a specialty among other medical specialties,
notably in Leipzig under Sudhoff. However, chairs were created in
France at the end of the eighteenth century (Ackerknecht 1967);
and in Vienna and Berlin and on an individual basis elsewhere the
subject was sufficiently established to experience a period of
danger in mid-century when scientific realism demanded a utilitarian rather than a literary or philosophical rationale (see references in Lesky 1965). At Vienna, posts in the history of medicine
were occupied in the nineteenth century by Seligmann, Puschmann and Neuburger; in Berlin by Hecker, Hirsch and J.L.
Pagel. Individual contributions to the literature were already
considerable and many research workers in medical subjects found
a historical perspective necessary to their work. However, the
argument that a historical survey taught the student of medicine a
prudent caution in the acceptance of new ideas and especially new
systems had already been formulated. Medical history was thus
early concerned with long spans of time and with indicating the
border between truth and error.

The 'space–time purview' became an essential aspect of the
utility of medical history. Fielding Garrison, whose single-volume
history of medicine (1913) continues to be regarded as the
standard reference in English, ascribed the introduction of this
technique to Osler, who had used it in the context of clinical
teaching in hospitals as a method enabling the medical student to
impose order on the mass of detail to which, owing to the massive
and increasing growth of medical knowledge, he was necessarily
subjected. The systematic selectivity of this approach is still well

illustrated by Garrison and Morton's *Medical Bibliography* (1943), which is based on a list compiled by Garrison at Osler's suggestion. By 1928 Garrison felt able to assert that 'there is hardly any good medical teacher today who does not supplement the detailed presentation of his subject by its historical milestones and landmarks, its triumphs and failures, its pathways and pitfalls' (Long 1928: vii). In addition to identifying the basic principles of the subject being taught, this teaching also sought to reconcile the student to the limits of certainty in medicine. Garrison's assertion is borne out by the number of histories of specialisms produced between 1900 and 1950 (Foster 1901; McHenry 1969; Long 1928; Pusey 1933; Bulloch 1938; Still 1931; Himes 1936; Ricci 1945; Sorsby 1948). Many of these were reprinted in the 1960s, a period of expansion that saw a few new examples – e.g. Valentin (1961), Parish (1965). William Osler organized his own library by combining the sort of selectivity referred to by Garrison with his own inclinations as a bibliophile and believer in the physician as a man of letters. His *Bibliotheca Osleriana* (Osler 1929) is divided into 'Bibliotheca Prima' – a comparatively small number of works, arranged in chronological order, representing the 'essential literature'; 'Bibliotheca Secunda' – the largest section, containing medical and scientific works of 'authors not of the first importance'; 'Bibliotheca Litteraria' – including what Osler called 'medicated novels' and 'medical works by laymen'; and further biographical, historical, and bibliographical categories. In the 'Prima' William Harvey (147 items) and his forerunners (79 items) are exceeded only by the section representing the confused rival claims to the introduction of anaesthesia (154 items) and rivalled only by Hippocrates (73 items).

Osler's influence on medical education was chiefly exerted during his period in Baltimore and was compatible with the utilitarian emphasis given to German conceptions of medical history after their transplantation into North America. English-language medical history has been well served by the contributions of emigrant European scholars, largely German-trained, in medicine and the humanities (Sigerist, Edelstein, Temkin, Ackerknecht). Although adopting a range of perspectives on methods, sources and the relations between history and medicine, these scholars had in common a classical, linguistic and philosophical erudition and an interest in primitive, classical and post-classical medicine that are difficult to match in any later generation. While maintaining a positivistic commitment and a sense of obligation towards present-day medical science, they did not see these as incompatible with a view of medicine as involving the wider dimension of healing and health. A conviction that medical thought was integrally related to cultural or intellectual developments allowed them to conduct studies in depth of limited periods of the kind advocated by Edelstein. These could take the form of intellectual biography, as with W. Pagel's studies of Paracelsus (1958), Harvey (1967) and Van Helmont (1982). Temkin's *Falling Sickness* (1945), a history of epilepsy, was intended to assist the difficulties of modern clinicians as well as to contribute to the history of concepts in medicine; but Sigerist, Temkin, Ackerknecht (1932) and later Rosen also published model studies demonstrating the place of medicine in reform movements in eighteenth-and nineteenth-century France and Germany. In this context medical history was seen as a semi-autonomous discipline that was best pursued or at least directed by full-time researchers and teachers and that could supply to medical education a 'culturizing, humanizing and liberalizing' influence that it was increasingly coming to lack. This point of view was identified with William Welch's foundation at Johns Hopkins, for many years the only Institute for the History of Medicine in America. Even in the United States medical history has never experienced the institutional explosion that took place in the history of science as a reflection of national policy after the Second World War.

A concern for the development of social welfare and the delivery of health care to all sectors of the population led Sigerist in the 1930s to link medical history with sociology and to stress the importance of the patient in the context of scientific as well as preventive medicine. A sociological approach to the subject was subsequently advocated by Sigerist's successor, Shryock, an American historian not trained in medicine, and has since received a great deal of attention, commensurate with the idea that the social sciences might provide the 'humanizing' element in medical education. However, the main emphasis has been not on social history of the kind advocated by Sigerist but on institutionalization, professionalization and transactional analysis, which reflect professional values, or the assumption of a polarity between practitioner and patient.

Shryock's important work provided both a synthesis of past and present trends and an acceptable blueprint for the future. *The Development of Modern Medicine* took account of the increasing emphasis being placed on the seventeenth-century scientific revolution as well as the nineteenth century and attempted to reconcile the positivist and relativist extremes by offering 'an historical or comparative approach to the problems of scientific method' (1936: viii). Shryock charted periods of methodological confusion in medicine, which he located as having occurred earlier in the history of physical sciences, and subsequently in the social disciplines. His two 'basic themes', the history of medicine and the history of public health, together reformulated for medical history the role of bridging the physical and the social sciences. Quantification was common to the development of medicine and to the present-day claim to legitimacy of sociology. The role of American medical historians in the evolution of a concept of social medicine as an applied discipline, 'concerned primarily with a mode of thought and only secondarily with the mechanics of action' (1936: ix), is exemplified by the collection edited by Galdston (1949) deriving from four years of work by a Committee on 'Medicine and the Changing Order' of the New York Academy of Medicine. Various historical perspectives were contributed by Temkin, Rosen, Shryock, Sigerist (a previously published paper) and Galdston. Other participants included John Ryle, the first professor of social medicine in England, and Lord Horder, who reflected on negotiations over the setting up of the National Health Service. Conflicting views were subdued to produce a historically based definition of social medicine as an 'anabolism of the biological, psychological and social sciences' (Galdston 1949: ix).

Shryock distanced himself from English writers on public health, who laid particular emphasis on the concept of prevention (Richardson 1887; Simon 1890; Bannington 1915; Newsholme 1927b and 1931; Frazer 1950), by regarding the concept of social medicine in England as having been deflected into public hygiene by the sanitarian movement. Rosen, whose volume of collected essays published between 1943 and 1973 (1974) emphasizes his influence in this area, saw social medicine 'as to a very large extent the history of social policy and action in relation to health problems' and as essentially a post-industrial development. Like Shryock, Rosen spoke of the history of social medicine rather than the social history of medicine, and of social medicine as being the more or less scientific study of the group rather than the individual. Of three component historical areas identified by Rosen – health in relation to the community, health as a social value, and health and social policy – later writers have continued to find the third the most accessible. The emphasis placed by historians of social medicine on the post-industrial period, on social policy and on the ground in common between medicine and the social sciences has confirmed the earlier emphasis on the nineteenth century as the period of most dramatic advance; it contrasts with the leaning of the German archival historians towards primitive and classical medicine as well as with the emphasis still placed on the Renaissance and the seventeenth century by historians of the medical specialisms.

In the continuing debate over the crisis in modern medicine, reference has in effect been made less to history than to the contemporary findings of anthropology and sociology (Rosen 1959; Hanlon *et al.* 1960), or to sociological studies using historical examples by way of illustration. Galdston's volume of 1949 may be compared with a later, British example (McLachlan and McKeown 1971) in which McKeown suggests that the most successful historian might be one who 'does not much care for history' but turns to it because of the necessity of understanding contemporary social problems (1971: 4). If medical history was earlier dominated by the perspectives of the emergent nineteenth-century medical professions, it has recently been affected by the authority increasingly asserted by the social science professions, by psychiatrists and psychologists and by paramedical groups. Social factors are thus admitted insofar as they are the subject matter of other scientific specialties. That the newer professions can find common ground with the older with respect to a limited definition of the central theme of the history of medicine is shown by Clarke (1971). Clarke urged that medical history itself should become a science and free itself from the literary and bibliographical mode still prevalent among British writers.

Emphasis is here being placed on British subjects and British sources, but it should be stressed that the literature of other countries could be similarly described, depending on the degree of their approximation to the structures of Western medicine. In the British literature, some access has been provided to most adjuncts of professional life, for example periodicals (LeFanu 1937–8) and societies (e.g. Dudfield 1906; Power 1939; McMenemey 1959). The voluntary hospitals were originally a conspicuous expression of civic pride and piety, and they subsequently became the basis for professional status among physicians and surgeons. The literature on them is consequently enormous and reflects their origins and later development (Gaskell 1964). For European and other perspectives see Howard (1789), Jetter (1966–72), Thompson and Goldin (1975), Webster (1978). For an indication of the range of records generated by charitable institutions see Marmoy (1977) and Kerling (1977). Highmore's *Pietas Londinensis* (1810) provides prospectus information for subscribers, comparable to that supplied by published annual reports. Burdett's later surveys (1891–3, 1896) of both private and public institutions in the English-speaking world represent a later stage of difficulty about finance and doubt as to the healthiness of hospitals. His *Yearbooks* (1890–1930) nonetheless place voluntary hospitals in their context of charities ranging from religious societies to vaccine lymph establishments; the substantial appendices of advertisements are intrinsic to Burdett's concerns. Most histories commemorate a single institution, in which any comparative approach is inappropriate, but some later sources reflect the need to assess the movement as a whole (Abel-Smith 1964) or to record later units of organization (National Health Service 1966; Ayers 1971).

Medical education is dealt with as a function of the hospitals and the universities (Brockbank 1936; Cope 1954; Newman 1957; Bellot 1929; Kirkpatrick 1912). The institutional figurehead of the profession, the (Royal) College of Physicians of London, found an apologist as early as 1684 (Goodall); the corresponding work for the modern period is Clark (1964–6; see also Widdess 1963; Creswell 1926). The London physicians were imitated by the surgeons, *Plarr's Lives* (1930; continued by Power and LeFanu in 1953 and Robinson and LeFanu in 1970) dating only from the institution of the order of fellows in 1843, and in due time by the younger colleges (e.g. Ricci 1945; Peel 1976). In the case of the College of Surgeons, the ordinary membership dated from 1800 and D'Arcy Power estimated that he was having to exclude between 10 000 and 15 000 individuals living at any one time (Power 1931: 98). Professional priorities have created an equivalent bias in the geographical coverage of the literature: London has received most attention; the medical schools and institutions of Scotland, some (see Comrie 1932; Ferguson 1948, 1958; Checkland 1980); Ireland far less (Cameron 1886), in spite of its goading and testing effect for British social policy in the nineteenth as in the seventeenth century; and Wales perhaps least of all (see Cule 1980). Only certain regions emerge strongly (Pickstone 1980). Areas such as pharmacy and nursing are now less neglected than previously, but this literature is in its turn reflecting an equivalent concern with professionalization, with an added emphasis on this as the social dimension of their subject (Kremers and Urdang 1940; Thatcher 1953; Thompson 1968; Baly 1973; Donnison 1977; Davies 1980). The same may be expected of other groups hitherto labelled as ancillary, or of rising status within the medical profession.

Recent historiography has tended to provide rationalizations for professional ambitions, rather than altering the terms of discussion historically. Concepts of social mobility (Parry and Parry 1976; Peterson 1978) and marginality (Inkster 1977) have been influentially employed, although it is notable that no satisfactory secondary account of the nineteenth-century 'medical reform' movement has yet been produced (see Simon 1887). The strength of the claims made by nineteenth-century physicians in particular and by their heirs finds its negative reflection in an emphasis on 'alternative' therapies such as homoeopathy, and in the use of such concepts as social control. Similarly much recent writing on women as patients is based on accepting as a general reality the image of middle-class women idealized by some of their male attendants. Stress is placed on women achieving professional status (Chaff *et al.* 1977). Attempts to estimate the full range of medical practitioners available to nineteenth-century patients are as yet tentative. Institutional or administrative histories collectivize the provision made for the poor; only F.B. Smith (1979) has attempted to estimate the experience of ill-health under nineteenth-century conditions from the patient's point of view. The personal testimony of Aronovitch (1974) is revealing for the present century.

Even within the definition of professional concerns there are many areas requiring further investigation: outpatient care; dispensaries (but see Loudon 1981), domiciliary care; smaller or specialist hospitals; private medical schools; the workings of the apprenticeship system. 'Casual' forms of instruction in health and medicine are now attracting notice. Except in its scientific, institutional or ideological aspect (Ackerknecht 1967; Poynter 1961; Foucault 1963), surprisingly little attention is paid to nineteenth-century clinical medicine, especially with respect to the daily preoccupations of the practitioner. These are not necessarily well represented in journals such as the *Lancet*, an extremely widely used source, but surely itself a subject for historical investigation (Sprigge 1897; Brook 1943). The nineteenth-century profession's reverence for its clinical teachers, and its bread-and-butter dependence upon comprehensive textbooks of clinical instruction, have found little echo in recent historiography. Although only partially considered, the hospital patient has received far more critical scrutiny than the much greater numbers of persons (including children) visited and operated upon at home. This is one of many aspects of the neglect of morbidity as opposed to mortality. An exaggerated emphasis on the infectious diseases has similarly obscured the importance of less well-defined causes of illness, or chronic rather than acute diseases and of *sequelae.* An awareness of the long-term complexities and dangers that the patient and the practitioner believed they faced in maintaining or restoring health – or what for the given individual had to be regarded as health – would do much both to reveal and explain the dependence of the nineteenth- and even the twentieth-century patient or practitioner on traditional explanations and remedies.

Moreover, there is much to be gained for any period in

accepting the validity of the patient's choice of practitioner. It is usually assumed that in the early modern period the tripartite division in medicine and surgery (physicians, surgeons, apothecaries) was strictly maintained, by mutual hostility if not on rational grounds. It is further assumed that the tiny numbers of physicians available left the bulk of the population 'at the mercy' of quacks, and drastically limited or even precluded the provision of medical poor relief (Oxley 1974; cf. Levy 1943, 1944; Fessler 1952). Raach (1962), in pointing to a surprisingly high incidence of academically educated physicians in country areas, nonetheless took these physicians at their own valuation. A broader view was suggested by Roberts (1962–4). It is now clear that the professionally ambitious physician coexisted with an extremely wide range of healers, that the barber-surgeons and surgeons carried the burden of general practice, that these 'general practitioners' included women as well as men, and that those wanting the services of a practitioner made a critical choice among the variety available according to their particular circumstances and the nature and phase of the illness. Municipal authorities chose freely from the same range of services in providing medical poor relief (Webb 1966).

These conclusions are borne out by both the exhaustive analysis of a single rich (but rare) source (MacDonald 1981) and the accumulation of data from an extremely wide range of sources, including wills, parish registers, freemen's rolls, municipal records and ecclesiastical visitations (Pelling and Webster 1979). Strictly occupational sources such as freemen's rolls or indentures must be supplemented by others to reach a true estimate of the size of the occupational group in towns; it cannot be assumed that guild restrictions (Vicary 1888; Parker 1914) were effective. Such investigations show a very high ratio of practitioners to patients in rural as well as urban areas. This is complemented by the finding that medical practice can be seen as one aspect of economic flexibility. One effect of the extrapolation backwards of modern concepts of professionalization has been the assumption that medical practitioners must have engaged in only one trade. The diverse economic activities even of nineteenth-century practitioners are often hinted at by contemporary biographers but this information has been ignored by later historians, or presented as a complicating factor in the process of professionalization. Similar assumptions are made with respect to the practitioner's intellectual, political or religious beliefs; these were perhaps better observed by the earlier generation of *Kulturgeschichte*-oriented historians. The notion of practitioners forming a single class in society has been varied only by reverting to the older view of tripartite division; that the physician, the surgeon and the apothecary have an *a priori* existence is assumed even in such controversial studies as Honigsbaum (1979).

Thus biographical sources for before the 1850s chiefly reflect less the real course of development of the profession than the profession's view of itself (Garrison 1928; Payne 1970; *Medical Register* 1779 etc.; Munk 1878; Plarr 1930; Smith 1932; Underwood 1977; Edinburgh University 1846, supplemented by the Edinburgh Royal College of Physicians Comrie Index; Drew 1968; Raach 1962; Bloom and James 1935; see also Raven-Hart and Johnston 1931–2; Partington 1961–70; J. Ferguson 1906 is less used but has more of interest) and must always exclude a large proportion of those engaged in practice, many of them formally qualified. For the period after 1800 and before the *Medical Register* beginning in 1858 there are in addition the National Library of Medicine's *Index Catalogue*, which lists obituaries; the Edinburgh Royal College of Physicians Card Index of obituaries in the *Edinburgh Medical Journal*; the (voluntary) *Medical Directories* beginning in 1845 (at first London only); and especially the lists published by the Society of Apothecaries (1840–), which are often the only means of locating those with basic qualifications between 1815 and 1845. The obituaries included in most issues of the *Directory* are intercalated in the Biographical section of the Wellcome Institute's published *Subject Catalogue* (1980). Nurses are recoverable only from Burdett's *Official Nursing Directory* (1898–1904). For 1750–1850 an index to all obituaries in medical journals and related sources is being prepared for publication by Mrs J. Loudon of the Wellcome Unit for the History of Medicine, University of Oxford. A cumulative card index from any source of all types of practitioner (including midwives) for Norfolk, Suffolk, Cambridgeshire, Essex and London for 1500–1640, and for some sources for these areas to 1720, also at the Oxford Unit, at present totals approximately 10 000 individuals. T.D. Whittet and Mrs J. Burnby are intending to transfer their indexes of English apothecaries and apprentices to the computer file of the Project for Historical Biobibliography (*Book Subscriptions Lists Project,* 1967–) at the University of Newcastle-upon-Tyne being directed by P.J. Wallis, which also includes eighteenth-century book subscription lists (see *Medical History*, 1976, Vol. 20, 323). In spite of their often high standing in towns in the early modern period, their participation in early capitalism and their function as general practitioners, apothecaries are generally ignored except by their own historians (Barrett 1905; Matthews 1962).

One approach to the unity of mental, physical and social effects has seemed to lie in the history of epidemiology. Hecker was convinced of the significance of collective experiences of disease in supplying insight into the phases of human history and the state of the human mind in society. He deplored contemporary medical science as having declined from the philosophical and moral spirit of the eighteenth century to become 'mechanical and defective', especially in England and France, and argued the claims of a 'higher law of nature uniting the utmost diversity of individual parts'. He regarded the recent, first incursion of cholera into Europe as symptomatic and stated that the present age demanded a 'historical pathology'. Babington, translating Hecker for the Sydenham Society (1844), rejected Hecker's notion of an organic universe but shared his taste for comprehensive theories and general laws to explain the causes of epidemics and their moral effects. Babington, like Ozanam (1817–23), saw the accumulation of information on epidemics as a contribution to exact knowledge, regarding such comprehensive quantification as the best legacy of *Encyclopédie* methodology and as a proper extension of the numerical method, then being applied to the equally inexact area of therapeutics. The moral, methodological and historiographical as well as the physical and scientific dimensions of epidemics have been variously emphasized by later authors (Frost 1936; Hirsch 1859–64; Creighton 1894; Prinzing 1916; Greenwood 1932; Zinsser 1935; Winslow 1943; McNeill 1977; Durey 1979).

Epidemics have been regarded alternately as causative and as symptomatic phenomena of human history. The bibliography of twentieth-century works added to the reprint of Creighton (1894) in 1965 shows, however, that more is required for satisfactory historical investigation than a conviction of the correctness of unifactoral germ theory. In making some just criticisms of Creighton, Roberts (1968) himself imposes a number of false dichotomies on nineteenth-century epidemiological thought, a tendency criticized by Pelling (1978). Discrete epidemics of identifiable diseases, supposed to have equally striking social effects, have distracted attention from endemic or less easily defined conditions; the best source on fevers remains Murchison (1862). An exception is Ackerknecht (1945). Only bubonic plague, arguably an endemic as well as epidemic disease, has seemed justifiably to demand treatment from literary, economic and social as well as medical historians (Gottfried 1978; Shrewsbury 1970; Hirst 1953). The strictly demographic treatment of Gottfried, which is based on a computer analysis of testamentary evidence, is methodologically in sympathy with the concept of 'subsistence crisis' produced by demographers and economic historians; this has been applied on the regional (Appleby 1978) and on the global level (Post 1977). The latter's comprehensiveness is reminiscent of the nineteenth-century sense of the importance of a range of factors such as meteorology in grand sequences of human events.

If quantitative criteria are applied to the history of medicine itself, it may seem to have changed little in the last twenty years. This is partly a matter of classification (Miller 1964; National Library of Medicine 1965–78). The largest categories continue to be 'diseases and injuries', 'medical education', drugs and hospitals, with almost equal interest being taken in medicine's connections with literature and religion as in its scientific aspects. An obvious growth area is the historical relations of psychology and psychiatry. Many would be prepared to regard this resort to history as a measure of present professional (including epistemological) uncertainties (Baruch and Treacher 1978). This field is freely interdisciplinary and the initiative in the present century has been taken by anthropologists and sociologists as well as by those practically concerned with mental illness (Sigerist 1931a; Galdston 1949; Bastide 1965; Rosen 1968). It has proved a relatively safe area for the rediscovery of cultural determinism and discrimination, although the most influential contributions (Foucault 1961; Szasz 1970) are concerned with the definitive defects of Western civilization and with major transitions within its course of development. The doctor or alienist has not lost his unique position but this is negatively rather than positively expressed. The value of these formulations will be tested by such intensive studies as MacDonald (1981).

Demography has come to provide some common ground for the social sciences and social, economic and medical history. The collectivity of human biological events and experiences offers the concept of 'vital revolutions', quantitatively expressed and representing major changes in human society as well as providing a reliable basis for comparisons (Glass and Eversley 1965; Glass and Revelle 1972; Imhof and Larsen 1975; Imhof 1980). The limitation of purely demographical history is that problems, sources and solutions can all be defined within a single set of terms provided by the discipline itself. Medical history has not hesitated to offer explanations (whether in terms of the mortality caused by hospitals, or the activities of relatively tiny professional groups) that are incommensurate with the problems so defined. A better balance of methods and sources has been inspired by the *Annales* school, created around that journal from the 1920s by its editors Marc Bloch and Lucien Febvre (Bloch 1924; Forster and Ranum 1975,

1980) and the rich archives of France; see for example Goubert (1974). Lebrun (1971) is an instance of the successful combination of demographical techniques with the concern of French historians for *mentalité*. The burgeoning field of English regional, urban and community studies for the early modern period extends to factors relating to population, mortality and 'life-course' without as yet venturing much beyond the quantitative and the structural, but see Webster, *Health, Medicine and Mortality* (1979) and Thomas (1971). Local studies are still required that treat the popular experience of illness and health, and the relation of this to the intellectual world of medicine, with the same breadth of materials and methods that have been used to examine poverty, literacy, crime and religion. The history of medicine, now defined as embracing all matters relating to health and illness, has everything to gain from the widest possible use of sources and techniques, brought to bear upon problems arising from the historical period chosen for study.

Bibliography

Abel-Smith, B. (1964). *The Hospitals, 1800–1948. A Study in Social Administration in England and Wales.* London; Heinemann
Ackerknecht, E.H. (1932). Beiträge zur Geschichte der Medizinalreform von 1848, *Sudhoffs Archiv*, Vol. 25, 61–109, 113–183
Ackerknecht, E.H. (1945). *Malaria in the Upper Mississippi Valley 1760–1900.* Bulletin of the History of Medicine Supplement, No. 4. Baltimore; Johns Hopkins Press
Ackerknecht, E.H. (1967). *Medicine at the Paris Hospital 1794–1848.* Baltimore; Johns Hopkins Press
Allbutt, C. (1905). *The Historical Relations of Medicine and Surgery to the End of the Sixteenth Century.* London; Macmillan. Reprinted (1978). New York; AMS Press
Appleby, A.B. (1978). *Famine in Tudor and Stuart England.* Liverpool; Liverpool University Press
Ariès, P. (1960). *L'Enfant et la Vie familiale sous l'ancien Regime.* Paris; Libraire Plon. English version (1962). *Centuries of Childhood: A Social History of Family Life.* London; Cape. Paperback (1973). Harmondsworth; Penguin
Aronovitch, B. (1974). *Give it Time: An Experience of Hospital 1928–1932.* London; André Deutsch
Artelt, W. (1949). *Einführung in die Medizinhistorik, ihr Wesen, ihr Arbeitsweise und ihre Hilfsmittel.* Stuttgart; Enke
Atwater, E.C. (1980). Medical Schools: How Should We Write their Histories?, *Bulletin of the History of Medicine*, Vol. 54, 455–460
Aveling, J.H. (1872). *English Midwives. Their History and Prospects.* London; Churchill. Ed. J.L. Thornton (1967). London; Hugh K. Elliott
Ayers, G.M. (1971). *England's First State Hospitals and the Metropolitan Asylums Board 1867–1930.* London; Wellcome Institute for the History of Medicine
Baillet, A. (1685–86). *Jugemens des scavans sur les principaux ouvrages des auteurs.*

4 tom. in 9 Vols. Paris; chez Antoine Dezallier. Revised edn by M. de la Monnoye (1722–30). 8 Vols. Paris; C. Moette

Bale, J. (1548). *Illustrium maioris Britanniae scriptorum, hoc est, Angliae, Cambriae ac Scotiae summarium.* [Ipswich]; per Theodoricum Plateanum.

Baly, M.E. (1973). *Nursing and Social Change.* London; Heinemann. 2nd edn (1980)

Bannington, B.G. (1915). *English Public Health Administration.* 2nd edn (1929). London; P.S. King and Son

Barrett, C.R.B. (1905). *The History of the Society of Apothecaries of London.* London; Elliot Stock

Baruch, G. and Treacher, A. (1978). *Psychiatry Observed.* London; Routledge and Kegan Paul

Bastide, R. (1965). *Sociologie des maladies mentales.* Paris; Flammarion. Trans. J. McNeil (1972) as *The Sociology of Mental Disorder.* London; Routledge and Kegan Paul

Bayle, P. (1710). *An Historical and Critical Dictionary ... with Many Additions and Corrections Made by the Author Himself.* 4 Vols. London; C. Harper, etc. 1st French edn (1697). Rotterdam; chez R. Leers

Bellot, H.H. (1929). *University College Londcn 1826–1926.* London; University of London Press

Billroth, T. (1876). *Über das Lehren und Lernen der medicinischen Wissenschaften an den Universitäten der deutschen Nation nebst allgemeinen Bemerkungen über Universitäten.* Vienna; C. Gerolds Sohn. Engl. edn (1924) as *The Medical Sciences in the German Universities: A Study in the History of Civilisation.* New York; Macmillan

Biographia Britannica (1747–66) (with a Supplement). 6 Vols, Vol. 6 in 2 Pts. London; W. Innys, etc. 2nd edn (1778–93). Ed. A. Kippis *et al.* Vols 1–5 [Aaron – Fastolff only]. London; C. Bathurst, etc.

Blake, J.B., Ed. (1968). *Education in the History of Medicine.* New York and London; Hafner

Blake, J.B. and Roos, C. (1967). *Medical Reference Works 1679–1966: A Selected Bibliography.* Chicago; Medical Library Association. Also *Supplement 1* (1970). Comp. M.V. Clark. Chicago; Medical Library Association

Bloch, M.L.B. (1924). *Les Rois thaumaturges.* Strasbourg; Librairie Istra. London; Oxford University Press. Trans. J.E. Anderson (1973) as *The Royal Touch: Sacred Monarchy and Scrofula in England and France.* London; Routledge and Kegan Paul. Montreal; McGill–Queen's University Press

Bloom, J.H. and James, R.R. (1935). *Medical Practitioners in the Diocese of London, Licensed ... 1529–1725.* Cambridge; Cambridge University Press

Bonser, W. (1963). *The Medical Background of Anglo-Saxon England: A Study in History, Psychology and Folklore.* London; Wellcome Historical Medical Library

Book Subscriptions Lists Project. (1967–). [Afterwards] *Project for Historical Biobibliography.* [Directed by P.J. Wallis]. Numbered Publications (1972–). Newcastle upon Tyne; Project for Historical Biobibliography at the University of Newcastle upon Tyne

Branca, P., Ed. (1977). *The Medicine Show: Patients, Physicians and the Perplexities of the Health Revolution in Modern Society* [essays from *Journal of Social History*]. New York; Science History Publications

Brieger, G.H. (1980). History of Medicine, in *A Guide to the Culture of Science, Technology and Medicine.* Ed. P.T. Durbin. New York; Free Press, 121–194

Brockbank, E.M. (1936). *The Foundation of Provincial Medical Education in England and of the Manchester School in Particular.* Manchester; Manchester University Press

Brook, C.W. (1943). *Carlile and the Surgeons.* Glasgow; Strickland Press

Brown, M.W. (1918). *Neuropsychiatry and the War: A Bibliography with Abstracts.* New York; War Work Committee. With *Supplement* (1918)

Brunfels, O. (1530). *Catalogus illustrium medicorum.* Strassburg; apud I. Schottū.

Buer, M.C. (1926). *Health, Wealth and Population in the Early Days of the Industrial Revolution.* London; Routledge and Sons. Reissued (1968). London; Routledge and Kegan Paul

Bulloch, W. (1938). *The History of Bacteriology.* Heath Clark Lectures. London; Oxford University Press. Reprinted (1960)

Burdett, H.C. (1890–1930). *Burdett's Hospital Annual and Yearbook of Philanthropy.* Different titles. London; The Scientific Press. Merged 1930 into *Report on the Financial Position of the Voluntary Hospitals*

Burdett, H.C. (1891–3). *Hospitals and Asylums of the World, Their Origin, History, Construction, Administration...* 4 Vols and portfolio. London; Churchill

Burdett, H.C. (1896). *Cottage Hospitals, General, Fever and Convalescent, Their Progress, Management and Work in Great Britain and Ireland, and the United States of America, with an Alphabetical List...*, 3rd edn. London; The Scientific Press. 1st edn 1877

Burdett, H.C. (1898–1904). *Burdett's Official Nursing Directory.* London; The Scientific Press

Burnett, J. (1966). *Plenty and Want: A Social History of Diet in England from 1815 to the Present Day.* London; Nelson

Bylebyl, J., Ed. (1979). *William Harvey and his Age: The Professional and Social Context of the Discovery of the Circulation.* Baltimore and London; Johns Hopkins University Press

Callisen, A.C.P. (1830–45). *Medicinisches Schriftsteller-Lexikon der jetzt lebenden Aerzte, Wundärzte, Geburtshelfer, Apotheker, und Naturforscher aller gebildeten Völker.* 33 Vols. Copenhagen; privately printed. Reprinted (1962–5). Nieuwkoop; B. de Graaf

Cameron, C.A. (1886). *History of the Royal College of Surgeons in Ireland and of the Irish Schools of Medicine, including a Medical Bibliography.* Dublin; Fannin. 2nd edn (1916). Dublin; Fannin. London; Baillière, Tindall and Cox

Cantlie, N. (1974). *A History of the Army Medical Department.* 2 Vols. Edinburgh; Livingstone. London; Churchill

Capp, B. (1979). *Astrology and the Popular Press. English Almanacs 1500–1800.* London and Boston; Faber

Catalogue of the Ferguson Collection of Books mainly relating to Alchemy, Witchcraft, and Gypsies in the Library of the University of Glasgow (1943). 2 Vols. [Glasgow]; R. Maclehose

Chaff, S., *et al.*, Ed. (1977). *Women in Medicine. A Bibliography of the Literature on Women Physicians.* Metuchen, NJ; Scarecrow

Checkland, O. (1980). *Philanthropy and Victorian Scotland: Social Welfare and the Voluntary Principle.* Edinburgh; John Donald

Cipolla, C.M. (1976). *Public Health and the Medical Profession in the Renaissance.* Cambridge; Cambridge University Press

Clark, G.N. (1964–6). *A History of the Royal College of Physicians of London.* 2 Vols. Oxford; Clarendon Press

Clarke, E., Ed. (1971). *Modern Methods in the History of Medicine.* London; Athlone Press

Comrie, J.D. (1932). *History of Scottish Medicine,* 2nd edn. 2 Vols. London; Wellcome Historical Medical Museum

Cope, Z. (1954). *The History of St. Mary's Hospital Medical School or a Century of Medical Education.* London; Heinemann

Copenhaver, B. (1978). *Symphorien Champier and the Reception of the Occultist Tradition in Renaissance France.* The Hague; Mouton

Cosenza, M.E. (1962). *Biographical and Bibliographical Dictionary of the Italian Humanists and of the World of Classical Scholarship in Italy, 1300–1800.* 6 Vols. Boston; G.K. Hall

Creighton, C. (1894). *A History of Epidemics in Britain.* London; Cambridge University Press. 2nd edn (1965), with additional material by D.E.C. Eversley, E.A. Underwood and L. Ovenall. 2 Vols. London; Frank Cass

Creswell, C.H. (1926). *The Royal College of Physicians of Edinburgh. Historical Notes from 1505 to 1905.* Edinburgh; The College

Crowley, C.G. (1885). *Dental Bibliography: A Standard Reference List of Books on Dentistry Published Throughout the World from 1536 to 1885.* Philadelphia; S.S. White Dental Mfg. Co. Reprinted (1968). Amsterdam; Liberac

Cule, J. (1980). *Wales and Medicine. A Source List for Printed Books and Papers Showing the History of Medicine in Relation to Wales and Welshmen.* [Aberystwyth; National Library of Wales]

Current Work in the History of Medicine; An International Bibliography (1954–). London; Wellcome Institute for the History of Medicine

Davies, C., Ed. (1980). *Rewriting Nursing History.* London; Croom Helm

De Kruif, P.H. (1926). *Microbe Hunters.* New York; Harcourt, Brace and Co. 24th printing (1950)

Delaunay, P. (1935). *La Vie médicale aux XVIe, XVIIe et XVIIIe siècles.* Paris; Editions Hippocrate

Delaunay, P. (1948). *La Médecine et l'église: Contribution à l'histoire de l'exercice médical par les clercs.* Paris; Editions Hippocrate

Dewhurst, K. (1963). *John Locke (1632–1704). Physician and Philosopher. A Medical Biography with an Edition of the Medical Notes in his Journals.* London; Wellcome Historical Medical Library

Dictionary of National Biography, The (1882–1900). Ed. L. Stephen and S. Lee. 63 Vols. London; Smith, Elder and Co. *Supplement* (1901). 3 Vols. Reprinted in 22 Vols (1908–9). *Index and Epitome* [i.e., *Concise D.N.B. to 1900*] (1903). Thereafter in 5 decennial vols, from 1901 (1920–71). London; Oxford University Press. See also Institute of Historical Research, London, *Corrections and Additions to the Dictionary of National Biography Cumulated from the Bulletin...1923–1963* (1966). Boston, Mass.; G.K. Hall

Donnison, J. (1977). *Midwives and Medical Men: A History of Interprofessional Rivalries and Women's Rights.* London; Heinemann

Dorwart, R.A. (1971). *The Prussian Welfare State before 1740.* Cambridge, Mass.; Harvard University Press

Drew, R. (1968). *Commissioned Officers in the Medical Services of the British Army 1660–1960* [incl. *Peterkin's Roll* and *Johnston's Roll*]. 2 Vols. London; Wellcome Historical Medical Library

Drummond, J.C. and Wilbraham, A. (1939). *The Englishman's Food: Five Centuries of English Diet.* London; J. Cape

Dudfield, R. (1906). History of the Society [of Medical Officers of Health], *Public Health*, Jubilee Number

Duncum, B.M. (1947). *The Development of Inhalation Anaesthesia, with Special Reference to the Years 1846–1900.* London; Oxford University Press

Durey, M. (1979). *The Return of the Plague: British Society and the Cholera 1831–2.* Dublin; Gill and Macmillan

Edinburgh, Royal College of Physicians. Card Index of Edinburgh MDs, 1705–1858. Comp. J.D. Comrie

Edinburgh, Royal College of Physicians. Card Index to Obituary Notices in *Edinburgh Medical Journal*, 1805–1954

Edinburgh University (1846). *Nomina Eorum qui Gradum Medicinae Doctoris in Academia Jacobi Sexti Scotorum Regis, quae Edinburgi...* [1705–1845]. Edinburgh; Neill

Éloy, N.F.J. (1755). *Dictionnaire historique de la médecine, contenant son origine, ses progrès, ses révolutions...l'histoire des plus célèbres médecins...anatomistes, chirurgiens, botanistes.* Brussels; chez J. vanden Berghen. 2nd edn (1778). 4 Vols. Mons; Hoyois

Eulner, H.-H. (1970). *Die Entwicklung der medizinischen Spezialfächer an den Universitäten des deutschen Sprachgebietes.* Vol. IV of *Studien zur Medizingeschichte des 19. Jahrhunderts.* Ed. W. Artelt and W. Rüegg. Stuttgart; F. Enke. Revision of Habilitationsschrift, Frankfurt am Main (1963)

Eyler, J.M. (1979). *Victorian Social Medicine: The Ideas and Methods of William Farr.* Baltimore and London; Johns Hopkins University Press

Farrell, G. (1956). *The Story of Blindness.* Cambridge, Mass.; Harvard University Press

Ferguson, J. (1906). *Bibliotheca Chemica: A Bibliography of Books on Alchemy, Chemistry and Pharmaceutics.* 2 Vols. Glasgow; J. Maclehose. Facsimile edn (1954). London; Derek Verschoyle

Ferguson, M. and Smith, D.B. (1930). *The Printed Books in the Library of the Hunterian Museum in the University of Glasgow; A Catalogue.* Glasgow; Jackson, Wylie and Co.

Ferguson, T. (1948). *The Dawn of Scottish Social Welfare: A Survey from Medieval Times to 1863.* London; Nelson

Ferguson, T. (1958). *Scottish Social Welfare 1864–1914.* Edinburgh and London; Livingstone

Fessler, A. (1952). The Official Attitude towards the Sick Poor in Seventeenth Century Lancashire, *Transactions of the Historic Society of Lancashire and Cheshire*, Vol. 102, 85–113

Filby, F.A. (1934). *A History of Food Adulteration and Analysis.* London; George Allen and Unwin

Finnegan, F. (1979). *Poverty and Prostitution: A Study of Victorian Prostitutes in York.* Cambridge; Cambridge University Press

Fischer, D.H. (1977). *Growing Old in America.* New York; Oxford University Press

Fleming, G. (1871–82). *Animal Plagues: Their History, Nature and Prevention.* 2 Vols. London; Chapman and Hall

Flinn, M.W. (1970). *British Population Growth 1700–1850.* London; Macmillan. Reprinted (1972)

Forster, R. and Ranum, O., Ed. (1975). *Biology of Man in History. Selections from the Annales.* Trans. E. Forster and P.N. Ranum. Baltimore and London; Johns Hopkins University Press

Forster, R., and Ranum, O., Ed. (1980). *Medicine and Society in France. Selections from the Annales.* Baltimore and London; Johns Hopkins University Press

Foster, M. (1901). *Lectures on the History of Physiology during the Sixteenth, Seventeenth and Eighteenth Centuries.* Cambridge Natural Science Manuals. Cambridge; Cambridge University Press. Reprinted (1924).

Foucault, M. (1961). *Folie et déraison: Histoire de la folie à l'âge classique.* Paris; Plon. Abridged edn (1964). Trans. (1965) as *Madness and Civilisation.* New York; Pantheon Books. 2nd edn (1971). English edn. (1967). London; Tavistock

Foucault, M. (1963). *Naissance de la clinique: une archéologie du regard médical.*

Paris; Presses Universitaires de France. Trans. A.M. Sheridan Smith (1973) as *The Birth of the Clinic*. London; Tavistock

Frank, R.G. (1980). *Harvey and the Oxford Physiologists: A Study of Scientific Ideas*. Berkeley; University of California Press

Frazer, W.M. (1950). *A History of English Public Health 1834–1939*. London; Baillière, Tindall and Cox

Frost, W.H., Ed. (1936). *Snow on Cholera: Being a Reprint of Two Papers by John Snow, M.D., Together with a Biographical Memoir by B.W. Richardson*. Harvard University Press. Facsimile edn (1965). New York and London; Hafner

Galdston, I., Ed. (1949). *Social Medicine: Its Derivations and Objectives*. The New York Academy of Medicine Institute on Social Medicine. New York; The Commonwealth Fund

Garrison, F.H. (1913). *An Introduction to the History of Medicine, with Medical Chronology, Suggestions for Study and Bibliographic Data*. Philadelphia and London; W.B. Saunders. 4th edn (1929). Philadelphia; Saunders. Reprinted (1960)

Garrison, F.H. (1928). Available Sources and Future Prospects of Medical Biography, *Bulletin of the New York Academy of Medicine*, Vol. 4, 586–607

Garrison, F.H. and Morton, L.T. (1943). *A Medical Bibliography (Garrison and Morton). An Annotated Checklist of Texts Illustrating the History of Medicine*. 3rd edn (1970). London; André Deutsch

Gaskell, E. (1964). Bibliography of Hospital History, in *The Evolution of Hospitals in Britain*. Ed. F.N.L. Poynter. London; Pitman, 255–279

Gesner, C. (1545–55). *Bibliotheca universalis*. 4 Vols. Zürich; apud C. Froschoverum

Glass, D.V. and Eversley, D.E.C., Ed. (1965). *Population in History: Essays in Historical Demography*. London; Edward Arnold. Reprinted (1969)

Glass, D.V. and Revelle, R., Ed. (1972). *Population and Social Change*. London; Edward Arnold

Goodall, C. (1684). *The Royal College of Physicians of London, Founded and Established by Law...* London; for Walter Kettilby

Gottfried, R.S. (1978). *Epidemic Disease in Fifteenth Century England: The Medical Response and the Demographic Consequences*. Leicester; Leicester University Press. New Jersey; Rutgers University Press

Goubert, J.-P. (1974). *Malades et médecins en Bretagne 1770–1790*. Rennes; Université de Haute-Bretagne

Greenwood, M. (1932). *Epidemiology, Historical and Experimental*. Baltimore; Johns Hopkins Press

Gurlt, E.J. (1898). *Geschichte der Chirurgie und ihrer Ausübung: Volkschirurgie, Alterthum, Mittelalter, Renaissance*. 3 Vols. Berlin; Hirschwald. Reprinted (1964). Hildesheim; Olms

Haller, A. von (1771–2). *Bibliotheca botanica*. 2 Vols. London; prostant apud C. Heydinger

Haller, A. von (1774–5). *Bibliotheca chirurgica*. 2 Vols. Berne; Haller. Basle; Schweighauser

Haller, A. von (1774–7). *Bibliotheca anatomica*. 2 Vols. Zürich; apud Orell, Gessner, etc.

Haller, A. von (1776–9). *Bibliotheca medicinae practicae*. 4 Vols. Berne; Haller

Hanlon, J.J., Rogers, F.B. and Rosen, G. (1960). A Bookshelf on the History and Philosophy of Public Health, *American Journal of Public Health*, Vol. 50, 445–458

Hecker, J.F.K. (1844). *The Epidemics of the Middle Ages*. Trans. B.G. Babington. London; The Sydenham Society

Heller, R. (1976). 'Priest-Doctors' as a Rural Health Service in the Age of Enlightenment, *Medical History*, Vol. 20, 361–383

Highmore, A. (1810). *Pietas Londinensis: The History, Design and Present State of the Various Public Charities in and near London.* London; for R. Phillips

Himes, N.E. (1936). *Medical History of Contraception.* Baltimore; Williams and Wilkins. Reprinted (1963). New York; Gamut Press

Hirsch, A. (1859–64). *Handbuch der historisch-geographischen Pathologie.* 2 Vols in 3. Erlangen. Stuttgart; F. Enke. Trans. of 2nd German edn by C. Creighton. (1883–6). 3 Vols. London; New Sydenham Society

Hirsch, A. (1884–8). *Biographisches Lexikon der hervorragenden Ärzte aller Zeiten und Völker.* 6 Vols. Vienna and Leipzig; Urban und Schwarzenberg. 3rd edn with J.L. Pagel (1901), to 1930. 8 Vols. Munich and Berlin; Urban und Schwarzenberg

Hirst, L.F. (1953). *The Conquest of Plague: A Study of the Evolution of Epidemiology.* Oxford; Clarendon Press

History of the Family (1971, 1975). *Journal of Interdisciplinary History*, Vol. 2 (1971), Vols 5 and 6 (1975), Special Numbers. The first enlarged and published (1973) as *The Family in History.* Ed. T.K. Rabb and R.I. Rotberg. New York; Harper Torchbooks

History of the Great War Based on Official Documents. Medical Services (1921–31). 12 Vols. London; HMSO

Honigsbaum, F. (1979). *The Division in British Medicine: A History of the Separation of General Practice from Hospital Care 1911–1968.* London; Kogan Page

Howard, J. (1789). *An Account of the Principal Lazarettos in Europe...with Further Observations on some Foreign Prisons and Hospitals: and Additional Remarks on the Present State of Those in Great Britain and Ireland.* Warrington and London; T. Cadell

Hufton, O. (1974). *The Poor of Eighteenth-Century France 1750–1789.* Oxford; Clarendon Press

Hughes, M.J. (1943). *Women Healers in Medieval Life and Literature.* New York; King's Crown Press

Hunter, R. and McAlpine, I. (1963). *Three Hundred Years of Psychiatry 1535–1860.* London; Oxford University Press. Reprinted (1970)

Hutchins, B.L. (1909). *The Public Health Agitation 1833–1848.* London; A.C. Fifield

Hutchinson, B. (1799). *Biographia Medica; or, Historical and Critical Memoirs of...the Most Eminent Medical Characters that have Existed from the Earliest Account of Time to the Present Period.* 2 Vols. London; for J. Johnson

Imhof, A.E., Ed. (1980). *Mensch und Gesundheit in der Geschichte.* Abhandlungen zur Geschichte der Medizin und der Naturwissenschaften, No. 39. Husum; Matthieson Verlag

Imhof, A.E. and Larsen, Ø. (1975). *Sozialgeschichte und Medizin: Probleme der quantifizierenden Quellenbearbeitung in der Sozial- und Medizingeschichte.* Oslo; Universitetsforlaget. Stuttgart; Gustav Fischer

Index Medicus, War Supplement: A Classified Record of Literature on Military Medicine and Surgery 1914–1917 [1918]. Washington; Carnegie Institute

Inkster, I. (1977). Marginal Men: Aspects of the Social Role of the Medical Community in Sheffield 1790–1850, in *Health Care and Popular Medicine in Nineteenth Century England.* Ed. J. Woodward and D. Richards. London; Croom Helm, 128–163

Jennett, S., Ed. (1963). *Journal of a Younger Brother: The Life of Thomas Platter as a Medical Student in Montpellier at the Close of the Sixteenth Century.* London; Frederick Muller

Jetter, D. (1966–72). *Geschichte des Hospitals.* 3 Vols. Wiesbaden; Franz Steiner Verlag

Jöcher, C.G. (1750–1). *Allgemeines Gelehrten-lexikon.* 4 Vols. Leipzig; J.F. Gleditschens Buchhandlung. Continued by J.C. Adelung and H.W. Rotermund, *Fortsetzung und Ergänzungen...* (1784–1819). 6 Vols. [A to Ri only]. Various places and publishers

Jourdain, A.J.L. (1820–5). *Dictionnaire des sciences médicales: Biographie médicale.* 7 Vols. Paris; Panckoucke

Keevil, J.J. (1952). *Hamey the Stranger* [Baldwin Hamey the elder, 1568–1640]. London; Geoffrey Bles

Keevil, J.J. (1957–8). *Medicine and the Navy 1200–1900.* 2 Vols. Edinburgh and London; Livingstone. See also C. Lloyd and J.L.S. Coulter (1961)

Keill, N. (1965). *Psychiatry and Psychology in the Visual Arts and Aesthetics: A Bibliography.* Madison; University of Wisconsin Press

Keill, N. (1966). Medicine and Art 1934–1964: A Bibliography, *Journal of the History of Medicine,* Vol. 21, 147–172

Kerling, N.J. (1977). *Report on the Records of Hospitals in the City of London and Borough of Hackney Health District, 1137–1974.* London; The Historical Manuscripts Commission

Kirkpatrick, T.P.C. (1912). *History of the Medical Teaching in Trinity College, Dublin, and of the School of Physic in Ireland.* Dublin; Hanna and Neale

Koch, C.R.E., Ed. (1909). *History of Dental Surgery.* 2 Vols. Chicago; National Art Publ. Co.

Kremers, E. and Urdang, G. (1940). *History of Pharmacy: A Guide and a Survey,* 2nd edn. Philadelphia; J.B. Lippincott

Laignel-Lavastine, M., Ed. (1936–49). *Histoire générale de la médicine, de la pharmacie, de l'art dentaire et de l'art vétérinaire.* 3 Vols. Paris; Albin Michel

Lambert, J. (1963). *Sir John Simon 1816–1904 and English Social Administration.* London; MacGibbon and Kee

Lebrun, F. (1971). *Les Hommes et la mort en Anjou aux 17ᵉ et 18ᵉ siècles.* Paris; Mouton

LeFanu, W.R. (1937–8). British Periodicals of Medicine: A Chronological List, *Bulletin of the Institute of the History of Medicine,* Vol. 5, 735–761, 827–846; Vol. 6, 614–648. Publ. sep. (1938). Baltimore; Johns Hopkins Press. Supplemented by A.M. Shadrake (1963). British Medical Periodicals, 1938–61, *Bulletin of the Medical Library Association,* Vol. 51, 181–196

Lesky, E. (1965). *The Vienna Medical School of the Nineteenth Century.* Trans. L. Williams and I.S. Levij (1976). Baltimore and London; Johns Hopkins University Press

Levy, H. (1943). The Economic History of Sickness and Medical Benefit before the Puritan Revolution, *Economic History Review,* Vol. 13, 42–57

Levy, H. (1944). The Economic History of Sickness and Medical Benefit since the Puritan Revolution, *Economic History Review,* Vol. 14, 135–160

Lewis, J. (1980). *The Politics of Motherhood: Child and Maternal Welfare in England 1900–1939.* London; Croom Helm

Lewis, R.A. (1952). *Edwin Chadwick and the Public Health Movement 1832–1854.* London; Longmans, Green and Co.

Lloyd, C. and Coulter, J.L.S. (1961). *Medicine and the Navy 1200–1900,* Vol. III: *1714–1815.* Edinburgh; Livingstone

Long, E.R. (1928). *A History of Pathology.* Baltimore; Williams and Wilkins. 2nd edn (1965). New York; Dover

Loudon, I.S.L. (1981). The Origin and Growth of the Dispensary Movement, *Bulletin of the History of Medicine,* Vol. 55, 323–342

McCleary, G.F. (1933). *The Early History of the Infant Welfare Movement.* London; Lewis

McCleary, G.F. (1935). *The Maternity and Child Welfare Movement.* London; King

MacDonald, M. (1981). *Mystical Bedlam: Madness, Anxiety and Healing in Seventeenth-Century England.* New York and Cambridge; Cambridge University Press

McHenry, L.C., Ed. (1969). *Garrison's History of Neurology* [1925] *Revised and Enlarged with a Bibliography...* Springfield, Ill.; Thomas

McLachlan, G. and McKeown, T., Ed. (1971). *Medical History and Medical Care: A Symposium of Perspectives.* London; Oxford University Press

McLaren, A. (1978). *Birth Control in Nineteenth Century England.* London; Croom Helm

Maclean, I. (1980). *The Renaissance Notion of Woman: A Study in the Fortunes of Scholasticism and Medical Science in European Intellectual Life.* New York; Cambridge University Press

McMenemey, W.H. (1959). *The Life and Times of Sir Charles Hastings, Founder of the British Medical Association.* Edinburgh; Livingstone

McNeill, W.H. (1977). *Plagues and Peoples.* Oxford; Blackwell

Malgaigne, J.F. (1840–1). *Oeuvres complètes d'Ambroise Paré.* 3 Vols. Paris; Baillière. Trans. and Ed. W.B. Hamby (1965) as *Surgery and Ambroise Paré.* Norman, Oklahoma; University of Oklahoma Press

Manget, J.J. (1731). *Bibliotheca scriptorum medicorum veterum et recentiorum.* 4 Parts in 2 Vols. Geneva; Perachon and Cramer

Marmoy, C.F.A. (1977). *The French Protestant Hospital: Extracts from the Archives of 'La Providence' relating to Inmates and Applicants for Admission 1718–1957...* 2 Vols. London; Huguenot Society

Matthews, L.G. (1962). *History of Pharmacy in Britain.* Edinburgh; Livingstone

May, J. O'Hara (1977). *Elizabethan Dyetary of Health.* Lawrence, Kansas; Coronado Press

Medical Directory, The London (1845–7). Then *London and Provincial Medical Directory* (1848–69); inclusive of Medical Directories for Scotland and for Ireland and of *General Medical Register,* 1861–9. Then *The Medical Directory ...and General Medical Register* (1870–)

Medical Register (1779, 1780, 1783). London; for J. Murray, for Fielding and Walker, for Joseph Johnson respectively

Miller, G. (1957). *The Adoption of Inoculation for Smallpox in England and France.* London; Oxford University Press

Miller, G. (1964). *Bibliography of the History of Medicine in the United States and Canada, 1939–1960,* 2nd edn. Baltimore; Johns Hopkins Press. Annual supplements continue in *Bulletin of the History of Medicine* (1962–6)

Miller, G., Ed. (1966). *A Bibliography of the Writings of Henry E. Sigerist.* Montreal; McGill University Press

Morris, C. (1934). *The Diary of a West Country Physician A.D. 1684–1726.* Ed. E. Hobhouse. London; Simpkin Marshall

Munk, W. (1878). *The Roll of the Royal College of Physicians of London ... 1518 to ... 1825* [Fellows and Licentiates], 2nd edn. 3 Vols. London; the College. Supplemented by G.H. Brown (1955). *Lives of the Fellows ... 1826–1925.* London; the College. Also R.R. Trail (1968). *Lives ... Continued to 1965.* London; the College

Murchison, C. (1862). *A Treatise on the Continued Fevers of Great Britain.* London; Parker, Son, and Bourn. 3rd edn (1884). Ed. W. Cayley. London; Longmans, Green and Co.

National Health Service (1966). *Birmingham Regional Hospital Board, 1947–1966.* [Birmingham]; NHS

National Library of Medicine, USA (1873–1961). *Catalogue of the Library of the Surgeon-General's Office* [authors]. Comp. J.S. Billings. 3 Vols. (1873–4). Washington; Government Printing Office. Then *Index-Catalogue...Authors and Subjects.* 16 Vols. (1880–95). *Alphabetical List of Abbreviations of Titles of Medical Periodicals...* (1895). Then *Index-Catalogue...* 2nd Ser. 21 Vols. (1896–1916); 3rd Ser. 10 Vols. (1918–32); 4th Ser. (Army Medical Library). 11 Vols. (1936–55); 5th Ser. (National Library of Medicine). 3 Vols. (1959–61). Washington; US Dept. of Health, Education and Welfare. Ser. 1–3 reprinted (1972). New York and London; Johnson Reprint Corporation. Also *Armed Forces Medical Library Catalog. A Cumulative List of Works Represented by Armed Forces Medical Library Cards 1950–1954.* 6 Vols. (1955). Ann Arbor, Mich.; J.W. Edwards. Then *National Library of Medicine Catalog. A List of Works Represented by National Library of Medicine Cards 1955–1959.* 6 Vols. (1960). Washington; Judd and Detweiler. Ditto, *1960–1965.* 6 Vols. (1966). New York; Rowman and Littlefield. Then *Current Catalog 1965–1970.* 7 Vols with 1 Vol., *Technical Reports 1968–1970* (n.d.). Bethesda; US. Dept. of Health, Education and Welfare. Also *Current Catalog. Annual Cumulation* (1966–). Bethesda; US Dept. of Health, Education and Welfare

National Library of Medicine, USA [1948?]. *A Catalogue of Incunabula and Manuscripts in the Army Medical Library.* Ed. D.M. Schullian and F.E. Sommer. New York; H. Schuman

National Library of Medicine, USA (1965–78). *Bibliography of the History of Medicine.* 1–4 (1965–8); Cumulative Volume (1964–9); 6–9 (1970–3); Cumulative Volume (1970–4); 11–14 (1975–8)

National Library of Medicine, USA (1967). *A Catalogue of Sixteenth Century Printed Books in the National Library of Medicine.* Ed. R.J. Durling. Bethesda; US Dept. of Health, Education and Welfare

National Library of Medicine, USA (1968). *A Summary Checklist of Medical Manuscripts on Microfilm held by the National Library of Medicine.* Bethesda; US Dept. of Health, Education and Welfare

National Library of Medicine, USA (1971). *A Catalogue of Incunabula and Sixteenth Century Printed Books in the National Library of Medicine, First Supplement.* Comp. P. Krivatsky. Bethesda; US Dept. of Health, Education and Welfare

National Library of Medicine, USA (1972). *Index of N.L.M. Serial Titles. A Keyword Listing of Serial Titles Currently Received.* Bethesda; US Dept of Health, Education and Welfare

National Library of Medicine, USA (1979). *A Short-Title Catalogue of Eighteenth Century Printed Books in the National Library of Medicine.* Comp. J.B. Blake, Bethesda; US Dept. of Health, Education and Welfare

Neumann, L.G. (1896). *Biographies vétérinaires.* Paris; Asselin and Houzeau

Newman, C. (1957). *The Evolution of Medical Education in the Nineteenth Century.* London; Oxford University Press

Newsholme, A. (1927a). *Health Problems in Organized Society. Studies in the Social Aspects of Public Health.* London; P.S. King and Son

Newsholme, A. (1927b). *Evolution of Preventive Medicine.* Baltimore; Williams and Wilkins

Newsholme, A. (1931). *International Studies on the Relation between Private and Official Practice of Medicine with Special Reference to the Prevention of Disease.* London; Allen and Unwin

Medicine since 1500 403

Osler, W. (1929). *Bibliotheca Osleriana: A Catalogue of Books Illustrating the History of Medicine and Science...Bequeathed to McGill University.* Oxford; Clarendon Press. 2nd edn (1969). Montreal and London; McGill–Queen's University Press

Oxley, G.W. (1974). *Poor Relief in England and Wales 1601–1834.* Newton Abbot; David and Charles

Ozanam, J.A.F. (1817–23). *Histoire médicale, générale et particulière des maladies epidémiques, contagieuses et epizootiques,* 1st edn. Paris, chez Mequignon-Marvis et à Lyon, chez l'auteur. 2nd edn (1835). 4 tom. in 2 Vols. Paris and Lyons; libraires pour la médecine et chez l'auteur

Pagel, J.L. (1898). *Historisch-medicinische Bibliographie für die Jahre 1875–1896.* Berlin; Karger.

Pagel, J.L. (1901). *Biographisches Lexicon hervorragender Ärzte des neunzehnten Jahrhunderts.* Berlin and Vienna; Urban und Schwarzenberg

Pagel, W. (1958). *Paracelsus: An Introduction to Philosophical Medicine in the Era of the Renaissance.* Basle; Karger

Pagel, W. (1967). *William Harvey's Biological Ideas: Selected Aspects and Historical Background.* Basle; Karger

Pagel, W. (1982). *Joan Baptista Van Helmont: Reformer of Science and Medicine.* Cambridge; Cambridge University Press

Parish, H.J. (1965). *A History of Immunization.* London; Livingstone

Parker, G. (1914). The History and Powers of the Barber-Surgeons in Great Britain, *International Congress of Medicine, History of Medicine,* Sect. 23, 285–295

Parry, N. and Parry, J. (1976). *The Rise of the Medical Profession: A Study of Collective Social Mobility.* London; Croom Helm

Partington, J.R. (1961–70). *A History of Chemistry.* 4 Vols. London; Macmillan. Vols 2, 3, 4 reprinted (1969), (1970), (1972) respectively

Pauly, A. (1874). *Bibliographie des sciences médicales.* Paris; Tross

Payne, J.F. (1900). *Thomas Sydenham.* London; T. Fisher Unwin

Payne, L.M. (1970). Materials for Medical Biography, in *Proceedings of the 3rd International Congress of Medical Librarianship, Amsterdam, 5–9 May 1969.* Ed. K.E. Davis and W.D. Sweeney. Amsterdam; Excerpta Medica, 251–257

Peel, J. (1976). *The Lives of the Fellows of the Royal College of Obstetricians and Gynaecologists 1929–1969.* London; Heinemann

Pelling, M. (1978). *Cholera, Fever and English Medicine 1825–1865.* Oxford; Oxford University Press

Pelling, M. and Webster, C. (1979). Medical Practitioners, in *Health, Medicine and Mortality in the Sixteenth Century.* Ed. C. Webster. Cambridge; Cambridge University Press, 165–235

Peterson, M.J. (1978). *The Medical Profession in Mid-Victorian London.* Berkeley; University of California Press

Pettigrew, T.J. [1840]. *Medical Portrait Gallery. Biographical Memoirs of the Most Celebrated Physicians, Surgeons...* 4 Vols. London; Fisher, Son and Co.; Whittaker and Co.

Pettigrew, T.J. (1844). *On Superstitions Connected with the History and Practice of Medicine and Surgery.* London; J. Churchill

Pickstone, J.V., Ed. (1980). *Health, Disease and Medicine in Lancashire 1750–1950. Four Papers on Sources, Problems and Methods.* Dept. of History of Science and Technology, UMIST, Occasional Publ. No. 2. Manchester; the Dept.

Plarr's Lives of the Fellows of the Royal College of Surgeons of England (1930). Revised by D'A. Power, W.G. Spencer and G.E. Gask. 2 Vols. Bristol; Wright. Continued by D'A. Power and W.R. LeFanu (1953). *Lives of the Fellows...1930–*

1951. London; the College. Also R.H.O.B. Robinson and W.R. LeFanu (1970). *Lives of the Fellows...1952–1964.* Edinburgh; Livingstone

Ploucquet, W.G. (1808–14). *Literatura medica digesta sive repertorium medicinae practicae, chirurgiae atque rei obstetriciae.* 4 Vols and Supplement. Tübingen; apud J.G. Cottam

Post, J.D. (1977). *The Last Great Subsistence Crisis in the Western World.* Baltimore and London; Johns Hopkins University Press

Power, D'A. (1931). *The Foundations of Medical History.* Baltimore; Williams and Wilkins

Power, D'A. (1939). *British Medical Societies.* London; Medical Press and Circular

Poynter, F.N.L., Ed. (1961). *The Evolution of Medical Practice in Britain.* London; Pitman

Poynter, F.N.L. Ed. (1963). *The Journal of James Yonge* [1647–1721], *Plymouth Surgeon.* London; Longmans

Poynter, F.N.L. (1972). The Evolution of Military Medicine, in *A Guide to The Sources of British Military History.* Ed. R. Higham. London; Routledge and Kegan Paul, 591–605

Poynter, F.N.L. and Bishop, W.T., Ed. (1951). *A Seventeenth Century Doctor and his Patients: John Symcotts 1592?–1662.* Bedfordshire Historical Record Society, Vol. 31. Streatley; the Society

Prinzing, F. (1916). *Epidemics Resulting from Wars.* Ed. H. Westergaard. Oxford; Clarendon Press

Proksch, J.K. (1895). *Die Geschichte der venerischen Krankheiten.* 2 Vols. Bonn; Peter Hanstein

Puschmann, T. (1891). *A History of Medical Education from the Most Remote to the Most Recent Times.* Ed. and trans. E.H. Hare. London; Lewis

Pusey, W.A. (1933). *The History of Dermatology.* London; Baillière, Tindall and Cox

Raach, J.H. (1962). *A Directory of English Country Physicians 1603–1643.* London; Dawsons

Ranum, O. and Ranum, P., Ed. (1972). *Popular Attitudes toward Birth Control in Pre-Industrial France and England.* New York; Harper and Row

Rather, L.J. (1965). *Mind and Body in Eighteenth Century Medicine: A Study based on Jerome Gaub's De regimine mentis.* London; Wellcome Historical Medical Library

Rather, L.J. (1978). *The Genesis of Cancer. A Study in the History of Ideas.* Baltimore and London; Johns Hopkins University Press

Raven-Hart, H. and Johnston, M. (1931–2). Bibliography of the Registers (Printed) of the Universities, Inns of Court, Colleges and Schools of Great Britain and Ireland, *Bulletin of the Institute of Historical Research,* Vol. 9, 19–30, 65–83, 154–170; Vol. 10, 109–113

Razi, Z. (1980). *Life, Marriage and Death in a Medieval Parish. Economy, Society and Demography in Halesowen 1270–1400.* Cambridge; Cambridge University Press

Ricci, J.V. (1945). *One Hundred Years of Gynaecology 1800–1900.* Philadelphia; The Blakiston Co.

Richards, P. (1977). *The Medieval Leper and his Northern Heirs.* Cambridge; D.S. Brewer

Richardson, B.W. (1887). *The Health of Nations: A Review of the Works of Edwin Chadwick, with a Biographical Dissertation.* 2 Vols. London; Dawsons. Reprinted (1965)

Roberts, R.S. (1962–4). The Personnel and Practice of Medicine in Tudor and Stuart England, *Medical History,* Vol. 6, 363–382; Vol. 8, 217–234

Roberts, R.S. (1968). Epidemics and Social History, *Medical History*, Vol. 12, 305–316

Rockey, D. (1980). *Speech Disorder in Nineteenth Century Britain: The History of Stuttering*. London; Croom Helm

Rosen, G. (1943). *The History of Miners' Diseases: A Medical and Social Interpretation*. New York; Schuman

Rosen, G. (1946). *Fees and Fee Bills: Some Economic Aspects of Medical Practice in Nineteenth Century America*. Baltimore; Johns Hopkins Press

Rosen, G. (1959). A Bookshelf on the Social Sciences and Public Health, *American Journal of Public Health*, Vol. 49, 441–454

Rosen, G. (1968). *Madness in Society: Chapters in the Historical Sociology of Mental Illness*. Ed. B. Nelson. London; Routledge and Kegan Paul. Chicago; University of Chicago Press

Rosen, G. (1974). *From Medical Police to Social Medicine: Essays on the History of Health Care*. New York; Science History Publications

Russell, K. (1947). A Checklist of Medical Books Published in English before 1600, *Bulletin of the History of Medicine*, Vol. 21, 922–958

Russell, K. (1963). *British Anatomy 1525–1800: A Bibliography*. Melbourne; Melbourne University Press

Sand, R. (1952). *The Advance to Social Medicine*. London; Staples Press. 1st French edn (1948)

Shrewsbury, J.F.D. (1970). *A History of Bubonic Plague in the British Isles*. Cambridge; Cambridge University Press

Shryock, R.H. (1936). *The Development of Modern Medicine: an Interpretation of the Social and Scientific Factors Involved*. Philadelphia; University of Pennsylvania Press. 2nd edn (1947). Paperback edn (1979). Madison; University of Wisconsin Press

Sigerist, H.E. (1931). Psychopathologie und Kulturwissenschaft, *Abhandlungen aus der Neurologie, Psychiatrie, Psychologie*, Vol. 61, 140–146

Sigerist, H.E. (1931). *Einführung in die Medizin*. Leipzig; Georg Thieme Verlag. Trans. M.G. Boise (1932) as *Man and Medicine. An Introduction to Medical Knowledge*. New York; W.W. Norton

Sigerist, H.E. (1951, 1961). *A History of Medicine*. Vol. I: *Primitive and Archaic Medicine*. Vol. II: *Early Greek, Hindu and Persian Medicine*. New York; Oxford University Press

Sigerist, H.E. (1960). *On the Sociology of Medicine*. Ed. M.I. Roemer. New York; MD Publications. See also G. Miller (1966)

Simon, J. (1887). *Public Health Reports*. Ed. E. Seaton. 2 Vols. London; J. and A. Churchill

Simon, J. (1890). *English Sanitary Institutions, Reviewed in their Course of Development and in some of their Political and Social Relations*. London; Cassell. Reprinted (1970). New York and London; Johnson Reprint Corporation

Smith, F. (1919–33). *The Early History of Veterinary Literature and its British Development*. 4 Vols. London; Baillière, Tindall and Cox

Smith, F.B. (1979). *The People's Health 1830–1910*. London; Croom Helm

Smith, R.W.I. (1932). *English-Speaking Students of Medicine at the University of Leyden* [1575–1875]. Edinburgh; Oliver and Boyd

Society of Apothecaries (1840). *A List of Persons who have Obtained Certificates of their Fitness and Qualification to Practise as Apothecaries, from August 1, 1815, to July 31, 1840*. London; the Society. Thereafter annually to 1883; then with changes to 1896

Sorsby, A. (1948). *A Short History of Ophthalmology*, 2nd edn. London; Staples Press. 1st edn (1933). London; J. Bale and Co.

Sprigge, S. Squire (1897). *The Life and Times of Thomas Wakley.* London; Longmans, Green and Co. Facsimile edn of 1899 reissue (1974). New York; Krieger

Stieb, E.W. (1966). *Drug Adulteration: Detection and Control in Nineteenth Century Britain.* With G. Sonnedecker. Madison; University of Wisconsin Press

Still, G.F. (1931). *The History of Paediatrics; the Progress of the Study of Diseases of Children up to the End of the XVIIIth Century.* London; Oxford University Press

Stone, L. (1977). *The Family, Sex and Marriage in England 1500–1800.* London; Weidenfeld and Nicolson

Sudhoffs Klassiker der Medizin und der Naturwissenschaften (1910–). 1–. Leipzig; Barth

Szasz, T. (1970). *The Manufacture of Madness: A Comparative Study of the Inquisition and the Mental Health Movement.* New York; Harper and Row

Talbot, C.H. and Hammond, E.A. (1965). *The Medical Practitioners in Medieval England. A Biographical Register.* London; Wellcome Historical Medical Library

Temkin, O. (1945). *The Falling Sickness: A History of Epilepsy from the Greeks to the Beginnings of Modern Neurology.* Baltimore; Johns Hopkins Press

Temkin, O. (1973). *Galenism: Rise and Decline of a Medical Philosophy.* Ithaca and London; Cornell University Press

Temkin, O. (1977). *The Double Face of Janus and Other Essays in the History of Medicine.* Baltimore and London; Johns Hopkins University Press

Temkin, O. and Temkin, C.L., Ed. (1967). *Ancient Medicine: Selected Papers of Ludwig Edelstein.* Baltimore; Johns Hopkins Press

Thatcher, V.S. (1953). *History of Anesthesia with Emphasis on the Nurse Specialist.* Philadelphia; Lippincott

Thomas, K. (1971). *Religion and the Decline of Magic. Studies in Popular Beliefs in Sixteenth and Seventeenth Century England.* London; Weidenfeld and Nicolson. New York; Charles Scribner's Sons. Paperback edn (1980). Harmondsworth; Penguin

Thompson, A.M.C. (1968). *A Bibliography of Nursing Literature 1859–1960, with an Historical Introduction.* London; The Library Association

Thompson, J.D. and Goldin, G. (1975). *The Hospital: A Social and Architectural History.* New Haven; Yale University Press

Thomson, J. (1859). *An Account of the Life, Lectures and Writings of William Cullen, M.D.* 2 Vols. Reissue with 2nd Vol., and biographical notice of the author, by J. and W. Thomson and D. Craigie. Edinburgh; Blackwood

Thornton, J.L. (1966). *Medical Books, Libraries and Collectors: A Study of Bibliography and the Book Trade in Relation to the Medical Sciences,* 2nd edn. London; André Deutsch

Thorwald, J. (1957). *The Century of the Surgeon.* London; Thames and Hudson. Paperback edn (1961). London; Pan Books

Titmuss, R. (1950). *Problems of Social Policy. History of the Second World War. United Kingdom Civil Series.* London; HMSO and Longmans, Green and Co.

Tuke, D. Hack (1882). *Chapters in the History of the Insane in the British Isles.* London; Kegan Paul, Trench and Co.

Underwood, E.A. (1977). *Boerhaave's Men: at Leyden and After.* Edinburgh; Edinburgh University Press

Valentin, B. (1961). *Geschichte der Orthopaedie.* Stuttgart; Georg Thieme

Vicary, T. (1888). *The Anatomie of the Bodie of Man* [1577]. Ed. F.J. and P. Furnivall, with appendices. London; Early English Text Society

Webb, J., Ed. (1966). *Poor Relief in Elizabethan Ipswich.* Suffolk Records Society, Vol. 9. Ipswich; the Society

Webb, S. and B. (1910). *The State and the Doctor.* London; Longmans

Webb, S. and B. (1927–9). *English Local Government: English Poor Law History:* Part I, *The Old Poor Law.* Part II [in 2 Vols], *The Last Hundred Years.* 3 Vols. London; Longmans, Green and Co.

Webster, C. (1975). *The Great Instauration: Science, Medicine and Reform, 1626–1660.* London; Duckworth

Webster, C. (1978). The Crisis of the Hospitals during the Industrial Revolution, in *Human Implications of Scientific Advance.* Ed. E.G. Forbes. Edinburgh; Edinburgh University Press, 214–223

Webster, C. (1979). Alchemical and Paracelsian Medicine, in *Health, Medicine and Mortality in the Sixteenth Century.* Ed. C. Webster. Cambridge; Cambridge University Press, 301–334

Wellcome Historical Medical Library (1954). *A Catalogue of Incunabula in the Wellcome Historical Medical Library.* Comp. F.N.L. Poynter. London; the Library

Wellcome Historical Medical Library (1962, 1966, 1976). *A Catalogue of Printed Books in the Wellcome Historical Medical Library. I: Books Printed before 1641. II: Books Printed from 1641 to 1850, A–E; ...F–L.* 3 Vols. Comp. H.R. Denham. London; the Library

Wellcome Historical Medical Library (1962, 1973). *Catalogue of Western Manuscripts on Medicine and Science in the Wellcome Historical Medical Library. I: MSS Written before 1650 AD. II: MSS Written after 1650 AD.* 2 Vols. Comp. S.A.J. Moorat. London; the Library

Wellcome Institute for the History of Medicine (1973). *Portraits of Doctors and Scientists in the Wellcome Institute of the History of Medicine.* By R. Burgess. London; the Institute

Wellcome Institute for the History of Medicine (1980). *Subject Catalogue of the History of Medicine and Related Sciences.* 18 Vols [Subject Section, 9 Vols; Biographical Section, 5 Vols; Topographical Section, 4 Vols]. Munich; Krause International

Westergaard, H.L. (1932). *Contributions to the History of Statistics.* London; King

Whitteridge, G. (1969). *William Harvey and the Circulation of the Blood.* London; Macdonald. New York; Elsevier

Wickersheimer, C.A.E. (1906). *La médecine et les médecins en France à l'époque de la renaissance.* Paris; A. Maloine

Wickersheimer, C.A.E. (1936). *Dictionnaire biographique des médecins en France au moyen âge.* 2 Vols. Paris; Droz. *Supplement* (1979). Ed. D. Jacquart. Geneva; Droz. Paris; Champion

Widdess, J.D.H. (1963). *A History of the Royal College of Physicians of Ireland, 1654–1963.* Edinburgh; Livingstone

Wilson, A.T. and Levy, H. (1939, 1941). *Workmen's Compensation.* 2 Vols. London; Oxford University Press

Winslow, C-E. A. (1943). *The Conquest of Epidemic Disease. A Chapter in the History of Ideas.* Princeton; Princeton University Press. Reprinted (1980)

Wood, A. a (1721). *Athenae Oxonienses...to which are added the Fasti or Annals of the said University,* 2nd edn. 2 Vols. London; for R. Knaplock, D. Midwinter and J. Tonson

Woodward, J. (1974). *To Do the Sick no Harm: A Study of the British Voluntary Hospital System to 1875.* London; Routledge

Woodward, J. and Richards, D., Ed. (1977). *Health Care and Popular Medicine in Nineteenth Century England: Essays in the Social History of Medicine.* London; Croom Helm

Young, S. (1890). *Annals of the Barber-Surgeons of London, Compiled from their Records.* London; Blades, East and Blades. Reprinted (1978). New York; AMS Press

Zinsser, H. (1935). *Rats, Lice and History.* Boston, Mass.; Little, Brown

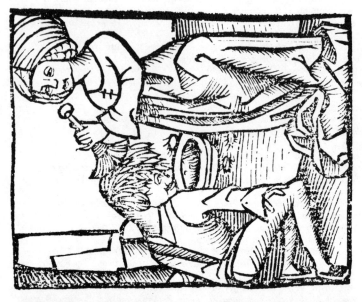

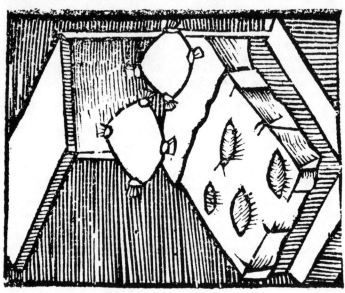

PART IV

20

The history of American science and medicine

Edward H. Beardsley

Introduction

In 1944 George Sarton summed up a long-held belief about the nature of science and its history. Science, he said, 'is essentially international or supranational. There are no scientific problems which are exclusively American. There is no American Science....' (Jaffe 1944: xiii). Sarton, and indeed most Americans who considered themselves historians of science or medicine before the 1940s, took exception to national labelling because for them the history of these fields was essentially intellectual history, whose proper concern was the ideas, or content, of science and medicine, without reference to place of origin.

Despite Sarton's insistence, I make no apology for the title of this chapter. Except for the presumptuousness of using the term 'American' for a discussion that ignores the history of Canadian and Latin American developments, this title accurately reflects the emphasis of the scholars who have come to dominate the historiography of science and medicine in the United States since the 1960s. To those scholars Sarton's definition is both overly narrow and ahistorical, for in their view the history of science and medicine involves more than content. It is a matter of context as well and is posited on the assumption that there are political, economic and cultural dimensions to this history that are not only uniquely American but also as integral a part of the history of the two fields as the development of ideas themselves.

It was a mounting concern with context, then, that gave rise to the present-day specialties known as the history of American sicence and the history of American medicine. In many respects, of course, these two fields share common boundaries and a common history but, in order to summarize their development as academic specialties, it will be convenient (and, in part, necessary) to treat them as distinct entities, at least for the period up to about 1950.

The evolution of two new historical specialties

The history of American medicine had its origins in the 1920s with the founding of the American Association for the History of Medicine in 1925 and the Johns Hopkins Institute of the History of Medicine in 1926. By the late 1930s the Institute and its publication, the *Bulletin of the History of Medicine* (which also served as the organ of the Association), were emerging as centres of scholarly research and publication. Although primary emphasis was given to European developments, both were receptive to American topics and to projects stressing the social dimensions of medical history. This was so largely because of the influence of Institute director and *Bulletin* editor, Henry E. Sigerist, easily the most dynamic figure in medical history scholarship in the period. An outspoken socialist, Sigerist stressed the relevance of a host of non-scientific factors – political, religious, philosophic, as well as economic – to the understanding of success and failure in medical history.

Outside the small band at the Hopkins, however, most of those writing medical history before the Second World War were amateur historians, nearly all practising or academic physicians. American topics received some attention, but the great bulk of writing was internal history, focused largely on Europe and mostly biographical in form. Professional historians or physicians with training in history were, with a few exceptions, conspicuously absent.

If medical history up to 1940 was essentially a story by, about and for physicians, the boundaries of the field began to shift noticeably in the immediate post-war years, as an increasing number of general American historians were attracted to the subject. Not only were they aware of the large part medicine played in the Allied victory, but the vigorous debate over national health insurance created additional interest in the role of medicine in America's past. Besides the force of events, individual historians also played a role, as they urged their colleagues to explore the possibilities of the new field. Most influential among them was Richard Shryock, who had himself shifted to medical history (in the 1930s) from the more traditional field of Reconstruction history. A pioneering and productive scholar, he had an influence beyond scholarship. At meetings of national historical organizations beginning in the 1940s Shryock was conspicuous in stressing the role of medicine in American history and calling on his colleagues to give more attention to the subject.

Little by little the historical fraternity began to respond. A sign of awakening interest was a report to the 1944 meeting of American historians listing areas 'untilled or further tillable', which suggested medical history as one field historians might profitably cultivate. Although the late 1940s witnessed no rush of professionals into the new area (only one PhD dissertation was completed in the field between 1945 and 1950), no longer did historians view American medical history as the insignificant preserve of retired physicians. As more historians enlisted in Shryock's cause, they found a new outlet for their work in *The Journal of the History of Medicine and Allied Sciences*, established in 1946 by the respected academic physician and public health historian, George Rosen.

While historians of American medicine found some encouragement of their work in an earlier tradition of general medical history, no such welcome was extended to the pioneer historians of American science. In fact the established community of general historians of science in the US was frankly sceptical of American science history, particularly if written by non-scientists. The centre of this community in the pre-war period (as now) was the History of Science Society and its journal, *Isis*, under the editorship of George Sarton. Sarton's view, a position that was endorsed by most Society members, was that only working scientists were equipped to write the history of science. That position, along with the belief that the only legitimate history was 'internal' history, effectively blocked attention to American topics, whether by general historians or historians of science. The former believed themselves ill-equipped for the task, while the latter, viewing the American record as mostly barren of major scientific achievement, felt the subject unworthy of their attention. Accordingly, the literature of American science history was miniscule. In 1939, the *Isis Critical Bibliography* contained only eight items on American science out of a total of over 1100 entries.

But, just as in the case of American medical history, the Second World War, with its dramatic demonstration of the influence of science on human affairs, altered historians' perspective on the history of science and brought them a new confidence in their fitness to enter the field. Once more, it was Shryock who alerted historians to the possibilities at hand. Writing a year before the A-bomb drop, Shryock told colleagues that the contemporary significance of science was reason enough to begin tracing its historic relationship to American society. No matter that American scientists had generally failed to make major contributions to research before the mid-twentieth century. Science had always been important to the American people, and its history thus had much to contribute to general American history. Two years later, when the attention of historians and everyone else was riveted to issues of science and society, leading historian Arthur Schlesinger (1946: 163) sounded Shryock's challenge even more strongly. Though a solid grounding in science, Schlesinger conceded, would aid the historian, even without it historians had a valuable contribution to make, for they 'can often perceive social implications and interrelations which specialists in [science]... are unaware of or disregard'.

By the late 1940s, then, a handful of American historians were beginning to press the claims of American science and medicine for acceptance as legitimate specialties in general American history. The next two decades saw a slow but steady growth not only in other historians' recognition of the two fields but also in their bodies of literature, which came increasingly to emphasize an 'external' rather than an 'internal' approach.

One sign of professional acceptance was the growing number of PhD dissertations in the two areas awarded by departments of history. During the 1950s the total rose from ten in the first half of the decade to twenty-seven in the period 1955–60, with American medicine and American science topics about equally represented. Of course, formal programmes in the history of science were also awarding the PhD for science and medical topics, but indications were that their students had little interest in American subjects. According to one survey of such programmes in the early 1970s, only six of seventy-five degree candidates indicated a preference for American science history.

Although a small band, historians and others who turned to the history of American science and medicine in the 1945–65 period generated a body of literature of signal importance. Truly seminal works, they not only filled in the boundaries of an hitherto unexplored terrain but also suggested several themes that would engage the attention of later scholars.

In the history of American medicine, Shryock remained the most influential worker. His study of American medical research (1947), the first general treatment of the subject, was also a further exploration of Shryock's major concern with the way social and economic forces interacted with medicine. Later, Shryock (1960) took as his theme the emerging American medical profession during the 1660–1860 period, as well as the struggling national effort to secure the public health. The capstone of Shryock's effort was a collection of essays (1966) dealing with American medicine in the nineteenth and twentieth centuries, which treated a number of issues of interest to later workers, such as the medical care of slaves and American indifference to basic research.

Another important scholar, a physician as well as historian, was Erwin Ackerknecht. His study of malaria in the American Mid-West (1945) showed how disease was fundamentally altered by patterns of settlement and economic development. Social dimension of disease was also the subject of Charles Rosenberg's investigation (1962) of cholera in America. Rosenberg's book commanded wide interest, for it showed the potential of using medical history as a mirror on American life, to reflect subtle social changes that might otherwise be overlooked by historians.

An important contribution to medical biography, in that it focused on the most influential figure in America's medical past, was Donald Fleming's study of William Henry Welch (1954). With Welch as his vehicle, Fleming was also able to describe the creation of the Johns Hopkins medical tradition and to assess its influence on medical developments elsewhere.

Although there were a few broad-gauged histories of American science in the post-war era comparable to Shryock's, early scholarship in American science history, by contrast to the work of medical historians, tended to emphasize individual careers and the relations between government and science. In certain respects that emphasis merely reflected different historical traditions: more American scientists than physicians achieved eminence in research in the pre-1900 period, and science made deeper inroads than medicine into federal government bureaucracy.

The first wide-ranging study of America's scientific past was Dirk Struik's examination (1948) of the evolution of science and technology in New England. Though he peered at events through a Marxist lens, mathematician Struik succeeded in unearthing a considerable record of scientific achievement, much of which was indeed connected to the economic requirements of a maturing society. Brook Hindle's study (1956) of colonial American science (and medicine), on the other hand, had no such ideological bias. What caused colonial science to assume a more independent stance was not the needs of the economic order but the high-blown optimism and nationalism of the American Revolution.

Two important early efforts to rehabilitate the reputation of nineteenth-century scientists were Joseph Coulson's biography (1950) of Joseph Henry and Donald Fleming's biography (1950) of John W. Draper. Although Coulson's account verged on an apologetic, it persuasively argued Henry's claim to international standing in nineteenth-century physics. Fleming's study did more than establish Draper's reputation in physiology and physics; it also revealed the high standards and status of science in late nineteenth-century America.

An important milestone in the history of American science was reached with the publication of Hunter Dupree's study (1957) of the historical relations between science and the federal government. The first, and still the best, history of the growth of a national scientific bureaucracy, Dupree's account also revealed the crucial role that Washington played, sometimes unwittingly, in promoting basic research.

Two biographies that charted one of the great rivalries in American science were Dupree's study (1959) of Asa Gray and Edward Lurie's biography (1960) of Louis Agassiz. Important accounts of the professionalization of American science in the middle nineteenth century, they were also a valuable source for the American debate over evolution, for on that issue Agassiz and Gray were natural and bitter opponents.

One of the first efforts by a historian of American science to trace the impact of science on American social thought was William Stanton's study (1960) of pre-Civil War scientific racism. Focusing on an assortment of professional and amateur investigators known as the 'American School of Anthropology', Stanton showed that these pre-Darwinian pluralists posed a stern challenge to the unitary, Biblical view of creation and in the process provided a new scientific underpinning to slavery.

A final product of the emergent period of American science history deserving mention was Nathan Reingold's collection (1964) of primary documents, selected from the published and manuscript sources of nineteenth-century science. Valuable in its own right in highlighting what Reingold termed the geophysical tradition in American science, the collection was perhaps more significant for what it revealed about the status of the discipline by the mid-1960s. As an index of the developmental stage of a historical specialty, a primary source book signals, first, that a sufficient body of secondary literature exists to allow scholars to interpret the significance of the proferred documents. It suggests, second, that the level of interest and sophistication among scholars in a new field has reached the point at which they are ready to move beyond traditional interpretations to a consideration of alternative viewpoints that the basic sources might imply.

The period of maturity, 1965–

Indeed, a host of signs pointed to the mid-1960s as the start of a new phase in the emergence of the history of American science and American medicine. One was the marked increase in the number of recruits from graduate programmes in history. Between 1966 and 1972 the number of dissertations in the two fields (a total of fifty-one, nearly all written within history departments) was about twice as large as for any comparable, earlier period and helped explain historians' dominance of the two areas. In terms of the sheer bulk of published material there was also impressive growth. In the period 1950–65, some forty-two monographs in the history of American science were reviewed in *Isis*. By 1966–80 that total had climbed to ninety-eight. In American medicine there were similar increases, as the number of reviews rose from fifteen to thirty-six across the two periods.

Certainly one important measure of the 'arrival' of American science and medical history by 1970 was the recognition of established historical and scientific groups. *The Journal of American History*, a major professional quarterly, had long featured a listing of articles from other periodicals, and its categories were a good measure of what the mainstream profession regarded as legitimate scholarly fields. Up to 1970 they included such areas as business and economic history, foreign affairs, and colonial history. In June 1970 the *Journal* added a new category: 'science and medicine'. Other groups accorded similar recognition. In 1976, in connection with the American Bi-Centennial, there were a host of scholarly celebrations of America's past, with science and medicine coming in for their share of attention. Both major medical history quarterlies (*The Bulletin of the History of Medicine* and *The Journal of the History of Medicine and Allied Sciences*) gave special attention to American medicine, but even more noteworthy was an American Association for the Advancement of Science (AAAS) conference on science in the American context whose sponsors included not only the National Science Foundation but the History of Science Society as well.

The surest sign of heightened maturity and professionalism within the two fields was the willingness of scholars to take a more critical stance toward their collective effort. In the initial decades after the Second World War so little was known about the history of science or medicine in America that every contribution added something of value. But once the pioneering work was done – and it was essentially completed by the mid-1960s – scholars began to sense a need to pause, reflect and take stock. Out of that process have come a sharper definition of objectives, shifts in subjects, new methodologies and a revision of earlier scholarship. As a by-product of this kind of critical questioning, contention and division have also arisen within the scholarly community.

A major concern of historians of American science was whether they were fulfilling their primary and distinctive task of relating science to the broader American social framework. One scholar who worried about this was Nathan Reingold (1968: 216), who noted a sharp division between those historians of science who emphasized the development of scientific ideas and those, a group dominated by Americanists, who focused on scientists operating within a certain national context. Occasionally, attempts were made by each group to invade the other's domain, but generally such efforts were not successful. Historians of American science, it was true, were seriously concerned to show how science and scientists had affected society, but too often – in studies of scientific institutions and education, for example – they succeeded merely in 'extending the boundary of "internal" history of the immediate environment of the scientists'. Furthermore (Reingold 1967), scholars had not yet defined exactly what they meant by society (whether social organizations, ideas or groupings) when they referred to science–society relationships, nor had they analysed the process by which science had exerted its wider influence. As for demonstrating the reverse impact – i.e., the influence of society on science – barring the Marxist historians, there had been almost no discussion of those possibilities. One other gap in the literature that concerned a number of historians of American science was the absence of studies focusing on the social milieu of the European scientist. Not until historians of American science understood how science had developed within the context of other national cultures could they say anything definitive about the uniqueness of American science.

Because the social connections of medicine had always been much more direct and obvious than those of science, American medical historians did not worry as much about definitions as they did about the subjects they were investigating. Ackerknecht, for example, suggested that historians had focused too much on the medical practice of élite doctors. More needed were studies of average physicians who treated the masses and of whether their practice conformed to accepted ethical standards. In the 1970s, younger medical historians began to argue for an even more basic shift in focus: physicians of whatever calibre should be taken from the centre stage and more attention paid to patients. Influenced by the growing interest of general American historians in the history of the common people and in women's history, a number of

American medical historians sought to open their field to this 'new social history' and to examine medical history from the standpoint of patients, whether found in hospitals, asylums or at home.

As the history of American science and medicine merged with general American history, one result was a wider application of new research methodologies that had proved their value in the larger field. Quantitative approaches seemed particularly promising. One of the first to adopt them was historian of science George Daniels (1968), who in his study of the Jacksonian period used statistical analysis to re-examine issues of scientific productivity and professionalization. Another technique was the use of oral history. Though only applicable to recent topics, taped interviews proved valuable in gathering historical material usually absent from the written record. This approach was put to good use in Nuel Pharr Davis's study (1968) of American nuclear physicists, Kenneth Ludmerer's examination (1972) of the tie between genetics and eugenics, and Garland Allen's biography (1978) of T.H. Morgan.

The innovation that produced the greatest historiographic shift and stirred most controversy, however, was the introduction into American medical history of the techniques of the 'new social history'. Taking their cue from French historians of the *Annales* school, who pioneered in the use of quantitative techniques and conceptual models from the behavioural sciences, social historians of medicine likewise brought a new kind of source material into play. Focusing on population groups who left few personal records, these historians mined their data largely from manuscript censuses, tax lists, demographic statistics and hospital patient records. Their work has been marked not only by a shift in emphasis from physician to patient but also by an interest in the structure and transformation of medical institutions and the social responses to disease.

These efforts have not met with universal approval. More traditional historians of medicine have charged that what was being offered was not medical history at all. If it was, said historical editor Leonard Wilson (1980: 7), 'it is medical history without medicine'. Also, said critics, much of the new writing had an adversarial quality: too often, doctors and medical institutions were depicted as villains bent on controlling, sometimes brutalizing, their patients, especially females. Even proponents of the new approach raised notes of caution. In a recent and useful collection of representative writing, Gerald Grob (1977: 402) discussed the problems facing the social history of medicine. Noting the lack of exposure to 'internal' history of many of his younger colleagues,

Grob warned that if the new field was to achieve its potential, scholars must 'begin with a firm understanding of the evolution of medical theory...'.

One inevitable consequence of the critical questioning and new research approaches in the history of American science and medicine was the revision of many earlier interpretations. In the history of American science, revisionism has focused on the nineteenth century and has centred in some way upon America's supposed indifference to basic research. The history of American medicine has shown a similar tendency in the re-examination of such topics as the relation between physicians and female patients, nineteenth-century asylum treatment, and the health and medical care of Negroes.

By the late 1970s, then, the history of American science and the history of American medicine had fully earned their credentials as legitimate scholarly fields. Their vitality was measured not only in a substantial and increasingly sophisticated literature but equally in the revisionist tendencies that had become a habit in both specialties. In addition, workers in each area met a ready acceptance from mainstream historians, enjoyed frequent opportunities for exchange of views, and found ample outlets for their research. The two fields had become, in a phrase, fully professional.

Issues and themes in the history of American medicine since 1965

The pitfall of any categorization of recent writing, particularly one that emphasizes the monographic literature, is that a number of significant efforts will fall outside the chosen framework. But in the belief that even a partial survey will be of use to beginning medical historians and to interested general historians, the following is offered as a summary guide.

Disease in America

Most of the work in this area has focused on infectious epidemic disease. For the colonial period John Duffy's study (1959) is still the best survey. Besides cholera and malaria, whose histories have been noted (Rosenberg 1962; Ackerknecht 1945), the other major epidemic malady in pre-industrial America was yellow fever, which has been examined by John B. Blake (1968) for the eighteenth century and John Duffy (1966) for the nineteenth. Considerable interest has also developed in America's more recent experience with influenza. Alfred Crosby (1976) explores the impact of the 1918 pandemic on Wilsonian diplomacy, while June Osborne's edited volume (1977) looks at influenza since the First World War and contains a useful chapter by Arthur J. Viseltear on the history of swine flu legislation.

The history of poliomyelitis has received attention as well, mostly from those who participated in its conquest. Saul Benison (1967) has edited the oral biography of the man who headed the Rockefeller virology programme. The most comprehensive treatment, though, is that of John R. Paul (1971) who contends that the National Foundation for Infantile Paralysis, by concentrating on the Salk vaccine, retarded development of the more effective Sabin vaccine.

Far less work has been done on important industrial, nutritional and parasitic diseases. There are, for example, no satisfactory accounts of byssinosis or hookworm. Elizabeth Ethridge's history (1972) of Southern pellagra, however, is an important exception whose particular value lies in its insights into the relation between disease and socioeconomic conditions.

The care of the mentally ill in America

Historians of the nineteenth-century asylum have divided, ofttimes sharply, over such questions as the origin of asylum care, the motives of early and later superintendents, and the cause of the mid-century shift in asylum function from curing patients to merely holding them in custody. One student has been Gerald Grob, whose major writings include a biography (1978) of a leading psychiatrist and medical statistician in the 1800s and studies (1971, 1973) of the social policies of nineteenth-century asylums. In Grob's view (1973) the asylum originated in certain demographic changes that made earlier forms of treatment ineffective. Eventually, the humanitarian aims and reasonably successful therapy of early superintendents were frustrated by the growth of a custodial function, but that was a change over which they had little control.

Grob's position has met strong opposition from more radical social historians. The most extremely divergent view is that of Christopher Lasch (1973: 3–17), who believes that the asylum originated not in humanitarian concern but in a desire to enforce uniform behaviour. Using the concept of a 'total' institution, Lasch argues that all institutional confinement was inherently repressive. Thus, there was no shift in asylum function at mid-century; it was a totalitarian institution from the start. David

Rothman (1971) tends toward a middle position. Conceding the benevolent motives of medical superintendents, but questioning the value of their therapy, Rothman places the origin of the asylum in the contemporary belief that social mobility was causing widespread mental disorder. The shift to custody was in turn due to new social perceptions, notably a rising nativism and a readiness to confine any foreigners showing signs of deviance.

Medical care in America

Another interest of American medical historians has been the treatment of somatic illness, especially in the nineteenth century. William G. Rothstein's study (1972) of American physicians, while primarily concerned with the struggle of regular practitioners for professional dominance, puts patient–physician relationships at the centre of the story and argues that it was the advent of science that ended sectarian medicine and gave rise to a rational and unitary therapy. Martin Kaufman's history of homoeopathy (1971) covers much of the same ground, but from the vantage point of the major group of 'irregular' practitioners. Gert H. Brieger's edited collection of articles (1972) from the *Bulletin of the History of Medicine* is more eclectic but gives considerable attention to nineteenth-century medical care, with selections on the Lewis and Clark expedition, the Civil War and the development of anaesthesia.

The eighteenth and twentieth centuries have also received attention. Whitfield Bell's collection (1975) of his pieces on the eighteenth-century contains a useful portrait of the colonial physician, selections on leading practitioners and an essay on Benjamin Franklin's medical interests. Rosemary Stevens' study (1971) of the twentieth century shows that the rise of specialization and technical excellence have altered existing patterns of medical care and led to the current health care crisis.

A general history of American hospitals has yet to be written, but there are histories of individual institutions, as well as a growing periodical literature on the basic changes in hospital–patient relationships beginning in the late 1800s. Susan Reverby and David Rosmer's edited collection (1979: 105–31) of essays in the social history of medicine shows how those relationships were affected by changing economic conditions. Also important is the work of Charles Rosenberg, who in one article (1977) examines institutional care from the patient's perspective and in a second (1979a) looks at an important transitional period in American hospitals.

Finally, considerable attention has been paid to the medical care of black Americans. Marion Torchia (1975) examines the impact of racism on public health programmes in the era of segregation, but it is the health and medical care of slaves that has attracted the greatest attention. One question still unresolved is whether slaves received as good care as whites. Kenneth and Virginia Kiple argue (Branca 1977: 21–46) that the poor diet of slaves was a major contributor to high child mortality. On the other hand, Todd Savitt's investigation of Virginia slavery (1978) finds that, where physician care was involved, blacks and whites got comparable attention. Savitt shows, though, that slavery itself had a worsening effect on illness and that Southern doctors often used slaves, free Negroes and poor whites for experimental and demonstration purposes.

Professional organization

Several historians have recently enlarged our understanding of this topic. Shryock's account of medical licensing (1967) shows that success or failure of such movements has always been influenced as much by social attitudes as by medical needs. Joseph Kett (1968) has taken a broader view. Focusing on medical education and licensing, medical societies and sectarianism before 1860, Kett concludes that it was probably a good thing that élite urban doctors were unable to impose high licensing standards. Otherwise there would have been a severe doctor shortage.

For the twentieth century, the progressive era has held a particular fascination. James Burrow (1977) examines the key medical changes of that period in science, education, economics and public health and shows how the American Medical Association (AMA) adjusted to them. Ronald Numbers (1978) narrows his focus to one major issue, compulsory health insurance. According to Numbers, the AMA's shift from apathy to outright opposition was the result of rising physician income and the related fear that such a programme would be the entering wedge of socialism.

Public health history

There is no good general history of American public health, although chapters on the subject in John Duffy's overview history (1976) of American medicine provide a broad outline of major events and trends. The writings of George Rosen (1958, 1974, 1976), if collected in one place, would come closest to a general survey. In all his work Rosen strove to measure the social dimension of public health issues, and his influence is reflected in Charles Rosenberg's edited collection (1979b) of articles in honour of Rosen, which contains additional pieces of the American story.

Specialized studies of American health history abound. A large portion of the monographic literature focuses on the local scene. Stuart Galishoff's account (1975) of Newark from 1895 to 1918 describes how one industrial city responded to health crises left in the wake of major economic change. John Duffy's two-volume history (1968–74) of health developments in New York City is the most thorough study of its kind and carries the story to about 1970. Barbara Gutman Rosenkrantz's examination (1972) of Massachusetts during the century after 1840 is more than just a look at policies and programmes of the nation's first state board of health. It examines as well how important groups such as physicians and politicians were able to set the limits of permissible public health work.

Besides local histories, which centre mostly on the Northeast, biographies also help piece the story together. Ethridge's study (1972) is as much a biography of federal health officer Joseph Goldberger as it is a history of pellagra. James Cassedy's biography (1962) of Charles V. Chapin presents the career of the most important local health officer of the early 1900s, while Margaret Wolfe's account (1978) of Lucius Polk Brown reveals the intensity of health politics in New York City in the progressive period.

Industrial and environmental health have thus far received only scant attention. One exception is James Whorton's account (1975) of the early debate over the dangers of arsenical insecticides and of early efforts at regulation, both set in the context of agricultural commercialization in the late 1800s. Valuable to anyone working in the twentieth century is Monroe Lerner and Odin Anderson's compilation (1963) of key mortality and morbidity data, with notes on major health trends and their social implications.

Women and medicine

With the rise of contemporary feminism and the 'new social history', American medical historians began to pay more attention to the role and place of women in medical history. Interest has focused primarily on women as patients, professionals and lay reformers. When historians of a more radical stamp have viewed women in the first two roles, they have often cast the male doctor as villain, showing him as one who sought to control or oppress his patients or to restrict women's entry into a predominantly male profession. According to John and Robin Haller (1973), nineteenth-century doctors, frightened by the prospect of female liberation and willing to bend science to the task of containing it, united in a campaign to keep women in the home (and out of the world of men), where the dictates of their sex more properly put them. If the Hallers' physicians acted out of social and political concern, G.H. Barker Benfield's doctors (1976) sought to bind women to the fireside because of a general hostility toward females that sprang from their own sexual insecurities. Focusing on early professional gynaecologists, Benfield argues that this profession, with its unnecessary surgery and experimentation, was at base a system of female oppression. Several medical historians, however, have taken issue with such accounts. Regina Markell Morantz (1974) argues that they are marred by presentism and that their picture of women-hating male doctors is a caricature.

Even though well known, problems of women practitioners continue to attract interest. Mary Roth Walsh (1978) recounts discrimination against female doctors in nineteenth-century Boston, while Judy Barrett Litoff (1978) discusses the campaign of twentieth-century males to drive women from the field of midwifery.

Historians have also examined the role of women in health and medical reform. Morantz (1977) focuses on female leadership of the self-help medical movement of the pre-Civil War era and relates it to women's changing social status. For a slightly later period Ronald Numbers (1976) discusses the health reform activities of the leader of the Seventh-day Adventist movement. Finally, James Reed's history (1978) of birth control emphasizes the 1900s and looks primarily at Sanger's efforts to win acceptance of contraceptives.

Issues and themes in the history of American science since 1965

Science in the eighteenth century

While this period is now rather out of fashion, good work continues. For many years, owing largely to the writing of I.B. Cohen (1941, 1953, 1956), scholarly interest centred on the work of Benjamin Franklin. Then, in the 1950s, Whitfield Bell (1955), in what is still a useful guide to unexplored topics, called historians' attention to other areas in need of study and listed some fifty scientists whose contributions justified fuller treatment.

Several of them have found their biographers (for example, Hindle 1966), but others await attention. Probably the most comprehensive study of the colonial period to date is that by Raymond Phineas Stearns (1970). Winner of the National Book Award in science, Stearns' history was highly praised for its abundance of new material and for positioning American science squarely within the international scientific framework of the 1700s. The influence of the Royal Society of London, heavily stressed by Stearns, is also one theme of Alexandra Oleson and Sanford Brown's collection of essays (1976) on the general scientific and learned society in America. Before the advent of scientific specialization these groups had a sizeable impact on the growth of knowledge and culture in the US.

Nineteenth-century American science

Until recently, historians emphasizing the American context regarded the 1800s as a time of scant popular or even professional interest in basic science. Taking their cue from Alexis de Tocqueville, scholars like Shryock and Cohen argued that American society, with its emphasis on immediate results, was indifferent to basic research and esteemed only men of practical genius. But in the 1970s that view came under fire. One early sign of an interpretive shift was the collected papers (Daniels 1972) of a 1970 conference called to reassess such earlier views. Particularly suggestive was the article by Reingold (Daniels 1972: 38–62), which argues that later historians accepted too uncritically the complaints of nineteenth-century scientists. The correct picture was not that of a decline from an eighteenth-century high but one showing steady, if slow, growth from the 1700s.

Since 1970 a number of specialized studies have continued the reassessment. Two broad conclusions to emerge were that the American public was more interested in and supportive of basic research than formerly imagined and that the relationship between pure and applied science was basically harmonious, not antagonistic. Bruce Sinclair's study (1974) of the Franklin Institute sees a commonality of interest among scientists, engineers and mechanics, along with a general agreement that technical education should stress theory as well as application. The close relationship between pure and applied science is also one theme running through the published edition of the Joseph Henry papers (Reingold 1972–5). In his first two volumes Reingold recreates in detail the world of the nineteenth-century scientist, showing that, while an emerging professional community pulled away from American society, it also maintained a multitude of ties to it. Margaret Rossiter (1975) focuses on the relationship between America's agricultural chemists and her practical farmers and shows that the latter, though insistent on results, were eager to embrace the scientific approach, which was being institutionalized by the 1870s in the federally sponsored state agricultural colleges.

The place of science in higher education has also been re-evaluated (Guralnik 1975). Before, liberal arts colleges were seen as the preserve of classicists and theologians; Guralnik shows that science was an integral part of the pre-Civil War curriculum. To say that a large part of the public put a premium on scientific understanding is not to say, of course, that the goals of professional scientists and laymen were identical. Sally Gregory Kohlstedt (1976) clarifies this in her study of the early AAAS. Whereas lay members sought to popularize science, working scientists desired to orient the AAAS toward research.

One reason usually given to explain America's failure in basic science was the hostility of organized religion and theology. But latter-day scholars have found not warfare, but a large measure of harmony between the two areas. Theodore Dwight Bozeman (1977) examines the attitudes of Old School Presbyterians before 1860 and finds that at least one Protestant sect, via its acceptance of the Baconian method, was highly tolerant of science as an intellectual enterprise. Charles Rosenberg (1976: 135–52) has examined the supposedly antagonistic relationship from another angle and finds that unfulfilled religious enthusiasm was what provided much of the scientific idealism and drive of America's early agricultural chemists.

Relations between science and government

An underlying and recurring theme in the writing of historians and others who have focused on the relationship between science, scientists and the federal government has been the continuing struggle between a scientific élite and the people's representatives over the terms of government support of science. George Daniels' examination (1967) of the growing tension between the pure science ideal and the values of a democratic culture provides a useful introduction to the nineteenth-century story. An early treatment of this battle focusing on a specific episode is Wallace Stegner's biography (1954) of geologist John Wesley Powell, who was unable to reform arid land policy because of a politically motivated Congress. More recently, Dean Allard, Jr. has returned to the theme in a biography (1978) of Spencer F. Baird, which depicts Baird's frustration as he attempted to extend federal regulation to the private fishing industry.

Major interest has centred on the twentieth century, particularly on the uneasy partnership between government and scientist in the development of the atomic bomb and on the later elaboration of a policy of nuclear deterrence. The best general treatment of these issues is Richard Hewlett, Oscar Anderson and F. Duncan's history of the US Atomic Energy Commission (Hewlett and Anderson 1962; Hewlett and Duncan 1969), the first volume of which contains an account of the efforts of scientists to set the terms of national and international control of atomic energy. The policy role of individual scientists and the way that role was shaped by the interaction of personal politics and national political mood are the subject of Nuel Pharr Davis's dual biography (1968) of E.O. Lawrence and Robert Oppenheimer. A related work is Herbert York's study (1976) of the superbomb, which shows that Oppenheimer was not as 'dove-ish' as traditionally portrayed.

Not all recent histories have been concerned with security issues. James L. Penick *et al.* (1965) focus on domestic science questions and by the use of contemporary documents show how federal science policy was the result of an interaction of various interests. Daniel Greenberg (1967), on the other hand, emphasizes primarily the internal politics of American science and shows how that community has operated to get what it wants from government.

Science and Western exploration

This story is in some respects merely another chapter in the history of the science–government relationship. It was public support that enabled scientists to venture into these uncharted regions, yet that support carried with it a pressure for public accountability and practical results that often frustrated purely professional goals. Even so, the explorations generated abundant new knowledge and enhanced the reputation of American science.

In the pre-Civil War period, natural science owed a large debt to the Army Corps of Topographical Engineers and its handful of civilian scientist advisers who classified America's Western treasures. The story of that achievement had been told by William Goetzmann (1959), who returned to the subject again a few years later (1966) with a Pulitzer Prize-winning account of the whole nineteenth-century experience of Western exploration. This took as its central themes the role of science in American nationalism and the struggle between civilian and military science for dominance in the West.

Landed exploration did not monopolize American activity. The government's first truly scientific expedition, in fact, was the 'Wilkes Expedition', an exploration of the Pacific Ocean (and the American Northwest) in the early 1840s, described most recently by William Stanton (1975). While discovery was just one purpose of the voyage, its scientific achievement was perhaps most important, for it established the credibility of American intellect and stimulated the activity of a generation of later American scientists.

Science and race

American scientists and the historians who study them have, like all their countrymen, shown considerable interest in the Negro. Following Stanton's account (1960), more recent writing has examined scientists' racial ideas as they emerged under the influence of evolutionary concepts. John Haller's review (1971) of the 1860–1900 period argues that evolution only strengthened a prevailing racist ideology by providing a more scientific rationale for Negro inferiority. In fact, the consensus of physicians, ethnologists and sociologists was that evolution had stopped working for Negroes, who would one day be extinct. That consensus began to weaken by the early 1900s, however, and according to George Stocking (1968) it was the work of Franz Boas that catalysed the shift in thinking. Boas's writing, which argued a separation of culture and race, not only undermined the earlier racist position but also helped establish anthropology and, later, other social sciences on a firmer scientific basis. The emergence of biology in the early 1900s provided a new rationale for racial inferiority, of course. But, as Hamilton Cravens (1978) shows, hereditarian ideas were themselves eventually overturned by what was primarily an environmentalist argument drawn from evolution.

Scientific disciplines in America

The recent period has seen the appearance of a number of histories of individual disciplines, whose perspectives are as diverse as their subjects. E.H. Beardsley's history (1964) of the nineteenth-century chemistry profession is almost entirely 'external' history, emphasizing the development of major institutions and showing the impact of industrialization on professional growth. Daniel Kevles (1978) uses a far wider lens in looking at American physicists. Surveying the profession from its post-Civil

War beginnings to the era of Vietnam, Kevles's account is a comprehensive history not only of institutions and public relations but also of American contributions to the concepts of modern physics.

Other disciplines have been presented through the medium of biography. Perhaps no American field was so dominated by the work of a single individual as was genetics by the work of Thomas H. Morgan, who established the chromosome theory and helped raise America to a leading position in genetics research. There are two recent biographies of Morgan. Ian Shine and Sylvia Wrobel's small volume (1976) is valuable for its view of Morgan's relations with students and colleagues. The most definitive study, however, one falling squarely within the 'internal' tradition, is Garland Allen's biography (1978), which is a tribute both to Allen's ability to deal with complex scientific ideas and to his skills in historical research, for Morgan routinely destroyed all his letters and other papers.

'External' histories of genetics have been chiefly concerned with the rise and decline of American eugenics. Mark Haller (1963) provided the earliest general treatment of that movement. William Pickens (1969), who looks at eugenics in the progressive period, finds a convergence between its goals and the values of progressive reformers. By contrast to those studies, Kenneth Ludmerer (1972) examines the relationship between eugenics and genetics and thus tries to connect 'internal' and 'external' history. Garland Allen has surveyed (1976) the whole body of this literature from a frankly Marxist perspective that views the rise and decline of eugenics in terms of the needs of American corporate capitalism.

Bibliography

Ackerknecht, E.H. (1945). *Malaria in the Upper Mississippi Valley, 1760–1900*. Bulletin of the History of Medicine Supplement, No. 4. Baltimore; Johns Hopkins University Press

Allard, C. (1978). *Spencer Fullerton Baird and the United States Fish Commission*. New York; Arno Press

Allen, G.E. (1976). Genetics, Eugenics and Society: Internalists and Externalists in Contemporary History of Science, *Social Studies of Science*, Vol. 6, 105–122

Allen, G.E. (1978). *Thomas Hunt Morgan. The Man and His Science*. Princeton, NJ; Princeton University Press

Beardsley, E.H. (1964). *The Rise of the American Chemistry Profession, 1850–1900*. Gainesville; University of Florida Press

Bell, W. (1955). *Early American Science. Needs and Opportunities for Study*. Williamsburg; Institute of Early American History and Culture

Bell, W. (1975). *The Colonial Physician and Other Essays*. New York; Science History Publications

Benfield, W.J.B. (1976). *The Horrors of the Half-Known Life: Male Attitudes Toward Women and Sexuality in Nineteenth Century America.* New York; Harper and Row

Benison, S. (1967). *Tom Rivers: Reflections on a Life in Medicine and Science.* Cambridge, Mass.; MIT Press

Blake, J. (1968). Yellow Fever in Eighteenth-Century America, *Bulletin of the New York Academy of Medicine*, Vol. 44, 673–686

Bozeman, T.D. (1977). *Protestants in An Age of Science.* Chapel Hill; University of North Carolina Press

Branca, P., Ed. (1977). *The Medicine Show: Patients, Physicians and the Perplexities of the Health Revolution in Modern Society* (essays from *Journal of Social History*). New York; Science History Publications

Brieger, G.H. (1972). *Theory and Practice in American Medicine.* New York; Science History Publications

Burrow, J. (1977). *Organized Medicine in the Progressive Era.* Baltimore; Johns Hopkins University Press

Cassedy, J. (1962). *Charles V. Chapin and the Public Health Movement.* Cambridge, Mass.; Harvard University Press

Cassedy, J., comp. (1979). *Research in Progress.* Baltimore; American Association for the History of Medicine. (Circulated to membership)

Cohen, I.B., Ed. (1941). *Benjamin Franklin's Electrical Experiments.* Cambridge, Mass.; Harvard University Press

Cohen, I.B. (1953). *Benjamin Franklin: His Contribution to the American Tradition.* Indianapolis; Bobbs-Merrill

Cohen, I.B. (1956). Franklin and Newton; an Inquiry into Speculative Newtonian Experimental Science and Franklin's Work in Electricity as an Example thereof, *Memoirs of the American Philosophical Society*, Vol. 5, No. 43. 2nd edn (1966). Cambridge, Mass.; Harvard University Press

Coulson, J. (1950). *Joseph Henry. His Life and Work.* Princeton; Princeton University Press

Cravens, H. (1978). *The Triumph of Evolution: American Scientists and the Heredity–Environment Controversy.* Philadelphia; University of Pennsylvania Press

Crosby, A. (1976). *Epidemic and Peace, 1918.* Westport; Greenwood Press

Daniels, G. (1967). The Pure Science Ideal and Democratic Culture, *Science*, Vol. 156, 1699–1705

Daniels, G. (1968). *American Science in the Age of Jackson.* New York; Columbia University Press

Daniels, G., Ed. (1972). *Nineteenth Century American Science.* Evanston; Northwestern University Press

Davis, N.P. (1968). *Lawrence and Oppenheimer.* New York; Simon and Schuster

Duffy, J. (1959). *Epidemics in Colonial America.* Baton Rouge; Louisiana State University Press

Duffy, J. (1966). *Sword of Pestilence. The New Orleans Yellow Fever Epidemic of 1853.* Baton Rouge; Louisiana State University Press

Duffy, J. (1968–74). *A History of Public Health in New York City.* 2 Vols. New York; Russell Sage Foundation

Duffy, J. (1976). *The Healers. The Rise of the Medical Establishment.* New York; McGraw Hill

Dupree, A.H. (1957). *Science in the Federal Government. A History of Policies and Activities to 1940.* Cambridge, Mass.; Harvard University Press

Dupree, A.H. (1959). *Asa Gray, 1810–88.* Cambridge, Mass.; Harvard University Press

Ethridge, E. (1972). *The Butterfly Caste. A Social History of Pellagra in the South.* Westport; Greenwood Press

Fleming, D. (1950). *John William Draper and the Religion of Science.* Philadelphia; University of Pennsylvania Press

Fleming, D. (1954). *William Henry Welch and the Rise of Modern Medicine.* Boston; Little, Brown

Galishoff, S. (1975). *Safeguarding the Public Health: Newark, 1895–1918.* Westport; Greenwood Press

Goetzmann, W. (1959). *Army Exploration of the American West, 1803–63.* New Haven, Conn.; Yale University Press

Goetzmann, W. (1966). *Exploration and Empire: The Explorer and Scientist in the Winning of the West.* New York; Knopf

Greenberg, D. (1967). *The Politics of Pure Science: An Inquiry into the Relationship between Science and Government in the United States.* New York; New American Library. Also (1969) as *The Politics of American Science.* London; Penguin Books

Grob, G., Ed. (1971). *Insanity and Idiocy in Massachusetts.* Cambridge, Mass.; Harvard University Press

Grob, G. (1973). *Mental Institutions in America. Social Policy to 1875.* New York; The Free Press

Grob, G. (1977). The Social History of Medicine and Disease in America: Problems and Possibilities, *Journal of Social History*, Vol. 10, 391–409

Grob, G. (1978). *Edward Jarvis and the Medical World of Nineteenth Century America.* Knoxville; University of Tennessee Press

Guralnik, S. (1975). *Science and the Ante-Bellum American College.* Philadelphia; American Philosophical Society

Haller, J. (1971). *Outcasts from Evolution. Scientific Attitudes of Racial Inferiority, 1859–1900.* Urbana; Illinois University Press

Haller, J. and Haller, R. (1973). *The Physician and Sexuality in Victorian America.* New York; W.W. Norton Co.

Haller, M. (1963). *Eugenics: Hereditarian Attitudes in American Thought.* New Brunswick; Rutgers University Press

Hewlett, R.G. and Anderson, O.E. (1962). *The New World, 1939–1946.* Vol. 1 of *A History of the United States Atomic Energy Commission.* University Park, Pa.; The Pennsylvania State University Press

Hewlett, R.G. and Duncan, F. (1969). *Atomic Shield, 1947–1952.* Vol. 2 of *A History of the United States Atomic Energy Commission.* University Park, Pa. and London; The Pennsylvania State University Press

Hindle, B. (1956). *Pursuit of Science in Revolutionary America.* Chapel Hill; University or North Carolina Press

Hindle, B. (1966). *David Rittenhouse.* Princeton; Princeton University Press

Jaffe, B. (1944). *Men of Science in America. The Role of Science in the Growth of Our Country.* New York; Simon and Schuster

Kaufman, M. (1971). *Homeopathy in America. The Rise and Fall of a Medical Heresy.* Baltimore; Johns Hopkins University Press

Kett, J. (1968). *The Formation of the American Medical Profession. The Role of Institutions.* New Haven; Yale University Press

Kevles, D. (1978). *The Physicists: The History of a Scientific Community in Modern America.* New York; Knopf

Kohlstedt, S. (1976). *The Formation of the American Scientific Community: The AAAS, 1849–60.* Urbana; Illinois University Press

Lasch, C. (1973). *The World of Nations: Reflections on American History, Politics, and Culture.* New York; Knopf

Leavitt, J. and Numbers, R. (1978). *Sickness and Health in America. Readings in the History of Medicine and Public Health*. Madison; University of Wisconsin Press

Lerner, M. and Anderson, O. (1963). *Health Progress in the United States, 1900–60*. Chicago; Chicago University Press

Litoff, J. (1978). *American Midwives, 1860 to the Present*. Westport; Greenwood Press

Ludmerer, K. (1972). *Genetics and American Society. A Historical Appraisal*. Baltimore; Johns Hopkins University Press

Lurie, E. (1960). *Louis Agassiz. A Life in Science*. Chicago; University of Chicago Press

Morantz, R.M. (1974). The Perils of Feminist History, *Journal of Interdisciplinary History*, Vol. 6, 649–660

Morantz, R.M. (1977). Making Women Modern. Middle-Class Women and Health Reform in Nineteenth Century America, *Journal of Social History*, Vol. 10, 490–507

Numbers, R. (1976). *Prophetess of Health: A Study of the Life of Ellen G. White*. New York; Harper and Row

Numbers, R. (1978). *Almost Persuaded. American Physicians and Compulsory Health Insurance, 1912–20*. Baltimore; Johns Hopkins University Press

Oleson, A. and Brown, S., Ed. (1976). *The Pursuit of Knowledge in the Early American Republic*. Baltimore: Johns Hopkins University Press

Osborne, J., Ed. (1977). *History, Science and Politics: Influenza in America, 1918–76*. New York; Prodist

Paul, J.R. (1971). *A History of Poliomyelitis*. New Haven; Yale University Press

Penick, J., Purcell, C., Sherwood, M. and Swain, D., Ed. (1965). *The Politics of American Science: 1939 to the Present*. Chicago; Rand McNally

Pickens, W. (1969). *Eugenics and the Progressives*. Nashville; Vanderbilt University Press

Reed, J. (1978). *From Private Vice to Public Virtue. The Birth Control Movement and American Society Since 1830*. New York; Basic Books

Reingold, N. (1964). *Science in Nineteenth Century America. A Documentary History*. New York; Hill and Wang

Reingold, N. (1967). Review of D. Van Tassel and M. Hall, *Science and Society in the United States* (Homewood; Dorsey Press, 1966), *Isis*, Vol. 58, 257

Reingold, N. (1968). Social Relations of Science, *Isis*, Vol. 59, 216

Reingold, N., Ed. (1972–5). *The Papers of Joseph Henry*. 2 Vols. Washington; The Smithsonian Institution

Reverby, S. and Rosner, D., Ed. (1979). *Health Care in America. Essays in Social History*. Philadelphia; Temple University Press

Rosen, G. (1958). *A History of Public Health*. New York; MD Publications

Rosen, G. (1974). *From Medical Police to Social Medicine: Essays on the History of Health Care*. New York; Science History Publications

Rosen, G. (1976). *Preventive Medicine in the U.S., 1900–1975. Trends and Interpretations*. New York; Science History Publications

Rosenberg, C. (1962). *The Cholera Years: 1832, 1849, and 1866*. Chicago; University of Chicago Press

Rosenberg, C. (1976). *No Other Gods: On Science and American Social Thought*. Baltimore; Johns Hopkins University Press

Rosenberg, C. (1977). 'And Heal the Sick.' The Hospital and the Patients in Nineteenth Century America, *Journal of Social History*, Vol. 10, 428–447

Rosenberg, C. (1979a). Inward Vision and Outward Glance: The Shaping of the American Hospital, 1880–1914, *Bulletin of the History of Medicine*, Vol. 53, 346–391

Rosenberg, C. (1979b). *Healing and History. Essays for George Rosen*. New York; Science History Publications

Rosenkrantz, B.G. (1972). *Public Health and the State. Changing Views in Massachusetts, 1842–1936*. Cambridge, Mass.; Harvard University Press

Rossiter, M.W. (1975). *The Emergence of Agricultural Science: Justis Liebig and the Americans, 1840–80*. New Haven and London; Yale University Press

Rothman, D. (1971). *Discovery of the Asylum. Social Order and Disorder in the New Republic*. Boston; Little, Brown

Rothstein, W. (1972). *American Physicians in the Nineteenth Century. From Sects to Science*. Baltimore; Johns Hopkins University Press

Savitt, T. (1978). *Medicine and Slavery: The Diseases and Health Care of Blacks in Ante-Bellum Virginia*. Urbana; University of Illinois Press

Schlesinger, A. (1946). An American Historian Looks at Science and Technology, *Isis*, Vol. 35, 162–166

Sherwood, M. (1965). *Exploration of Alaska, 1856–1900*. New Haven, Conn.; Yale University Press

Shine, I. and Wrobel, S. (1976). *Thomas Hunt Morgan. Pioneer of Genetics*. Lexington; University of Kentucky Press

Shryock, R. (1936). *The Development of Modern Medicine: An Interpretation of the Social and Scientific Factors Involved*. Philadelphia; University of Pennsylvania Press. 2nd edn (1947). Paperback edn (1979). Madison; University of Wisconsin Press

Shryock, R. (1947). *American Medical Research, Past and Present*. New York; The Commonwealth Fund

Shryock, R. (1960). *Medicine and Society in America, 1660–1860*. New York; New York University Press

Shryock, R. (1966). *Medicine in America. Historical Essays*. Baltimore; Johns Hopkins University Press

Shryock, R. (1967). *Medical Licensing in America, 1650–1965*. Baltimore; Johns Hopkins University Press

Sinclair, B. (1974). *Philosopher Mechanics. A History of the Franklin Institute, 1824–65*. Baltimore; Johns Hopkins University Press

Stanton, W. (1960). *The Leopard's Spots. Scientific Attitudes Toward Race in America*. Chicago; University of Chicago Press

Stanton, W. (1975). *The Great United States Exploring Expedition, 1839–42*. Berkeley; University of California Press

Stearns, R.P. (1970). *Science in the British Colonies of North America*. Urbana; University of Illinois Press

Stegner, W. (1954). *Beyond the Hundredth Meridian: John Wesley Powell and the Second Opening of the West*. Boston; Houghton Mifflin

Stevens, R. (1971). *American Medicine and the Public Interest*. New Haven, Conn.; Yale University Press

Stocking, G. (1968). *Race, Culture, and Evolution*. New York; The Free Press

Struik, D. (1948). *Yankee Science in the Making*. Boston; Little, Brown

Torchia, M. (1975). The Tuberculosis Movement and the Race Question, 1890–1950, *Bulletin of the History of Medicine*, Vol. 49, 152–168

Van Tassel, D. and Hall, M. (1966). *Science and Society in the U.S.* Homewood; Dorsey Press. (Has a useful bibliography)

Walsh, M. (1978). *'Doctors Wanted: No Women Need Apply.' Sexual Barriers in the Medical Profession, 1835–1975*. New Haven, Conn.; Yale University Press

Whorton, J. (1975). *Before Silent Spring: Pesticides and Public Health in Pre-DDT America*. Princeton, NJ; Princeton University Press

Wilson, L.G. (1980). Medical History Without Medicine, *Journal of the History of Medicine and Allied Sciences*, Vol. 35, 5–7

Wolfe, M.R. (1978). *Lucius Polk Brown and Progressive Food and Drug Control.* Lawrence; Regents Press of Kansas
York, H. (1976). *The Advisers. Oppenheimer, Teller, and the Superbomb.* San Francisco; W.H. Freeman

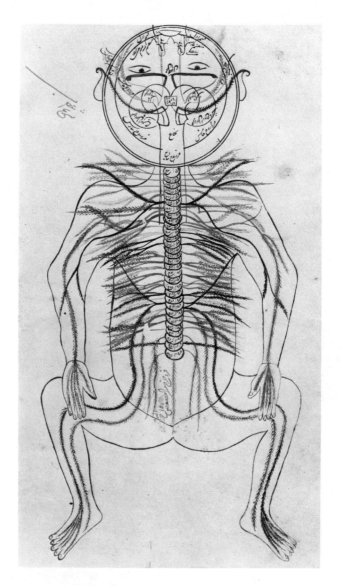

Plate 9. The nervous system. One of a set of anatomical drawings that illustrate arteries, veins, nerves, bones, muscles, and, frequently, a pregnant woman. This illustration is bound with a copy of the *Canon* of Ibn Sīnā, Wellcome MS Or. 155, fol. 123v (dated AD 1632). By courtesy of the Wellcome Trustees

21

Islamic science and medicine

Emilie Savage-Smith

In the Islamic world the Arabic word *'ilm*, usually translated as 'science', was and still is very broadly used for any attempt to understand, explain, control or influence events and relationships in the realm of human affairs as well as that of nature. Consequently, 'science' encompasses astrology–astronomy, arithmetic, geometry, algebra, alchemy, the interpretation of dreams, cosmology and cosmogony, medicine, pharmacology, botany, agricultural practices, farriery, hawking, geography, the military arts, physiognomy, divinatory practices and magical procedures as well as the disciplines concerned with Qur'ānic exegesis, jurisprudence, rhetoric, grammar, philosophy, logic, ethics and the writing of history. Various writers classified the sciences into different groupings such as the 'religious sciences' including jurisprudence, exegesis and the traditions of the Prophet (*ḥadīth*), and the 'foreign sciences' or 'sciences of the ancients', which included among other topics mathematics, medicine and astronomy. The classification of the sciences and the recognition of those topics considered legitimate to investigate differed from one scholar to another (see, for example, Gardet and Anawati 1948).

For the purposes of this chapter, the definition of 'science' will exclude Qur'ānic exegesis, jurisprudence, grammar and related topics, and will concentrate on those subjects that today we refer to as the exact sciences and the biological sciences and medicine, along with the ancillary fields of alchemy, divination and magic, which are sometimes referred to in the West as 'pseudo-sciences'.

For many centuries Arabic was the main vehicle of communicating ideas on all these topics among Muslims, Christians and Jews from Spain through North Africa and the Near East to Persia and Western India, although a distinct literature written in the Persian language using the Arabic alphabet did also develop. There were also some Hebrew treatises of considerable importance, particularly in Spain, but these will not be included in this chapter.

In approaching a topic in the history of Islamic science for the first time a non-specialist will inevitably confront certain difficulties, such as the transliteration of words, the various forms of Arabic names, and the conversion of dates. Convenient guides to begin with are the essays by Hodgson (1974) and Lewis (1951) and the article on Islamic proper names in the *Encyclopaedia of Islam* (1960–, iv: 179–81). Probably the most usable set of tables for converting a Muslim date to a Christian one is that by Freeman-Grenville (1963), which gives complete instructions for interpolating to determine a precise day equivalent. A basic bibliographic reference guide to general Islamic studies is Grimwood-Jones, Hopwood and Pearson (1977).

Prior to the nineteenth century there was no significant research into the history of Islamic science. In the last century the early biobibliographical study of Islamic physicians and natural scientists by Wüstenfeld was published in 1840, while Islamic astronomy profited from the early work of Sédillot (1844, 1845–9). Islamic medicine received attention with the still useful English translation by Greenhill of Rhazes' important treatise on smallpox and measles (al-Rāzī 1848) and the general but uncritical history of Islamic medicine by Leclerc (1876). Anatomical and medical terminology was studied by Hyrtl, Favrot, Sanguinetti and van Vloten in the latter half of the nineteenth century; see Savage-Smith (1976: 261–4).

At the end of the nineteenth and beginning of the twentieth century several studies were produced that are useful to investigators today. The monumental history of Arabic ophthalmological practice by Hirschberg (1908) is still a major source, although some aspects are outdated by more recently discovered material and the numerous publications of Meyerhof (see Schacht 1950). The standard biobibliographical source for the history of Islamic astronomy and mathematics is still the study by Suter (1900, 1902). The investigations of Steinschneider (1889, 1904–5) on the transmission of treatises into Arabic and from Arabic into Latin are still fundamental studies. The numerous writings and translations in the first part of this century by E. Wiedemann on many different aspects of Islamic science are for the most part quite reliable and still provide a rich source of information for modern historians. A bibliography of his studies has been compiled by H.J. Seemann in the reprint of Wiedemann's 69-part series of studies published in the *Sitzungsberichte der Physikalische-medizinische Sozietät zu Erlangen* from 1902 to 1928 (Wiedemann 1970). Historians today could well profit from a reprint of his remaining historical works, which were sometimes published in journals most difficult to locate today (all these are listed by Seemann in the reprint mentioned above); his private library was given to the University of Leyden, which consequently has an extensive collection of some of his rare studies with occasional corrections by the author.

The first three volumes of the widely influential bibliographical study of sources for the history of science by G. Sarton (1927–48) cover many aspects of Islamic science. This source is, however, to a considerable extent outdated and somewhat limited in its scope by its logical positivist approach to the history of science. Unfortunately, the broader approach of an historian of ideas, as so admirably exemplified in the examination of Western sources by Thorndike (1923–58), has not been undertaken for the comparable aspects of Islamic thought, although Thorndike's study does have chapters of interest to historians of Islamic sciences such as astrology.

While these early studies can still prove useful, there are some particularly important bibliographical sources that touch on nearly all aspects of Islamic science and medicine. While being of particular value to the specialist, they can be of great assistance to the non-specialist as well. Foremost among them is the extensive work of Brockelmann (1889–1936, 1937–42, 1943–9), listing by author manuscripts, printed works as well as secondary studies, and recently supplemented by Sezgin (1970, 1971, 1974, 1978, 1979). Sezgin has grouped the material into subject categories, with secondary divisions by author, and has limited the material to treatises written before the middle of the eleventh century AD. For some reservations and critical comments regarding the work of Sezgin see Plessner (1972), Rosenfeld (1978) and King (1979c). The comparable source for Persian writings is the biobibliography by Storey (1958, 1971, 1977). Any investigator in the history of Islamic science should be cognizant of the relevant material in these volumes.

In addition to these volumes, the researcher will find useful various series of bibliographical listings such as the *Index Islamicus* (J.D. Pearson 1958, 1961–77), which covers studies printed between 1906 and 1975; publications after 1975 are surveyed in its continuation, *The Quarterly Index Islamicus* (J.D. Pearson 1977–).

A number of journals provide bibliographies of recently printed secondary sources some of which pertain to various aspects of Islamic science. They include the annual *Critical Bibliography* published by *Isis*, the *Bibliographie* published as part of *Cahiers de Civilisation Médiévale x^e–xiie siècles*, the Bibliography of Periodical Literature appended to each issue of *The Middle East Journal*, and the review of Oriental literature, *Orientalistische Literaturzeitung*. Since these bibliographies are drawn from different sources they should each be consulted if a thorough search of the literature is to be made. On the other hand, *Abstracta Islamica*, which is issued occasionally as a supplement to *Revue des études islamiques*, is not generally helpful for the present purposes since it does not concern itself with the sciences. The *Mélanges de l'Institut Dominician d'Études Orientales* (Cairo) publishes in its annual issue a full description of books printed and manuscripts edited in Egypt.

For the specialist wishing to examine manuscript material, a guide to catalogues of the numerous collections of Arabic manuscripts is Huisman (1967) and Sezgin (1967: 706–69; 1970: 383–410; 1974 :433–58; 1978: 311–469). The *Revue de l'Institut des Manuscrits Arabes (Majallah Ma'had al-makhṭūṭāt al-'arabîyah)* published in Cairo (in Arabic) is useful, for besides occasional editions of texts it publishes catalogues of particular Middle Eastern manuscript collections, many now recorded on microfilm by the League of Arab States in Cairo. For Arabic archival sources, Berque and Chevalier (1976) should be consulted. In addition to the extensive microfilm collection assembled by the League of Arab States, there are several microfilm projects that have material of interest to historians of Islamic science. The Vatican Film Library at St Louis University, St Louis, Missouri, has on microfilm the entire Arabic collection of manuscripts at the Vatican, except for the Sbath manuscripts. The Hill Monastic Manuscript Library (HMML) of St John's Abbey, Collegeville, Minnesota, has microfilmed manuscripts from seventy-three Austrian libraries, including all the Arabic and Hebrew manuscripts at the Österreichische Nationalbibliothek in Vienna, and also smaller libraries and monastic collections in Spain. The microfilms of manuscripts in Istanbul collected by H. Ritter are now on deposit at the University of Uppsala (see Bjorkmann 1971). The pharmaceutical and medical manuscript material in the microfilm collection developed by M. Levey is now at the University of Utah.

For an introduction to a particular topic or author, a rich source and starting point is the *Encyclopaedia of Islam*, especially the more recent but still incomplete second edition (hereafter abbreviated EI²). A knowledge of the Arabic term, in the German system of transliteration, is, however, necessary to find the entry for a topic, but the reader is assisted by an index to the first three volumes of the second edition by H. and J.D. Pearson (1979). *The Dictionary of Scientific Biography* (Gillispie 1970–8) is a secondary biographical source of somewhat uneven value, sometimes providing quite detailed bibliographies. The recent bibliography by Nasr (1975–8) of Islamic sciences, of which only the first two volumes devoted to general works have appeared, is quite inadequate and disappointing (see Hall 1978).

In 1977 the *Journal for the History of Arabic Science* was established with an international board of editors for the purpose of publishing articles in English, French or Arabic, and editions of texts, on topics in Islamic science including Persian, Turkish and Urdu as well as Arabic materials. It is hoped that the journal, published twice yearly by the Institute for the History of Arabic Science at the University of Aleppo, will become a major forum for historians of Islamic science. The founding institution is also sponsoring a series of monographs devoted to catalogues of manuscript collections and editions of lengthy texts, as well as international conferences on the history of Islamic science.

For someone wanting a general introduction to the field, there are surprisingly few essays that present such an overview of Islamic science. Among those that are available, the essays by Plessner (1974) and Vernet (1974) in the second edition of the *Legacy of Islam* are among the best, although they are brief. Unfortunately, the quite extensive and well-documented history prepared by F.R. Maddison and A.J. Turner as a text to accompany the exhibition held at the Science Museum in London in 1976 as part of the Festival of Islam was never published (Oxford, Museum of the History of Science). The essay by Sabra (1976) in a volume published at the time of the Festival of Islam is rewarding though also quite short. In the first edition of the *Legacy of Islam*, the contributions of Meyerhof (1931) and Carra de Vaux (1931) can still be useful despite their more simplistic approach. The *Cambridge History of Islam* contains a chapter by Anawati (1970) which is well written, as is also the section by Kennedy (1968) in the *Cambridge History of Iran*, whereas the somewhat longer essay by Arnaldez and Massignon (1957) is rather superficial and disappointing. As for monographs that can serve as general introductions, that by Mieli (1938) is unsatisfactory and outdated, although the bibliography by A. Mazahéri appended to the reprinted version (Mieli 1966) can be of some use. The slender volume by Winter (1952) touches upon some highlights of Islamic science but does not place them within a cultural or historical context. The well-illustrated book on Islamic science by Nasr (1976) is inaccurate and misleading; see, for example, King (1978) for a critical review. Nasr's earlier collection of annotated readings in Islamic science (Nasr 1968) can be useful in a classroom, but all of Nasr's writings are highly personal essays, infused with Ṣūfī attitudes and marred by numerous inaccuracies.

For specific areas of Islamic science, some very useful and thorough bibliographic guides have appeared in recent years. The field of Islamic medicine and pharmacology has been particularly well served by the exhaustive bibliographical history by Ullmann (1970) with a *Nachträge* by Ullmann (1972: 452–63). This thorough guide to printed and manuscript materials completely replaces the faulty bibliography of printed secondary literature by Ebied (1971), while for some of the early physicians additional manuscript material is mentioned by Sezgin (1970). For studies appearing after 1970, the *Current Work in the History of Medicine* and the *Bibliography of the History of Medicine* should be consulted under the particular topic or author, as well as the more general bibliographical aids previously mentioned. Persian medical literature has received much less attention than the Arabic sources, although the Persian materials are numerous and deserve detailed attention. The standard guide to such literature is Storey (1971), while the detailed catalogue by Richter-Bernburg (1978) is extremely useful.

Islamic medicine has received more attention from historians than any other aspect of Islamic science. A recent and very rewarding contribution is that by Ullmann (1978), which is solidly based on written sources, but is not completely comprehensive in that it omits certain topics such as surgery and ophthalmology. The lecture by Browne (1921) still has merit and is reliable although much has been done by historians since its composition. The history of Arabic and Persian medicine by Elgood (1951) can still be recommended, though it is not overly concerned with the complexities of the subject, while the study by Elgood (1970) of Ṣafavid (seventeenth-century Persian) practices is rich in material but woefully lacking in specific identification of sources. The early two-volume history by Leclerc (1876) is now quite outdated, while Campbell (1926) is highly unreliable.

Two medical topics have received particular attention from historians, namely pharmacology and ophthalmology. The pharmacological literature, both on simple drugs and compound remedies, has received much attention from Meyerhof (see Schacht

1950), P. Sbath, M. Levey and others. Yet much remains to be done, for many influential *aqrābādhīn* have yet to be analysed; see Ullmann (1970: 257–320). The field of Islamic ophthalmology is still indebted to the history by Hirschberg (1908) and the work of Meyerhof (Schacht 1950); see Ullmann (1970: 204–14). Meyerhof edited and translated all or parts of a number of important ophthalmological treatises, in collaboration with several orientalists, including P. Sbath who was himself a collector of Arabic medical manuscripts. Three-quarters of the large collection of Sbath manuscripts are now at the Vatican; if the present location of the remainder of his private collection as well as the extremely important medical manuscripts in private collections in Syria that he catalogued (Sbath 1938–9), could now be ascertained, the history of Islamic medicine would be greatly assisted.

The last several decades have seen the publication of many editions and translations of medical texts that may serve as a foundation for future histories. The Arabic translation of Greek medical texts has benefited especially from two series of monographs devoted to just these topics, the Oriental Supplement to the *Corpus Medicorum Graecorum* and the *Arabic Technical and Scientific Texts*. During the past fifty years the Osmania Oriental Publication Bureau (Dā'irat al-ma'ārif al-'uthmānīyah) in Hyderabad has issued editions of several medical texts, in addition to a few astronomical ones; the texts have been very useful to historians although they have no accompanying translation and seldom are annotated.

Yet with all this attention to textual material there still remains a great need for critical editions and annotated Western translations, as well as historical comparisons and analyses. Many of the major early compositions still await a translation into a Western language with a good commentary and a reliable edition of the text. For example, the enormously influential *al-Hāwī* by al-Rāzī (Rhazes) has no translation into a modern Western language, and only one book of the *Qānūn* by Ibn Sīnā (Avicenna) is available in a Western language other than Latin, while the most reliable Arabic text of the *Canon* is still a printing made in Rome in 1593. A similar state of affairs pertains to the tenth-century medical encyclopaedia of al-Majūsī (Haly Abbas). Furthermore, little written after the eleventh century AD has been studied.

In recent years a few topics, such as plague tracts (see Dols 1977), have attracted renewed attention, but there remain a large number of subjects that need careful examination. Foremost among these is the design and administration of Islamic hospitals; for what little has been done see the entry *bīmāristān* in EI[2] (i: 1222–6), 'Īsā Bey (1928), and Terzioğlu (1968). Other topics include the medical training and examination of physicians, the relation of the *ḥisba* system to the maintenance of standards (see EI², iii: 485–93), the various levels of medical care available in a society, and the role of divinatory practices in the diagnosis and prognosis of disease and of magical procedures in prevention and cure. Moreover, more attention might be given to the extant, unfortunately rather small, collections of medieval Islamic medical instruments in museums, as well as the Hilton-Simpson collection of nineteenth-century North African instruments (in the Pitt-Rivers Museum, Oxford), and their relation to the illustrations and descriptions of such instruments in medieval manuscripts; for a bibliography of studies and reports on Greco-Roman and Islamic medical instruments see Savage-Smith (1976: 256–60).

With regard to the fields of zoology and animal lore, original sources and secondary studies are listed by Ullmann (1972) and for the early period by Sezgin (1970). For lapidology Ullmann (1972) is again useful, while for writings on plants and agriculture, including geoponica, Ullmann (1972) and Sezgin (1971) should be consulted. Other useful guides are the related subject entries in EI² of which the following are particularly significant contributions: *ḥayawān* (the animal kingdom) iii: 304–15; *faras* and *khayl* (farriery) ii: 784–7 and iii: 1143–6; *bayzara* (hawking) i: 1152–5; *ibil* (camel) iii: 665–8; *fahd* (cheetah) ii: 738–43, *bayṭār* (veterinary surgeon) i: 1149; and *filāḥa* (agriculture) ii:899–910. Many texts in the natural sciences have yet to be analysed, however, and no satisfactory history of these subjects exists.

There is considerable current activity in the fields of Islamic astronomy–astrology and mathematics, but there is no up-to-date survey in a European language. Consequently there is need for a comprehensive and critical historical study of the development and interaction of these disciplines in the Islamic world. The standard general history of astronomy and astrology in Islam is still 'Astro-logie–astronomia–geographia' comprising the fifth volume of Nallino (1939–48). This volume is an Italian translation of his earlier Arabic essay (Nallino 1911). Though outdated by numer-ous individual studies since its appearance, this Italian translation, which is not easily accessible, perhaps warrants a reprint. Also still quite useful is the short English essay by Nallino (1921) on Islamic astronomy and astrology. A new general survey of Islamic astro-nomy is currently being prepared by D.A. King and B.A. Rosen-feld as a contribution to a general history of astronomy to be published by Cambridge University Press. The only monograph devoted to a history of Arabic mathematics is that by Yuschke-vitch (1976), which is a French translation of the chapter on

Islamic mathematics taken from his earlier history of medieval mathematics written in Russian and translated into German (Yuschkevitch 1961), with additions by the author and an updated bibliography.

This century has seen many short studies, however, and some editions and translations of mathematical and astronomical texts. A basic biobibliographical tool is still Suter (1900, 1902) supplemented by Renaud (1932). A rich bibliographic source for secondary studies of Islamic mathematics and mathematical astronomy is the *Mathematical Reviews*, which include summaries of studies by Russian scholars such as Rosenfeld. For manuscript and secondary sources for mathematical tracts written before the middle of the eleventh century AD, the most important source is Sezgin (1974); see also King (1979c) and Rosenfeld (1978). For astronomical writings of the same time period, see Sezgin (1978). Sources for Islamic astrology are discussed by Ullmann (1972), while Persian sources for the history of mathematics, astronomy, astrology and geography are dealt with by Storey (1958). Useful introductions to recent work on Islamic arithmetical and algebraic texts are the relevant articles in EI², such as *ḥisāb al-'akḍ* (iii: 466–8), *ḥisāb al-ghubār* (iii: 468–9), *'ilm al-ḥisāb* (iii: 1138–41) and *al-djabr wa 'l-muḵābala* (ii: 360–2). For short introductions to the literature on astronomy the articles in EI², *'ilm al-hay'a* (iii: 1135–8), *falak* (ii: 761–3) and *asṭurlāb* (i: 722–8), are convenient.

An interesting essay surveying the present state of scholarship in the history of Islamic astronomy and mathematics has been written by King (1980). For a guide to the numerous Islamic star charts (*zij*es) see the survey by Kennedy (1956), which is currently being revised with the collaboration of D.A. King. A guide to the work of the school of Maragha is Kennedy (1966). For Byzantine and Pahlavi (Sasanian) interactions see the various studies by Pingree (e.g., 1970). The collected papers of Hartner (1968) cover iconographic as well as other aspects of Islamic astronomical work. Star names have received much recent attention with the work of Tibbetts (1971) and Kunitzsch (1959, 1961), who is also responsible for a long-needed study of the Arabic version of Ptolemy's *Almagest* (Kunitzsch 1974). A detailed catalogue by D.A. King (1981) of the extensive holdings of astronomical and mathematical manuscripts in the Egyptian National Library (Dār al-Kutub) in Cairo should provide a rich source for future historians.

Artifacts related to Islamic astronomy have been much better preserved than medical instruments and have been studied in much greater detail. A comprehensive historical study by F.R.

Maddison and A. Brieux of all types of Islamic astronomical instruments that are signed or dated is nearing completion and will provide a very valuable research tool. The undertaking will replace the earlier more limited listings by Price (1955), Mayer (1956) and Gunther (1932), and will include instruments in addition to astrolabes. For a detailed comparative and historical study of Islamic celestial globes see the forthcoming study by E. Savage-Smith.

The related field of optics received considerable scholarly attention from, among others, E. Wiedemann (see Seemann in Wiedemann 1970) and, more recently, A.I. Sabra whose long-awaited critical edition of Ibn al-Haytham's *Kitāb al-manāẓir* will be appearing soon. A bibliography of printed and secondary sources for the history of Islamic optics and ophthalmology will form part of the forthcoming volume on sources for Byzantine, Islamic and Latin optics and ophthalmology compiled by J. Neu, E. Savage-Smith, and D. Lindberg.

The numerous studies by E. Wiedemann are an important source for the history of Islamic technology (see Wiedemann 1970). In recent years the engineer and Arabist D.R. Hill has translated and commented extensively on a series of three major technological texts: al-Jazarî (1974), Archimedes (1976), and the Banū Mūsā (1979). For critical evaluations of these studies see King (1975, 1977). An important study of medieval Persian metal technology is that by Allan (1979).

Astrology was such an integral part of most medieval astronomical thought that the separation of the two approaches is frequently difficult and leads to distortions. Much more historical work has been done on treatises or parts of treatises that deal with mathematical and observational aspects of astronomy and far less on astrology. While the edition and translation of the astrology written in the eleventh century by al-Bîrūnî (1934) is extremely useful and the recent edition and translation of the Arabic version of Dorotheus (1976) most welcome, they represent only a very small fraction of the astrological literature and cannot be used as a reliable guide to all the attitudes and methods. Only one Persian astrology has attracted scholarly attention (Elwell-Sutton 1977). An almost overwhelming amount of material remains untouched by scholars and some of the most popular Islamic astrological compendia, such as those written in the thirteenth century by Aḥmad ibn 'Alî al-Būnî, have been virtually ignored as historical sources, except for some interest shown in the sections on magic squares.

Ullmann (1972) attempted a preliminary survey of sources for

Islamic astrological thought, but no survey has ever been undertaken comparable to the *Catalogus Codicum Astrologorum Graecorum* for Byzantine material. No attempt has been made to analyse the development of different astrological methods, lines of influence, the comparative nature of the contents of the treatises, and other historical problems, while employing sound historical and philological methods.

A similar state of affairs exists for the history of Islamic alchemy. While receiving early attention from J. Ruska, P. Kraus and more recently M. Plessner, only a small part of the contents of alchemical tracts have been published, with the result that a thorough and reliable history of Arabic alchemy is not yet possible; for a discussion of the present state of the field see the entry *kimiyā'* in EI² (iv: 110–15). For a list of manuscript sources as well as secondary studies see Sezgin (1971) and Ullmann (1972, 1974–6).

If the areas of astrology and alchemy are in need of a great deal of serious historical attention, this is even more true of the areas of divination and magic. Again, Ullmann (1972) has surveyed some of the sources for magical practices and Fahd (1966) for divinatory practices, although his accompanying historical comments are inadequate. For Persian sources in the occult sciences see Storey (1977). See also Anawati (1972) for a good bibliography on talismans and Savage-Smith and Smith (1980) for the practice of geomancy. Moreover, the accounts of the tricks of conjurers, forgers and beggars by writers such as the eighth-century al-Jāḥiz, the twelfth-century Ibn al-Jauzî and the thirteenth-century al-Jaubarî merit renewed attention from historians of science, following some of the early studies by Wiedemann (see Wiedemann 1970).

There are still other areas of Islamic science that deserve more attention. For example, a historical study of the cosmographical literature is needed. Even the important and frequently cited thirteenth-century cosmography by Zakariyā' ibn Muḥammad al-Qazwînî has never received proper historical attention, or for that matter a complete translation into a European language, and it stands in need of a good critical edition to replace the very inadequate one prepared in 1848 (al-Qazwînî 1848–9). Such cosmographical literature is rich in information on zoology, stars, geology, plants and other natural phenomena. The treatises concerned with descriptive and mathematical geography and cartography merit careful attention; see the article *djughrāfiyā* in EI² (ii: 575–90) and Storey (1958). For example, to name only two, the geography written by al-Qazwînî in the thirteenth century and the geographical tract by the eleventh-century Andalusian Abū 'Ubaid al-Bakrî could both use a complete critical edition and systematic study. For the processing of geographical data from astronomical sources see Kennedy and Haddad (1971) and King (1980: note 15).

General encyclopaedic literature has to a large extent been overlooked by historians of science. This is a vast and potentially rich source; for a bibliography of Persian encyclopaedias see Storey (1977). The importance and role of pseudepigraphy – writings spuriously attributed to others – in Islamic scientific literature deserves more attention from modern scholars. A preliminary study of Islamic pseudepigraphical literature was undertaken by Steinschneider (1862). More recently two important studies have been the edition and translation of the 'Picatrix', which circulated under the name of the tenth-century mathematician and astronomer al-Majrîtî when in fact it was composed a century later (al-Majrîtî 1933, 1962), and the demonstration by Lemay (1978) that the 'Centiloquium' attributed to Ptolemy was actually written in the tenth century by Aḥmad ibn Yūsuf. For the important fabricated accounts by Abū Ma'shar of early chronologies and Hermes Trismegistus see Pingree (1968) and Plessner (1954), and for a general guide to work on the Hermetic literature see the article *Hirmis* in EI[2] (iii: 463–5).

As can be seen from this survey, although scholarly interest in the history of medieval Islamic science has increased enormously in recent years, there remains much to be done before a truly comprehensive and coherent picture can emerge. Only a small percentage of the available written documents have been examined, and many non-written sources need further study and integration with the written documents. Possible originality and modernity ought not to be the sole criteria for examining a given topic or treatise. The general aim of understanding thoroughly the prevailing concerns of the scholarly community and their function within that particular society and culture will in the long run be more productive of the integrative historical analyses now needed of medieval Islamic science.

Bibliography

Oxford, Museum of the History of Science. Unpublished typescript. Maddison, F.R. and A.J. Turner (1976). Science and Technology in Islam: Catalogue of an Exhibition held at the Science Museum, London, April–August 1976, in Association with the Festival of Islam

Oxford, Pitt-Rivers Museum. The Hilton-Simpson Collection of North African Medical Instruments

Allan, J.W. (1979). *Persian Metal Technology, 700–1300 AD*. With an Appendix by A. Kaczmarczyk and R.E.M. Hedges. Oxford Oriental Monographs, No. 2. London; Ithaca Press for the Faculty of Oriental Studies and the Ashmolean Museum, University of Oxford

Anawati, G.C. (1970). Science, in *The Cambridge History of Islam*. Ed. P.M. Holt, A.K.S. Lambton, and B. Lewis. 2 Vols. Cambridge; Cambridge University Press, Vol. 2: 741–779

Anawati, G.C. (1972). Trois talismans musulmans en arabe provenant du Mali (marché de Mopti), *Annales islamologiques*, Vol. 11, 287–339

Arabic Technical and Scientific Texts (1966–). 8 Vols published. Cambridge; Heffer for Cambridge Middle East Centre

Archimedes (1976). *On the Construction of Water-Clocks: Kitāb Arshimidas fī 'amal al-binkamat*. Ed. and Trans. D.R. Hill. London; Turner and Devereux

Arnaldez, R. and Massignon, L. (1957). La Science arabe, in *La Science antique et médiévale*. Vol. 1 of *Histoire générale des sciences*. Ed. R. Taton. 4 Vols. (1957–64). Paris; Presses Universitaires de France, 430–471. English trans. (1963). Arabic Science, in *Ancient and Medieval Science from the Beginnings to 1450*. Ed. R. Taton. Trans. A.J. Pomerans. New York; Basic Books, 385–421

Banū Mūsā ibn Shākir (1979). *The Book of Ingenious Devices (Kitāb al-Ḥiyal) by the Banū (sons of) Mūsā bin Shākir*. Trans. and Annotated by D.R. Hill. Dordrecht and Boston, Mass.; D. Reidel

Berque, J. and Chevalier, D., Ed. (1976). *Les Arabes par leurs archives (xvie – xxe siècles)*. Colloques Internationaux du Centre National de la Recherche Scientifique, No. 555. Paris; Éditions du Centre National de la Recherche Scientifique

Bibliography of the History of Medicine (1966–). Washington, DC; National Library of Medicine

al-Bîrûnî, Abū al-Raiḥān Muḥammad ibn Aḥmad (1934). *The Book of Instruction in the Elements of the Art of Astrology. Written in Ghaznah, 1029 A.D*. Ed. and Trans. R. Ramsay Wright. London; Luzac

Bjorkmann, W. (1971). Mikrofilmsammlung in Uppsala, *Der Islam*, Vol. 41, 298

Brockelmann, C. (1889–1936). *Geschichte der arabischen Litteratur*, 1st edn. 2 Vols. Leyden; Brill

Brockelmann, C. (1937–42). *Geschichte der arabischen Litteratur, Supplement*. 3 Vols. Leyden; Brill

Brockelmann, C. (1943–9). *Geschichte der arabischen Literatur*, 2nd edn. 2 Vols. Leyden; Brill

Browne, E.G. (1921). *Arabian Medicine*. Cambridge; Cambridge University Press. Reprinted (1962). Cambridge; Cambridge University Press

Campbell, D. (1926). *Arabian Medicine and its Influence on the Middle Ages*. 2 Vols. London; Kegan Paul, Trench, and Trübner

Carra de Vaux, Baron (1931). Astronomy and Mathematics, in *The Legacy of Islam*, 1st edn. Ed. T. Arnold and A. Guillaume. Oxford; Clarendon Press, 376–397

Catalogus Codicum Astrologorum Graecorum (1898–1951). Ed. F. Boll, F. Cumont, *et al*. 12 Vols. Brussels; Lamertin

Corpus Medicorum Graecorum Supplementum Orientale (1963–70). 3 Vols. Berlin; Akademie-Verlag

Current Work in the History of Medicine; An International Bibliography (1954–). London; Wellcome Institute for the History of Medicine

Dieterici, F. (1876). *Die Philosophie der Araber im X. Jahrhundert n. Chr.; Gesamtdarstellung und Quellenwerke*. 14 Vols. Leipzig; J.G. Hinrichs'sche Buchhandlung. Reprinted (1969). Hildesheim; Olms

Dols, M.W. (1977). *The Black Death in the Middle East*. Princeton, NJ; Princeton University Press

Dorotheus of Sidon (1976). *Dorothei Sidonii Carmen astrologicum.* Ed. D. Pingree. Leipzig; Teubner

Ebied, R.Y. (1971). *Bibliography of Mediaeval Arabic and Jewish Medicine and Allied Sciences.* Wellcome Institute for the History of Medicine, Occasional Series 2. London; Wellcome Institute for the History of Medicine

Elgood, C.L. (1951). *A Medical History of Persia and the Eastern Caliphate.* Cambridge; Cambridge University Press. Reprinted (n.d.). Amsterdam; APA-Philo

Elgood, C.L. (1970). *Safavid Medical Practice, or The Practice of Medicine, Surgery and Gynaecology in Persia between 1500 A.D. and 1750 A.D.* London; Luzac

Elwell-Sutton, L.P. (1977). *The Horoscope of Asadullāh Mîrzā: A Specimen of Nineteenth-Century Persian Astrology.* Nisaba, Vol. 6. Leyden; Brill

Encyclopaedia of Islam (1911–38), 1st edn. Ed. M.Th. Houtsma, A.J. Wiensinck, *et al.* 4 Vols. Leyden; Brill

Encyclopaedia of Islam (1960–), 2nd edn. 4 Vols published. Leyden; Brill

Fahd, T. (1966). *La Divination arabe, études religieuses, sociologiques et folkloriques sur le milieu natif de l'Islam.* Strasburg; Université de Strasbourg. Leyden; Brill

Freeman-Grenville, G.S.P. (1963). *The Muslim and Christian Calendars, being tables for the conversion of Muslim and Christian dates from the Hijra to the year A.D. 2000.* London, New York and Toronto; Oxford University Press

Gardet, L. and Anawati, M.-M. (1948). *Introduction à la théologie musulmane, essai de théologie comparée.* Études de Philosophie Médiévale, 37. Paris; Librairie Philosophique J. Vrin

Gillispie, C.C., Ed. (1970–8). *Dictionary of Scientific Biography.* 15 Vols. New York; American Council of Learned Societies, Charles Scribner's Sons

Goldstein, B.R. (1965). On the Theory of Trepidation, *Centaurus*, Vol. 10, 232–247

Goldstein, B.R. (1979). Medieval Observations of Solar and Lunar Eclipses, *Archives Internationales d'Histoire des Sciences*, Vol. 29, 101–156

Goldstein, B.R. and Pingree, D. (1979). Astrological Almanacs from the Cairo Geniza, *Journal of Near Eastern Studies*, Vol. 38, 153–175, 231–256

Grignaschi, M. (1976). L'Origine et les métamorphoses du 'Sirr al-asrār', *Archives d'histoire doctrinale et littéraire du Moyen-Age*, Vol. 43, 7–112

Grimwood-Jones, D., Hopwood, D. and Pearson, J.D., Ed. (1977). *Arab Islamic Bibliography. The Middle East Library Committee Guide Based on Giuseppe Gabrieli's* Manuale di bibliographia musulmana. Hassocks, Sussex; The Harvester Press. Atlantic Highland, NJ; The Humanities Press

Gunther, R.T. (1932). *The Astrolabes of the World.* 2 Vols. Oxford; Oxford University Press

Hall, R.E. (1978). Book Review of S.H. Nasr (1975–8), *Isis*, Vol. 69, 457–461

Hartner, W. (1968). *Oriens–Occidens. Ausgewählte Schriften zur Wissenschafts-und Kulturgeschichte. Festschrift zum 60. Geburtstag.* Collectanea, Vol. 3. Hildesheim; G. Olms

Hau, F.R. (1978–9). Die Bildung des Arztes im Islamischen Mittelalter, *Clio Medica*, Vol. 13, 95–124, 175–200

Hirschberg, J. (1908). *Geschichte der Augenheilkunde, Buch II: Geschichte der Augenheilkunde im Mittelalter.* Vol. 13 of *Handbuch der gesamten Augenheilkunde*, 2nd edn. Ed. A. Graefe and E.T. Saemisch. 15 Vols. (1899–1919). Leipzig; Engelmann. Reprinted (1977). Vol. 2 of J. Hirschberg, *Geschichte der Augenheilkunde.* 7 Vols. Hildesheim; G. Olms

Hodgson, M.G.S. (1974). Introduction to the Study of Islamic Civilization, in *The*

Classical Age of Islam. Vol. 1 of *The Venture of Islam*, M.G.S. Hodgson. Chicago and London; University of Chicago Press, 3–69

Huisman, A.J.W. (1967). *Les Manuscrits arabes dans le monde: une bibliographie des catalogues.* Leyden; Brill

'Īsā Bey, Aḥmad (1928). *Histoire des bimaristans (hôpitaux) à l'époque islamique. Discours prononcé au Congrès international de médecine tropicale et d'hygiene tenu au Caire, Décembre 1928.* Cairo; Paul Barbey

Iskandar, A.Z. (1976). Bibliographical Studies in Medical and Scientific Arabic Work, *Oriens*, Vol. 25–26, 133–147

Jachimowicz, E. (1975). Islamic Cosmology, in *Ancient Cosmologies*. Ed. C. Blacker and M. Loewe. London; Allen and Unwin, 143–171

al-Jazarî, Ibn Razzāz (1974). *The Book of Knowledge of Ingenious Mechanical Devices (Kitāb fī ma'rifat al-ḥiyal al-handasiyya).* Ed. and Trans. D.R. Hill. Dordrecht and Boston, Mass.; Reidel

Kennedy, E.S. (1956). *A Survey of Islamic Astronomical Tables.* Transactions of the American Philosophical Society, N.S., Vol. 46, Pt. 2. Philadelphia; American Philosophical Society

Kennedy, E.S. (1966). Late Medieval Planetary Theory, *Isis*, Vol. 57, 365–378

Kennedy, E.S. (1968). The Exact Sciences in Iran under the Saljuqs and Mongols, in *The Cambridge History of Iran.* Ed. J.A. Boyle. 5 Vols. Cambridge; Cambridge University Press, Vol. 5: 659–679

Kennedy, E.S. and Haddad, F. (1971). Geographical Tables of Medieval Islam, *al-Abḥāth*, Vol. 24, 87–102

King, D.A. (1975). Medieval Mechanical Devices, *History of Science*, Vol. 13, 284–289

King, D.A. (1977). On Arabic Water-Clocks, *History of Science*, Vol. 14, 295–298

King, D.A. (1978). Book Review of S.H. Nasr (1976), *Journal for the History of Astronomy*, Vol. 9, 212–219. Reprinted (1978) in *Bibliotheca Orientalis*, Vol. 35, 339–342

King, D.A. (1979a). Islamic Mathematics, *History of Science*, Vol. 17, 295–296

King, D.A. (1979b). Ibn Yūnus and the Pendulum: A History of Errors, *Archives Internationales d'Histoire des Sciences*, Vol. 29, 35–52

King, D.A. (1979c). Notes on the Sources for the History of Early Islamic Mathematics, *Journal of the American Oriental Society*, Vol. 99, 450–459

King, D.A. (1980). The Exact Sciences in Medieval Islam: Some Remarks on the Present State of Research, *Bulletin of the Middle East Studies Association*, Vol. 14, 10–26

King, D.A. (1981). *A Catalogue of the Scientific Manuscripts in the Egyptian National Library. Part 1: A Critical Handlist of the Scientific Collections. Indexes of Copyists and Owners.* Cairo; General Egyptian Book Organization in Collaboration with the American Research Center in Egypt and the Smithsonian Institution

Kunitzsch, P. (1959). *Arabische Sternnamen in Europa.* Wiesbaden; Harrassowitz

Kunitzsch, P. (1961). *Untersuchungen zur Sternnomenklatur der Araber.* Wiesbaden; Harrassowitz

Kunitzsch, P. (1974). *Der Almagest: die Syntaxis mathematica des Claudius Ptolemäus in arabisch–lateinischer Überlieferung.* Wiesbaden; Harrassowitz

Kunitzsch, P. (1976). Eine bilingue arabisch–lateinische Lostafel, *Revue d'Histoire des Textes*, Vol. 6, 267–304

Leclerc, L. (1876). *Histoire de la médecine arabe; exposé complet des traductions du Grecs; les sciences en Orient, leur transmission à l'occident par les traductions Latines.* 2 Vols. Paris; Leroux. Reprinted (1963). Burt Franklin Research & Source Work Series, No. 18. New York; Burt Franklin

Lemay, R. (1978). Origin and Success of the Kitāb Thamara of Abū Ja'far Aḥmad ibn Yūsuf ibn Ibrāhīm from the tenth to the seventeenth century in the world of Islam and the Latin West, in *Proceedings of the First International Symposium for the History of Arabic Science, April 5–12, 1976*. Vol. 2, Papers in European Languages. Ed. A. al-Hassan, G. Karmi and N. Namnun. Aleppo; Institute for the History of Arabic Science, 91–107

Lewis, B. (1951). The Near and Middle East, in *Handbook of Oriental History by Members of the Department of Oriental History, School of Oriental and African Studies, University of London*. Ed. C.H. Philips. London; Offices of the Royal Historical Society, 1–46. Reprinted (1963)

Maddison, F.R. (1963). Early Astronomical and Mathematical Instruments. A Brief Survey of Sources and Modern Studies, *History of Science*, Vol. 2, 17–50

al-Majrīṭī, Maslama ibn Aḥmad [spurious] (1933). *Picatrix 'Das Ziel des Weisen'*. Ed. H. Ritter. Studien der Bibliothek Warburg, Vol. 12. Leipzig and Berlin; Teubner

al-Majrīṭī, Maslama ibn Aḥmad [spurious] (1962). *'Picatrix' Das Ziel des Weisen von Pseudo-Maǧrīṭī*. Trans. H. Ritter and M. Plessner. Studies of the Warburg Institute, Vol. 27. London; Warburg Institute, University of London

Manzalaoui, M. (1974). The Pseudo-Aristotelian Kitāb sirr al-asrār. Facts and Problems, *Oriens*, Vol. 23–24, 146–257

Matthews, N. and Wainright, M.B. (1980). *A Guide to Manuscripts and Documents in the British Isles Relating to the Middle East and North Africa*. Ed. J.B. Pearson. Oxford; Oxford University Press

Mayer, L.A. (1956). *Islamic Astrolabists and Their Works*. Geneva; Kundig

Meyerhof, M. (1931). Science and Medicine, in *The Legacy of Islam*, 1st edn. Ed. T. Arnold and A. Guillaume. Oxford; Oxford University Press, 311–355

Mieli, A. (1938). *La Science arabe et son rôle dans l'évolution scientifique mondiale*. Leyden; Brill. Reprinted (1966), with Bibliographical Appendix by A. Mazahéri. Leyden; Brill

Nallino, C.A. (1911). *'ilm al-falak, ta'rīkhuhu 'ind al-'arab fī al-qurūn al-wusṭā*. Rome. (In Arabic)

Nallino, C.A. (1921). Sun, Moon, and Stars (Muhammadan), in *Hastings Encyclopaedia of Religion and Ethics*. Ed. J. Hastings. 12 Vols. (1908–21). Edinburgh; T. & T. Clark, Vol. 12: 88–101

Nallino, C.A. (1939–48). *Raccolta di scritti editi e inediti*. Ed. and Trans. M. Nallino. 6 Vols. Rome; Pubblicazioni dell'Istituto per l'Oriente

Nasr, S.H. (1964). *An Introduction to Islamic Cosmological Doctrines*. Cambridge, Mass.; Harvard University Press. Revised edn (1978). London; Thames and Hudson

Nasr, S.H. (1968). *Science and Civilization in Islam*. Cambridge, Mass.; Harvard University Press

Nasr, S.H. (1975–8). *An Annotated Bibliography of Islamic Sciences*. 2 Vols. Imperial Iranian Academy of Philosophy Pubs., Nos 17 and 36. Tehran; Offset Press

Nasr, S.H. (1976). *Islamic Science; An Illustrated Study*. London; World of Islam Festival Publishing Co.

O'Leary, De Lacy (1949). *How Greek Science Passed to the Arabs*. London; Routledge and Kegan Paul

Pearson, H. and J.D. (1979). *The Encyclopaedia of Islam, New Edition. Index to Volumes I–III*. Ed. E. van Donzel. Leyden; Brill. Paris; Maisonneuve & Larose

Pearson, J.D., Ed. (1958). *Index Islamicus; 1906–1955*. Cambridge; Heffer

Pearson, J.D., Ed. (1961–77). *Supplements to Index Islamicus*. 4 Vols. London; Mansell

Pearson, J.D., Ed. (1977–). *The Quarterly Index Islamicus.* 1 Vol. published. London; Mansell

Pingree, D. (1968). *The Thousands of Abū Ma'shar.* Studies of the Warburg Institute, Vol. 30. London; Warburg Institute, University of London

Pingree, D. (1970). The Fragments of the Works of al-Fazārī, *Journal of Near Eastern Studies,* Vol. 29, 103–123

Plessner, M. (1954). Hermes Trismegistus and Arab Science, *Studia Islamica,* Vol. 2, 45–59

Plessner, M. (1972). Essay Review: The History of Arabic Literature, *Ambix,* Vol. 19, 209–219

Plessner, M. (1974). The Natural Sciences and Medicine, in *The Legacy of Islam,* 2nd edn. Ed. J. Schacht and C.E. Bosworth. Oxford; Clarendon Press, 425–460

Price, D.J. (1955). An International Checklist of Astrolabes, *Archives Internationales d'Histoire des Sciences,* Vol. 8, 243–263, 363–381

al Qazwīnī, Zakarīyā' ibn Muḥammad (1848–9). *Kitāb 'ajā'ib al-makhlūqāt wa gharā'ib al-maujūdāt: al-Qazwīnī's Kosmographie.* Ed. F. Wüstenfeld. 2 Vols. Göttingen. Reprinted (1967). Wiesbaden; G. Olms

al-Rāzī, Abū Bakr Muḥammad ibn Zakarīyā' (1848). *A Treatise on the Small-Pox and Measles.* Trans. W.A. Greenhill. London; Sydenham Society

Renaud, H.P.J. (1932). Additions et corrections à Suter 'Die Mathematiker und Astronomen der Araber', *Isis,* Vol. 18, 166–183

Richter-Bernburg, L. (1978). *Persian Medical Manuscripts at the University of California, Los Angeles: A Descriptive Catalogue.* Humana Civilitas, Sources and Studies Relating to the Middle Ages and the Renaissance, Vol. 4. Malibu, Calif.; Undena

Rosenfeld, B.A. (1978). Mathématiques, *Archives Internationales d'Histoire des Sciences,* Vol. 28, 325–329

Sabra, A.I. (1976). The Scientific Enterprise: Islamic Contributions to the Development of Science, in *The World of Islam: Faith, People, Culture.* Ed. B. Lewis. London; Thames and Hudson, 181–200

Saidan, A.S. (1967). The Comprehensive Work on Computation with Board and Dust by Naṣir al-Dīn al-Ṭūsī, *al-Abḥāth,* Vol. 20, 91–163, 213–292

Sarton, G. (1927–48). *Introduction to the History of Science.* 3 Vols in 5 Pts. Baltimore; Williams and Wilkins

Savage-Smith, E. (1976). Some Sources and Procedures for Editing a Medieval Arabic Surgical Tract, *History of Science,* Vol. 14, 245–264

Savage-Smith, E. and Smith, M.B. (1980). *Islamic Geomancy and a Thirteenth-Century Divinatory Device.* University of California, Los Angeles, Studies in Near Eastern Culture and Society, No. 2. Malibu, Calif.; Undena

Sayili, A. (1960). *The Observatory in Islam and its Place in the General History of the Observatory.* Publications of the Turkish Historical Society, Ser. 7, No. 38. Ankara; Turkish Historical Society

Sbath, P. (1938–9). *Al-Fihris (Catalogue de manuscrits arabes).* 3 parts. Cairo; Al-Chark

Schacht, J. (1950). Max Meyerhof, *Osiris,* Vol. 9, 7–32

Sédillot, L.A. (1844). Mémoire sur les instruments astronomiques des arabes, *Mémoires de l'Academie Royale des Inscriptions et Belle-lettres de l'Institut de France,* Vol. 1, 1–229

Sédillot, L.A. (1845–9). *Matériaux pour servir à l'histoire comparée des sciences mathématiques chez les Grecs et les Orientaux.* 2 Vols. Paris; Firmin Didot Frères

Sezgin, F. (1967). *Qur'ānwissenschaften, Ḥadīth, Geschichten, Fiqh, Dogmatik, Mystik bis ca 430 H.* Vol. 1 of *Geschichte des arabischen Schrifttums.* Leyden; Brill

Sezgin, F. (1970). *Medizin–Pharmazie–Zoologie–Tierheilkunde bis* ca *430 H.* Vol. 3 of *Geschichte des arabischen Schrifttums*. Leyden; Brill

Sezgin, F. (1971). *Alchemie–Chemie–Botanik–Agrikultur bis* ca *430 H.* Vol. 4 of *Geschichte des arabischen Schrifttums*. Leyden; Brill

Sezgin, F. (1974). *Mathematik bis* ca *430 H.* Vol. 5 of *Geschichte des arabischen Schrifttums*. Leyden; Brill

Sezgin, F. (1978). *Astronomie bis* ca *430 H.* Vol. 6 of *Geschichte des arabischen Schrifttums*. Leyden; Brill

Sezgin, F. (1979). *Astrologie – Meteorologie und Verwandtes bis* ca *430 H.* Vol. 7 of *Geschichte des arabischen Schrifttums.* Leyden; Brill

Steinschneider, M. (1862). *Zur pseudepigraphischen Literatur insbesondere der geheimen Wissenschaften des Mittelalters.* Wissenschaftliche Blätter aus der Veitel Heine Ephraim'schen Lehranstalt (Beth ha-Midrasch) in Berlin, I,3. Berlin; Rosenthal

Steinschneider, M. (1889). *Die arabischen Übersetzungen aus dem Griechischen.* A collection of 4 articles reprinted (1960). Graz; Akademische Druck- u. Verlagsanstalt

Steinschneider, M. (1904–5). *Die Europäischen Übersetzungen aus dem Arabischen bis Mitte des 17 Jahrhunderts.* 2 Vols. Sitzungsberichte der Kaiserlichen Akademie der Wissenschaften in Wien, phil.-hist. Klasse, nos. 149 and 151. Reprinted (1956). Graz; Akademische Druck- u. Verlagsanstalt

Storey, C.A. (1958). *Mathematics, Weights and Measures, Astronomy, and Astrology, Geography.* Vol. II, Part 1 of *Persian Literature: A Bio-bibliographical Survey.* London; Luzac

Storey, C.A. (1971). *Medicine.* Vol. II, Part 2 of *Persian Literature: A Bio-bibliographical Survey.* London; Luzac for the Royal Asiatic Society

Storey, C.A. (1977). *Encyclopaedias and Miscellanies, Arts and Crafts, Science, Occult Arts.* Vol. II, Part 3 of *Persian Literature: A Bio-bibliographical Survey.* Leyden; Brill for the Royal Asiatic Society of Great Britain

Strohmaier, G. (1969). Arabisch als Sprach der Wissenschaft in den frühen medizinischen Übersetzungen, *Mitteilungen des Institut für Orientforschung*, Vol. 15, 77–85

Suter, H. (1900). *Die Mathematiker und Astronomen der Araber und ihre Werke.* Abhandlungen zur Geschichte der mathematischen Wissenschaften, 10. Leipzig; Teubner. Reprinted (1963). Ann Arbor, Mich.; University Microfilms

Suter, H. (1902). Nachträge und Berechtigungen, *Abhandlungen zur Geschichte der mathematischen Wissenschaften*, Vol. 14, 157–185

Terzioğlu, A. (1968). Mittelalterliche islamische Krankenhäuser unter Berücksichtigung der Frage nach den ältesten psychiatrischen Anstalten, Berlin, Technische Universität, Dissertation

Thorndike, L. (1923–58). *A History of Magic and Experimental Science.* 8 Vols. New York; Columbia University Press

Tibbetts, G.R. (1971). *Arab Navigation in the Indian Ocean before the Coming of the Portuguese, being a translation of Kitāb al-Fawā'id fī uṣūl al-baḥr wa'l-qawā'id of Aḥmad b. Mājid al-Najdī together with an introduction on the history of Arab navigation, notes on the navigational techniques and on the topography of the Indian Ocean, and a glossary of navigational terms.* Oriental Translation Fund, New Series, 42. London; Luzac for the Royal Asiatic Society

Ullmann, M. (1970). *Medizin im Islam.* Handbuch der Orientalistik, Abteilung I, Ergänzungsband VI, Abschnitt 1. Leyden; Brill

Ullmann, M. (1972). *Die Natur- und Geheimwissenschaften im Islam.* Handbuch der Orientalistik, Abteilung I, Ergänzungsband VI, Abschnitt 2. Leyden; Brill

Ullmann, M. (1974–6). *Katalog der arabischen alchemistischen Handschriften der Chester Beatty Library.* 2 Vols. Wiesbaden; Harrassowitz

Ullmann, M. (1978). *Islamic Medicine*. Islamic Surveys, 11. Edinburgh; Edinburgh University Press

Vernet, J. (1974). Mathematics, Astronomy, Optics, in *The Legacy of Islam*, 2nd edn. Ed. J. Schacht and C.E. Bosworth. Oxford; Clarendon Press, 461–488

Wiedemann, E. (1970). *Aufsätze zur arabischen Wissenschaftsgeschichte*. Collectanea VI. 2 Vols. Hildesheim; G. Olms

Winter, H.J.J. (1952). *Eastern Science. An Outline of its Scope and Contribution*. The Wisdom of the East Series. Ed. J.L. Cranmer-Byng. London; John Murray

Wüstenfeld, H.F. (1840). *Geschichte der arabischen Aerzte und Naturforscher*. Göttingen; Vandenhoeck & Ruprecht

Yuschkevitch, A.P. (1961). *Istoriya matematiki v srednie veka*. Moscow. German Trans. (1964). *Geschichte der Mathematik im Mittelalter*. Basle; Pfalz-Verlag. Leipzig; Teubner

Yuschkevitch, A.P. (1976). *Les Mathématiques arabes (viiie–xve siècles)*. Trans. M. Cazenave and K. Jaouiche. Preface by R. Taton. Collection d'Histoire des Sciences, No. 2. Paris; Librairie Philosophique J. Vrin

22

Science and medicine in India

T.J.S. Patterson

Introduction

Indian scientific works were mostly written in Sanskrit, the cultural language, as summaries of oral teachings, very much condensed into couplets; this technique was established by 500 BC (Filliozat 1963a: 133, 141). There was considerable interchange of scientific information with the Arabs from the seventh century AD, and in this way some Indian knowledge reached the West in the Middle Ages. But most Indian science remained unknown in Europe until the end of the eighteenth century, when the first translations into European languages were made (S.N. Sen 1972: 44).

This chapter deals only with writings in, or translations into, English. The works quoted are, as far as possible, by Indian authors.

Good general surveys of the history of science and medicine in India, with extensive bibliographies, are Bose, Sen and Subbarayappa (1971) and Jaggi (1969–80). For bibliographies on all subjects connected with India, see Besterman (1975); Kalia and Jain (1975); Kaul (1975); Mahar (1964); Pearson (1979 – especially pp. 240–4: *Traditional Sciences and Technology* by J.P. Losty).

Additional bibliographies on special subjects are:

Alchemy – Ray (1967)
Anatomy – M. Roy (1967)

Biology – Kapil (1970)
Botany – Swamy (1973)
Chemistry – Ray (1956)
Glass manufacture – Govind (1970)
Mathematics – Bag (1979)
Mathematical astronomy – Pingree (1978)
Medicine
    Indian medicine – Mukhopadhyaya (1923–9)
    Indian Medical Service – Crawford (1914)
    in the nineteenth century – Subba Reddy (1975)
    tropical – Scott (1942)
Mineralogy – Lahiri (1968)
Paper technology – Ghori and Rahman (1966)
Pharmacy – Srivastava (1954)
Physics – Sen (1966a)
Pottery – Kashikar (1969)

For biographical dictionaries, see Buckland (1906), covering the period from about AD 1750; Keene (1894), Muhammadan; S.P. Sen (1972), 1800–1947. Baxter (1979) has given a guide to biographical sources, to be used with the general biographical index of the India Office Library and Records (IOLR), listing the entries by occupation and date. The extensive holdings of IOLR are voluminously catalogued. Wainwright and Matthews (1965) list the Western manuscripts in all subjects, including the sciences, in the British Isles, excluding IOLR.

For the history of Indian medical periodicals, see Neelameghan (1963). Indian scientific periodicals current up to the end of 1963 are covered by Arora (1964).

Walker (1968) is an encyclopaedia of all aspects of Hinduism, and Hobson-Jobson (Crooke 1903) is a useful glossary of Anglo-Indian words and phrases.

The Indus Valley Civilization (2500–1500 BC)

The history of science in India starts with the Indus Valley Civilization – the Harappan Culture. Excavations at Harappa and Mohenjo-daro in 1921–2 showed large, well-planned cities with an efficient system of public and private water-supply and drainage. The people were literate, although the script has not yet been deciphered. They were expert potters and metal-workers, but did not use iron, glass or the horse and plough. This was an urban civilization; the Vedics, who succeeded them, were primarily agricultural (Deshpande 1971: 1–22; Jaggi 1969–80, I; Subbarayappa 1971: 568).

The Vedic period (1500–500 BC)

From about 1500 BC the Indus Valley was invaded by the Vedic Aryans from the north-west. From then until the eleventh–twelfth centuries AD, science in India was based on their thoughts, arts, crafts and religious practices. The four Vedas, collections of their sacred songs and rituals, were given their final form about 1500–1000 BC. The Vedic people had an instinctive conviction of the natural order of the world as governed by a cyclical law, referring 'not only to the natural but also to the moral order' (Filliozat 1963a: 134). They held the doctrine of the five elements as the basis of matter, as well as of the composition of the human body (Subbarayappa 1971: 572).

There was no rigid division between mathematics and astronomy (Srinivasiengar 1967). Vedic priests made astronomical studies to ensure that sacrifices were performed at auspicious times, to coincide with given moments in the cosmic cycle (Filliozat 1963a: 138). They used a lunar zodiac, with a 'lunar day', which was peculiar to Indian astronomy; the Vedas describe twenty-eight constellations that formed the basis of their luni-solar calendar. The Vedas contain the same number of metrical divisions (10 800) as there are 'moments' in the year, and the number of divisions and the number of syllables (432 000) were also the bases of the cosmic cycles of later Indian and foreign astronomers (Filliozat 1963a: 136–8; Pingree 1978; Sen 1965). To the Vedics, 'numbers and their reckoning had a special appeal'. They used, and had names for, large numbers – up to 10^{12} and even larger (Subbarayappa 1971). They were familiar with many mathematical operations; much of their work with permutations and combinations was derived from the metrical pattern of their Sanskrit verse (Bag 1966; Jaggi 1969–80, II: 124). Their geometry was applied to the siting and construction of sacrificial altars (Jaggi 1969–80, II: 139), which were often of complicated patterns – e.g. a falcon with outstretched wings. The altar had to combine fixed dimensions with a fixed number of bricks, and the surface area had to be such that it could be increased without change of shape (Filliozat 1963a: 148). They had formulae for these manipulations, but these seem to have been 'particular cases of an empirical nature and not the result of a systematic theory of geometry' (Winter 1952: 18).

No astrological material is found in any Indian texts before the Christian era; 'it was only under the influence of the Greeks that horoscopic astrology made its debut in India, thereafter to achieve quick popularity' (Filliozat 1963a: 139).

Indian alchemy developed continuously from the Vedic period

until the end of the sixteenth century AD, when it faded out without changing into the science of chemistry. At first it was concerned more with the spiritual side (immortality); *soma* was important to increase vitality and longevity. The virtues of gold were appreciated, but there were no attempts at transmutation of metals (Subbarayappa and Roy 1968), which only appeared later, with the rise of Tantrism (fourth–sixth centuries AD).

In the earliest stage of Vedic medicine (the magico-empirical), verses were used as charms for warding off and treating diseases. In conjunction with these, many plant and some mineral remedies were used (Sharma, Seerwani and Shastry 1972). The Vedic texts contained anatomical and physiological information, although this was not classified. Anatomical dissections were carried out, with careful observations of the human body as well as of a number of animals – particularly the horse, the main victim of Vedic sacrifices (Filliozat 1963a: 152; Hoernle 1907; Jaggi 1969–80, II: 166; M. Roy 1967). Diseases were carefully described, but there was no attempt at classification. Studies were made of the morphology of plants, which were classified by their medicinal properties (Swamy 1973: 61–98).

In the Vedic period ploughing was started, and horses were used; crops of wheat, barley and, later, rice, were raised, and the land was improved by a system of rotation of crops. Rapid progress was made in the use of iron from about 1000–800 BC, and pottery reached a highly sophisticated form in the Painted Grey Ware (Kashikar 1969; Lahiri 1968; Raychaudhuri 1964).

From about 500 BC the Vedic religion 'assumed features which today are recognised as Hinduism' (Thapar 1966: 131) – although this term was not used until very much later – which has continued up to the present day.

Fifth century BC – fifth century AD

From about the seventh century BC began the development of the formal philosophical systems that were the basis of Indian physical ideas: 'the atomic nature of matter, and the union and collocation of the atoms to form larger aggregates of molecules, both homogeneous and heterogeneous, constitutes the basic and fundamental postulates guiding the Indian thought in their attempt to find out a rational explanation of the nature of the universe and of cosmic evolution' (Ray 1966). These ideas were particularly developed from the fifth century AD and continued to receive support up to the eighteenth century (Jaggi 1969–80, II: 52; B.N. Seal 1915: 24).

The Indian doctrine of the five elements – earth, water, fire, air and a non-material ubiquitous substance – was established by the seventh century BC. These terms have a wider connotation than the modern 'element', and each is only to be understood in relation to the other four; the first four are considered to be atomic (Subbarayappa 1966).These ideas were slightly modified by the Jainas and the Buddhists (Jaggi 1969–80, II: 59; B.N. Seal 1915: 92–3; Sikdar 1970: 199). The rise of Buddhism from the fifth century BC was very much accelerated from the middle of the third century BC under the Emperor Asoka (Winter 1952: 17), leading to contacts with China (Needham 1954: 206).

Number symbols were officially adopted from the middle of the third century BC; the decimal notation using nine figures and a special zero-sign came into use in the fifth century AD (Filliozat 1963a: 142, 150). The impetus theory, to describe the continued motion of a projectile, was developed in about the third century BC (B.N. Seal 1915: 129; Sen 1966a: 34). The binomial theorem was also developed at this time, in association with the metrical problems of metre in Sanskrit language (Bag 1966: 68). There was particular concern with phonetic studies, on which the method of reciting Vedic hymns was based.

From about the sixth century BC medical practice began to be codified into *Ayurveda* – 'the science of life' (Kutumbiah 1962; Filliozat 1949; Mukhopadhyaya 1923–9; *Theories and Philosophies of Medicine* 1973: 255; Zimmer 1948; Gupta 1977). The basic doctrines came down through two main schools: Caraka of Kashmir, primarily concerned with internal medicine (Mehta 1949; Ray and Gupta 1965), and Susruta of Benares, primarily concerned with surgery (Bishagratna 1907–16; Singhal and colleagues 1972–81). They codified the earlier doctrines, and are still the authorities for much of the practice of Indian medicine today.

Ayurveda is based on the classical Indian doctrine of the five elements to describe the constitution of the human body and of all medicaments. The elements act in the body in the form of three humours: *vata*, *pitta* and *kapha* (breath, bile and mucus). Blood is recognized as a vital factor in disease, but is not regarded as a fourth humour (Subbarayappa 1966). The proportion of the three humours varies from person to person; in good health they are in equilibrium, and disease is a result of imbalance of the three. Treatment is designed to restore equilibrium. At first only vegetable materials were used for treatment. Large numbers of plant remedies were described, and botany became systematized with

detailed classifications and morphology as the basis for pharmaceutical studies (Sircar 1950: 123). Later, minerals were introduced, based on the earlier alchemical practices (Filliozat 1963a:
155–6), the most important contributor of metallic preparations to
the pharmacopoeia being Nagarjuna (Ray 1970: 94).

There were high standards of training and practice, particularly
in surgery, where a wide range of operations was performed, using
many skilfully made instruments (Sarkar 1918: 54; Zimmerman
and Veith 1961: 56). Human dissections were carried out, but the
knowledge of anatomy so obtained was limited. The circulation of
the blood was not understood, and it was thought that venous
blood was converted to arterial in the liver. The heart was the
central organ of consciousness, until, with the rise of Tantrism,
this was transferred to the brain and spinal cord (B.N. Seal 1915:
208–17).

Ayurveda has branches dealing with veterinary science, particularly the cow, horse and elephant, and also with trees and plants
(Majumdar 1971: 254–6).

Filliozat (1949) shows the parallels of Indian medicine with
Greek medicine, and (1970: 326) discusses the relation of Greek
and Indian medicine before Alexander's invasion in 327–5 BC. He
suggests that there were earlier contacts, with Persia as the
intermediary. Although the classical Indian texts were written
later than the Greek, their sources are older, and India has not
borrowed her medicine from Greece (Filliozat 1963a: 156).

At this period there was further development of mining and
agriculture, with a system of irrigation, and recipes for fertilizing
the soil and nourishing plants (B.N. Seal 1915: 126). The manufacture of glass started later in India than elsewhere, but then reached
a high state of perfection (Govind 1970: 281). The use of bellows
allowed the production of high-quality iron and steel objects.
Between 600 and 500 BC, the notable Northern Black Polished
Ware (NBP) appeared. By the first century AD the Indians had
also developed bleaching, dyeing with fast dyes (and the extraction
of indigotin from the indigo plant), calico-printing, tanning,
soap-making, and the preparation of the strong cements used in
building temples (Sarkar 1918: 44; B.N. Seal 1915: 64).

Sixth–eleventh centuries AD

Astronomy and mathematics, particularly algebra, were further
developed by the great Indian astronomers of the fifth – seventh

centuries AD – Aryabhata, Varahamihira and Brahmagupta – who codified and added to the earlier work.

Medical writers such as Madhava (c. AD 700) (Meulenbeld 1974) and Vagbhata (c. AD 650; Vogel 1965) were still working on the principles of Caraka and Susruta, and largely agreeing with them. Metals, minerals and their compounds were studied, particularly mercury, sulphur and mica. The combination of mercury with sulphur as cinnabar was the main life-prolonging essence of the Tantrists.

With the rise of Tantrism, which dominated the Indian scene between AD 700 and 1300 (Ray 1967: 1–21), alchemy became concerned with transmutation, and there were many advances in the knowledge of different metals, particularly mercury. The early medicinal use of metals is associated with the *Siddha* system of medicine, still practised in South India and, possibly, the oldest indigenous system of medicine (Kutumbiah 1973: 21; Subba Reddy 1973: 182). Complicated processes were developed to 'kill' or purify the metals, and make them suitable for internal use by combining them with various medicinal plants, as well as using them for rejuvenation and prolonging life (Jaggi 1969–80, V: 131).

From the seventh century, Arabs trading along the Malabar Coast brought about the exchange of scientific and medical knowledge between Indians and Arabs. The Indian ideas were translated and incorporated into Arabic texts. Rhazes (AD 865–925) had extensive knowledge of Indian medicine, which he incorporated into his writings; these were translated into Latin in the thirteenth century, and became the standard texts in Europe (Singer 1943).

Paper-making was introduced in the eleventh century, probably from China via Nepal (Ghori and Rahman 1966: 133).

This period in India was ended by the repeated Muslim invasions from the north-west, which started in the eleventh century and continued up to the establishment of the Moghul Empire by Babur in 1526.

Twelfth – fifteenth centuries

From the twelfth century AD science in India began to wane; most of the writings were simply commentaries on, and elaborations of, earlier work. Hindu learning was dominated by the Muslim rulers, and became withdrawn and secretive to defend it from the invaders (Filliozat 1963b: 602). Furthermore, the rigidity of the caste system was now firmly established. This led to separation of the intellectuals in the community from the lower castes who carried out the techniques of the arts and crafts; theory was divided from practice, and the spirit of enquiry gradually died out (P.C. Ray in P. Ray 1956: 240; P. Ray 1966).

The Muslims gave official support only to their own sciences, and Gopal (1969) even suggests that some Mughal noblemen were actively concerned in the suppression of scientific knowledge. Rahman (1975), however, thinks that the number of manuscripts of this period now available is a measure of considerable scientific activity in medieval India, especially if the Indian knowledge that had earlier spread to the Arabs and was brought back with the Muslims is included.

With the rising power of the Muslims, their system of medicine, *Unani Tibb* ('*Unani*' means 'Greek'), began to compete with *Ayurveda* (Siddiqui 1971: 268; *Theories and Philosophies of Medicine* 1973: 83). Although there was always a good deal of interchange, *Unani* medicine was practised mainly in the cities and in the courts and palaces, and *Ayurveda* mainly in country districts and among the poor.

Sixteenth – seventeenth centuries

Astronomical studies were now limited to commentaries on earlier works, and 'were mainly intended to help in astrological computation which had become more and more popular and complex' (Filliozat 1963b: 602). In mathematics there were no new developments after the middle of the sixteenth century (Saraswathi 1969), and in chemistry all the writings were based on earlier works.

In medicine, contacts with Arabs since the ninth century, when there had been Indian physicians at the Arab courts, had introduced pulse-lore and insistence on the importance of diagnosis (Jaggi 1969–80, IV: 217; Kutumbiah 1967: 11). During the Mughal period, well-organized hospitals were set up in all the main cities, with free treatment for the people. Muslim and Hindu practitioners were appointed equally to these, and worked side by side, with no distinction made between them (Verma 1970: 347). The majority of the Indian medical writings in the sixteenth century were commentaries on the classical authors. The most notable and original writer was Bhavaprakasa, who described syphilis and its treatment with mercury (Jaggi 1969–80, IV: 41; Ray 1970: 97).

From the beginning of the sixteenth century Indian science began to come under the influence of European science, which was transmitted by travellers and traders. François Bernier MD, a graduate of Montpellier who travelled extensively in the East in the middle of the seventeenth century, was well received by the Emperor and noblemen in India, and was able to explain to them the contemporary work in Europe of Gassendi, Harvey and Pecquet (Chevers 1854: 219). European astronomical ideas began to be introduced in the seventeenth century, and the Maharaja Sawai Jai Singh II of Jaipur collected astronomical documents from India, Arabia and Europe, and established five observatories in different parts of India (Filliozat 1963b: 603).

But with the general decline of Indian science, science in India became more and more the science of the Europeans, introduced and largely practised by them. The Portuguese were the first in India; by 1510 they were established on the west coast, with their capital at Goa (Neelameghan 1961: 52). The Dutch followed in 1595, making the centre of their empire in the East Indies (Honig and Verdoorn 1945). The English East India Company set up its first trading post in India in 1608 (Woodruff 1953). The early traders had little knowledge of tropical conditions and diseases. John Woodall, the first Surgeon-General of the East India Company, published a manual for the surgeons of the Company in 1617, in which he set out the available information, including the causes, prevention and treatment of scurvy (Kirkup 1978). At first the Europeans were keen to learn as much as they could from local practitioners and their knowledge of indigenous drugs (K.K. Roy 1974: 697; Subba Reddy 1940: 49). Garcia da Orta of Portugal, in the sixteenth century in Goa (Boxer 1963; Markham 1913), and Bontius, the Dutch physician in the East Indies in the early seventeenth century (Schoute 1937: 28), studied and catalogued the local medicinal plants. John Marshall, a trader in Bengal from 1668 to 1677, described the systems of Hindu science and medicine that he had learned from local practitioners. He and his contemporaries often tried the local remedies, and proved their efficacy (Khan 1927). The European surgeons slowly learned to modify the heroic methods of treatment that they had brought with them (bleeding, purging and the excessive use of mercury). They soon noticed that Indians were relatively immune to some of the local diseases, and there were attempts to increase the resistance of Europeans by the process of 'indianization' (bleeding or starving, followed by a diet exclusively of Indian food) to make their blood more like that of the Indians (Goodeve 1837: 124).

Agriculture continued in the traditional Indian pattern, with the addition of new species introduced by the Europeans.

As the Europeans became more powerful towards the end of the seventeenth century they became less dependent on Indians and

Indian medicine, and increasingly scornful of their science. John Fryer, who was in India from 1673 to 1682, gave a full description in 1698 of all that he had seen (Fryer 1979: 175); he was very critical of what he regarded as their 'primitive' methods.

The eighteenth century

By the end of the seventeenth century, the English, with their greater sea-power, had defeated the Portuguese and the Dutch. With the defeat of the French on land by 1762, the (British) East India Company became the largest and most powerful trading company in the East, until, by the beginning of the nineteenth century, it was effectively the government of British India.

For the greater part of the eighteenth century most Europeans were contemptuous of Indian science and medicine, although some industrial processes continued at a very high level: reports from India in the eighteenth century showed that their standard of cotton materials and printing was higher than anything in Europe, and the Indian skills in iron and steel work were greater than the British (Dharampal 1971). Much of this technology was suppressed in the nineteenth century by the British policy of supporting British industry and making India the consumer (Blanpied in Dharampal 1971: xix, xxii).

Indian medicine continued on traditional lines, but there was no longer any enthusiasm to learn from it, although the traditional Indian method of inoculating for small-pox was described in detail and highly commended by Holwell in his report to the College of Physicians in London in 1767 (Dharampal 1971: 143).

Indian surgery, which had been so highly developed under Susruta (Jaggi 1969–80, IV: 167, 177), had steadily declined and was now confined to scattered families, which handed down a particular craft from father to son, often in conditions of great secrecy. This decline was associated with the rise of Buddhism with its emphasis on non-violence, and the rigidity of the caste-system; contact with blood was defilement for the higher castes who had been the practitioners of surgery. There were three operations in particular: cutting for stone – this technique was well known in Europe from the earliest times; couching for cataract – the Indian method was occasionally successful, but was soon overtaken by the improved methods introduced by the Europeans; grafting skin for deformities of the face – here the Indians showed great skill, and reports of their success which reached Europe towards the end of the eighteenth century were the starting point for the modern specialty of plastic surgery (Patterson 1974: 694).

For the wars with the French, the East India Company developed a regular army with a regular medical service, which continued until Independence in 1947 (Beatson 1902–3; Crawford 1914; McDonald 1950). The Company began to recruit Indians into its armies, and the Company surgeons became responsible for their health. The first hospital, in Madras in 1664, was for Europeans only (Subba Reddy 1947: 22). The first hospital for Indian soldiers in the Company's service was not opened until 1760, and the first for Indian civilians in 1792. These civilian hospitals were often founded by individual Company surgeons.

Contact with Indian physicians was mainly at the courts of rulers and noblemen who requested consultation with European practitioners, particularly when some surgical operation was required, for the Indians had no general surgeons at this time. This was encouraged by the Company in the interests of good trading.

With the social, political and industrial changes in Europe at the end of the eighteenth century, the British in India began to take some interest in, and responsibility for, the people who now came under their charge in increasing numbers. Stimulated by Sir William Jones, Europeans learned, with astonishment, of the antiquity of Indian culture, its science and medicine. Sanskrit works, particularly on astronomy, mathematics and medicine, were translated into European languages (S.N. Sen 1972: 44–70). Jones had founded the Asiatick Society in 1784, and started publishing *Asiatick Researches* to make these new findings more widely known. There was a revival of interest in Indian medicine at a time when Europeans had nothing new to offer for the treatment of tropical diseases (see Ainslie 1826; and Johnson 1815, whose very successful textbook reached its sixth edition in 1841 with 'very few original doctrines subverted, or practices exploded'). There was a general feeling that such an advanced state of civilization and culture should not be interfered with, but as much as possible should be learned from it. As part of this policy, towards the end of the eighteenth century the East India Company set up colleges and medical schools for Indians to study the sciences, including medicine, in the vernaculars.

This was the time of the start of the great botanical collections by Company surgeons and others. The publication of this botanical knowledge, and the correspondence between interested collectors, led to the formation of the first medical societies and the publication of the first medical journals (Neelameghan 1963).

The French had started surveying and producing maps in the

early eighteenth century, and the British in the second half of the century; James Rennell, the Surveyor General, produced the first 'Map of Hindoostan' in 1783. By the end of the century many land and coastal surveys had been carried out, but these were scattered and uncoordinated until the Trigonometrical Survey was set up in 1818 (Subbarayappa 1971).

The nineteenth century

During the first half of the nineteenth century there was growing criticism in Britain of the management of Indian affairs by the East India Company, whose trading monopoly was terminated in 1813. After the Mutiny (the Sepoy Rebellion), the power of the Company was transferred to the Crown in 'An Act for the Better Government of India' of 1858.

Up to 1830 further institutions were opened by the Company to educate Indians in science, with teaching partly in the vernacular and partly in English. The teachers were mainly European, many of them drawn from the Company's service. But the drive for 'Westernization', both secular and religious, had been growing. The only course for India was thought to lie in abandoning Indian ways and arranging for all education to be on Western lines. There was thus a complete reversal of the earlier liberal attitude of Europeans to Indian culture.

As the result of the report of the Grant Committee, set up in 1833 under Governor Lord William Bentinck, all the native colleges were closed to make way for teaching in science and medicine on wholly Western lines, with the teaching in English (Subba Reddy 1975: 1–34). This was reinforced by the adoption of English as the official language of India in 1835, as recommended by Macaulay in his 'Great Minute' of 2 February 1835. Increasing numbers of medical schools were then set up on Western lines. In 1839 the first Indian students graduated from the new Calcutta Medical School. After 1835 there was no official or general support for Indian medicine. There was some support by individuals, and small local schemes were set up to make use of Indian practitioners when it was realized that theirs was the only medicine that could reach many of the villages. But most Europeans became increasingly opposed to Indian medicine (Jaggi 1977: 320–47). Although there had been attempts to improve the state of public health (Ranken 1827: 300), all the major public health reforms came after 1858 (S.C. Seal 1971: 25).

The first Indian universities were founded in 1857, but, even after the reform of the educational system of 1854, there was relative neglect of the teaching of science to Indians by the government, and a failure to appoint, as had been recommended, scientific teachers to the universities. European scientific work in India tended to be limited to the field-sciences – for military, political and commercial purposes. Indians were restricted to membership of the official Surveys, often in relatively subordinate posts, and there were very limited facilities for independent research (Sen 1966b: 112–22). The Trigonometrical Survey was set up in 1818, and the major central scientific departments followed throughout the nineteenth century: Geological (1851), Meteorology (1875) and Botanical (1890) (Subbarayappa 1971). Roxburgh's *Flora indica* appeared in 1820–4, and Hooker's *The Flora of British India* in 1872–97 (Leroy 1965: 375), and the first Indian pharmacopoeias were published (see Dutt 1877; Dymock, Warden and Hooper 1890–3; Burkhill 1965). The first official Pharmacopoeia by Waring (1868) contained all the information in the British Pharmacopoeia of practical use in India, together with all local products that had been proved to be of value.

Scientific work was slow to be taken up by Indians; at first they were excluded from, for example, any sort of surveying. Teaching of Indian medicine was now confined entirely within the family. Its practitioners were continuing along the same lines as the classical authors of a thousand years before (Jolly 1901), but were responsible for the treatment of the greater part of the population, particularly in the rural areas. The middle and richer classes of Indians came to make increasing demands for European medicine (Maclean 1886).

By the end of the nineteenth century, however, important scientific work was started by men such as Asutosh Mukherji in mathematics, J.C. Bose and C.V. Raman in physics, and P.C. Ray in chemistry.

The twentieth century

The Indian Institute of Science was founded in 1909 and the Indian Council of Medical Research in 1912 (Filliozat 1963c: 592). Between 1912 and 1917 a number of Medical Acts set up Medical Councils in the various provinces, and laid down qualifications for registration of medical practitioners that excluded traditional physicians and made it illegal for a registered practitioner to be associated with Indian medicine (Hehir 1923: 96).

From 1920, however, increasing Indian nationalism began to change the position of science and medicine: before 1920, scientific research had been mainly a monopoly of the scientific services; after 1920 the leadership passed over largely to the universities. In medicine, the first Committee on Indigenous Systems of Medicine was set up in Madras. It reported in 1923, with the recommendation that, as Indian medicine was the best way of reaching the majority of the people, it should be developed by taking into account recent advances in medical science, and with proper training schemes and facilities for research. No action was taken on this. The Bhore Committee – The Health Survey and Development Committee – which reported in 1946, dealt only with 'modern' (Western) medicine. After widespread criticism, the Chopra Committee on Indigenous Systems of Medicine was set up, and reported in 1948. It urged the integration of Indian with Western medicine so that the student should be taught those aspects of Western medicine that were not part of Indian medicine (Jaggi 1977: 344).

After Independence in 1947, the Council of Scientific and Industrial Research was set up to support research in chemistry, metallurgy, electro-chemistry and drugs; there is now a state department of atomic energy. Between 1947 and 1959, fifteen new universities and four higher institutions, empowered to award degrees, were established (as against nineteen between 1857 and 1947; Sen 1966b: 119). In 1959 the National Institute of Sciences in India constituted a Board to write an authoritative history of science in India and to encourage the general study of the history of science in Indian universities; since 1966 it has published the *Indian Journal of History of Science.*

In 1969 the Central Council for Research in Indian Medicine and Homoeopathy was established with particular responsibility for the evaluation and standardization of traditional drugs (Chopra 1969). In 1971 the Central Council of Indian Medicine was set up to regulate the standards of education and to control practice in the traditional systems. Central government now supports six separate medical systems: modern, *Ayurvedic* and *Siddha, Unani,* homoeopathy (Kishore 1973: 76), Yoga (now being investigated scientifically; Jaggi 1969–80, V: 53, 74) and naturopathy (the system favoured by Gandhi). Each of these has its own training schools and hospitals. But the majority of trained practitioners, modern and Indian, remain in the cities, and many rural areas are served by the type of folk-medicine that has persisted in India since Vedic times, with its charms, herbal remedies and offerings to the gods. This is so deeply rooted in the villages and among the scheduled castes that it is a barrier to the acceptance of modern medicine, which is regarded as alien because it appears to run counter to all tradition (Jaggi 1969–80, III: 213).

Bibliography

Ainslie, W. (1826). *Materia Indica: or, some Account of those Articles which are Employed by the Hindoos, and other Eastern Nations, in their Medicine, Arts, and Agriculture.* 2 Vols. London; Longman, Rees, Orme, Brown, and Green

Arora, G.K. (1964). *Directory of Indian Scientific Periodicals 1964.* Delhi; Indian National Scientific Documentation Centre

Bag, A.K. (1979). *Mathematics in Ancient and Medieval India.* Varanasi; Chaukhambha Orientalia

Bag, A.K. (1966). Binomial Theorem in Ancient India, *Indian Journal of History of Science*, Vol. 1, 68–74

Baxter, I.A. (1979). *A Brief Guide to Biographical Sources.* London; India Office Library and Records

Beatson, W.B. (1902–3). *Indian Medical Service. Past and Present.* London; Simpkin, Marshall, Hamilton, Kent and Co.

Besterman, T. (1975). *A World Bibliography of Oriental Bibliographies.* Oxford; Blackwell

Bhaduri, J.L., Tiwari, K.K. and Biswas, B. (1971). Zoology, in *A Concise History of Science in India.* Ed. D.M. Bose, S.N. Sen and B.V. Subbarayappa. New Delhi; Indian National Science Academy, ch. 8: 403–444

Bhishagratna, K.K.L. (1907–16). *An English Translation of the Susruta Samhita Based on Original Sanskrit Texts.* 3 Vols. Calcutta; Bhaduri

Bose, D.M., Sen, S.N. and Subbarayappa, B.V. (1971). *A Concise History of Science in India.* New Delhi; Indian National Science Academy

Boxer, C.R. (1963). *Two Pioneers of Tropical Medicine: Garcia d'Orta and Nicolas Monardes.* London; Wellcome Historical Medical Library

Buckland, C.E. (1906). *Dictionary of Indian Biography.* London; Swan Sonnenschein

Burkhill, J.H. (1965). *Chapters on the History of Botany in India.* Delhi; Government of India Press

Chevers, N. (1854). Surgeons in India – Past and Present, *Calcutta Review*, Vol. 23, No. 45, 217–254

Chopra, R.N. (1969). *Glossary of Indian Medicinal Plants.* New Delhi; Publications and Information Directorate

Crawford, D.G. (1914). *A History of the Indian Medical Service 1600–1913.* 2 Vols. London; W. Thacker

Crooke, W. (1903). *New Edition of Hobson-Jobson. A Glossary of colloquial Anglo-Indian Words and Phrases, and of Kindred Terms, Etymological, Historical, Geographical and Discursive.* By H. Yule and A.C. Burnell. London; John Murray

Deshpande, M.N. (1971). Archaeological Sources for the Reconstruction of the History of Sciences of India, *Indian Journal of History of Science*, Vol. 6, 1–22

Dharampal, S. (1971). *Indian Science and Technology in the Eighteenth Century. Some Contemporary European Accounts.* Delhi; Impex India

Dutt, U.C. (1877). *The Materia Medica of the Hindus, Compiled from Sanskrit Medical Works.* With a glossary of Indian plants by G. King. Calcutta; Thacker Spink

Dymock, W., Warden, C.J.H. and Hooper, W. (1890–3). *Pharmacographia Indica. A History of the Principal Drugs of Vegetable Origin, Met with in British India.* 3 Vols. London; Kegan Paul. Reprinted (1972). Karachi; Institute of Health and Tibbi Research

Filliozat, J. (1949). *La Doctrine classique de la médicine indienne, ses origines et ses parallèles grecs.* Paris; Imprimerie Nationale. Trans. D.R. Chanana (1964) as *The Classical Doctrine of Indian Medicine. Its Origins and its Greek Parallels.* New Delhi; M. Manoharlal

Filliozat, J. (1963a). Ancient Indian Science, in *A General History of the Sciences.* Ed. R. Taton. Trans. A.J. Pomerans. 4 Vols. London; Thames and Hudson, Vol. 1, ch. 4: 133–160

Filliozat, J. (1963b). Indian Science from the 15th to the 18th Century, in ibid., Vol. 2, ch. 2: 602–604

Filliozat, J. (1963c). Indian Science in 1800–1960, in ibid., Vol. 4, ch.6: 591–593

Filliozat, J. (1970). Influence of Mediterranean Culture Areas on Indian Science, *Indian Journal of History of Science*, Vol. 5, 326–331

Fryer, G. (1979). John Fryer, F.R.S. and his Scientific Observations, Made chiefly in India and Persia between 1672 and 1682, *Notes and Records of the Royal Society of London*, Vol. 33, 175–206

Ghori, S.A.K. and Rahman, A. (1966). Paper Technology in Medieval India, *Indian Journal of History of Science*, Vol. 1, 133–149

Goodeve, H.H. (1837). A Sketch of the Progress of European Medicine in the East, *Quarterly Journal of the Calcutta Medical and Physical Society*, Vol. 2, 124–156

Gopal, S. (1969). Social Set-up of Science and Technology in Mughal India, *Indian Journal of History of Science*, Vol. 4, 52–58

Govind, V. (1970). Some Aspects of Glass Manufacturing in Ancient India, *Indian Journal of History of Science*, Vol. 5, 281–308

Gupta, S.P. (1977). *Psychopathology in Indian Medicine (Ayurveda) with Special Reference to its Philosophical Bases.* Aligarh; Ajaya Publishers

Hehir, P. (1923). *The Medical Profession in India.* London; Oxford Medical Publications

Hoernle, A.F.R. (1907). *Studies in the Medicine of Ancient India.* Vol. 1, *Osteology.* Oxford; Clarendon Press

Honig, P. and Verdoorn, F. (1945). *Science and Scientists in the Netherlands Indies.* New York; Board for the Netherlands Indies, Surinam and Curacao

Jaggi, O.P. (1969–80). *History of Science and Technology in India.* Delhi; Atma Ram and Sons. Vol. I, *Dawn of Indian Technology (pre- and proto-historic period)* (1969). Vol. II, *Dawn of Indian Science (Vedic and Upanishadic period)* (1969). Vol. III, *Folk Medicine* (1973). Vol. IV, *Indian System of Medicine* (1973). Vol. V, *Yogic and Tantric Medicine* (1973). Vol. VII, *Science and Technology in Medieval India* (1977). Vol. VIII, *Medicine in Medieval India* (1977). Vols XII–XV, *Western Medicine in India* (1979–80). (Vol. VI, *Indian Astronomy and Mathematics*, and Vols IX–XI, *Modern Science and Technology* in preparation)

Jaggi, O.P. (1977). Indigenous Systems of Medicine during British Supremacy in India, *Studies in History of Medicine*, Vol. 1, 320–347

Johnson, James (1815). *The Influence of Tropical Climates, more especially the Climate of India on European Constitutions.* London; Thomas and George Underwood. 6th edn (1841) with J.R. Martin

Jolly, J. (1901). *Medicin.* Strasburg; Karl J. Trübner. Trans. C.G. Kashikar (1951) as *Indian Medicine.* Poona; C.G. Kashikar. 2nd edn (1977). Delhi

Kalia, D.R. and Jain, M.K. (1975). *A Bibliography of Bibliographies on India.* Delhi; Concept Publishing Co.

Kapil, R.N. (1970). Biology in Ancient and Medieval India, *Indian Journal of History of Science*, Vol. 5, 119–140

Kashikar, C.G. (1969). Pottery in the Vedic Literature, *Indian Journal of History of Science*, Vol. 4, 15–26

Kaul, H.K. (1975). *Early Writings on India. A Union Catalogue of Books on India in the English Language Published up to 1900 and Available in Delhi Libraries*. London; Curzon Press

Keene, H.G. (1894). *An Oriental Biographical Dictionary, founded on materials collected by the late T.W. Beale*. London; W.H. Allen

Khan, S.A. (1927). *John Marshall in India. Notes and Observations in Bengal 1668–1672*. London; Humphrey Milford

Kirkup, J. (1978). *The Surgions Mate by John Woodall. A Complete Facsimile of the Book Published in 1617*. Bath; Kingsmead Press

Kishore, J. (1973). About Entry of Homoeopathy into India, *Bulletin of the Institute of History of Medicine (Hyderabad)*, Vol. 3, 76–78

Kutumbiah, P. (1962). *Ancient Indian Medicine*. Bombay; Orient Longmans

Kutumbiah, P. (1967). The Pulse in Indian Medicine, *Indian Journal of History of Medicine*, Vol. 12, 11–14

Kutumbiah, P. (1973). The Siddha and Rasa Siddha Schools of Indian Medicine, *Indian Journal of History of Medicine*, Vol. 18, 21–33

Lahiri, D. (1968). Mineralogy in Ancient India, *Indian Journal of History of Science*, Vol. 3, 1–8

Leroy, J.F. (1965). Botany, in *Science in the Nineteenth Century*. Ed. R. Taton. London; Thames and Hudson, 375–389

McDonald, D. (1950). *Surgeons Twoe and a Barber. Being Some Account of the Life and Work of the Indian Medical Service (1600–1947)*. London; Heinemann

Maclean, W.C. (1886). *Diseases of Tropical Climates*. London; Macmillan

Mahar, J.M. (1964). *India. A Critical Bibliography*. Tucson; University of Arizona Press

Majumdar, R.C. (1971). Veterinary Sciences, in *A Concise History of Science in India*. Ed. D.M. Bose, S.N. Sen and B.V. Subbarayappa. New Delhi; Indian National Science Academy, 254–256

Markham, C.R. (1913). *The Simples and Drugs of India*. Trans. of Garcia d'Orta (1563). *Coloquios dos simples e drogas e consas medicinais da India*. London; Sotheran

Mehta, P.M. (1949). *The Caraka Samhita*. 6 Vols. Jamnagar; Shree Gulabkunver-ba Ayurvedic Society

Meulenbeld, G.J. (1974). *The Madhavanidana and its Chief Commentary*. Leyden; Brill

Mukhopadhyaya, G.N. (1923–9). *History of Indian Medicine*. 3 Vols. Calcutta; Calcutta University Press

Needham, J. (1954). Chinese–Indian Cultural and Scientific Contacts, in *Science and Civilisation in China*. Cambridge; Cambridge University Press, Vol. 1: 206

Neelameghan, A. (1961). The Royal Hospital at Goa as Described in Some Seventeenth Century Travel Accounts, *Indian Journal of History of Medicine*, Vol. 6, 52–56

Neelameghan, A. (1963). *Development of Medical Societies and Medical Periodicals in India, 1780 to 1920*. Calcutta; Oxford Book and Stationery Company

Patterson, T.J.S. (1974). The Transmission of Indian Surgical Techniques to Europe at the End of the Eighteenth Century, *Proceedings of XXIII International Congress of the History of Medicine*, Vol. 1, 694–696

Pearson, J.D. (1979). *South Asian Bibliography*. Sussex; Harvester Press

Pingree, D. (1970–6). Census of the Exact Sciences in Sanskrit, *Memoirs of the American Philosophical Society*, Vol. 81, 1–60; Vol. 86, 1–147; Vol. 111, 1–208

Pingree, D. (1978). History of Mathematical Astronomy in India, in *Dictionary of Scientific Biography*. Ed. C.C. Gillispie. New York; American Council of Learned Societies, Charles Scribner's Sons, Vol. 15, supplement 1: 533–633

Rahman, P. (1975). *Bibliography of Source Material on History of Science and Technology in Medieval India*. New Delhi; Indian National Science Academy

Ranken, J. (1827). On Public Health in India, *Transactions of the Medical and Physical Society of Calcutta*, Vol. 3, 300–350

Ray, P. (1956). *History of Chemistry in Ancient and Medieval India* (incorporating *History of Hindu Chemistry* by P.C. Ray). Calcutta; Indian Chemical Society

Ray, P. (1966). The Theory of Chemical Combination in Ancient Indian Philosophies, *Indian Journal of History of Science*, Vol. 1, 1–14

Ray, P. (1967). Origin and Tradition of Alchemy, *Indian Journal of History of Science*, Vol. 2, 1–21

Ray, P. (1970). Medicine – as it Evolved in Ancient and Mediaeval India, *Indian Journal of History of Science*, Vol. 5, 86–100

Ray, P. and Gupta, H.N. (1965). *Caraka Samhita (a Scientific Synopsis)*. New Delhi; National Institute of Sciences of India

Raychaudhuri, S.P. (1964). *Agriculture in Ancient India*. New Delhi; Indian Council of Agricultural Research

Roy, K.K. (1974). Early Relations between the British and Indian Medical Systems, *Proceedings of XXIII International Congress of the History of Medicine*, Vol. 1, 697–703

Roy, M. (1967). Anatomy in the Vedic Literature, *Indian Journal of History of Science*, Vol. 2, 35–46

Saraswathi, T.A. (1969). Development of Mathematical Ideas in India, *Indian Journal of History of Science*, Vol. 4, 59–78

Sarkar, B.K. (1918). *Hindu Achievements in Exact Science. A Study in the History of Scientific Development*. London; Longmans, Green

Schoute, D. (1937). *Occidental Therapeutics in the Netherlands East Indies during Three Centuries of Netherlands Settlement (1600–1900)*. Batavia; Netherlands Indian Public Health Service

Scott, H.H. (1942). *A History of Tropical Medicine*, 2nd edn with appendix. 2 Vols. London; Edward Arnold

Seal, B.N. (1915). *The Positive Sciences of the Ancient Hindus*. London; Longmans, Green

Seal, S.C. (1971). A Short History of Public Health in India, *Indian Journal of History of Medicine*, Vol. 16, 25–41

Sen, S.N. (1965). *A Bibliography of Sanskrit Works in Astronomy and Mathematics*. New Delhi; National Institute of Sciences of India

Sen, S.N. (1966a). The Impetus Theory of the Vaisesikas, *Indian Journal of History of Science*, Vol. 1, 34–45

Sen, S.N. (1966b). The Character of the Introduction of Western Science in India during the Eighteenth and the Nineteenth Centuries, *Indian Journal of History of Science*, Vol. 1, 112–122

Sen, S.N. (1972). Scientific Works in Sanskrit, Translated into Foreign Languages and Vice-versa in the 18th and 19th Century A.D., *Indian Journal of History of Science*, Vol. 7, 44–70

Sen, S.P. (1972). *Dictionary of National Biography*. 4 Vols. Calcutta; Institute of Historical Studies

Sharma, A.L., Seerwani, A.B. and Shastry, V.R. (1972). Botany in the Vedas, *Indian Journal of History of Science*, Vol. 7, 38–43

Siddiqui, M.Z. (1971). The *Unani Tibb* (Greek Medicine) in India, in *A Concise History of Science in India*. Ed. D.M. Bose, S.N. Sen and B.V. Subbarayappa. New Delhi; Indian National Science Academy, 268–273

Sikdar, J.C. (1970). Jaina Atomic Theory, *Indian Journal of History of Science*, Vol. 5, 199–218

Singer, C. (1943). *A Short History of Science to the Nineteenth Century*. Oxford; Clarendon Press

Singhal, G.D. and colleagues (1972–81). *Ancient Indian Surgery Series*. 10 Vols. Varanasi; Singhal Publications, Banaras Hindu University

Sircar, N.N. (1950). An Introduction to the Vrksayurveda of Parasara, *Journal of the Royal Asiatic Society of Bengal*, Vol. 16, 123–139

Srinivasiengar, C.N. (1967). *The History of Ancient Indian Mathematics*. Calcutta; World Press

Srivastava, G.P. (1954). *History of Indian Pharmacy*. Calcutta; Pindars

Subbarayappa, B.V. (1966). The Indian Doctrine of Five Elements, *Indian Journal of History of Science*, Vol. 1, 60–67

Subbarayappa, B.V. (1971). In *A Concise History of Science in India*. Ed. D.M. Bose, S.N. Sen and B.V. Subbarayappa. New Delhi; Indian National Science Academy, 568

Subbarayappa, B.V. and Roy, M. (1968). *Matrkabhedatantram* and its Alchemical Ideas, *Indian Journal of History of Science*, Vol. 3, 42–49

Subba Reddy, D.V. (1940). Medicine in India in the Middle of the XVI Century, *Bulletin of the History of Medicine*, Vol. 8, 49–67

Subba Reddy, D.V. (1947). *The Beginnings of Modern Medicine in Madras*. Calcutta; Thacker, Spink and Company (1933) Limited

Subba Reddy, D.V. (1973). History of Siddha Medicine, *Bulletin of Institute of History of Medicine, Hyderabad*, Vol. 3, 182–185

Subba Reddy, D.V. (1975). Medical Literature of India, Ancient, Medieval and Modern, *Annals of Indian Academy of Medical Sciences*, Vol. 9, 1–34

Swamy, B.G.L. (1973). Sources for a History of Plant Sciences in India, *Indian Journal of History of Science*, Vol. 8, 61–98

Thapar, R. (1966). *A History of India. Volume I*. Harmondsworth; Penguin Books

Theories and Philosophies of Medicine (1973). With particular reference to Greco-Arab medicine, Ayurveda and traditional Chinese medicine. Compiled by Department of Philosophy of Medicine and Science, Institute of History of Medicine and Medical Research, New Delhi

Verma, R.L. (1970). The Growth of Greco-Arabian Medicine in Medieval India, *Indian Journal of History of Science*, Vol. 5, 347–363

Vogel, C. (1965). *Vagbhata's Astanganghrdayasamhita*. Wiesbaden; Franz Steiner

Wainwright, M.D. and Matthews, N. (1965). *A Guide to Western Manuscripts and Documents in the British Isles relating to South and South East Asia*. London; Oxford University Press

Walker, B. (1968). *Hindu World. An Encyclopedic Survey of Hinduism*. 2 Vols. London; George Allen and Unwin

Waring, E.J. (1868). *Pharmacopoeia of India, Prepared Under the Authority of Her Majesty's Secretary of State for India in Council*. London; W.H. Allen

Winter, H.J.J. (1952). *Eastern Science. An Outline of its Scope and Contributions*. The Wisdom of the East Series. Ed. J.L. Cranmer-Byng. London; John Murray

Woodruff, P. (1953). *The Men who ruled India*. Vol. I, *The Founders*. London; Jonathan Cape

Zimmer, H.R. (1948). *Hindu Medicine*. Baltimore; Johns Hopkins Press

Zimmerman, L.M. and Veith, I. (1961). Surgery of the Orient. India: Sushruta, Ch. 5 in *Great Ideas in the History of Surgery*. Baltimore; Williams and Wilkins, 56–67

23

Science and medicine in China

Christopher Cullen

Introduction

The academic study of the history of science in China is a field of relatively recent growth, and in Europe and America at least the number of scholars properly equipped for original work is still small. In the present state of the study there would be little point in casting this chapter in the form of a condensed *vade mecum* for the researcher. My aim is rather to begin to satisfy the curiosity of users of this book who may wish to know something of the form and content of present-day scholarship and to be guided to an introductory selection of Western-language material. With this purpose in mind this introduction is devoted to a description of Chinese source materials and the means of access to them. There follows a brief outline of certain topics in Chinese philosophy, after which the main areas of Chinese science are discussed in order. The bibliography is not intended as a comprehensive guide to all the basic material in Western languages; this task has already been admirably fulfilled in Nakayama and Sivin (1973: 279–314), which provides useful guidance on general questions of Chinese history, culture and bibliography in addition to reviewing literature on Chinese science. In what follows it is inevitable that references to the work of Joseph Needham will occur with equal or greater frequency than to any other author's writings; an elementary acquaintance with the literature will show that this is simply a reflection of the magnitude and significance of his contribution to the subject. With all due credit to his collaborators and to the high quality of the specialist work his initiative has stimulated elsewhere, it is still to the East Asian History of Science Library in Cambridge that one must look for the major growth point of scholarship on Chinese science in the West. Since learning is ultimately dependent on the funding of individuals and institutions, it may not be out of place to note that the long-term future of Needham's institute is precarious: at the time of writing (1980) it has neither permanent endowment nor any formal connection with a university department of sinology or the history of science. The fact that this situation has persisted so long is a standing reproach. The eventual dispersal of the research environment that has produced what is probably the most significant British contribution to humane learning this century would be nothing short of a tragedy and a disgrace.

Three oriental languages are indispensable requirements for access to all the material of interest to the would-be researcher. Two of them, modern Chinese and Japanese, are the media of a rich body of sinological scholarship produced during the present century. For the greater part of the last 3000 years however, the language of the primary documents and of all scholarly annotations to them was classical Chinese, sometimes called literary Chinese. This is, roughly speaking, a written form of the vernacular tongue of the second half of the first millennium BC, the period from which date the classical exemplars of literary style. As the spoken language continued to evolve, the written idiom clung to the ancient models, with the eventual result that it became unintelligible to those without a classical education. To this obstacle to literacy we must add the difficulty of the Chinese script itself. Learning to write a word involves committing to memory a written sign that has no direct connection with the sound or the sense of the word represented; despite common misconceptions, Chinese characters are neither ideograms nor pictograms, and their phonetic components are now of historical significance only. The literate class in pre-modern China was relatively small, consisting largely of the landowning gentry who ran affairs at the local level and provided recruits for the governing élite of the imperial civil service. The bulk of extant Chinese literature is however vast. One reason for this is simply the great time-span covered by Chinese civilization, which is certainly the longest-lived literate culture, despite the fact that its origins in the second millennium BC are fairly recent compared to those of the ancient Near Eastern civilizations. Again, printing has been in use in China for the best part of the last 1000 years. Most significant of all, however, is the overwhelmingly literary and humanistic bias of traditional élite culture. For most of China's history the values of this culture were embodied in a corpus of classical literature that, as the basis of the civil service examinations, was intensively studied by all those who aspired to élite membership. Confucius (c.551–479 BC) was honoured as the greatest exponent of the cultural and moral tradition; he himself claimed to be 'a transmitter, not a maker, one who knows and loves the ancients'. Despite the many profound changes that have overtaken Chinese society over the last three millennia, the power of the Confucian tradition was rarely challenged until the present century.

The historian of science and technology cannot afford to neglect any part of the written records of a civilization. This is particularly true in the case of a modern Westerner studying a complex and alien culture such as China, where any attempt to evaluate a document out of context is likely to prove disastrous. What follows is an attempt to outline some of the main categories of literature recognized by traditional Chinese scholarship. The first resort for the reader in search of further information on this as on all other topics discussed in this chapter must inevitably be Joseph Needham's multi-volumed pioneering survey *Science and Civilisation in China*, which has been appearing at a steady rate since 1954. All Needham's volumes have a three-part bibliography: (A) for Chinese and Japanese books before 1800, (B) for post-1800 oriental-language material, and (C) for Western-language material. The first of these fills a great need for the non-sinologist faced with the title of a pre-modern Chinese work. Under the romanized title he will find the title in Chinese characters, with a translation and if required an additional indication of contents. There follows a dating, details of authorship, references to secondary scholarship and to translations if any. In addition, each section of Needham's work is preceded by a careful evaluation of the relevant literature. The comprehensive and systematic documentation provided by Needham makes it pointless to go into much detail in the present survey, beyond what is required to give an introductory outline. As for other Western-language bibliographies, Wylie (1867) may still be useful for Chinese literature as a whole, although much of its scholarship has been overtaken and its romanization is now obsolete. (On romanization of Chinese see Nakayama and Sivin 1973: 310ff.) Watson (1962) is a good beginner's survey of the literature of the classical period and a handbook edited by Loewe and Boltz (in advanced preparation) will give detailed accounts of all significant books up to the third century AD. Balazs and Hervouet (1978) sets out to cover the Sung dynasty (AD 960

−1279); despite the uneven quality of its entries it is an invaluable source. For the Ming dynasty (AD 1368–1644) and the Ch'ing dynasty (AD 1644–1911) respectively, recourse must be had to the biographical dictionaries of Goodrich and Fang (1976) and Hummel (1943–4), which index references to works under the entries for their authors. Some idea of the richness of Chinese-language bibliographical material may be gained from Teng and Biggerstaff (1971: 1–82).

The core of the Confucian tradition was a body of works bearing the title *ching* ('canon' or 'classic'). By the beginning of the second millennium AD, thirteen of these were officially recognized: (1) *Chou i*, or *I ching* (Book of Change), originally a book of divination of the early or middle first millennium BC, structured around sixty-four hexagrams each composed of six broken or unbroken lines. Its explanatory material made it the basis of an elaborate metaphysics. (2) *Shang shu*, or *Shu ching* (Book of Documents), containing records of imperial enactments and pronouncements from legendary times to c.1000 BC. (3) *Mao shih*, or *Shih ching* (Book of Poetry), an anthology compiled around the time of Confucius. (4) *Chou li* (Ritual of the Chou dynasty), an idealized description of the state organization of the Western Chou dynasty (c.1100–771 BC). (5) *I li* (Book of Ritual), a guide to the proper conduct of all kinds of ceremonial, public and private, perhaps c.200 BC. (6) *Li chi* (Record of Ritual), a varied collection of material, often non-ritual, compiled from earlier sources at the end of the first millennium BC. (7) *Tso chuan*, (8) *Kung-yang chuan* and (9) *Ku-liang chuan*, three works connected with the *Ch'un ch'iu* (Spring and Autumn Annals), a briefly worded chronicle of the state of Lu traditionally said to have been edited by Confucius. The first of these is a rich collection of early historical material, while the other two are commentaries on the philosophical significance of the wording of the original annals. (10) *Lun yü* (Selected discourses, or Analects), a collection of material comprising sayings of Confucius and his disciples, and anecdotes about them. (11) *Hsiao ching* (Book of Filial Piety), perhaps a school text of the first/second centuries BC. (12) *Erh Ya* (Literary Expositor), a glossary of terms in the classics, of the same period. (13) *Meng Tzu*, the works of the Confucian philosopher Meng K'o (Mencius, *fl.* 320 BC). Good translations of most of these works are available by scholars such as Biot (1851), Legge (1893–5), Waley (1935, 1937, 1938) and Lau (1963, 1976, 1979).

It is dangerous to view China through solely Confucian spectacles, and until recent decades Western sinologists were perhaps a little too inclined to be conditioned by traditional élite conceptions of Chinese culture. Nevertheless it remains true that a basic acquaintance with the canonical corpus is as essential for understanding Chinese history and society as an acquaintance with the Bible is important for the study of the last 2000 years in Europe. Apart from their importance as background material, some of the classics contain primary evidence for the historian of science and technology. The historical works (particularly the *Tso chuan*) yield important data on ancient calendrical science, as well as records of phenomena such as solar eclipses (see below), and the final section of the *Chou li* (entitled *K'ao kung chi*, The Artificers' Record) lists and describes the activities of the varieties of craftsmen and technical specialists in state employ. An important point in using the classics is that a very brief reference to a topic in the original text may well have provoked a flood of exegesis and additional material from later scholars, which in standard editions appears as a running commentary in smaller characters. Such commentaries, especially those of the first millennium AD, may contain much valuable material from works otherwise lost, and familiarity with them is therefore indispensable.

For the Confucian scholar-official it was inconceivable that one could succeed in dealing with the problems of the present without having assimilated the lessons of the past. The writing of history from the approved moral standpoint was felt to be of such crucial importance that it was brought under the control of the imperial government at an early stage; for a review of the Chinese historiographical tradition see the essay by Pulleyblank in Dawson (1964). As a result, sinologists now have at their disposal an unbroken series of standard histories of successive dynasties from the Han (202 BC to AD 220) onwards. Official history, like all other kinds of history, must be read with an eye for bias and omission, but by any standards the Chinese material is superior to that available for other ancient civilizations. All the histories follow the same general pattern: the core of the work is the *pen chi* (Basic Annals), a chronological account of the events of the reigns of successive emperors, often with long quotations from edicts and other official documents. In addition there are the *lieh chuan* (Ordered Accounts), for the most part biographies of noteworthy persons categorized under such headings as ministers, scholars, etc. For our present purpose, however, perhaps the greatest interest lies in the *chih* (Monographs). Some of these are devoted to accounts of the structure of the imperial bureaucracy, state ritual, the administrative divisions of the Empire or matters of finance.

Some histories include (to the delight of modern scholars) a bibliographical account of the holdings of the imperial library, but the historian of science will be particularly drawn to the accounts of calendrical astronomy prepared by the State Observatory, the review of mathematical harmonics as connected with ritual music and weights and measures, and the records of striking phenomena observed in the heavens or on the earth. Heavenly portents noted range from comets to aurorae and parhelia, while terrestrial phenomena include such things as earthquakes and even sex-changes in humans. Much of this material, particularly in the field of astronomy, retains its value for modern scientists; for examples see Clark and Stephenson (1977). A full sinological guide to the standard histories as well as to many other important sources of historical data is provided in Wilkinson (1974).

Another important form of officially sponsored compilation was the *lei shu*, or topically arranged encyclopaedia. The last and greatest of these is the *T'u shu chi ch'eng*, completed in 1726. The edition of 1888 runs to over 1700 volumes. Like its predecessors it consists of quotations from relevant works with a minimum of editorial comment; in some cases entire books have been copied into the text. The *T'u shu chi ch'eng* was the last of a long line; one of the earliest *lei shu* extant is the *T'ai p'ing yü lan* completed in AD 983. Works such as these can often serve as an invaluable means of first access to material on almost any subject, and some have been indexed for convenience of reference.

Traditional China was, as the reader will have gathered, a culture given to the planning and execution of great literary projects, and this proclivity for large-scale organization has affected the way in which works by individual authors circulate. As elsewhere, single works were separately printed and published, either as a commercial undertaking or at the initiative and expense of patrons of scholarship. It is however very common to find that a work of scholarly importance has found a place in one of the great *ts'ung shu* collections, in which numbers of books having some common feature were published together. Several modern *ts'ung shu* set out to include all books of major importance and constitute a complete basic library in themselves. What may be thought of as one of the earlier *ts'ung shu*, the *Yung lo ta tien*, was completed by an imperial commission of over 2000 scholars in AD 1407 and contained 11 095 chapters arranged in encyclopaedic form. It was however too large to print, and after the disasters of five centuries only 370 volumes survive. A similar project was mounted in the late eighteenth century under the patronage of the emperor Ch'ien-lung. The resulting collection was entitled *Ssu k'u ch'üan shu* (The Complete Library of the Four Treasuries), a reference to the division of the work into the four categories of *ching* (classics), *shih* (history), *tzu* (philosophers, very broadly interpreted) and *chi* (belles-lettres). Two copies of the complete manuscript survive, and the associated critical bibliographies are among the basic tools of all classical sinologists. While scholars owe Ch'ien-lung a debt of gratitude, it should not be forgotten that he took advantage of this great review of all known literature to suppress nearly 3000 books in whole or in part on ideological grounds. On the subject of collectanea it is impossible not to mention the *Tao tsang*, or Taoist Patrology, a collection of 1464 works mostly with a direct connection with Taoist philosophy or religion, first collected and printed under the Sung in AD 1019. Needham has always held that the Taoists were a key group in the development of scientific thought in China, and although scholars have not been unanimous in their assent it is certainly true that the Taoist corpus contains a great deal to interest the historian of science, including works on alchemy, yogic practices and techniques of geomancy.

Much more space than this introduction affords would be required to give anything like a balanced picture of the literary resources available to the researcher. I have therefore concentrated on trying to convey some of the special characteristics of Chinese literature, principally its huge extent and the depth and quality of the scholarship it has attracted over many centuries. The historian of science and technology need have no fear of running out of fresh material for generations to come, and in recent years there have been exciting additions to the corpus of ancient literature through the discoveries of substantial quantities of manuscript material from tombs of the first few centuries BC.

Some aspects of Chinese philosophy

Full-scale scholarly introductions to Chinese philosophy in English are provided by Fung (1952–3) and Chan (1963); the latter is perhaps a little more accessible to the unprepared reader. For the historian of science however, it is inevitable that one should turn first of all to the survey of the development of philosophy that occupies the second volume of Needham's *Science and Civilisation in China*. It is now twenty-five years since it appeared, and it is fairly safe to say that no subsequent publication in the field has excited equal interest. The reader should however be warned that no other part of Needham's work has aroused so much disagreement; much of the controversial reaction is not of abiding interest, but a useful survey of the various ways in which Needham's work has been received is given by Nakayama (1973). Essential as general surveys are, it is often more fruitful in the long run to begin by reading the words of the philosophers themselves, even if this has to be done through translations. The skeleton outline of the historical development of Chinese philosophy that follows is given solely as a context for an introductory sample of basic works.

The Warring States period (fifth century BC to the beginning of the Ch'in dynasty in 221 BC) was an age of increasingly ruthless warfare that ended when one feudal state finally overcame all the others and unified China under a rule that was as oppressive as it was short-lived. This time of political chaos was perhaps the most creative and certainly the most varied period of Chinese thought, the time of what the Chinese call the *pai chia* (the Hundred Schools of Thought). One of these schools, that of the *fa chia* (Legalists), taught a ruthless *Realpolitik* that was adopted by the state of Ch'in during its rise to power. During the short period of Ch'in imperial rule (221–207 BC) all other schools of thought were suppressed; it is of interest that the *fa chia* was the only group of ancient thinkers approved by the ideologues of the Cultural Revolution (1966–9). In itself, legalism had little to say on natural philosophy; one basic text of the school, the *Book of Lord Shang*, is translated in Duyvendak (1928).

While the Han dynasty (202 BC to AD 220) continued the political practices of the Ch'in in many ways, it adopted Confucianism as the state ideology, and in so doing gave it a pre-eminent position that it retained for most of the next 2000 years. The extent of the Confucian canon has already been indicated above. Two essential texts, the Analects of Confucius and works of Mencius, have been translated and excellently discussed by Lau (1976, 1979). While these two thinkers represent the core of the humanistic and highly moral Confucianism that plays such a major part in Chinese intellectual history, one should not ignore the development represented by Hsün Tzu (*fl.*298–238 BC). Whereas other Confucians held that the supreme spiritual entity T'ien (by this time stripped of the attributes of personal deity) was vitally concerned with morality and might demonstrate its judgements through natural portents, Hsün Tzu took a sceptically naturalistic view that envisaged the control of nature by rational manipulation. There is a partial translation by Watson (1967). From his writings it is clear that Mencius regarded the school of thought founded by Mo Tzu (*fl.*479–438 BC) as a principal opponent of Confucianism, and although Mohism did not survive the Ch'in suppression it is of great interest for the historian of science. Mo Tzu's moral philosophy was utilitarian, and his followers pursued studies in logic, physical science and techniques of defensive siege warfare. Mo Tzu's basic works are translated in Watson (1967), and the science and logic of the Mohist canon are thoroughly studied in Graham (1978). One claim made by Graham is that the successes of the Mohists refute any suggestion that the nature of the Chinese language could have had an inhibiting effect on scientific development.

Apart from the Confucians however, it was the Taoists who exerted an enduring influence on the Chinese world-view. Whereas Confucians centred their attention on the order of human society as a microcosm of the order of the universe, Taoists were inclined to regard man as a rather insignificant entity involved in the vast flux of universal change behind which lay the unchanging reality of the *tao* (the Way). Without doing too much violence to a complex phenomenon, it may be said that the Taoist thinkers of the Warring States period left their mark on later Chinese culture in two ways. In the first place, however much élite culture might stress the claims of human society on its members, the sense of the importance of the natural world as an alternative source of value and significance was never wholly absent. Needham is prepared to see a fairly sharp antithesis between nature-centred Taoists (scientific) and man-centred Confucians (at best uninterested in science, at worst anti-scientific); one of the dangers of applying this approach to individuals is that one becomes entrapped in circularities in trying to decide which of the two camps a particular person belongs to. The picture is complicated by the fact that although, philosophically speaking, Taoism became one of the many strands composing élite culture, it also gave rise to popular movements of a religious nature. The theological content of these cults was partly derived from early Chinese folk beliefs but was greatly influenced by elements derived from Buddhism, which began its missionary activity in China in the first few centuries AD. Religious Taoism became an important vehicle for attempts to attain physical immortality through the practice of alchemy or through yogic techniques. Two basic works of Warring States Taoism are the *Tao te ching*, translated with full introductory material by Lau (1963), and the *Chuang Tzu*, translated by Watson (1968). The alchemical and religious dimensions of later Taoism are well represented by Ware's (1966) translation and study of an early fourth-century AD work, the *Pao p'u tzu* of Ko Hung. Sivin (1968) is an intensive study of the evidence relating to Sun Ssu-mo, a seventh-century AD Taoist alchemist, while Schafer (1977) has much material on Taoist views of the structure of the universe under the T'ang dynasty (AD 618 – 906). Here, as for all other topics treated in this survey, the relevant volumes of *Science and Civilisation in China* are a vital source of information and analysis.

In the earlier years of Western sinology the study of Chinese philosophy tended to focus almost exclusively on the thinkers of the Warring States period. This bias was perhaps encouraged by the way in which even the most innovative thinkers of later times made a practice of claiming support for their views from ancient authorities. One area in which the non-sinologue student of Chinese philosophy may most fruitfully redress the balance is through the study of the so-called neo-Confucian philosophers of the Sung (AD 960–1279) and subsequent dynasties. It must be said that this term, though customary, is almost as misleading as would be the term 'neo-Christian' applied to Thomas Aquinas and other Schoolmen of the medieval West. In the same way that Aquinas set out to assimilate Aristotelian philosophy to Christian thought, the neo-Confucians attempted a synthesis between the ethical and humanistic tradition of Confucianism and the metaphysics of Taoism and Buddhism. The greatest figure of the movement was Chu Hsi (AD 1130–1200), whose work was regarded as the standard expression of Confucian thought for the major part of the last five centuries. Chan (1967) translates an important philosophical anthology compiled by Chu Hsi, but perhaps the most accessible introduction to neo-Confucian philosophy is provided by Graham (1958). The strand of neo-Confucianism represented by Chu Hsi stressed the necessity for methodical self-cultivation and the rational investigation of all things. Needham has found Chu's world-view, which he characterizes as 'organic' in the Whiteheadian sense, of great interest in relation to the development of scientific thought, and it is certainly true that the Sung period was marked by a flowering of Chinese natural philosophy; see for example the biography of Shen Kua (AD 1031–95) by Nathan Sivin in the *Dictionary of Scientific Biography* (Gillispie 1970–8). An early critique of Needham's interpretation of neo-Confucianism is Chan (1957); Peterson (1980) is the most recent review of the question. Graham (1973) is an important discussion of a number of points relating to developments in philosophy and science in China and the West.

The main areas of Chinese science

In a volume of the present kind there is no need to insist on the dangers of unthinking attempts to apply modern divisions of knowledge to the intellectual development of ancient non-European cultures. Anyone who sets out to write a history of (say) Chinese biology will find plenty of fascinating material scattered through the literature, but the fact remains that the corpus so assembled will not relate to any single entity in the Chinese intellectual universe. Some of it may relate to medical theory, some to the discipline of 'internal alchemy', some to neo-Confucian philosophy of nature, some to pharmacognosy and some to the agricultural arts, while material on uncommon phenomena in the world of animals and plants may be dealt with in treatises on divination. In the outline that follows I have adopted the subject division proposed by Nathan Sivin in Nakayama and Sivin (1973: xix–xxv), which has the advantage of attempting to use discipline boundaries as they actually existed in traditional China. Another caution that must be entered is cogently put by Sivin (1977: xvi). Noting 'the traditional Chinese unconcern for integrating all the sciences', Sivin points out that there was simply no forum in which practitioners of the various disciplines devoted to a rational understanding of aspects of the natural world could meet on common ground. A mathematical astronomer would not see his concerns as in any way connected with those of an alchemist, and there was no Academy or Lyceum to bring them together: the first was part of the palace civil service, while the second might spend his life in a remote mountain abbey. Needham's strong commitment to the universality of science sometimes leads him to speak with intellectual hindsight, but his careful documentation and strong sense of historical context preserves his work from scientistic crudities. The same cannot be said for some less scholarly studies, particularly in the field of Chinese medicine, which is a rich area of misleading popularization.

The quantitative sciences

MATHEMATICS

At some time near the beginning of the first century AD an unknown author or authors compiled a comprehensive treatise on mathematics under the title *Chiu chang suan shu* (Nine Chapters of Mathematical Arts). In a number of ways it was to set the pattern for subsequent developments in Chinese mathematics, both as a model that was consciously imitated and in its strengths and limitations. Typically a problem is stated, a numerical answer is given, and in conclusion the text gives a step-by-step account of the process of calculation required, without any attempt at rationale or proof. The subjects treated include arithmetic of the sort required by bureaucrats engaged in calculating tax liability, problems of area from land surveying and the calculation of volumes of material required for variously shaped fortifications and dykes. Methods are given for ascertaining unknown heights, depths and distances by the use of sighting rods. In modern terms the arithmetical examples given involve the solution of problems in elementary algebra up to the level of quadratic and simul-taneous linear equations; these are solved by the systematic manipulation of counting rods on a rectangular grid. The telemet-rical problems involve the use of similar triangles and Pythagoras' theorem. In succeeding centuries mathematical writers continued, ostensibly at least, to phrase their problems in practical terms, and at no time was there interest in deductive argument of the Euclidean type. Geometry remained relatively undeveloped, and there was nothing that could be called trigonometry. The Chinese mathematical genius was essentially arithmetico-algebraic: under the Sung, the counting-board manipulations of the old handbooks were being used to solve equations of up to the ninth degree as well as indeterminate equations. On the whole it must be said that as a science in itself mathematics remained the preserve of relatively lowly ranking specialists and was not perceived as an important part of élite culture. Metaphysical speculations of a numerological kind are found in connection with the discipline of mathematical harmonics discussed below.

Until fairly recently Western scholarship on Chinese mathema-tics was, to say the least, of very variable quality. The only really useful book on the subject in English (Mikami 1913) was by a Japanese. In his work on mathematics published in the third volume of *Science and Civilisation in China*, Needham collabo-rated with the scientifically and classically trained scholar Wang Ling, and the result is a stimulating survey with the wealth of detail and insight one expects from such combination. Needham's treat-ment is not however free from defects; some of its faults of interpretation or emphasis may be related to a failure to make the fullest use of modern scholarship in Chinese and Japanese, and there are sometimes frustrating failures to explain just how a particular technique was used. It must nevertheless be counted as a most successful contribution to the field, not simply when viewed in comparison with what preceded it, but also in the light of the increasing volume of specialist studies it has continued to provoke. One scholar who acknowledges the initial stimulus to his studies provided by Needham is Libbrecht, whose review article (1980) gives an accurate and up-to-date conspectus of the state of research. Libbrecht (1973) is a detailed study of a mathematical text by Ch'in Chiu-shao, who worked in the thirteenth century when Chinese mathematics was at its peak; it can be confidently recommended for its thoroughness and lucidity. Vogel (1968) is a translation, with the minimum of introduction, of the *Chiu chang suan shu* largely based on Berezkina (1957). Other Chinese mathematical works have been studied by Lam (1977) and Ang (1969).

MATHEMATICAL HARMONICS

From early times music played a central role in state ceremonial, and the use of music of the correct form was regarded as vital for the well-being of the state. Since the state was held to be the human expression of the order of the universe, it was natural for music to be seen as intimately related to the structure of the cosmos. A phenomenon such as musical resonance struck the Chinese as a particularly telling instance of a universal principle that 'things of the same category respond to one another'. This principle, elaborated by the Han Confucian Tung Chung-shu (c.179–104 BC), was the basis of a scheme of non-causative correlation of types of event in the human and natural worlds. Thus, the playing of a particular musical mode held to be correlated with the qualities of damp and cold might be expected to 'call forth' unseasonably dank weather in the height of summer. Any suggestion of a mechanical connection between the actions of the players and the gathering of clouds would, however, have been foreign to Chinese thinking. Given the significance attached to music, it is not surprising to find the early development of studies seeking to examine the laws connecting the physical dimensions of objects with the pitch of the sound produced, and the instrument most intensively studied was the notched pitch-pipe. The relations between the sizes of standard pitch-pipes were made the basis of an elaborate cosmic numerology, and during the Han dynasty attempts were made to use the pitch-pipes as the starting point for a universal metric scheme. Perhaps the peak of Chinese studies in this field was the work of the Ming prince Chu Tsai-Yü in the sixteenth century. Needham argues strongly that his discoveries may be the source of the idea of equal temperament introduced in Europe not long after. Whatever the truth of the matter, the rationale of Chinese harmonics and its role in the cosmic order is a subject deserving of attention. At present, the best introduction to the topic is still the treatment given by Needham (with the collaboration of Kenneth Robinson) in *Science and Civilisation in China* (4,I: 126–228).

MATHEMATICAL ASTRONOMY

As far back as the evidence goes (the late second millennium BC) the traditional Chinese calendar has been of the luni-solar type. In an agricultural society an adequate correspondence between seasonal activity and the cycle of twelve lunations can be maintained by the *ad hoc* insertion of an intercalary month in any year when the month-count seems to be noticeably ahead of the progress of the crops. From early times, however, Chinese calendrical specialists sought to reduce their work to rules applicable in the long term, and refinement continued far beyond any practical social requirement. Planetary ephemerides were incorporated in calendrical treatises after the first century BC, and efforts were made to represent correctly the anomalous motions of the sun and moon. Such detail may seem pointless until it is realized that the Chinese emperor was in a sense responsible for and expressed in his person the harmony of the entire cosmos. Accuracy in astronomical matters was thus an important part of imperial prestige, and it was felt that a calendar reform was an appropriate accompaniment to dynastic change. Whereas in the Hellenistic world any mathematical attempt to predict celestial phenomena involved the use of a geometricized conception of the structure of the cosmos, Chinese calendrical science produced a strong tradition of algebraic–arithmetical astronomy largely independent of physical cosmology.

It is unfortunate that Needham's treatment of this topic is deliberately brief and summary. His description of Chinese astronomical instrumentation and systems of celestial coordinates in *Science and Civilisation in China*, Vol. 3, is fascinating, but may leave the reader wondering quite why the Chinese state regarded such matters as important enough to be the province of a principal department of government. At present it is still the case that the most important scholarship on the topic of calendrical astronomy is in Japanese; a glimpse of its content may be had from Yabuuti (1963). An important discussion of the computational techniques of early mathematical astronomy and their relation to metaphysical assumptions about the cosmos is given in Sivin (1969), which may be recommended as the best introduction to the subject at present available. The situation will be transformed in a few years' time with the appearance of a full study and translation of the *Shou shih li*, a thirteenth-century treatise on mathematical astronomy, which represents the peak of the Chinese achievement in this field; the study is the product of a collaborative effort led by Nathan Sivin. References to recent scholarship in the general area of Chinese astronomy will be found in the review article by Cullen (1980).

The qualitative sciences

MEDICINE

Despite the mushrooming growth of literature devoted to Chinese medical science in recent years it must still be said that the amount of serious scholarship worth the name is relatively small so far as Western languages are concerned. Traditional Chinese medical theory differs from modern Western thinking in a number of crucial ways. In the first place the universe within which the human microcosm operates is considered in terms of concepts that have no real Western parallel, although misleading resemblances are inevitably seized on by the ill-informed. There is also the problem that the use of technical terms by Chinese medical specialists may differ significantly from their more general philosophical application. Concepts such as *yin-yang*, *wu-hsing* and *ch'i* will be mentioned in the section on physical studies below, but a few loci of specifically medical confusion may be outlined here. In the first place it must be realized that the dictionary definition of (say) the word *kan* as 'liver' may be dangerously misleading in a medical context as opposed to a culinary one: the names of things we now recognize as physical organs are used in Chinese medicine to refer to functional systems of which the liver of our example is merely the physical substrate. One functional system, the *san-chiao*, has no physical substrate at all. This does not however mean that the Chinese were so bad at anatomy that they imagined an organ where there was none, rather that they were not really talking about anatomy as we would recognize it.

One not uncommon way of paying the Chinese dubious compliments has been to extol the power of their allegedly empirically based therapeutics at the expense of a supposed lack of medical theory. For some reason it has also tended to be assumed that acupuncture was usually the therapy of first resort. Both misconceptions are not unconnected with the political role allotted to traditional medicine in China over the past few decades. Chinese therapeutics is in fact a theoretical discipline of great complexity, and much of its significance will be missed if it is not realized that the disease entities it sets out to treat are often far from corresponding to those recognized in modern Western medicine. It is worth noting, by the way, that much of what passes for traditional Chinese medicine in both China and the West is simply the application of traditional Chinese *materia medica*, acupuncture and moxa, to diseases diagnosed and classified according to totally non-Chinese criteria. Interesting as this may be for the development of medical science, it renders contemporary practice a very dubious guide for the historian.

Needham's main work on Chinese medicine is still to come. In the interim there is a book-length study of the history of acupuncture and moxa (Lu Gwei-Djen and Needham 1980). A number of short essays have been collected in Needham (1970). The study by Porkert (1974) fully deserves its editor's description as 'the first truly scholarly book on Chinese medicine in a Western language'. Porkert confines himself to the task of elucidating the underlying theoretical framework of Chinese medical thought, while Unschuld (1973, 1979) has begun to consider a wider range of social and historical issues connected with Chinese medical practice at all levels of society. One cannot as yet recommend any translations of Chinese medical works without considerable reservations. One of the most common of these, Veith (1949), has been reprinted at least twice and is on the shelves of many libraries and booksellers; it is nevertheless so misleading that it is better avoided completely. In default of anything better, Chamfrault and Ung (1954–) contains a useful and interesting selection of material.

ALCHEMY

The reader in search of material on the history of chemical techniques in China will find no lack of sources in the literature; until the relevant sections of *Science and Civilisation in China* appear, a view of chemical technology may be gained from Li (1948) and Sun (1966). It would, however, be something of a distortion to approach the subject of alchemy through the perspective of the history of chemistry, for although China was not lacking in sooty empiricks their purposes were not strictly chemical as we would recognize it, and their preoccupations need to be understood in a much wider context. The ultimate purpose of the adept was to attain a state of perfection and unity with the cosmic process, so that he too would become as enduring as heaven and earth, an immortal. He might set out to attain this aim through the 'external alchemy' (*wai tan*) of the laboratory. If he took this route he would attempt to produce elixirs by recapitulating, on a telescoped scale of time, the processes by which natural substances were thought to mature in the depths of the earth. The ingestion of the perfected drug would produce a parallel refinement of the adept himself. Or alternatively he might resort to *nei tan* (internal alchemy), in which his own body served as the alchemical vessel while it underwent the disciplines of meditation, breath control and special sexual practices. *Nei tan* naturally shades off into the more general field of dietetics, hygienics and callisthenics of the sort still in evidence amongst health enthusiasts in the parks of Peking at dawn.

Alchemy was closely connected with Taoist religion, and many important alchemical texts are to be found in the *Tao tsang* patrology mentioned earlier. Serious study of Chinese alchemical literature began in the 1930s under the leadership of Tenney L. Davis at MIT; the translations and other studies of Davis's group are listed in Leicester and Klickstein (1950). The useful translation of the fourth-century AD *Pao p'u tzu* by Ware (1966) has already been mentioned. There is no doubt, however, that Sivin (1968) set standards of scholarship beyond anything reached by its predecessors. Anyone who wants an example of the literary, philological, historical and scientific skills that must be deployed to attack the tangled thickets of early alchemical texts could do no better than to turn to this book. Over the last few years the resources available in English have been massively increased by the publication of parts II, III and IV of Volume 5 of *Science and Civilisation in China*, which with the impending part V will complete the survey of alchemy. In addition to Needham's collaboration with Lu Gwei-Djen and Ho Peng-yoke, it should be noted that Vol. 5:IV contains a substantial contribution by Sivin on the theoretical background of elixir alchemy. One is glad to be able to say that a similar picture is emerging in subsequent volumes of the project, which is increasingly becoming a cooperative endeavour drawing in scholars from all parts of the world.

ASTROLOGY

Inscribed oracle bones of the second millennium BC bear records of eclipses and, in one possible case, a supernova seen as a 'new star'. Observation of celestial portents played an important political role for most of the life of the traditional Chinese state, and was the province of a group of civil servants whose task was to record and interpret anything unusual seen in the sky. Everything that happened in the heavens was linked to earthly events through an elaborate scheme of correlation: celestial disorder was a reflection of faults in the political order of the human world. At a time when direct criticism of the ruler was too dangerous, an official might well make use of a discussion of recent astrological omens to get his point across. One example of how this was done is discussed in de Crespigny (1976), which studies a set of memorials submitted to the emperor by the second-century AD scholar Hsiang K'ai. The borderline between the regular and the ominous was not always fixed: thus in early times lunar eclipses were ominous, but as they became predictable they diminished in significance. It was never possible to make completely reliable predictions of solar eclipses, even at the peak development of Chinese calendrical mathematics. The difficulty was to some extent resolved by over-prediction: only an unexpected eclipse was ominous, and a predicted eclipse that did not materialize was an occasion for congratulating the emperor on the success of his moral influence in warding off the ill omen. Transient and unpredictable phenomena such as comets, meteor showers and aurorae were always ominous, and the value of the lengthy series of such records in the astrological monographs of the dynastic histories is very great. A representative specimen of one of these monographs has been translated and discussed by Ho (1966), and several examples of the use of ancient Chinese data by modern astronomers will be found in Clark and Stephenson (1977). A brief general characterization of Chinese astrology is given by Nakayama (1966), while Schafer (1977) performs the essential task of setting out the full and rich cultural context of the way the ancient Chinese looked at the stars.

GEOMANCY

In the present state of studies, the inclusion of geomancy in this listing can do little more than point to its existence and importance as a future area of study. Geomancy (*feng shui*, literally: 'wind and water') was a discipline that set out to lay down rules for the proper and felicitous siting of houses and tombs in the landscape. Its results were certainly successful from the aesthetic point of view, but the geomancer was much more than a Chinese Capability Brown, and would certainly never have thought of resorting to drastic modification of natural features. He may tentatively be characterized as a terrestrial physiologist, who analysed the configuration of hills and rivers in terms of the concepts of Chinese natural philosophy. One aid used by later geomancers in the attempt to trace the flow-patterns of the *ch'i* through the landscape was the magnetic compass. There is a brief treatment of geomancy in *Science and Civilisation in China* (2: 359–63), and the studies of March (1968) and Feuchtwang (1974) may also be consulted. An important recent contribution is Bennett (1978). Real progress will demand an assault on the scale of the one that has been mounted on alchemy, and similar difficulties of understanding may be expected to present themselves.

PHYSICAL STUDIES

The modern Chinese term for physics, *wu li*, is a borrowing from the usages of pre-modern natural philosophy, and the relations between the ancient and modern meanings parallel the history of the English word. *Wu li* (literally: 'the pattern-principles of things') referred to the attempt to make coherent sense of the natural world through the application of basic philosophical concepts. The object of this endeavour was the deepening of insight rather than success in making predictions. The one quantitative Chinese science to achieve a fair measure of predictive success, mathematical astronomy, tended to discard its metaphysical substructure as it refined its predictive techniques. It is worth emphasizing the point that whatever the interest and sophistication of the thought-schemes of Chinese natural philosophy, it is far safer to make comparisons with (say) Stoic thought than with any of the vocabulary of modern science. Thus in his study of natural philosophy in Vol. 2 of *Science and Civilisation in China* Needham expresses a strong negative judgement about the influence of the classificatory scheme of the *Book of Change* on the development of Chinese scientific thought (1956, 2: 336). It is uncertain how far such a judgement is unfair to the *Book of Change* or overgenerous to other aspects of Chinese thought in comparison. There is also the question of emphasis to be considered: a neo-Confucian thinker might insist that insight into the structure of reality could be gained by the intensive study of the natural world, but the centre of his attention would always be directed to the ethically organized world of human beings as the most perfect expression of the universal order.

   It may be helpful to add a few brief notes on certain Chinese concepts in natural philosophy that lack parallels in Western thought. Apart from Needham's works, further discussions will be found in Graham (1958) and in Porkert (1974); the latter is particularly valuable for the detailed philological and historical background it supplies. Outside of this context, the characterizations given below may have a limited value in indicating possible areas of interest and perhaps in acting as a prophylactic against the confusion produced by philosophasters who enjoy the creative misuse of a sprinkling of Chinese terms.

   Yin–yang: the use of this formulation rather than 'the *yin* and the *yang'* is deliberate, for it is not rare to find misleading parallels drawn with (say) negative and positive electric charge. Such expressions convey the false impression that *yin* and *yang* are two separately existing components or forces making up the totality of things. It is more accurate to say that thinking in *yin–yang* terms involves a readiness to analyse the cosmos in terms of sets of complementary polar oppositions. Such pairings might include dark/light, cold/hot, female/male, decay/growth, earth/heaven and moon/sun. It is rare for the words *yin* and *yang* to appear alone as syntactic elements without at least an implied nominal entity for them to qualify.

Wu hsing: the translation of this phrase as 'the five elements' has spread much confusion. The impression is not uncommon that the Chinese used the five 'elements' of wood, fire, earth, metal and water in the same way that the ancient and medieval West thought of the four elements of earth, air, fire and water. The philologically accurate rendering 'five phases' is much more illuminating: as with the case of *yin–yang* we are dealing with function rather than substance. It is unfortunate that Needham has continued the older usage, despite full consciousness of the risks involved. The typical Chinese question in natural philosophy was not so much 'what is it made of?' but rather 'what is happening here?' The use of various cyclically repeating sequences of the five phases provided a rich conceptual repertoire for the analysis of processes of all kinds, which could be linked to the standard phases through a process of categorical correlation. Thus, for instance, in terms of direction the order of the phases given above could be linked to the sequence east, south, centre, west and north. The use of five-phase analysis underwent a highly specialized development in medical theory.

Ch'i: one historian of Chinese science has advanced the view in private that in any published work one is entitled to leave up to three technical terms as untranslated transliterations. This word and its successor would be prime candidates for such treatment. Faced with the problem of finding a single English word to represent *ch'i*, Graham (1958) chooses 'ether' on the disarmingly frank grounds that 'it means so little in English that it can hardly cause confusion'. Other candidates have included 'pneuma', 'vital breath' and 'material force'. The last of these is the choice of Chan (1963), and the tension implicit in its wording points to the problem involved. *Ch'i* partakes at times of the properties of a subtle vapour pervading (or even composing) everything. On the other hand it is far from being mere matter – the concept of 'dead matter' is in any case not a part of Chinese physical thinking.

Needham's formulation 'matter-energy' conveys something of the right flavour, as does Porkert's 'configurational energy'. In both cases the word 'energy' has been seized on by writers lacking the philological and historical sensitivity of either author, and there is simply no substitute for an acquaintance with the usage of this term in the texts themselves.

Li (to be distinguished from an identically pronounced but differently written word meaning 'ritual, proper conduct'): this concept was of ancient lineage, but was first given a central role in the neo-Confucian synthesis under the Sung. *Li* is the pattern of organizing principle that constitutes the essential structure of the cosmos. *Li* is non-coercive and non-causative, and it would not be accurate to think of it as 'laws' of nature. The concept of *li* seems to be strongly related to the Chinese ideal of a well-ordered hierarchical social structure, whose members know their place and perform their duties without the need for explicit exercise of authority. The universal order as a whole is an expression of *li*, but each particular thing may also be said to have its own *li* that makes it what it is. It is significant that when Chu Hsi said that one could discover the *li* in inanimate matter he did so in order to point out that even something so insignificant as a stick or stone is not entirely devoid of a place in the pattern of things. The fullest expression of *li* is to be found in human beings, the more so as their moral perfection increases. *Li* is not ultimately an object of scientific thought but rather of mystical contemplation, even though the progressive realization of *li* might start from the process of *ko wu*, the investigation of things.

Bibliography

Ang, T.S. (1969). *A Study of the Mathematical Manual of Chang Ch'iu-chien*. Kuala Lumpur; University of Malaya

Balazs, E. and Hervouet, Y. (1978). *A Sung Bibliography*. Hong Kong; Chinese University Press

Bennett, S. (1978). Patterns of the Sky and Earth: a Chinese Science of Applied Cosmology, *Chinese Science*, 3, 1–26

Berezkina, E.I. (1957). Drevnekitajskij Traktat *Matematika v devjati Knigach*, *Istoriko-matematiceskie issledovaniia*, Vol. 10, 423–584

Biot, E. (1851). *Le Tcheou-Li ou Rites de Tcheou*. 3 Vols. Paris; Imprimerie Nationale

Chamfrault, A. and Ung, K.S. (1954–). *Traité de médecine Chinoise*. 5 Vols. Angoulême; Coquemard

Chan, Wing-tsit (1957). Neo-Confucianism and Chinese Scientific Thought, *Philosophy East and West*, Vol. 6, 309–332

Chan, Wing-tsit (1963). *A Source Book in Chinese Philosophy*. Princeton, NJ; Princeton University Press

Chan, Wing-tsit (1967). *Reflections on Things at Hand: The Neo-Confucian Anthology.* New York; Columbia University Press

Clark, D.H. and Stephenson, F.R. (1977). *The Historical Supernovae.* Oxford; Pergamon Press

Crespigny, R. de (1976). *Portents of Protest in the Later Han Dynasty: the Memorials of Hsiang K'ai to the Emperor Huan in 166 A.D.* Canberra; Australian National University Press

Cullen, C. (1980). Joseph Needham on Chinese Astronomy, *Past and Present*, No. 87, 39–53

Dawson, R. Ed. (1964). *The Legacy of China.* Oxford; Clarendon Press

Duyvendak, J.J.L. (1928). *The Book of Lord Shang.* London; Probsthain

Feuchtwang, S.D.R. (1974). *An Anthropological Analysis of Chinese Geomancy.* Vientiane, Laos; Vithagna

Fung, Yu-lan (1952–3). *A History of Chinese Philosophy.* 2 Vols. Trans. D. Bodde. Princeton, NJ; Princeton University Press

Gillispie, C.C., Ed. (1970–8). *Dictionary of Scientific Biography.* 15 Vols. New York; American Council of Learned Societies, Charles Scribner's Sons

Goodrich, L. and Fang, C.Y. (1976). *A Dictionary of Ming Biography.* New York; Columbia University Press

Graham, A.C. (1958). *Two Chinese Philosophers: Ch'eng Ming-tao and Ch'eng Yi-ch'uan.* London; Lund Humphries

Graham, A.C. (1973). China, Europe and the Origins of Modern Science, in *Chinese Science: Explorations of an Ancient Tradition.* Ed. S. Nakayama and N. Sivin. Cambridge, Mass.; MIT Press, 45–69

Graham, A.C. (1978). *Later Mohist Logic, Ethics and Science.* Hong Kong; Chinese University Press

Ho, Peng-yoke (1966). *The Astronomical Chapters of the Chin Shu.* Paris; Mouton

Hummel, A.W. (1943–4). *Eminent Chinese of the Ch'ing Period. 1644–1912.* 2 Vols. Washington DC; Library of Congress

Lam, Lay-yong (1977). *A Critical Study of the Yang Hui Suan Fa.* Singapore; Singapore University Press

Lau, D.C., Trans. and Ed. (1963). *Lao Tzu: Tao Te Ching.* Harmondsworth; Penguin

Lau, D.C., Trans. and Ed. (1976). *Mencius.* Harmondsworth; Penguin

Lau, D.C., Trans. and Ed. (1979). *Confucius: The Analects.* Harmondsworth; Penguin

Legge, J. (1893–5). *The Chinese Classics*, 2nd edn. 7 Vols. Oxford; Clarendon Press

Leicester, H.M. and Klickstein, H.S. (1950). Tenney Lombard Davis and the History of Chemistry, *Chymia*, Vol. 5, 1–16

Li, Ch'iao-p'ing (1948). *The Chemical Arts of Old China.* Easton, Pa.; Journal of Chemical Education

Libbrecht, U. (1973). *Chinese Mathematics in the Thirteenth Century: The Shu-shu-chiu-chang of Ch'in Chiu-shao.* Cambridge, Mass.; MIT Press

Libbrecht, U. (1980). Joseph Needham's Work in the Area of Chinese Mathematics, *Past and Present*, No. 87, 30–39

Lu Gwei-Djen and Needham, J. (1980). *Celestial Lancets. A History and Rationale of Acupuncture and Moxa.* Cambridge; Cambridge University Press

March, A.L. (1968). An Appreciation of Chinese Geomancy, *Journal of Asian Studies*, Vol. 27, 253–267

Mikami, Y. (1913). *The Development of Mathematics in China and Japan.* Leipzig; B.G. Teubner. New York; G.E. Stechert

Nakayama, S. (1966). Characteristics of Chinese Astrology, *Isis*, Vol. 57, 442–454

Nakayama, S. (1973). Joseph Needham, Organic Philosopher, in *Chinese Science: Explorations of an Ancient Tradition.* Ed. S. Nakayama and N. Sivin. Cambridge, Mass.; MIT Press

Nakayama, S. and Sivin, N., Ed. (1973). *Chinese Science: Explorations of an Ancient Tradition.* Cambridge, Mass.; MIT Press

Needham, J. (1954–). *Science and Civilisation in China.* Cambridge; Cambridge University Press. Vol. 1, Sections 1–7, with Wang Ling, *Introductory Orientations* (1954). Vol. 2, Sections 8–18, with Wang Ling, *History of Scientific Thought* (1956). Vol. 3, Sections 19–25, with Wang Ling, *Mathematics and the Sciences of Heavens and the Earth* (1959). Vol. 4, *Physics and Physical Technology.* Section 26, with K.G. Robinson, *Part I. Physics* (1962). Section 27, *Part II. Mechanical Engineering* (1965). Sections 28–29, with Wang Ling and Lu Gwei-Djen, *Part III. Civil Engineering and Nautics* (1971). Vol. 5, *Chemistry and Chemical Technology.* Section 33, *Part II. Spagyrical Discovery and Invention: Magisteries of Gold and Immortality* (1974). Section 33 continued, with Ho Ping-yoke and Lu Gwei-Djen, *Part III. Spagyrical Discovery and Invention: Historical Survey, from Cinnabar Elixirs to Synthetic Insulin* (1976). Section 33 continued, with Ho Ping-yoke, Lu Gwei-Djen and Nathan Sivin, *Part IV. Spagyrical Discovery and Invention: Apparatus, Theories and Gifts* (1980)

Needham, J. (1970). *Clerks and Craftsmen in China and the West.* Cambridge; Cambridge University Press

Peterson, W. (1980). 'Chinese Scientific Philosophy' and Some Chinese Attitudes Towards Knowledge about the Realm of Heaven and Earth, *Past and Present,* No. 87, 20–30

Porkert, M. (1974). *The Theoretical Foundations of Chinese Medicine: Systems of Correspondence.* Cambridge, Mass., MIT Press

Schafer, E.H. (1977). *Pacing the Void: T'ang Approaches to the Stars.* Berkeley; University of California Press

Sivin, N. (1968). *Chinese Alchemy: Preliminary Studies.* Cambridge, Mass.; Harvard University Press

Sivin, N. (1969). Cosmos and Computation in Early Chinese Mathematical Astronomy, *T'oung Pao,* Vol. 55, 1–73

Sivin, N. (1977). *Science and Technology in East Asia.* New York; Science History Publications

Sun, E-tu Zen, Trans. and Ed. (1966). *T'ien-kung K'ai-wu. Chinese Technology in the Seventeenth Century.* University Park, Pa; Pennsylvania State University Press

Teich, M. and Young, R. (1973). *Changing Perspectives in the History of Science: Essays in Honour of Joseph Needham.* London; Heinemann

Teng, S.Y. and Biggerstaff, E. (1971). *An Annotated Bibliography of Selected Chinese Reference Works,* revised edn. Cambridge, Mass.; Harvard University Press

Unschuld, P.U. (1973). *Die Praxis des traditionellen Chinesischen Heilsystems.* Wiesbaden; Steiner

Unschuld, P.U. (1979). *Medical Ethics in Imperial China.* Berkeley; University of California Press

Veith, I. (1949). *The Yellow Emperor's Classic of Internal Medicine.* Berkeley; California University Press (see comment on p.491)

Vogel, K. (1968). *Neun Bücher Arithmetischer Technik.* Brunswick; Vieweg

Waley, A., Trans. and Ed. (1935). *The Way and its Power.* London; G. Allen and Unwin

Waley, A., Trans. and Ed. (1937). *The Book of Songs.* London; G. Allen and Unwin

Waley, A., Trans. and Ed. (1938). *The Analects of Confucius.* London; G. Allen and Unwin

Ware, J.A., Trans. and Ed. (1966). *Alchemy, Medicine, Religion in the China of AD 320. The Nei P'ien of Ko Hung.* Cambridge, Mass.; MIT Press

Watson, B. (1962). *Early Chinese Literature.* New York; Columbia University Press

Watson, B. (1967). *Basic Writings of Mo Tzu, Hsün Tzu and Han Fei Tzu.* New York; Columbia University Press

Watson, B. (1968). *The Complete Works of Chuang Tzu.* New York; Columbia University Press

Wilkinson, E. (1974). *The History of Imperial China: a Research Guide.* Cambridge, Mass.; Harvard University Press

Wylie, A. (1867). *Notes on Chinese Literature.* Shanghai; American Presbyterian Press. Reprinted (1939). Peiping; Vetch

Yabuuti, K. (1963). Astronomical Tables in China from the Han to the T'ang Dynasties, *Chūgoku chūsei gijutsushi no kenkyū.* Tokyo; Heimarusha, 455–492. Continued (1963) in *Japanese Studies in the History of Science*, Vol. 2, 94–100

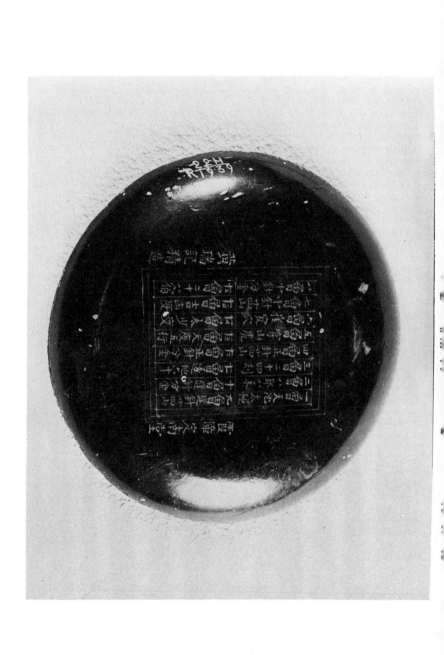

Bibliography of journals

This bibliography contains English-language and major international journals that commenced publication subsequent to the listing by Sarton and Mayer (G. Sarton, *Horus. A Guide to the History of Science. A First Guide for the Study of the History of Science with Introductory Essays on Science and Tradition.* New York; Ronald Press, 1952). In addition, journals covered by *Historical Abstracts* (Hist. Abs.) are indicated (see Chapter 9).

AAHM Newsletter. American Association for the History of Medicine, No. 1–, 1979–. Los Angeles

The Academy Bookman. Friends of the Rare Book Room, Library, New York Academy of Medicine, Vol. 1, No.1–, 1948–. New York

Acta Cartographica, from Periodicals, Vols. 1–25, 1967–1977. Amsterdam

Acta Historiae Rerum Naturalium nec non Technicorum (Czechoslovak Studies in the History of Science), Vol. 1, No.1–, 1965–. Prague

Acta Mathematica, 1882–. Stockholm

Acta Medicae Historiae Patavina, Vol. 1, No.1–, 1954–. Padua

Acta Musei Moraviae. Scientia Naturales: Folia Mendeliana, Vol.1–, 1966–. Brno

Acta Pharmaciae Historiae de l'Académie Internationale d'Histoire de la Pharmacie, Vols 1–5, 1959–1968. The Hague

Adīy àt Hàlàb. An Annual Devoted to the Study of Arabic Science and Civilisation, Vol. 1–, 1975–. Aleppo

Adler Museum Bulletin, Vol. 1, No. 1–, 1975–. Johannesburg

Aesculape. Revue mensuelle illustré, Vol. 1, No. 1 – Vol.51, No.6, 1911–1968. Paris. (1923–1940 official organ of the Société internationale d'histoire de la médecine)

Aesculapius, Medical Heritage Society, Vol. 1–, 1972–. Chicago

Agricultural History, Vol. 1, No.1–, 1927–. Washington DC

Agricultural History Review, Vol. 1, No.1–, 1953–. Reading

AIAA History Newsletter, No.1–, 1976–. Houston; American Institute of Aeronautics and Astronautics

AIHP Notes. American Institute of the History of Pharmacy, Vol. 1, No.1–, 1955–. Madison, Wisc.

AIP Newsletter. Center for the History of Physics, No.1–, 1964–. New York

Ambix, being the Journal of the Society for the Study of Alchemy and Early Chemistry, Vol. 1, No.1–, 1937–. Also known as the Society for the History of Alchemy and Chemistry. London

American Journal of Chinese Medicine, Vol.1, No.1–, 1973–. New York

Analecta Medico-Historica, Academiae Internationalis Medico-Historica, Nos 1–4, 1966–1968. Oxford

Annales de la Société Belge d'Histoire des Hôpitaux, Vol.1–, 1963–. Brussels

Annali dell'Instituto e Museo di Storia della Scienze di Firenze, Vol.1, No.1–, 1976. Florence

Annals of the History of Computing, Vol.1, No.1–, 1979–. Arlington, Va. Hist. Abs. 1979–

Annals of Medical History, Vols 1–10, N.S. 1–10, 3 Ser. 1–4, 1917–1942. New York

Annals of Science, Vol.1, No.1–, 1936–. London. Hist. Abs. 1955–

Apeiron. A Journal for Ancient Philosophy and Science, Vol.1, No.1–, 1966–. Monash University, Clayton

The Apollonian, Vol. 1–, 1926–. Boston, Mass.

Archaeoastronomy Bulletin, Vol.1, No.1–, 1977–. Maryland

Archeion. Founded 1919 by Aldo Mieli. Original title: *Archivo di Storia della*

Scienze. Title changed in Vol. 8, 1927. In 1948 became *Archives Internationales d'Histoire des Sciences*
Archiv Istorii Nauki i Techniki, No.1–, 1933–. Leningrad
Archive for History of Exact Sciences, Vol.1, No.1–, 1960–. West Berlin
Archives Internationales d'Histoire des Sciences, Vol.1–, 1948–. Paris. Vols 1–9 also numbered *Nouvelle série d'Archeion* 27–35. Hist. Abs. 1967–
Archives of Natural History, Vol.10, No.1–, 1981–. London. Formerly *Journal of the Society for the Bibliography of Natural History,* Vol.1, No.1–, 1936–
Australian Association for the History and Philosophy of Science. Newsletter, No.1–, 1968–. Sydney

Bibliography of the History of Medicine, Vol.1–, 1965–. Bethesda, Ma.
Biographical Memoirs of Fellows of the Royal Society, Vol. 1–, 1955–. London. Formerly *Obituary Notices of Fellows of the Royal Society,* Vols 1–9, 1932–1955
Biological Abstracts, 1926–. Menasha, Philadelphia. From 1939 issued in sections: A, General biology; B, Basic medical sciences; C, Microbiology, immunology, public health, and parasitology; D, Plant sciences; E, Animal sciences. During 1941–53 further sections issued: F, Animal production and veterinary sciences; G, Food and nutrition research; H, Human biology; J, Cereals and cereal products. Formerly *Abstracts of Bacteriology,* 1917–25. Baltimore; and *Botanical Abstracts,* 1918–26. Baltimore
Biological Journal of the Linnean Society, Vol.1–, 1969–. London. Formerly *Proceedings of the Linnean Society,* 1868–1968. London
Bollettino di Storia della Scienze Matematiche, Vol. 1–, 1981–. Unione Matematica Italiana
Books and Astronomers. Monthly Essays, Vol. 1, No.1–, 1978. New York
British Journal for the History of Science, Vol. 1, No. 1–, 1962–. London, currently Chalfont St Giles. Hist. Abs. 1967–
The British Journal for the Philosophy of Science, Vol.1, No.1–, 1951–. Aberdeen. Until 1959 journal of the Philosophy of Science Group of the British Society for the History of Science
British Society for the History of Science Newsletter, No.1–, 1980–. Chalfont St Giles
BSBI Abstracts. Abstracts of Literature relating to the Vascular Plants of the British Isles, 1971–. London
Bulletin of the British Museum (Natural History), Historical Series, Vol.1, No.1–, 1953–. London
Bulletin of the British Society for the History of Science, Vol.1, No.1 – Vol.2, No.19, 1949–1958. London. Vol. 2 issued as supplements to *Annals of Science.* Hist. Abs. 1955–1960
Bulletin of the Cleveland Medical Library, Vol.1, No.1–, 1954–. Cleveland
The Bulletin of the History of Dentistry, Vol.1, No.1–, 1953–. Chicago, then Batavia NY
Bulletin of the History of Medicine, Vol. 7, No.1–, 1939–. Baltimore. Continuation of *Bulletin of the Institute of the History of Medicine, Johns Hopkins University,* Vols 1–6, 1933–1938. Hist. Abs. 1963–
Bulletin of the Hunt Institute for Botanical Documentation, Vol. 1, No.1–. 1979–. Pittsburgh
Bulletin of the Indian Institute of History of Medicine, Vol. 1–, 1963–. Hyderabad
Bulletin Signalétique 522 Histoire des Sciences et des Techniques, 1969–. Paris
Bulletin de la Société Française d'Histoire des Hôpitaux, No.1–, 1959–. Paris
Bulletin of the Society of Medical History of Chicago, Vol.1, No.1 – Vol.6, No.1, 1911–1948. Chicago

Cauda Pavonis: the Alchemy and Literature Newsletter, No.1–, 1977–. Las Cruces, New Mexico; Association for the Study of Alchemy and Literature
Centaurus. International Magazine for the History of Science, Medicine and Technology, Vol.1, No.1, 1950–. Copenhagen. Hist. Abs. 1963–
The Charles Babbage Institute Newsletter, No.1–, 1979–. Palo Alto, Calif.
Chemistry, 1927–. Washington
Chemistry in Britain, 1965–. London
Chinese Journal of History of Science. K'O Hsueh Shih Chi K'an, 1958–.
The Chinese Journal of Medical History, Vol. 1, No. 1–, 1947–. Shanghai, currently Peking
Chinese Medical Journal, Vols 1–2, 1973–1974. N.S. Vol. 1–, 1975–. Peking
Chinese Science, Vol.1, No.1–, 1975–. Cambridge, Mass., currently Philadelphia
Chymia. Annual Studies in the History of Chemistry, Vols 1–12, 1948–1967. Philadelphia
Clio Medica. Acta Academiae Internationalis Historiae Medicinae, Vol. 1, No.1–, 1965–. Oxford, then Amsterdam
Communicationes de Historia Artis Medicinae, Vol.1–, 1955–. Budapest. Until Vol. 43, 1968, *Communicationes ex Biblioteca Historiae Medicae Hungaricae*
Contemporary Scientific Archives Centre. Progress Report, No.1–, 1973–. Oxford
The Council on Botanical and Horticultural Libraries. Newsletter, No.1–, 1972–. New York
Cuadernos de Historia de la Medicina Espanola, Vol.1–, 1962. Salamanca. Hist. Abs.
Cuadernos de Historia Sanitaria, Vols 1–16, 1952–1960. Havana. Hist. Abs. 1955–1960
Current Work in the History of Medicine, An International Bibliography, Vol. 1–, 1954–. London; Wellcome Institute for the History of Medicine

De Historia Medicinae (Alabama Society of Medical History), Vol. 1, No.1 – Vol. 5, 1956–1963. Birmingham, Ala.
Dynamis. Acta Hispanica ad Medicinae Scientiarumque Historiam Illustrandam. Vol. 1. No. 1–, 1981–. Granada

Endeavour. A Quarterly Review Designed to Record the Progress of the Sciences of Mankind, Vol. 1, No. 1–, 1942–. London
Energy History Report, No. 1– [Unconfirmed]. Washington DC; Dept. of Energy
Entomologist's Record and Journal of Variation, 1890–. London
Episteme, Rivista Critica di Storia delle Scienze Mediche e Biologiche, Vols 1–10, 1967–1976. Milan
EPS. The Ethno-Pharmacology Society Newsletter, Vol. 1, No. 1–, 1977–. Irvine, Calif.
Equilibrium. Quarterly Journal of the International Society of Antique Scale Collectors, No. 1–, 1978–. Chicago, Ill.

Fabula. Zeitschrift für Erzählforschung/Journal of Folklore Studies/Revue des Etudes sur le Conte Populaire, Vol. 1, No. 1–, 1958–. West Berlin
Friends of the P.I. Nixon Medical Historical Library Annual Bulletin, No. 1–, 1972–. San Antonio, Texas

Ganita Bhāratī. Bulletin of the Indian Society for History of Mathematics, Vol. 1, No. 1/2–, 1979–. Mesra, Ranchi
Gesnerus, Vol. 1, No. 1–, 1943–. Aarau

Hannah Institute for the History of Medicine, Vol. 1, No. 1–, 1977–. Toronto
Historia Hospitalium, Vol. 1–, 1966–. Düsseldorf
Historia Mathematica, Vol. 1, No. 1–, 1974–. New York
Historia Medicinae Veterinariae, Vol. 1, No. 1–, 1976–. Copenhagen
Historia Scientiarum. International Journal of the History of Science Society of Japan, No. 19–, 1980–. Tokyo. Formerly *Japanese Studies in the History of Science*, Vol. 1–, 1962. Hist. Abs. 1971–
Historical Bulletin. Notes and Abstracts dealing with Medical History, Vols 1–22, 1936–1958. Calgary
Historical Studies in the Physical Sciences, Vol. 1–, 1969–. Philadelphia
History of Anthropology Newsletter, Vol. 1, No. 1–, 1974–. Chicago
The History of Astronomy Resource Center Quarterly Newsletter, Vol. 1, No. 1–, 1980–
History of the Behavioral Sciences Newsletter, Nos 1–7, 1960–1964. New York
History of Medicine, Vol. 1, No. 1 – Vol. 7, Nos 1–2, 1968–1976; Vol. 8, No. 1–, 1980–. London
History and Philosophy of the Life Sciences. Pubblicazioni della Stazione Zoologica di Napoli, Section 2, Vol. 1–, 1979–. Naples
History and Philosophy of Logic, Vol. 1–, 1980–. Tunbridge Wells
History of Science, Vol. 1–, 1962–. Cambridge. Hist. Abs. 1967–
History of Science in America: News and Views, No. 1–. 1980–. Cambridge, Mass.
History of Science Society Newsletter, Vol. 1, No. 1–, 1972–. Minneapolis, then New York
History of Technology, Vol. 1–, 1976–. London. Hist. Abs. 1976–
HSTC Bulletin, Vol. 1, No. 1–, 1976–. Downsview, Ontario. From 1980 subtitled *Journal of the History of Canadian Science, Technology and Medicine*
Huntia, a Yearbook of Botanical and Horticultural Bibliography, Vol. 1–, 1964–. Pittsburgh

IA: The Journal of the Society for Industrial Archeology, Vol. 1, No. 1–, 1975–. Morgantown, W. Va.
IASTAM Newsletter. International Association for the Study of Traditional Asian Medicine, No. 1–, 1982–. Delaware
Imago Mundi. The Journal of the International Society for the History of Cartography, Vol. 1–, 1935–. Berlin, currently Amsterdam. Subtitle varies
The Impact of Science on Society, Vol. 1, No. 1–, 1950–. Paris; UNESCO
Indian Journal of the History of Medicine, Vol. 1–, 1956–. New Delhi/Madras
Indian Journal of History of Science, Vol. 1, No. 1–, 1966–. New Delhi
International Union of the History and Philosophy of Science. Division of the History of Science. Bulletin, No. 1–, 1975–. From 1978 *International Union of the History and Philosophy of Science. Division of the History of Science. Newsletter.*
Iranian Society of the History of Science and Medicine, Vol. 1, 1962. Teheran
Irish Naturalists' Journal, 1925–. Belfast. Formerly *Irish Naturalist*, 1892–1924. Dublin
Isis. Revue consacrée à l'histoire de la science, Vol. 1, No. 1–, 1913–. Wondelem-lez-Gand, currently Philadelphia as *Journal of the History of Science Society.* Hist. Abs. 1954–
Iz Istorii Biologicheskikh Nauk, Vol. 1–, 1966–. Moscow

Jahrbuch über die Fortschritte der Mathematik Vol. 1–68, 1871–1944. Berlin
Janus, revue internationale de l'histoire des sciences, de la médecine, de la pharmacie et de la technique, Vol. 1–, 1896–. Leyden
Journal of Chemical Education, 1924–. Easton, Pa.

Journal of Chinese Medicine, No. 1–, 1979–. Lewes, Sussex
Journal for the History of Arabic Science, Vol. 1, No. 1–, 1977–. Aleppo
Journal for the History of Astronomy, Vol. 1, No. 1–, 1970–. Currently Chalfont St Giles. Annual supplement: *Archaeoastronomy*, 1979–
Journal of the History of the Behavioral Sciences, Vol. 1–, 1965–. Boston, Mass. Hist. Abs. 1970–
Journal of the History of Biology, Vol. 1, No. 1–, 1968–. Cambridge, Mass. Hist. Abs. 1968–
Journal of the History of Ideas, Vol. 1, No. 1–, 1940–. Lancaster, Pa., currently Philadelphia. Hist. Abs. 1954–
Journal of the History of Medicine and Allied Sciences, Vol. 1, No. 1–, 1946–. New Haven, Conn. Hist. Abs. 1954
Journal of the History of Sociology, Vol. 1, No. 1–, 1978–. Boston, Mass.
Journal of the Japanese Society for the History of Pharmacy, Vol. 1–, 1966–. Tokyo
Journal of the Korean Academy of the History of Dentistry, Vols 1–3, 1960–1962. Seoul
Journal of the Society for the Bibliography of Natural History, 1936–. London
Journal of the Warburg and Courtauld Institutes, Vol. 1, No. 1–, 1937–. London

Koroth. A Bulletin devoted to the History of Medicine and Science, Vol. 1, No. 1/2–, 1952–. Jerusalem
Kwartalnik Historii Nauki i Techniki, Vol. 1–, 1956–. Warsaw. Hist. Abs. 1964–

Lettre d'Information du Centre Européen d'Histoire de la Médecine, Newsletter of the European Centre of the History of Medicine, No. 1–, 1979–. Strasbourg
The Locke Newsletter, No. 1–, 1970–. York
Lychnos, Vol. 1–, 1936–. Uppsala and Stockholm

Mathematical Reviews, 1940–. Lancaster
Medical Anthropology, Vol. 1, No. 1–, 1977–. Pleasantville, NY
Medical Anthropology Newsletter, Vol. 1, No. 1–, 1968–. South Birmingham, Ala., currently San Francisco
Medical History, Vol. 1, No. 1–, 1956–. London. Hist. Abs. 1967–
Medical History Review, No. 1–, 1971–. Nottingham
Medical Leaves; a Review of the Jewish Medical World and Medical History, Vols 1–5, 1937–1943. Chicago
Medizinhistorisches Journal, Vol. 1, No. 1–, 1966–. Hildesheim, then Stuttgart
Mendel Newsletter, No. 1–, 1969–. Philadelphia
Minerva: a Review of Science, Policy and Learning, Vol. 1, No. 1–, 1962–. London

National Academy of Engineering of the United States of America. Memorial Tributes, Vol. 1–, 1979–. Washington DC
National Academy of Sciences Biographical Memoirs, Vol. 1–, 1977–. Washington, DC
National Catalog of Sources for History of Physics. Report, No. 1–, 1969–. New York
The Natural Philosopher, Vols 1–3, 1963–1964. New York and London
Naturalist, 1864–. London
Newsletter, American Academy of the History of Dentistry, Vol. 1, No. 1, 1967. Chicago, then Batavia, NY
Newsletter. Historical Metallurgical Society. [Unconfirmed]
Newsletter/Nouvelles. La Société Canadienne d'Histoire de la Médecine/The Canadian Society for the History of Medicine, No. 1–, 1979–. Quebec

Newsletter of the International Commission on the History of Women in Science, Technology and Medicine, Vol. 1, No. 1 and 2–. Budapest and Berkeley, Calif.
Newsletter of the Optometric Historical Society, No. 1–, 1970–. St Louis, Mo.
Newsletter of the Scottish Society for Industrial Archaeology, No. 1–, 1969–. Glasgow
Nordisk Medicinhistorisk Årsbok, Vol. 1–, 1968–. Stockholm. Hist. Abs. 1960–
North Carolina Newsletter, No. 1–, 1980–. Durham; Medical History Program and the Trent Collection, Duke University
Notae de Historia Mathematica, Vol. 1, No. 1 – Vol. 3, No. 2, 1971–1973. Toronto
Notes and Records of the Royal Society of London, Vol. 1, No. 1–, 1938–. London
NTM. Zeitschrift für Geschichte der Naturwissenschaften, Technik und Medizin, Vol. 1, No. 1–, 1960–. Leipzig

Organon, No. 1–, 1964–. Warsaw
Osiris, Vols 1–15, 1936–1968. Bruges
Osler Library Newsletter, No. 1–, 1969–. Montreal

Paleopathology Newsletter, No. 1–, 1973–. Detroit
Perspectives in Biology and Medicine, Vol. 1, No. 1–, 1957–. Chicago
Pharmaceutical Historian; Newsletter of the British Society for the History of Pharmacy, Vol. 1, No. 1–, 1967–. London
Pharmaceutical Society of Great Britain. History of Pharmacy Committee. Newsletter. Nos 1–6, 1956–1960. London
Pharmacy in History, Vol. 4, No. 1–, 1959–. Madison, Wisc. Continued AIHP Notes
Philosophy of Science, Vol. 1, No. 1–, 1936–. East Lansing, Mich.
Philosophy of Science Association Newsletter, No. 1–, 1977–. East Lansing, Mich.
Physis. Rivista di Storia della Scienza, Vol. 1, No. 1–, 1959. Florence. Hist. Abs. 1964–
Polish Medical Sciences and History Bulletin, Vols 1–4, 1973–1976. Warsaw. Continued as Polish Medical Science and History Bulletin, Vols 1–14, 1956–1971. Chicago
Pratique. Quarterly Newsletter of the Disinfected Mail Study Circle, Vol. 1, No. 1–, 1974–. London
Price-Priestley Newsletter, No. 1–, 1977–. Aberystwyth
Proceedings of the Charaka Club, Vols 1–11, 1902–1947. New York
Proceedings of the Royal Society of Medicine, Section of the History of Medicine, Vol. 6, Part 2–, 1912–. London
Project on the History of Recent Physics in the United States. Newsletter. Formed part of AIP Newsletter

Radical Science Journal, No. 1–, 1974–. London
Revista de la Sociedad Cubana de Historia de la Medicina, Vols 1–6, 1958–1963. Havana. Hist. Abs. 1958–1962
Revue d'Histoire des Sciences et de leurs Applications, Vol. 1, No. 1–, 1947–. Paris. Hist. Abs. 1955–1962, 1966–1967
Revue d'Histoire de la Pharmacie, Vol. 1–, 1913–. Paris
Revue Semestrielle des Publications Mathématiques, 1893–1934. Amsterdam and Leipzig
Rivista di Storia Critica delle Scienze Mediche e Naturali, Vol. 1, No. 1 – Vol. 47, 1910–1956. Florence
Rivista di Storia della Medicina, Vol. 1, No. 1 – Vol. 21, No. 2, 1957–1977. Rome

Science of Science, Vol. 1, No. 1–, 1980–. Warsaw and Dordrecht. Continues *Problems of the Science of Science*, Vol. 1–, 1970–. Warsaw

Science and Society, Vol. 1, No. 1–, 1936–. Chelmsford

Science Studies, Vol. 1, No. 1 – Vol. 4, No. 4, 1971–1974. London

Science, Technology, and Human Values, No. 1–, 1972–. Cambridge, Mass.

Scottish Society of the History of Medicine Newsletter, No. 1–, 1972–. Edinburgh

The Scottish Society of the History of Medicine. Report of Proceedings, 1948–. Edinburgh. From: 1971 published in *Medical History*, Vol. 26, No. 2– ·

Scripta Mathematica, Vol. 1, No. 1 – Vol. 24, No. 4, 1932–1973. New York

Smithsonian Annals of Flight, Vol. 1, No. 1–, 1964–. Washington DC

Smithsonian Institution. Archives and Special Collections of the Smithsonian Institution, Vol. 1, No. 1–, 1971–. Washington, DC

Smithsonian Journal of History, Vol. 1, No. 1 – Vol. 3, No. 4, 1966–1969. Washington, DC

Smithsonian Opportunities for Research and Study in History, Art, Science, No. 1–, 1964–. Washington, DC

Smithsonian Studies in History and Technology, 1966–1968. Washington DC. Hist. Abs. 1966–1968

Social Science and Medicine, Vol. 1, No. 1–, 1967–. Oxford and New York. Superseded in part in 1968: *Part A: Medical Psychology and Sociology. Part B: Medical Anthropology. Part C: Medical Economics. Part D: Medical Geography*.

Social Science History, Vol. 1, No. 1–, 1976–. Pittsburgh

Social Studies of Science, Vol. 5, No. 1 –, 1975–. London. Continues *Science Studies*, Vol. 1, No. 1– Vol. 4, No. 4, 1971–1974. Hist. Abs. 1975–

Society for Ancient Medicine Newsletter, No. 1–, 1976–. Hawaii, then Kentucky

Society for the Bibliography of Natural History. British Newsletter, Nos 1–7, 1977–1978. London

Society for the Bibliography of Natural History. Newsletter, No. 1–, 1979–. London

Society for the Bibliography of Natural History, London. North American Newsletter, No. 1, 1977. New York

Society for the History of Discoveries. Annual Report. No. 1–, 1961–. Columbia, MD

Society for the History of Technology. Newsletter, [unconfirmed]. Cleveland

Society for Industrial Archeology. Data Sheet, No. 1–, 1973–. Washington DC

Society for Industrial Archeology. SIA Newsletter, No. 1–, 1972–. Harrisburg, Pa.

Society for the Social History of Medicine. Bulletin, No. 1–, 1970–. London, then Nottingham

Society for Social Studies of Science Newsletter, Vol. 1, No. 1–, 1975–. Carbondale, Ill.

Sociology of the Sciences: A Yearbook, Vol. 1–, 1977–. Dordrecht

STSA Newsletter. Science, Technology and Society Association, 1979–. Manchester. Continues *SISCON Newsletter*, Nos 1–5, 1976–1978

STTH: Science/Technology and the Humanities, Vol. 1, No. 1–, 1978–. Melbourne, Fl.

Studi di Storia Ospitaliera, Vols 1–3, 1963–1965. Reggio Emilia

Studia Copernicana, Vol. 1–, 1970–. Wroclaw, Warsaw and Cracow

Studia Leibnitiana, Vol. 1, No. 1–, 1969–. Wiesbaden

Studies in the History of Biology, Vol. 1–, 1977–. Baltimore and London

Studies in the History of Medicine, Vol. 1, No. 1–, 1977–, New Delhi

Studies in History and Philosophy of Science, Vol. 1, No. 1–, 1970–. London. Hist. Abs. 1977–

Sudhoffs Archiv. Zeitschrift für Wissenschaftsgeschichte, Vol. 1, No. 1–, 1907–. Leipzig, currently Wiesbaden. Original title *Archiv für Geschichte der Medizin*. Hist. Abs. 1963–

Survey of Sources for the History of Biochemistry and Molecular Biology. Survey of Sources Newsletter, Vol. 1, No. 1–, 1975–. Philadelphia
Synthesis, Vol. 1, No. 1–, 1972–. Cambridge, Mass.

Teaching the History and Sociology of Pharmacy, No. 1, 1977–. Madison, Wisc.
Technikgeschichte, Vol. 1, No. 1–, 1909–. Berlin, currently Düsseldorf
Technology and Culture. The International Quarterly of the Society for the History of Technology, Vol. 1, No. 1–, 1959–. Chicago. Hist. Abs. 1960–
Technology in Society, Vol. 1, No. 1–, 1979–. New York and Oxford
Traditional Medical Systems, Vol. 1, No. 1–, n.d. 1980?–. Calcutta
Transactions of the British Society for the History of Pharmacy, Vol. 1, No. 1–, 1970–. London
Transactions. The Newcomen Society for the Study of the History of Engineering and Technology, Vol. 1, No. 1–, 1920–. London
Transactions and Studies of the College of Physicians of Philadelphia. Medicine and History, Ser. 5, Vol. 1, No. 1–, 1979–. Philadelphia

UMHP Bulletin (Union Mondiale des Sociétés d'Histoire Pharmaceutique), Nos 1–3, 1962–1963. Rotterdam and Washington DC
Utrecht Biohistorical Review, No. 1–, 1970–. Utrecht.

Veterinary History. Bulletin of the Veterinary History Society, Nos 1–12, 1973–79; N.S. Vol. 1, No. 1–, 1979–. London
Victorian Studies. Journal of the Humanities, Arts and Sciences. Vol. 1, No. 1–, 1957–. Bloomington, Ind.
Voprosy Istorii Yestesttvoznania i Techniki, Vol. 1–, 1956–. Moscow

The Watermark: Newsletter of the Association of Libraries in the History of the Health Sciences, Vol. 1, No. 1–, 1977–. Philadelphia

Zeitschrift für Mathematik and Physik, Vols 1–64, 1856–1917. Leipzig
Zentralblatt für Mathematik, 1931–. Berlin
Zoological Record, 1865–. London
Zygon. Journal of Religion and Science, Vol. 1, No. 1–, 1966–. Chicago. Hist. Abs. 1967–

Index

Major headings are subdivided as follows:

(i) by type of information source (e.g. bibliography, dictionary, survey), in alphabetical order;
(ii) by country or culture, in alphabetical order;
(iii) by period, in chronological order;
(iv) miscellaneous subdivisions, in alphabetical order.

Titles followed by '(j)' are periodicals. This indication has not been used where this is self-evident from the title.

Abhandlungen zur Geschichte der Mathematik, 260, 261
Abstract journals, 162, 177, 354
    development, 159
    dissertation, 149
Abstracta Islamica, 440
Abstracting services, 157
Academy of Natural Sciences of Philadelphia, Catalog of the Library of, 146
Ackerknecht, E.H., 61–62, 383, 384, 415, 418
Acta Mathematica, 261, 274
Acupuncture, 490–491
Adam, Melchior, 31
Adams, S., 141
Adelung, Johann Christoph, 32
Aepinus, Franz Ulrich Theodor, 295, 300
Aeschylus, 201, 202
Agassi, Joseph, 119, 127
Agassiz, Louis, 416

Agriculture, histories of, 45, 48
    in the Third World, 54
    Museum of English Rural Life, 50
Air pumps, 247, 289
Albion (computing device), 244
Alchemy, 223, 319, 320
    bibliographies, 319, 320
    Chinese, 491–492
    Indian,
        bibliography, 457
        in Vedic period, 459–460
        500–1100 AD, 463
    Islamic, 447
        symbolism, 320
        terminology, 320–321
Alexandria, Museum of, 209–210, 216
Algebra, 265
    19th century developments, 269–270
    notation, 265
    surveys of texts, 266
    (*see also* Mathematics)
Algebraic geometry, 270

509

Al-Khowarizmi, 264
Ambix (j), 160, 165–166, 317
America: History of Life (j), 162
American Association for the
    Advancement of Science, 427
American Association for the History
    of Medicine, 166, 412
American Historical Review, 161
American Medical Association, 423
American Men and Women of Science,
    141
American Museum of Natural History,
    Research Catalog, 144
American Philosophical Society,
    Transactions and Proceedings, 164
Ampère, André Marie, 271, 300
Anaesthesia, 383
Anatomy
    classical research, 216
    Indian,
        bibliography, 457
        to 5th century AD, 462
Annales, 164
Annales de Chimie, 329
Annals of the History of Computing,
    262
Annals of Science, 149, 163, 165, 354
*Annotated Bibliography in the History
    of Mathematics*, 275
Annual Review of Anthropology, 67
Anthropology, 175, 363
    guides to current thought, 66–67
    in history of science and medicine,
        61–80
        bibliographies, 70, 77–80
            guide to, 67
        reviews, 70
Anti-vivisection movement, 368
Apothecaries, biographies, 390
Arabic Technical and Scientific Texts,
    443
Archaeology, and economic history, 49
Archeion (j), 165
Archibald, R.C., 261
Archimedes of Syracuse, 210, 211, 265,
    287
    influence on later works, 222
    writings recovered, 228
Archive for History of Exact Sciences,
    165, 262
Archives,
    guides to, 180, 182–183
    US, 178
    (*see also* Manuscripts)

*Archives Internationales d'Histoire des
    Sciences*, 149, 160, 165
Archives Nationales (Paris), 180
Archives of Natural History, 166, 350,
    354
Archivio di Storia delle Scienze, 165
Aristarchus, 199
Aristotelianism, 5–6, 225, 228, 229, 232
Aristotle, 206–207, 227
    importance to scientific rationality,
        208 209
    influence on later work, 222, 231
    on superiority of science to
        technology, 204
    peripatetic physics, 213–214
    removal of forgeries from canon, 228
    survival of unpublished works, 222
Art galleries, technological exhibitions,
    50
Art, works of, 176
    (*see also* Illustrations)
Artefacts, 176
Arts and Humanities Citation Index, 162
Asiatick Researches (j), 467
Astrarium, 243–244
Astrolabes, 243, 244
    mariner's, 245
Astrology, 5, 212, 223
    Chinese, 481, 492–493
    Indian, 464
    (*see also* Astronomy)
Astronomical clocks, 243–244
Astronomy, 6
    bibliography, 274

    Arabic, bibliography, 438
    Chinese, 481, 489–490
    classical, 201, 211–212
    Indian,
        bibliography, 458
        in Vedic period, 459
        6th to 11th century AD, 462–463
        in 17th century, 465
    Islamic, 444, 445, 446–447
        biobibliographies, 445
        pseudepigraphical texts, 448

    Medieval and Renaissance, 229–230
    in late 16th century, 8, 290–291
    in 17th century, 8
    in early 19th century, 300–301
    in 20th century, 302

    academic study of, 294–295
    early relationship with astrology, 223
    instruments, 243–244

Astronomy,
  instruments (*cont.*)
    development in 19th century, 301
    mathematical models, 205–206,
      211–212
    observatories, 243
    sacred tradition, 205
    (*see also* Physical sciences)
Atomic bomb, 103–104
  political implications, 104–105
Atomic physics, 326, 428
Atomic weights, 326, 327
Auctions,
  natural history, register of, 351
  (*see also* Sale catalogues)
Avogadro, Amadeo, 326

Baas, J.H., 31–32, 36, 40
Babington, A.M., 352, 391
Bachelard, Gaston, 3, 7–8, 299
Bacon, Francis, 230, 245–246, 285, 288,
  321
Baconianism, 16
Bacteriology,
  advanced by improved microscopes,
    251
  experimental, 363
Baird, Spencer F., 427–428
Balances, chemical, 247
  accuracy, 250
Baldi, Bernardino, 260
Banks, Sir Joseph, 352
Barbaro, Ermolao, 226
Barchusen, Johann Conrad, 32
Barlow, P., 44
Barometric tube, 289
Beg, Ulugh, 245
Bell, Charles, 368
Benedetti, Giambattista, 267, 287
Berger, P.L., 86
Berkeley, Miles, 368
Bernal, J.D., 38, 100, 101, 108, 366
Bernard, Claude, 365
Bernier, François, 464–465
Bernoulli, Jakob, 295
Berthollet, Claude Louis, 324, 326, 328
Bertrand, Joseph Louis François, 271
Berzelius, J.J., 325, 326–327
Bessel, Friedrich Wilhelm, 296
Besterman, Theodore, 139
Bibliographical aids, 137–141
  bibliography of sources, 150–156
  data-bases, 149–150

Bibliographies,
  Greek, compilation, 208
  limitations, 177
  of bibliographies, 139
  subject, guide to, 253
  (*see also under individual subject
    headings*)
*Bibliography of the History of
  Medicine*, 147, 442
Bibliotheca Mathematica, 261, 274
Bibliotheca universalis, 30, 31
Biennial Review of Anthropology, 67
Billingsley, Henry, 288
Biobibliography, Project for Historical, 390
Biochemistry,
  survey of sources, 181
  (*see also* Life sciences)
Biogeography, 356
Biographical dictionaries, 141–143,
  187, 275, 382, 441
Biographie Universelle, 382
Biographies, 186
  (*see also* Prosopography, *and under
    individual subjects*)
*Biographisch-Literarisches
  Handwörterbuch zur Geschichte
  der exacten Naturwissenschaften*,
  141–142
Biological Abstracts, 354
*Biological Journal of the Linnean
  Society*, 354
Biology, history of, 110
  surveys, 362–363
  of sub-disciplines, 362–363
  Indian, bibliography, 458
  contributions by biologists, 364
  identification with history of
    medicine, 38
  philosophy, 365
  Romantic school, 365
  three phases of development, 361
  works written in crisis periods,
    364–365
  (*see also* Life sciences)
Biot, Jean Baptiste, 296
Bishop, J.L., 44
Black, Joseph, 323
Blake, William, 298
Bloch, Marc, 392
Bloor, D., 86
Boas, Franz, 429
Boë, Franz de le, *see* Sylvius,
  Franciscus

Boerhaave Museum, Leyden, material
on scientific instruments, 253
Bohr, Niels, 104
Bois, Franz du, *see* Sylvius, Franciscus
Bolles, A.S., 44
*Bollettino di bibliografia e storia delle
scienze matematiche*, 261
*Bollettino di storia delle scienze
matematiche*, 262
Bombelli, Rafael, 264, 266
Boncompagni, Baldassare, 260, 261
Bontius, 465
Boorstin, D., 49
Borel, Emile, 271
Born, Max, 6
Botanical Society of London, 356
Botanists, biographical dictionaries,
142, 350–351
Botany,
county Floras, 351
general history, 354
Indian, bibliography, 458
precision of information, 188
(*see also* Life sciences)
Boulger, G.S., 350–351
Bourbaki School, 271
Bower, Frederick Orpen, 368
Boyer, Carl, 261, 263
Boyle, Robert, 246, 291
biographies, 322
Bradwardine, Thomas, 224
Brahe, Tycho, 244
Braunmühl, Anton von, 271
Brecht, Bertolt, 184
Bridges, history of, 45
The Bridgewater Treatises, 18
British Association for the
Advancement of Science, 18, 109,
297
study of origins, 187
British Humanities Index, 159, 163
*British Journal for the History of
Science*, 163, 166
*British Journal for the Philosophy of
Science*, 166
British Library
catalogue, 145
Department of Manuscripts, 177
New Periodical Titles, 162
Serials in the British Library, 161
British Medical Journal, 168
British Museum (Natural History),
accessions lists, 144
Bulletin, Historical Series, 166, 354

British Museum Catalogue, 145
British Society for the History of
Medicine, 167
Bulletin, 166
British Union Catalogue of Periodicals,
161
Britten, J., 350–351
Brodman, E., 140
Brown, Lucius Polk, 424
Brunfels, Otto, 30, 273
Brunschvig, Léon, 6–7, 8, 10
BSBI Abstracts, 354
Bubonic plague, 391–392
Buckland, William, 17
Buddhism,
in China, 484
in India, 461
surgery, 466
Buffon, Georges Louis Leclerc, 295
Bulletin Analytique. Philosophie (j),
139–140
*Bulletin of the British Museum (Natural
History), Historical Series*, 166, 354
Bulletin of the History of Medicine, 160,
166, 412, 417, 422
Bulletin Signalétique (j), 139–140, 148,
274
*Bulletino di bibliografia e storia delle
scienze matematiche e fisiche*,
260–261
Buridan, Jean, 224
Burkett, J., 141
Burtt, E.A., 11–12
Business history, 48
Butterfield, Herbert, 12, 102

Cabanis, P.J.G., 35
*Cahiers de Civilisation Médiévale x^e-xii^e
siècles, Bibliographie*, 440
Calculus, 265, 270
Calendars, 243
Callisen, A.C.P., 381
Cambridge Economic History, 49
*Cambridge Monographs on the History
of Medicine*, 162
Camera obscura, 248
Cameras, 248
in stellar astronomy, 301
Canals, 47
Candolle, Alphonse de, 13
Cannizzaro, Stanislao, 327
Cannon, Susan F., 17
Cantor, Moritz, 259, 260, 261, 263, 271

Cardano, Girolamo, 264
Carnap, Rudolf, 117
Carnot, Nicolas Léonard Sadi, 299
Catalogues,
  libraries, 177
  museums scientific collections, 252
  of scientific instruments, 249
  of source materials, 176
  (*see also* Exhibition catalogues;
    Museums: catalogues; Sale
    catalogues)
Catalogus illustrium medicorum, 30
Cauchy, Augustin-Louis, 271
Caus, Salomon de, 287
Cavendish, Henry, 295
Centaurus (j), 160, 165
Center for Cartographic and
  Architectural Archives (US), 178
Center for the History of Physics (US),
  181
Center for Polar and Scientific Archives
  (US), 178
Centre for the Study of Medieval
  Mathematics (Italy), 273
Centre Internationale de Synthèse
  (France), 7, 165
Chalmers, G.K., 10
Champier, Symphorien, 273
Chapin, Charles V., 424
Charitable institutions, medical, guides
  to, 386–387
Charles, J.A.C., 298
Charleton, Walter, 290
Chasles, M., 260
Chaucer, Geoffrey, astrolabe treatise,
  244
Chemical industry, 110
  bibliography, 331
Chemical News, 329
Chemical Society of London, 329
Chemistry, history of, 317–346
  bibliography, 331–346
  encyclopaedias, 318
  institutions, 329, 330
  journals, 317
    history of, 329–330
  key to laboratory terminology, 319
  Greek, 319
  Indian, bibliography, 458
  early, 318–321
  in 17th and 18th centuries, 322–325
  in 19th century, 325–330
    in US, 429

Chemistry, history of (*cont.*)
  in 20th century, 330
  apparatus, 319
  organic, 327–328
  Paracelsianism, 321–322
  philosophy of, 318
  physical, 328–329
  (*see also* Biochemistry; Physical
    sciences)
Chemistry in Britain (j), 317
Ch'i concept, 495–496
Cholera, 415, 420
Chromatography, 330
Chronometers, 247
Chu Hsi, 485
Church of Jesus Christ of Latter-day
  Saints: parish register project, 179
Chymia (annual), 317
Cipolla, C.M., 49
Citation indexes, 157, 162
Civilization, role of scientific ideas in,
  12
Clairaut, Alexis Claude, 295
Clark, G.N., 102
Clark, Stuart, 67
Clark, V.S., 44
Classification of knowledge, 67
  considerations of library of Museum
    of Alexandria, 209
Clausius, Rudolf Julius Emmanuel,
  327
Clio Medica (j), 160, 167
Clocks, accuracy of, 250
Cohen, I.B., 426
Cohen, M.R., 197–199
Collison, R.L., 139, 143
Combustion, 323, 324
Comité International et Centre
  International d'Histoire des
  Sciences, 7
Commission pour l'inventaire mondial
  des appareils scientifiques d'intérêt
  historique, 252
Compass, 245
Computer analysis of data, 189
Computerized information retrieval
  systems, 149–150
Computing,
  Annals of the History of Computing,
    262
  archives, 181
Comte, Auguste, 4, 16, 118
Conceptual analysis, 8, 9, 14

Confucianism, 483
  core works, 479–480
  neo-Confucians, 485
Confucius, 478
  Analects, translation, 483
Contemporary Medical Archives
    Centre, 182
Contemporary Scientific Archives
    Centre, 180–181
Continuity thesis of Duhem, 6, 12
Cook, Captain James, zoological
    specimens, 352
Copernicanism, 288
Copernicus, Nicholas, 229–230, 244
Corpus Medicorum Graecorum, 443
Cosalli, Pietro, 260
Cosmography, Islamic, 447
Coulomb, Charles Augustin de, 296,
    300
County record offices, 179
*Courtauld and Warburg Institutes,
    Journal of*, 164
Craft processes, 50
  in Greek technology, 201
  (*see also* Technology)
Creighton, C., 40
'Critical idealism', 7
Crowther, J.G., 100
Crum Brown, Alexander, 328
Crystallography, 330
Culture,
  history of, periodical literature, 164
  sociology of, 88
*Current Work in the History of
    Medicine*, 148, 161, 354, 442
Curtze, Maximilian, 260
Cytology, 188, 363

D'Alembert, Jean le Rond, 117, 295
Dalton, John, 298, 326
Damerow, H., 33
Dams, history of, 45
Daremberg, Charles, 35–36
Darmstaedter, L., 187
Darwin, Charles, 17, 18, 186, 356, 367
  and natural theology, 19–20
  life and letters, 352
  research methods, 184
Darwinism, 367, 416
  Popper's views, 120–121, 122–123
  social, 110
D'Aubisson, J.F., 44
Daumas, M., 45

da Vinci, Leonardo, 224, 230, 266
Davis, Natalie, 61
Davis, Tenney L., 492
Davy, Humphrey, 297, 325
Dee, John, 285, 288
Defence research, *see* Military science
Democritus, 202
Demography, 189, 392–393
Department of Scientific and Industrial
    Research (UK), 178
Descartes, René, 265, 289, 290
  studies on, 267
Diaries, 176
Dictionaries,
  bibliography of, 143
  biographical, 141–143, 187, 275, 382,
    441
*Dictionary of British and Irish
    Botanists*, 142
Dictionary of National Biography, 143,
    187, 382
Dictionary of Scientific Biography,
    142–143, 275, 441
Dictionary of the History of Science, 138
Diepgen, P., 37
Differential equations, 19th century
    development of, 269
Diogenes Laertius, writings recovered,
    228
Diophantus, 199, 265
Directories, bibliography of, 253
  see also under individual subjects
Disciplinary matrices, 121, 123
Disease,
  cultural variations, 71–72
  ecological studies, 70, 71
  magical beliefs, 72–73
  sociological aspects, 70
  value of chronicling course of, 35
  (*see also* Epidemiology; Medicine)
Dissertation abstracts, 149
Distillation, history of, 319
Dondi, Giovanni de', 243–244
Douglas, Mary, 86
Drabkin, I.E., 197–199
Draper, John W., 416
Drawings, 176
  (*see also* Illustrations)
Drebbel, Cornelius, 287
Drug jars, 248
Drug safety, experimental approach to,
    363
Duhem, Pierre, 5–6, 12, 117, 224–225,
    229, 230

Dunn, Margaret, 182
Durkheim, Émile, 86
Dutt, R., 44
Dyestuffs industry, 331

East Asian History of Science Library, 477
East India Company, 465, 466, 468
Ecclesiastical records, 179
École Normale, 268
École Polytechnique, 268, 271, 324–325
Ecological studies of disease, 70, 71
Ecology, 356
Economic histories, 48–49
    limitations, 50
Edelstein, Ludwig, 197–199, 215
Edinburgh school of sociologists of knowledge, 119
Einstein, Albert, 6, 302
Eisenstein, Elizabeth, 68
Electrical engineering, histories of, 45
Electricity, 293, 299
    social status of research, 300
    (*see also* Physical sciences)
Electrochemistry, 325
Electrolysis, 325
Electronics industry, history of, collections on, 181
Electrostatic generators, 247
Elements, theories of, 322–323, 327
    Chinese, 495
    Indian, 461
Empedocles, 202, 206, 207
Encyclopaedia of Islam, 440–441
Encyclopaedias, 177
    bibliography, 143
    (*see also under individual subjects*)
Encyklopädie der mathematischen Wissenschaften mit Einschluss ihrer Anwendungen, 270
Energy, conservation of, 299
Erneström, Gustav, 261
Engels, Friedrich, 81
Engineering,
    during Renaissance, 45, 46–47
    Galileo's achievements, 46–47
    in antiquity, 45
    (*see also* Electrical engineering; Electronics industry; Mechanical engineering)
Engineers, biographies, 44–45
English Rural Life, Museum of, 50
Entomologists, index to obituaries, 351

Entomologist's Record, 354
Environmental health, in USA, 424
    (*see also* Public health)
Epicureans, 199
    physics, 213
Epidemiology, 70–71, 185, 189, 391
    bibliography, 391
    in USA, 420–421
Equatorium (medieval planetary computer), 244
Equilibrium, chemical, 328
Ethology, 363
Euclid, 211, 265, 288
    influence on later work, 222
Eudemus of Rhodes, 259
Eudoxus, 211
Eugenics, 110, 367, 419
    in USA, 430
Euler, Leonhard, 266, 268, 295
    bibliographies, 268
Evans-Pritchard, E.E., 65–66
Evolution debate, 416
    and racism, 429
Exhibition catalogues, technological, 50
Experimentalism in life sciences, 361–378
    bibliography, 368–378
Experiments, repetition of, 183–184
Exploration, American, 428

Fabian Society, 99
Fabula (j), 164
Falsification, 118, 119
Faraday, Michael, 300, 325
Farey, J., 44
Farrington, Benjamin, 100, 198, 199
Febvre, Luciien, 392
Fermat, Pierre, 265, 267, 290
Feyerabend, Paul, 119, 123–124
Fichte, Johann Gottlieb, 297
Films, 176
Fiore, Antonio Maria, 270
Fischer, A., 40
Flamsteed, John, 245
Flora Europaea, 188
Food processing industry, 331
Foster, Sir Michael, 35
Foucault, Michel, 88, 175
Fourcroy, Antoine François, 324
Fourier, Jean Baptiste Joseph, 296, 299
Fox Talbot, William, 248
Frank, P., 10

Frankfurt School, 185
Frankland, Edward, 328
Franklin, Benjamin, 422, 425
Franklin Institute, 426
Fraunhofer, Joseph von, 248
Freind, John, 31

Galdston, I., 385, 386
Galen, 74, 75, 199, 202, 208, 215
   anatomical observations, 216
   influence on later works, 222
   linkages in biological systems, 207
   studies of, 216–217
   writings recovered, 228
Galileo Galilei, 119, 224, 226, 265, 287,
   288
   experimental methods, 184
   significance to engineering, 46, 290
   studies of methodology, 231
   transition from medieval to modern
      science, 230
Galvani, Luigi, 296
Ganita Bhāratī (j), 262
Garrison, F.H., 37, 140, 188
Gaseous state theory, 322, 323
Gassendi, Pierre, 290
Gauss, Carl Friedrich, 266, 296, 297
Gay-Lussac, Joseph Louis, 298, 324
Geertz, Hildred, 65–66, 68
Genetic engineering, 111
Genetics, 181, 363, 366–367, 419
   in USA, 430
   (*see also* Eugenics)
Geography,
   historical, 175
   Islamic texts, 447–448
   of India, 468
Geology,
   archives, 181
   library collections, 146
   theological approach, 17
   use of grid references, 188
Geomancy, Chinese, 493–494
Geometry, 265
   19th century revival, 269
   (*see also* Mathematics)
Gesner, Conrad, 30–31, 273
Gesnerus (j), 160, 165
Giere, R.N., 126–127
Gilbert, William, 288
Gillispie, C.C., 142
Ginsburg, Jekuthiel, 261
Ginzburg, Carlo, 61, 69

Glassware,
   chemical, 248
   Indian, bibliography, 458
Goldberger, Joseph, 424
Goody, Jack, 68
Goodyer, John, 352
Government records, 177–178
   bibliography, 253
   (*see also* Public records; State
      papers)
Gowing, Margaret, 51, 180
Grainger, R.D., 368
Grand Dictionnaire Universel, 143
Graph theory, 270
Grattan-Guinness, Ivor, 262
Gray, Asa, 416
Greece (classical), *see* Chemistry,
   history of: Greek; Medicine:
   history of: Greek; Science: history
   of: Greek
Greenberg, D., 107
Gregory, James, 248
Gresham College, 288
Grimaldi, F.M., 289
Grove, Sir William Robert, 299
Grünbaum, A., 127
Guerlac, Henry, 9
Günther, S., 261
Guyton de Morveau, Louis Bernard,
   323

Haeser, Heinrich, 34, 35, 40
Hakluyt Society, 158
Haldane, J.B.S., 366
Hales, Stephen, 323
Hall, A.R., 14
Haller, Albrecht von, 32, 381
Halley's Comet, 295
*Handbook of Social and Cultural
   Anthropology*, 67
Hanson, N.R., 118, 126, 127
Harriot, Thomas, 267
Harrison, John, 245
Harvard College, scientific instrument
   collection, 246
Harvey, William, 229, 230, 245, 383,
   384
   research methods, 184
Haüy, René, 326
Heat research, 299
Hecker, J.F.K., 33–34, 40, 382, 391
Heisenberg, Werner Karl, 6
Helmholtz, Hermann Ludwig, 297, 299

Helmont, J.B., Van, 321, 322, 384
Hempel's 'covering-law' model,
  127–128
Henle, Jakob, 366
Henry, Joseph, 416, 426
Herasistratus, 216
Herbarum vivae icones, 30
Hermeticism, 288, 325
Hermite, Charles, 271
Hero, 214, 265
Herophilus, 216
Herschel, Sir William, 298, 301
Hesiod, 202
Hessen, Boris, 8–9, 100
Hinduism, 460
  encyclopaedia, 458
Hipparchus, 245
Hippocrates, 35, 383
  Corpus Hippocraticum, 209
Hippocratic medicine, studies of,
  216–217
Hirsch, August, 34–35, 40, 382
HISTLINE (computer program), 147
Historia animalium, 30
Historia Mathematica (j), 262, 274
  'Sources' section, 273
Historical Abstracts, 162
Historical geography, 175
Historical Journal, 161
Historical Society of Science, 158
History and Philosophy of Logic
  (annual), 262
History of Education (j), 164
History of Science (j), 160, 161
History of Science, 15th International
  Congress (1978), 182
History of Science and Technology, 2nd
  International Congress (1931), 38,
  100
History of Science Society, 99, 160,
  165, 413
Hobbes, Thomas, 285
Hoff, Jacobus Hendricus van't, 328
Hogben, Lancelot, 366
Hohenheim, Theophrastus Bombastus
  von, *see* Paracelsus
Homoeopathy, 422
  Indian, 470
Hooke, Robert, 246, 289
Hooker, Joseph, 352
Horder, Lord, 385
Horton, Robin, 68
Horus (j), 272

Hospitals, 188
  Indian, 464
    in 18th century, 467
  Islamic, 443–444
  United States, 422
  voluntary, 386–387
Hsiang K'ai, 493
Hsün Tzu, 483
Human dissection, 216
Humanism,
  contribution to recovery of scientific
    texts, 228
  delaying scientific development, 226,
    228
Humanities Index, 163
Husserl, Edmund, 8
Huxley, Aldous, 352
Huygens, Christiaan, 245, 267, 289,
  290, 291
Hydrogen bomb, 105
Hydrostatics, 288

Illustrations, bibliography, 253
  (*see also* Art, works of; Drawings)
Imperial Chemical Industries, 331
Impetus theory, Indian, 461
Index Islamicus, 439
Index Medicus, 147
Index to British Literary Bibliography,
  146
Indexes to data, in research, 189
India Office Library and Records, 458
Indian Council of Medical Research,
  469
Indian Institute of Science, 469
Indian Journal of History of Science,
  470
Indian Society for the History of
  Mathematics, Bulletin, 262
Indicators, chemical, 328
Industrial archaeology, 49–50, 176
Industrial surveys, 44, 110
Influenza epidemics, 421
Ingold, Christopher Kelk, 330
Institutions,
  documents as source material, 177
  histories of, use of biographical
    information, 187–188
  history of changes, 48
  (*see also under individual subjects*)
International Academy of the History
  of Medicine, 166–167

International Academy of the History of Science, 165
International Bibliography of Dictionaries, 143
International Catalogue of Scientific Literature, 274
International Congress of Mathematicians, 268–269
International Index, 163
International Journal of Oral History, 186
International Society for the History of Medicine, 166
International Union of the History and Philosophy of Science, national inventories of scientific instruments, 252
Interviews, 186
(*see also* Oral record)
Inventions, 50
Inventors, biographies, 44, 45
Ionic theory, 325–326
Irish Naturalists' Journal, 354
Ironbridge Museum, 50
Iron-founding, 46
Irving, J.D., 10
Idensee, E., 33
Isis (j), 10, 30, 99, 160, 165, 261, 413
  Critical Bibliography, 139, 140, 148, 161, 261, 274, 354, 440
  Cumulative Bibliography, 139, 161, 263, 275
  Directory of Members and Guide to Graduate Students, 149
  News of the Profession section, 149
Islam, *see* Medicine: history of: Islamic; Science: history of: Islamic
Istoriko-matematicheskie issledovaniia (j), 262

Jacobi, Carl Gustav Jacob, 271
Jahrbuch über die Fortschritte der Mathematik, 274
Janus (j), 165
Jarvis, Edward, 421
Johns Hopkins Institute for the History of Medicine, 39, 412
Joule, James Prescott, 299, 329
Journal des Sçavans, 159
Journal of American History, 417
Journal of Botany, 351
Journal of Chemical Education, 317

Journal for the History of Arabic Science, 441
Journal of the History of the Behavioral Sciences, 160
Journal of the History of Biology, 165, 350
Journal of the History of Ideas, 10, 12, 164
Journal of the History of Medicine, 160, 166
Journal of the History of Medicine and Allied Sciences, 159–160, 413, 417
Journal of Social History, 161

Karpinski, L.C., 261, 271
Keill, John, 246
Kepler, Johannes, 229, 230, 244, 265, 289, 291
  bibliography, 267
Klein, Felix, 271
Knowledge,
  classification of, 67, 209
  sociology of, 86–87
    Edinburgh school, 119
Koyré, Alexandre, 3, 7, 8–9, 12, 14, 99, 119
Kronecker, Leopold, 271
Kuhn, T.S., 20, 119–125, 181
Kummer, E.E., 271
Kurti, Nicholas, 180

Laboratory notebooks, 176
Labour history, 48
  effects of innovations, 52
Lagrange, Joseph Louis, 296
Lakatos, Imre, 20, 119, 121–122, 123, 126–127
Lambert, Johann Heinrich, 296
The Lancet, 388
Landau, L., 122, 124, 125, 126–127
Language of science, 5
Laplace, Pierre, Simon, Marquis de, 296, 297, 300
Lapland expeditions (1730s), 295
Larkey Committee, 141
Lavoisier, Antoine Laurent, 296, 299, 323–324
  bibliography of studies, 323
Lawrence, E.O., 428
Le Bel, Joseph Achille, 328
Leblanc process, 331

Leclerc, Daniel, 31
Lecourt, Dominic, 8
Legendre, Adrien Marie, 297
Le Goff, Jacques, 61
Leibniz, G.W., 265, 267–268, 293
    bibliography, 268
Lenses, 248
Leonardo of Pisa, 264
Le Roi Ladurie, Emmanuel, 61
Letters, 176
Lévi-Strauss, C., 67, 68
Levy, Hyman, 366
Li concept, 496
Library collections,
    catalogues of, 177
    guides to, 145–148
    on scientific instruments, 252–253
Library of Congress,
    bibliographical aids, 146
    L.C. Tracer Bullet, 148
    New Serial Titles, 162
    source material, 178
Libri, G., 177, 260
Liebig, Justus von, 297, 329
Life sciences,
    experimentalism in, 361–378
        bibliography, 368–378
    Indian,
        bibliographies, 457–458
        in Vedic period, 460
    institutions, 363, 368
    Islamic works, 444
    library collections, 146
    Medieval and Renaissance
        developments, 229
    in universities, 232
    sacred tradition in classical Greece,
        206
    in USA, 165
    (*see also* Biology; Botany; Natural
        history)
Light, research developments, 298
Linnaeus, Carolus (i.e. Carl von
    Linné), 352
Linnean Society, 354, 355
Literature, science-based, 185
Littré, Emile, 35, 36
Lockyer, Norman, 301
Logarithmic tables, 265
Logical empiricism, 118, 120
Longitude measurement, 245, 294
Loria, Gino, 261, 272
Lovejoy, Arthur, 12
Luckmann, T., 86

Lucretius, 202
Lunar Society, Birmingham, 293
Lyceum, 205, 209
Lyell, Charles, 17, 367
Lysenkoism, 330

Macfarlane, Alan, 61
Mach, Ernst, 5, 117
Machine tools, history, 45, 48
Machinery,
    early guides to, 44
    histories of, 48
Macrobiotics, 320–321
Magendie, François, 365
Magic,
    and medicine, 62
    beliefs on origins of disease, 72–73
    influence on science, 64–69
Magnetism, 288, 293, 299
    social status of research, 300
    (*see also* Physical sciences)
Maier, Anneliese, 119
Malaria, 415, 420
Malclès, L.-N., 139
Malinowski, Bronislaw, 65–66
Mannheim, Karl, 185
Manufactures, histories of, 44, 48
Manuscripts, 177
    bibliography, 253
    mathematical, 273
    (*see also* Archives)
Manzer, B., 159
Maps, 176
Marxism, 9, 100, 184, 330, 415, 429
    sociology of knowledge, 38
    technology, 52, 54
    view of social relations in science, 81,
        86–87
Mathematical physics, developments in
    19th century, 269
Mathematical Reviews, 274
Mathematicians,
    biographies, 260, 266
        and bibliographies, 19th century,
            269–270
Mathematics,
    historians of, directory, 262
    history of, 7, 259–284
        abstracts, 262, 274
        bibliographies, 259, 272, 273–275,
            275–284
        *Bibliography and Research Manual
            . . .*, 262

Mathematics,
  history of (*cont.*)
    biobibliographies, 268
    Centre for the Study of Medieval
      Mathematics, 273
    encyclopaedia, 270
    general works, 262–263
    guides, 272–273
    indexes, 274
    library collections, 273
    periodicals, 260–262
    resource file, 272
    source books, 263–264
    surveys, 259

    Arabic, biobibliography, 438
    Babylonian, 210
    Chinese, 486–488
      mathematical astronomy,
        489–490
      mathematical harmonics,
        488–489
    Greek, 210–211
    Indian,
      bibliography, 458
      in Vedic period, 459
      6th–11th centuries AD, 462–463
    Islamic, 444–445, 447
      biobibliographies, 445

  from Renaissance to end of 18th
    century, 264–268
  in 19th century, 268–270
    developments in analysis, 269

  history of education, 270–271
  in study of physics, 225
  (*see also* Algebra; Astronomy;
    Geometry)
Maud report (1941), 103
Maupertuis, Pierre Louis Moreau de, 295
Max-Planck-Gesellschaft archives, 182
Maxwell, James Clerk, 300, 327
May, Kenneth, 262
Mayer, Johann Tobias, 299
Measles, 438
Mechanical engineering, histories of, 45
Mechanics, 288
  Greek, 213, 214–215
  in Renaissance, 267
  in 17th century, 290
  rational, 295
  (*see also* Physical sciences)
Mechanics' institutes, 187, 249, 300
A Medical Bibliography, 140

*Medical Bibliography in an Age of
  Discontinuity*, 141
Medical Directory, 390
Medical History (j), 167
Medical records,
  preservation in UK, 182
    regional initiatives, 182
  quantification from studies of, 189
  surveys, Canadian, 182
Medical Register, 390
Medicine,
  historiography, 29–43
    overview, 29–30
  history of, 62
    bibliographies, 40–43, 137–141,
      147, 442
    bibliography of journals, 500–507
    biographical sources, 380, 384, 390
    guides to academic courses, 149
    guides to library collections,
      145–148
    guides to reference books and
      directories, 141
    periodical literature, 157–161,
      166–168
      guides, 386
    single-volume works, 382–383
    societies, 157, 158, 166
      guides, 386
    sources, 182–183
      bibliography, 190–194
    surveys, 138

  American, 384, 411–435
    bibliography, 430–435
    guides to periodical literature, 417
    medical care, 422–423
    professional organizations, 423
    public health, 423–424
    role of women, 424–425
    societies, 166, 412
    sociology, 414–415
    survey of research, 414
  Chinese, 490–491
    bibliography, 496–499
  Greek, 201, 215–217
    bibliography, 217–220
    compared with Indian, 462
    magical elements, 202
    mystical practices, 206
    plurality of centres, 215
  Indian,
    bibliography, 457, 458, 471–475

Medicine,
  Indian (*cont.*)
    educational institutions,
      468–469
    general surveys, 457
    in Vedic period, 460
    from 5th century BC to 5th
      century AD, 461–462
    in 16th–17th centuries, 464,
      465–466
    in 18th century, 466–468
    in 19th century, 468–469
    in 20th century, 469–471
    periodicals, 458
  Islamic, 438, 442
    bibliographies, 439–440, 442,
      448–455
    biobibliographies, 439
    practised in India, 464
    translated texts, 443
  Roman, 216

  period demarcations, 33, 34, 36, 37
  since 1500, 379–407
    bibliography, 393–407
    pre-18th century, 380
    in 18th century, 381
    in 19th century, 380
      biographies, 381–382
      subject indexes to periodicals,
        381
    in 20th century, 382–386
      influence of newer professions,
        386
      official histories of World War
        II, 178

  anthropology and, 70–75
    bibliographies, 70, 77–80
    reviews, 70
  cultural variety of healers, 74–75
  differentiated from history of
    science, 39
  doctor–patient interactions, 90,
    388, 389, 418
  education, 387, 388
  home treatment, 388
  institutionalization, 382
  limitations of modern works, 40
  Paracelsianism, 321–322
  primitive, 62
    folk healing methods, 73–74
    professionalization, 90
    quantification, 392

Medicine,
  primitive (*cont.*)
    reinterpretation of available
      sources, 174
    research methods, 183–190
      bibliography, 190–194
    sociological aspects, 90, 91, 174,
      384–386
      bibliography, 93–96
    role of doctors, 91–92
    specialisms, 383
    statistics of discoveries, 188
    teaching, 383
    traditional and biomedical
      systems, 70
    (*see also* Disease; Epidemiology;
      Public health; Social sciences:
      and history of science and
      medicine)
MEDLARS, 147, 148
Mélanges de l'Institut Dominican
  d'Études Orientales, 440
Mencius, 483
Mendel, Gregor, 366
Mendel Newsletter, 181
Mendeleev, Dmitri Ivanovich, 327
Mental illness, in USA, 421–422
  (*see also* Psychiatry)
Mersenne, Marin, 290
Merton, Robert K., 4, 13, 81, 102
Metallography,
  advanced by improved microscopes,
    252
  metal-refining, 49
Metaphysics, in cultural development,
  4
Meteorology,
  classical, 201
  instruments, 246
  observatories, 246
Metzger, Hélène, 119, 165
Meyerson, Émile, 7, 8, 119
Michell, John, 295
Microfiches, 157
Microscopes, 98, 245, 289
  accuracy, 184
  catalogue reprints, 248–249
  electron, 249
  history outline, 248
  home models, 247
  increasing power, 250–251
  survey of sources, 248
Microtomes, 249

Middle Ages, history of science in,
221–240
    bibliography, 233–240
    decline accelerated by humanism,
        226, 228
    innovation, 224
    level of scientific thought, 223
    linking with Renaissance science, 226
    manuscript sources, 224
    occult aspect, 231
    undefined group of disciplines,
        228–229
Middle East Journal, 440
Mieli, Aldo, 7, 165
Military science, 51
    domestic spin-off, 51
    funding US research, 107
    political ends, 102–103
Miller, Jonathan, 185
Millikan, Robert Andrews, 6
Mineralogy, Indian, bibliography of,
    458
Minerva (j), 164
Mining, 49
Mo Tzu, 483–484
Monge, G., 266, 271
Montucla, J.E., 260
Moore, Norman, 382
More, Henry, 9
Morgan, Thomas H., 419, 430
Mormon Church, parish register
    project, 179
Morton, L.T., 140
Mulligan, L., 14
Museum of Alexandria, 209–210, 216
Museum of English Rural Life, 50
Museum of the History of Science,
    library on scientific instruments,
    253
Museums,
    catalogues, 252
        of inventions, 50
    development from collections, 185
    extending expertise, 179
    guide to book and periodical
        collections, 144
    guide to publications of, 144
    guides to collections, 144
    industrial, 49–50
    scientific instruments, 252–253
Museums of the World, 144
Music,
    Chinese mathematical harmonics, 488
    time measurement, 184

Nairne, Edward, 248
Napier, John, 265
National Archives and Record Service
    (US), 178
National Health Service, 385
    preservation of records, 180, 182
National Historical Publications and
    Records Commission (US), 180
National Library of Medicine (US),
    147, 182
    Index Catalogue, 390
    Index of NLM Serial Titles, 147
    Office of Inquiries and Publications
        Management, 147
National Physical Laboratory (UK),
    178
National Register of Archives (UK),
    180, 182–183
National Union Catalog, 145
Natural history, 349–360
    abstract journals, 354
    Archives of Natural History, 166,
        350, 354
    bibliographies, 159, 350, 353,
        357–360
    biographical guides, 350–351, 352
    general histories, 354–355
    guides to collections, 351
    illustrations, surveys and
        bibliographies of, 353–354
    institutions, 355–356
    neglect by historians, 349–350
    periodicals, 354
    quantification studies, 356
    sociological approach, 355
    (*see also* Life sciences)
Natural philosophy, 292–294
Naturalist (j), 354
Nature (j), 160
Naturopathy, 470
Navigation,
    astronomical, 244
    instruments, 245
        chronometers, 247
Nazism, 110
Needham, Joseph, 38, 45, 100, 366,
    476–477
    Science and Civilisation in China,
        478, 482–483, 485
    on alchemy, 492
    on Chinese mathematics, 487
    on mathematical astronomy, 489
    on mathematical harmonics,
        488–489

Needham, Joseph,
  Science and Civilisation in China (cont.)
    on physical studies, 494
Negro race, 429
Neuburger, Max, 31, 36–37, 382
Neugebauer, Otto, 212
Neumann, John von, 271
Neurath, O., 10
Neurology, experimental basis, 362
*New Cambridge Bibliography of
    English Literature*, 140
New Sydenham Society, 158
New York Academy of Medicine:
    Committee on Medicine and the
    Changing Order, 385
Newcastle upon Tyne University,
    Project for Historical
    Biobibliography, 390
Newcomen Society, *Transactions* of,
    45, 165
Newton, Sir Isaac, 186, 265, 267
    alchemical manuscripts, 323
    bibliography, 267
    catalogue of library, 267
    impact on astronomy, 291–292
    optical instruments, 246, 248
Newtonianism, 16
Nicholson's Journal, 329
Nobert, Friedrich, 250
Nomina Anatomica, 188
Notae de Historia Mathematica, 262
NTM (j), 165
Nuclear armaments race, 104, 105
Nuclear physics,
    American, 419
    archives, 181
    official history, 178
    project histories, 106–107
Numbers,
    Indian symbols, 461
    19th century theory developments,
      269
Numeracy, 47
Nursing, 387
    biographies, 390
Nutrition, experimental approach to,
    363

Occult aspects of medieval science, 231
Oersted, Hans Christian, 297, 300
Official histories, 178
Official Museum Directory, 144
Official publications, 177–178

Oken, Lorenz, 297
Olbers, Wilhelm, 296
Online Review (j), 150
Ophthalmology,
    Arabic, 438
    Islamic, 443
      bibliography, 446
Oppenheimer, Robert, 428
Optical instruments, 246
    survey of sources, 248
Optics, 288
    developments in 17th century, 289
Oral History (j), 186
Oral History Society, 186
Oral record, 50, 186
Oresme, Nicole, 224
Organic chemistry, 327–328
Orientalische Literaturzeitung, 440
Orta, Garcia da, 465
Osiris (j), 165, 261
Osler, William, 32, 37, 382, 383
Osler Club of London, 167
Osmania Oriental Publication Bureau,
    443
Owen, Richard, 367
Oxford Review of Education, 164

Pacioli, Luca, 264
Padraig Walsh, S., 143
Pagel, J.L., 36, 382
Paley, William, 19
Paper-making, 46
    Indian, 463
      bibliography, 458
Pappus, 265
    writings recovered, 228
Paracelsianism, 31
Paracelsus (i.e. Theophrastus
    Bombastus von Hohenheim),
    321–322, 384
Parker, Irene, 13
Parmenides, 203
Pascal, Blaise, 290
Past and Present (j), 14, 160, 164
Patents, 50, 176
    chemical, 330
Patronage of science, 301
Payne, J.F., 382
Peiresc, Nicholas Claude Fabride, 290
Pellagra, 421, 424
Periodic law, 327
Periodical literature, 157–161,
    164–168, 177

Periodical literature (*cont.*)
  bibliographies of journals, 163,
    168–171, 500–507
  circulation, 160
  generated by societies, 158
  growth, 157
  guides, 159, 161–164
  limitations, 158
    of indexes to, 159
  refereeing system, 160
  timeliness, 160–161
Peripatetic physics, 213
Personal papers, 176–177
Peru, expeditions to (1730s), 295
Petrarch, 226
Pharmacology, 387
  Indian,
    bibliography, 458
    to 5th century AD, 462
    in 17th century, 465
    in 19th century, 469
  Islamic, 442–443
    bibliography, 442
  training, 329
Philolaus, 203
Philon of Byzantium, 214
Philosophical Transactions, 187
Philosophy,
  and science, bibliography of, 21–26
  Chinese, 482–485
  effects of modern scientific
    developments, 6
  history, 8, 31
  traditions in Greek physics, 213
Philosophy of Science (j), 10
Photography, collections,
  directory of, 248
  survey of sources, 248
Physical chemistry, 328–329
Physical sciences, history of, 9, 285–314
  academic studies, 294–297
  bibliography, 286, 303–314
  surveys of texts, 286

  Chinese, 494–496
  German, in late 18th century,
    297–301

  reorientation in 17th century, 288
  scientific revolution, 287
  at end of 19th century, 301–302

  professionalization, 296
  restructuring of British scientific
    community, 298

Physical sciences, history of (*cont.*)
  social status of practitioners, 299
  vocabularly development, 289
Physics, history of, 6, 7, 181
  Greek, 212–214
  Indian, bibliography, 458
  'law of inertia', 225
  mathematical, 19th century
    development, 269
  scientific instrument development,
    248
  US, 429–430
Physiology, experimentation in, 362
Pico, Giovanni, 226
Plans, 176
Plastic surgery, 467
Plato, 203
  conciliating 'truth' and 'opinion', 204
  use of polarities in biological systems,
    207
Platonism,
  in Koyré's work, 8, 9
  neo-Platonists, 11, 16
Ploucquet, W.G., 381
Pneumatics, 288, 298
  17th century, 289
Poggendorff, Johann Christian,
    141–142
Poincaré, Henri, 5, 271
Poisson, Simeon Denis, 296
Poliomyelitis, 421
Politics,
  in military science, 102–103
  involvement of scientific advisers,
    105–106
  relations with science and society,
    366–367
    analyses, 107
    bibliography, 111–115
    in non-US/UK countries, 110
    in US, 427–428
  views of historians of science,
    101–102
Polyvinyl chloride, 331
Poole's Index to Periodical Literature,
    159
Popper, Karl, 20, 68, 118–119, 120,
    122–123
Porcelain, 46
Positivism, 4–11
  effect on philosophy of science,
    117–118
  in cultural development, 4

Posters, 176
Pottery, Indian, bibliography of, 458
Powell, John Wesley, 427
Power, D'Arcy, 382
Preventive medicine, 385
Price, D.J. de Solla, 108
Price, Don, 107
Priestley, Joseph, 117, 286
Privy Council, Medical Department, 368
Probability theory, 267
Prony, Gaspard Riche de, 271
Prosopography, 186–187
Prout, William, 327
Psychiatric illness, 71, 72
    bibliography, 72
    therapy methods, 73
Psychiatry, 392
Psychology, 392
    applied to historical analysis, 185
    archives, 181
    experimentalism in, 362
Ptolemy, 199, 208
    astronomy, 212
    influence on later work, 222
Public health, in USA, 423–424
Public Record Office (UK), 178
Public records,
    preservation, 180
    (*see also* Government records; State papers)
Publications in Historical Bibliography, 159
Published papers, 176
Punched card indexes, 189
Puritan Revolution, 110, 365
    and development of science, 13–16
Puschmann, Theodor, 36, 40, 382
Pythagoreans, 203

Quadrant, 245
Quantification in research, 188–189
Quantum mechanics, 330
Quantum physics, archives in, 181
Quantum theory, 302
Quarterly Index Islamicus, 439

Racism, 429
Radar, 103
    official history, 178
Radical Science Journal, 162
Radio, history of, 45

Radioactivity, 330
Radioastronomy, 85
Rádl, E., 367
Rationality, 124–126
Ray, John, 352
Ray Society, 158
Reader, W.J., 110
Recipe books, 176
Redfield, Robert, 69
Regiomontanus, 265
Regnault, Henri Victor, 298
Reichenbach, Hans, 117
Relativity theory, 302
Religion,
    and science in 19th century, 16–20
    Greek,
        basis of scientific revelation, 203
        pre-scientific tradition, 205–207
        threat from technologists, 202
    influence on science, 64–69
        in India, 459
    primitive, 66
    scientists' affiliations, 13
    (*see also* Theology)
Remak, Robert, 366
Renaissance,
    history of science in, 221–240
        bibliography, 233–240
        occult aspects, 231
        undefined group of disciplines, 228–229
    library collections, 146
    mathematics, 264–265
    recovery of ancient sources during, 225
    retention of some 'medieval' science, 222, 226
Renouard, P.V., 35
Research methods, 183–190
    aids to precision, 188
    developments, 173
    entertainment aspect, 184–185
    of Aristotle, 208–209
Revue de synthèse (j), 165
Revue de synthèse historique (j), 165
Revue d'Histoire des Sciences (j), 149, 160, 165
Revue de l'Institut des Manuscrits Arabes (j), 440
Revue semestrielle des publications mathématiques, 274
Rey, Abel, 7, 165
Richard of Wallingford, 244
Richardson, Richard, 352

Ritter, Johann Wilhelm, 297, 298
Ritual, 67
Rosen, George, 61, 63, 384, 385, 413
Rosenberg, Charles, 415
Royal Botanic Gardens, Edinburgh,
    355
Royal Botanic Gardens, Kew, 178, 355
    Library, 146
Royal College of Chemistry, 329
Royal College of Physicians, 387
    Roll of the, 381
Royal College of Physicians,
    Edinburgh, card index of
    obituaries, 390
Royal College of Surgeons, *Plarr's
    Lives ...* , 387
Royal Greenwich Observatory, 178
Royal Institution,
    Christmas lectures, 185
    study of origins, 187
Royal Society, 101
    Catalogue of Scientific Papers,
        162–163, 274
    Contemporary Scientific Archives
        Centre, 180–181
    curator of experiments, 246
    influence on American science, 426
    motto, 246
    Notes and Records, 160, 166
    Philosophical Transactions, 159
    studies of origins, 14, 187
Royal Society of Medicine,
    Proceedings, 167
Rozier's Observations, 329
Ruska, Ernst, 249
Russell, Bertrand, 117
Russell, E.S., 37
Russo, F., 13, 138
Rutherford, Ernest, 330
Ryle, John, 385

Sale catalogues, 177
    guides to, 146
    (*see also* Auctions)
Salutati, Coluccio, 226
Sanderson, John Burdon, 368
Sarton, George, 10, 12, 39, 99, 118,
    165, 187, 261, 272, 411, 413
Sbath manuscript collections, 440, 443
Schelling, Friedrich Wilhelm, 297
Schleiden, M.J., 366
Schlesinger, Arthur, 414

Scholaticism, 232
Schott, Otto, 248
Schulze, Johann Heinrich, 32
Science,
    anthropological aspects,
        bibliography, 77–80
    area studies, 138
    as intellectual activity, 8
    costs of research, 107
    definitions in antiquity, Middle Ages
        and Renaissance, 223
    disciplinary matrices, 121, 123
    diversity of disciplines, 85
    economic importance in UK,
        107–108
    effect on research of institutional
        policies, 88
    government involvement, 109
    historians of,
        biobibliographies, 143
        ignoring politics, 106
    history of,
        academic courses, 149
        bibliographies, 21–26, 137–141,
            148
            of bibliographies, 139
            of journals, 500–507
        biographies, 141–143
        dictionaries, 138
        guide to sources, 137
        library collections, 145–148
        periodical literature, 149, 157–161,
            164–166
        reference books and directories,
            141
        societies, 157, 158
        sources and research methods,
            bibliography, 190–194
        surveys, 138
            of books, libraries and
                collections, 137
        teaching materials, 148–150

    American, 411–435
        AAAS conference, 417
        bibliography, 430–435
        evolution, 415
        exploration, 428–429
        guides to periodical literature,
            417
        in 18th century, 425–426
        in 19th century, 426–427
        individual disciplines, 429–430
        oral record, 419

Science,
  American (*cont.*)
    relations with government, 416, 427–428
    research methodologies, 419
  Chinese, 476–490, 491–496
    bibliographies, 476, 478, 482, 496–499
    encyclopaedic sources, 481–482
    general surveys, 478–479
    guide to bibliographies, 479
    historiography, 480
    language requirements, 477
    main divisions, 485–496
    Needham's survey, 478
    (*see also* Confucianism)
  Greek,
    bibliography, 217–220
    development of concept of systems, 207–208
    episteme as distinctive tradition, 203
    forerunner of 17th century achievements, 221
    in social context, 199
    primary sources, 197–198
    proliferation of anonymous treatises, 200
    survival of writings, 222
    treatises and teaching, 207–209
  Indian,
    Anglo-Indian glossary, 458
    bibliography, 471–475
    biographical dictionaries, 458
    educational institutions, 468–469
    general surveys, 457
    in Indus Valley Civilization, 458
    in Vedic period, 459–460
    in 5th century BC to 5th century AD, 460–462
    in 6th–11th centuries AD, 462–463
    in 12th–15th centuries, 463–464
    in 16th and 17th centuries, 464–466
    in 18th century, 466–468
    in 19th century, 468–469
    in 20th century, 469–470
    periodicals, 458
    Sanskrit summaries of oral teachings, 457

  Islamic, 437–448
    assimilation into European work, 222
    bibliographies, 439–440, 441, 448–455, 457
    bibliography of general encyclopaedias, 448
    biobibliographies, 438
    general surveys, 440–442
    guides, 438
    guides to manuscript collections, 440
    range of disciplines, 437
    study of pseudepigraphy, 448
  lacking for 15th century, 227
  medieval and Renaissance, 221–240
  and sociology, 81–96, 418, 419–420, 422
    analyses, 85–89
    bibliography, 93–96
  archive preservation, 181
  continuity thesis, 224
  cultural dimensions, 9–11
  influence of magic and religion, 64–69
    in 19th century, 16–20
  influence of primitive beliefs, 61
  limited to 'pure' research, 99–100
  'metaphysical research programmes', 120–121
  patterns of change, 122–124
  philosophy of science in relation to, 116–133
  reinterpretation of available sources, 174
  related to politics and political economy, 99–115
    bibliography, 111–115
  relationship to history of medicine, 29
  research methods, 121–122, 183–190
  research traditions, 122
  (*see also* Social sciences: and history of science and medicine)
  in cultural context, 68, 69
  philosophy of,
    bibliography, 128–133

Science,
    in cultural context (*cont.*)
        historical development, 116–120
        relationship with history of
            science, 126
        writings during 1970s, 120
    policy, 51, 88, 108–109
        diffusion into education,
            bibliography, 109
        government records, 177
        units of appraisal, 120–122
Science at the Cross Roads, 38, 100
Science Citation Index, 162
Science Museum,
    bibliography of publications, 144
    Book Exhibitions, 144
    camera collection, 248
    King George III collection, 246
    Library, 138
        material on scientific instruments,
            252–253
    scientific instrument inventory, 252
    Wellcome Medical Museum, 253
Science Studies (j), 81
Scientific American (j), 160
Scientific and Learned Societies, 145
Scientific Instruction and the
        Advancement of Science, Royal
        Commission on, 110
Scientific instruments, 176, 243–258
    bibliography, 253–258
    catalogues, 249
    encyclopaedias, 253
    general surveys, 243
    museums and libraries, 252–253
    national inventories, 252

    Renaissance developments, 289

    astronomical,
        Islamic, 446
        19th century developments, 301
    centres of manufacture, 245
    chemical, 329
    increasing accuracy, 249
    lecture-demonstrations, 246
    London trade, 247
    medical, Islamic, 444
    relationship to science, 8
    (*see also* Balances, chemical)
Scientific Manuscripts, Conference on
        (1962), 181
Scientific method, bibliography of, 120

Scientific theory,
    discussion of nature of, 5
    views of social scientists, 82
Scientists,
    analysis of activity, 88
    biographical dictionaries, 141–143
    in Museum of Alexandria, 209–210
    *Obituary Notices of Fellows of the
        Royal Society*, 163
    preservation of papers, 180–181
    study of religious affiliations, 13
Scott Barr, E., 142
Scottish Society of the History of
        Medicine, 167
Scripta Mathematica (j), 261
Sedgwick, Adam, 17
Serials in the British Library, 161
Set theory, 19th century development
        of, 269
's Gravesande, Willem, 246
Shamanism, 73, 74
Sheehy, E.P., 141
Shen Kua, 485
Short, James, 248
Shryock, Richard, 39, 384–385, 413,
        414–415, 426
Sidgwick, Neil Vincent, 330
Siemens, Sir William, 297
Sigerist, H.E., 31, 39, 61, 62, 166, 383,
        384, 385, 412
Simons, L.G., 262
Singer, Charles, 37, 38, 45, 99, 166
Slaves, medical care in USA, 423
Slocum, R., 141
Smallpox, 438, 466
Smith, Adam, 117, 285–286
Smith, David Eugene, 261, 271, 287
Smith, Sir James Edward, 352, 353
Smithsonian Institution,
    publications, 144–145
    Rare Books Library, on scientific
        instruments, 253
Snel, Willebrord, 289
Social history, 40, 89, 175
    effect of technology, 45, 47–48,
        53–54
    medicine in context of, 38, 39, 62, 63
Social Science and Medicine (j), 168
Social Science Citation Index, 159, 162
Social sciences,
    and history of science and medicine,
        70, 81–96, 174, 185–186,
        384–386, 418, 419–420, 422

Social sciences,
  and history of science and
  medicine (*cont.*)
    American, 414–415
    bibliography, 93–96
    studies in 1970s, 81, 82–83
    mistrust of scientific community,
      83–84
Social Sciences and Humanities Index,
  163
Social Studies of Science (j), 81, 162, 163
Societies, 157, 158, 165, 166
  encouraging scientific instrument
    making, 246
  proceedings as source material, 179
  studies of origins, 187–188
  (*see also under individual subjects*)
Society of Apothecaries, 167, 390
Society for the Bibliography of Natural
    History, 159, 350
  journals, 166
Society of Genealogists, 179
Society for the Social History of
    Medicine, 167, 180
Solvay Process, 331
Sorby, Henry, 252
Sources,
  cataloguing, 176
  covering plurality of disciplines, 175
  evaluation, 177
  preservation of material, 174,
    179–183
  types, 176–179
Sowerby family, 354
Spectrometers, 301
Spectroscopy, 329
Sprengel, Kurt, 32–33, 36
Staatsbibliothek Preissischer
    Kulturbesitz (Berlin), 180
Stanley, Thomas, 31
State papers, 176
  (*see also* Government records; Public
    records)
Statistics, 85
  caution in use, 188–189
Stereoisomerism, 328
Stevin, S., 265, 267
Stoics, 206–207
  philosophy of medicine, 216
  physics, 213
Stonehenge, 243
Straton of Lampsacus, 214
Structuralism, 175

*Studies in the History and Philosophy of
    Science* (j), 126, 163
Sudhoffs Archiv, 160, 166
Sun Ssu-mo, 484
Sun-dials, 244
*Surgeon-General's Office, Index
    Catalogue of the Library of*, 147
Surgery,
  Indian, in 18th century, 466–467
  instruments, 248
Surveying instruments, 245
Surveys, topographical, 49
Swineshead, Richard, 224
Sydenham, Thomas, 35
Sydenham Society, 158
Sylvius, Franciscus (i.e. Franz de le
    Boë, or du Bois), 322
Symbolism, 67

Tannery, Paul, 6
Tansley, Arthur George, 368
Tantrism, 463
Taoism, 482, 484
  alchemy in, 492
Tartaglia, Niccolò, 265, 266–267, 270,
    287
Tawney, R.H., 13
Taxonomy, theory of, 356
Teaching aids, guides to, 148–150
Technology, history of, 44–60
  bibliographies, 55–60, 253
  exhibitions, 50
  general works, 45
  oral record, 50

  Indian, 462
  Islamic, 446

  medieval and Rennaisance, 230

  aesthetic aspects, 51
  archaeology, 49
  definition in antiquity, 223
  developmental approach, 52–53
  effect of cultural transfer, 45–46
  identifiable movements, 53
  information dissemination, 47
  internalist treatments, 47, 48
  philosophy of, 54
  policies and institutions, 51
  related to science and academic
    learning, 8, 46
  transfer to Third World, 54
  (*see also* Craft processes)

Technology and Culture (j), 45
Telescopes, 245, 290
    home models, 247
    reflector, 248, 301
    survey of sources, 248
Television, 54
Telford, Thomas, 47
Temkin, O., 383, 384, 385
Tempier, Etienne, 6
Textiles, 46, 53, 54
Teyler's Museum, Haarlem, 246
    18th and 19th century scientific
        periodicals and books, 253
Thalès (j), 7
Thelwall, John, 174
Theodolite, 247
Theology,
    and puritanism, 13–16
    and science, bibliography, 21–26
    conflict with scientific thought, 6
    in cultural development, 4
    in scientific hypotheses, 5
    natural, 18
    (*see also* Religion)
Theophrastus, 206, 214
    influence on later works, 222
    writings recovered, 228
Thermodynamics, 329
Theses, guides to, 149
Thomas, Keith, 61, 65–66, 68
Thompson, Edward P., 61
Thomson, Thomas, 327
Thomson, William, 299
Thudichum, J.L.W., 368
Topology, 270
Toulmin, Stephen, 118, 121, 123, 125
*Transcultural Psychiatric Research
    Review*, 72
Travellers' writings, as information
    sources, 46
Treatises, Greek scientific, 208
Trigonometrical Survey (India), 468,
    469
Trigonometry, 265
Troeltsch, Ernst, 13
Truesdell, C.A., 262
Tugan-Baranovskii, M.I., 44
Tung Chung-shu, 488

Ubaldo, Guido, 267
*Ulrich's International Periodicals
    Directory*, 162
Underwood, E.A., 37

Unilever, 331
*Union List of Serials in the United States
    and Canada*, 162
United Kingdom Atomic Energy
    Authority, 106
United Nations Educational, Scientific
    and Cultural Organization
    (UNESCO), guides to
    bibliographical services, 139
United States Army Corps of
    Topographical Engineers, 428
United States Atomic Energy
    Commission, 106, 428
*United States Geological Survey
    Library, Catalog of*, 146
Universities,
    importance to medieval science, 232
    role in scientific training, 249

Valency, 328
    electronic theory, 330
Vatican manuscript collection, 440, 443
Venus expeditions (1760s), 295
Vesalius, Andreas, 229, 230, 244
Vienna Circle, 117, 118
Viète, F., 265, 267
Virchow, Rudolf, 366
Vitae Germanorum medicorum, 31
Vitruvius, 202, 214, 287
Vivisection, 216
Volta, Alessandro Guiseppe, 296, 325

War histories, 102–103
Warburg Institute Library, 146
Water conservation techniques, 49
Waterloo Directory, 159
Watt, James, 47
Weber, Max, 13, 185, 199
Webster, Charles, 15–16, 110
Weierstrass, Karl Theodor, 271
Welch, William Henry, 384, 415
Wellcome Historical Monographs, 167
Wellcome Institute for the History of
    Medicine, 167
    Contemporary Medical Archives
        Centre, 182
    Library, 147
    Subject Catalogue, 390
Wellcome Medical Museum, *see*
    Science Museum
Wellcome Unit (Oxford University),
    index to obituaries, 390
    Research Publications, 167

Wellesley Index, 159
Werner, Alfred, 328
Whewell, William, 117
Whipple Museum of the History of
    Science, library on scientific
    instruments, 253
Whitehead, Alfred North, 117
Who's Who, 141
Wiedemann, E., 438–439
Wiener, P.P., 10
Wilkes Expedition (1840s), 429
Williamson, Alexander W., 327
Witchcraft, *see* Magic
Withington, E.T., 37
Wittgenstein, Ludwig, 10, 118
Wohler, Friedrich, 328
Women, in American medical history,
    424–425
Woodall, John, 465
*World Directory of Historians of
    Mathematics*, 262

World List of Scientific Periodicals,
    161–162
Worrall, J., 127
Wu hsing concept, 495
Wunderlich, C.A., 34

Yellow fever, 420
Yin–yang concept, 494–495
Yoga, 470
Young, Robert, 185
Young, Thomas, 298

Zeitschrift für Mathematik und Physik,
    260, 261
    periodicals contents lists, 274–275
Zentralblatt für Mathematik, 274
Zoological Record, 354
Zoology, general histories of, 354–355